Bee

Ayotla

Bee

# The Natural Physician's Healing Therapies

## MARK STENGLER, N.D.
The Natural Physician™

Foreword by James F. Balch, M.D.

Prentice
Hall Press

QuA

**Library of Congress Cataloging-in-Publication Data**

Stengler, Mark.
    The natural physician's healing therapies : proven remedies that medical doctors don't
know  / Mark Stengler ; foreword by James F. Balch.
      p.  cm.
    Includes bibliographical references and index.
    ISBN 0-7352-0250-8 — ISBN 0-13-032041-2
    1. Naturopathy—Popular works.   I. Title.

RZ440 .S746 2001
615.5'35—dc21                                               2001021911

Acquisitions Editor: *Edward Claflin*
Production Editor: *Eve Mossman*
Formatting/Interior Design: *Robyn Beckerman*

© 2001 by Prentice Hall

Printed in the United States of America

10 9 8 7 6 5 4 3 2 1

**ISBN 0-7352-0250-8**

The Natural Physician™ is a trademark of Mark Stengler, N.D.

*This is a reference book based on research by the author, and the ideas, procedures, and suggestions in this book are
not intended as a substitute for the medical advice of your personal health professional. All matters regarding your
health require medical supervision. Consult your physician before adopting any of the suggestions in this book
(whether or not explicitly noted in the text), as well as about any condition that may require diagnosis or medical
attention. In addition, the statements made by the author regarding certain products and services represent the
opinions of the authors alone, and do not constitute a recommendation or endorsement of any product or service by
the publisher. The author and publisher disclaim any liability arising directly or indirectly from the use of the book,
or of any products mentioned herin.*

---

**ATTENTION: CORPORATIONS AND SCHOOLS**

Prentice Hall Press books are available at quantity discounts with bulk purchase for edu-
cational, business, or sales promotional use. For information, please write to: Prentice Hall
Special Sales, 240 Frisch Court, Paramus, New Jersey 07652. Please supply: title of book,
ISBN, quantity, how the book will be used, date needed.

---

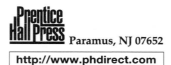 Paramus, NJ 07652

http://www.phdirect.com

# Contents

CONTENTS

# Foreword

In the introduction to the book *Prescription for Nutritional Healing*, I described the human body as being composed of "millions of tiny little engines." Some of those engines, I went on to say, work in unison while some work independently. All of them are "on call" 24 hours a day.

What I might have added is this: From time to time, some of those tiny engines may need a bit of "fixing." To fix them right, you need the right tools.

Now the tools have arrived, in this wonderfully detailed book, all described and explained by a naturopathic physician who uses those implements of healing with consummate skill every day. Mark Stengler, N.D., has treated thousands of people with the natural healing therapies he describes in this book, and his success as a healing physician has won him the respect of peers as well as patients.

I realize, of course, that some people who look through the sections of this book may wonder what I mean by describing these therapies as "healing tools." After all, many of us, when we think "medicine," think first of drugs, surgical tools, and all the high-tech paraphernalia of the operating room. How often do we consider that "acupressure," "coenzyme Q10," or "ginger root" could be healing therapies? Did you ever stop to think that "mental imagery," "prayer," soy," or "water" could help you preserve or recover your health? Can these healing therapies really help to repair the myriad tiny engines that power your body?

My reply: Absolutely.

In fact, in this book of 113 healing therapies, you'll find some of the oldest tools of healing that are known to humankind, alongside some of the newest that today's physicians are researching and exploring. Water, for example. For immunity, for mindpower, for energy, for alertness, for our daily nourishment, we depend on it. If you lack water, all the pharmaceuticals in the world will not be able to save you from the effects of dehydration. A battalion of surgeons wielding scalpels, lasers, X-rays, and cardiac monitors will not be able to rescue your organs from the effects of water depletion, nor can they restore cells that lose their most essential liquid components. Water is absolutely essential for all the engines of your body to work effectively.

Of course, now that I mention it, that may seem self-evident. But too often, the most obvious, natural, beneficial healing ingredients are neglected in favor of more complicated, and sometimes more harmful, modern implements of medical care. When was the last time a conventional medical doctor asked how many glasses of water you drink every day . . . or described to you the subtle effects of dehydration . . . or explained how substances like caffeine and caffeine-containing medicines can deplete your body of liquids?

"Water" is indeed a "healing therapy," and an important one at that.

But if some of the therapies in this book seem obvious, others are challenging our foremost medical researchers and biochemists to understand more precisely and definitely how the tiny engines in your body actually work. Take coenzyme Q10—more commonly called "CoQ10"—as an example. Here's a chemical substance smaller than the eye can see, almost obscured by myriad other components that power our cells and organs, recently revealed to be one of the most important power sources within and around the human heart. As Mark Stengler says so vividly, "When a heart doesn't have enough CoQ10 for proper electrical conduction, it suffers as it starves—and the whole circulatory system pays the price."

As with all the other healing therapies described in this book, Dr. Mark goes on to describe exactly what we know to date about CoQ10, how much you can take, when, for what conditions, and all the ways this essential tool of body maintenance can assist every part of your circulatory system. It's truly another "healing therapy." Though not so readily available as water, it's certainly just as important.

In addition to presenting us with an impressive array of healing therapies, this book performs another valuable service that speaks to the very essence of healing. It asks us to look outside the framework of conventional medicine for the assistance we need to maintain and improve our health. Too often, in the current healthcare environment, we begin to believe that physicians and surgeons can repair—even replace—the body parts that go wrong, get infected, act up, or refuse to work.

To take this attitude is to deny the body's most basic need, which is for attention and maintenance. "Fat reduction" is just one of the healing therapies in this book that contributes to the maintenance process—so, too, are "exercise," "fiber," "juicing," "phytonutrients," and all the vitamins, from A to E. If you follow the guidelines that Mark Stengler provides, you are doing more than fixing or repairing the parts that don't work. You're actually ensuring that you get the longest life and best use from the only body you'll ever have.

Even to a long-time proponent of natural medicine and nutritional healing, as I am, this book offers interesting surprises and remarkable fascinations. It draws on the healing traditions of numerous civilizations from around the world, and also reports practical applications of the healing process that come directly from the journals of a practicing "natural physician." Mark Stengler is to be applauded not only for his healing work, but for his persistent exploration of the real frontiers of natural medicine. With this book, we get a share of the knowledge offered by a truly dedicated healer who harmonizes the best of the art and science of healing.

James F. Balch, M.D.
Coauthor of *Prescription for Nutritional Healing*

# Health Begins with You

I have had a strong passion for natural healing therapies since I was a child. Though I never would have admitted it to my school friends, I actually preferred books about natural medicine and healing to the more usual fare of comic books, TV shows, and adventure movies. Not that I was just a bookworm, either. I always wanted to find out more about the herbs, supplements, or healing therapies that I was reading about. As I matured a bit, I also discovered that I very much wanted to help other people get over their illnesses—especially when I had heard about, or read about, a healing therapy that could work for them.

So my choice of studies led me to medicine. Fortunately, I began my studies at a time when alternative medicine was being integrated with mainstream and conventional medical practice in the United States. Following my premedical studies at the University of Calgary, I was accepted at one of the foremost naturopathic colleges in the U.S., the National College of Naturopathic Medicine in Portland, Oregon, where I received my doctorate in naturopathic medicine and certification in homeopathy, and became an associate clinical professor. Still later, when I was already in clinical practice, I continued my studies in nutrition, nutritional supplements, herbal therapy, and homeopathy, and am currently working on my master's degree in acupuncture and Oriental medicine. Today I enjoy helping people with all kinds of health ailments at my practice in La Jolla, California. I also educate people through my work with the media and through a class I teach at San Diego State University.

Holistic therapies made sense to me from the very beginning. I'm sure you have your own associations with that word, but to me it has a very exact meaning. Our bodies are infinitely complicated, elaborately designed arrangements of living tissues, organs, and myriad other substances that all function together in ways that can never be explained in "mechanical" terms—precisely because we *are* living, breathing human begins. Our bodies are genetically designed to be compatible with healing substances as found in nature. When helping people stay at the peak of good health, or recover from illness, a physician can't just treat one organ, one set of tissues, or one aching joint. The whole person deserves attention, since all the living parts of that person are so intricately related.

As you might expect from someone with those views, the therapies I describe in this book are holistic rather than mechanistic. In my practice, I encourage people to use natural substances and methods to aid the healing process, rather than relying on the kind of mechanistic "fix-its" that can sometimes be accomplished with pharmaceutical medications, surgical processes, and conventional medical procedures. These mechanistic methods have their place, but they also have their limitations—and one of their limiting factors is that they're done *by* someone else *to* you. When that happens, you're automatically depriving yourself of innate abilities that only you possess—the capacity, know-how, interest, inspiration, and motivation to use all your emotional, spiritual, and physical powers to heal yourself.

Which brings me to this book: All of the natural therapies in this book are healing methods that you can select for your own, personal healing.

As you look through the table of contents, you may be surprised by the apparent simplicity of some of these therapies.

In my view, a healing therapy is anything that contributes to good health and vitality. So you'll find sections on food and many sections that are concerned with nutrients. In addition, you can learn more about the healing power of such therapies as exercise, mental imagery, and prayer.

You'll also find information about substances that might be totally foreign to your experience: gugulipid, boswellia, spirulina, gymnema, and symphytum. I'm also introducing some breakthrough therapies—such as phytonutrients—that are just beginning to get the recognition they deserve. Whatever your familiarity with these healing therapies, I hope you will explore these sections to learn more about nature's incredible array of natural healing substances—for that's exactly what they are.

Some of these substances fall into the category of traditional herbs that have been known and used for hundreds or thousands of years by practical healers or ordinary physicians. You'll find ginkgo, along with echinacea, ginseng, aloe, dandelion, and dozens of others. Though the popularity of these remedies has waxed and waned over the centuries, many of them have specific healing properties that are well known to doctors and practitioners who are accustomed to using natural medicines and who see the results of these remedies every day. Many of these remedies belong to a vast unwritten lexicon of healing that dates back several millennia and includes the secrets of Chinese and Ayuverdic medicines.

Another category of healing therapies includes homeopathic remedies such as arnica, ferum phos, nux vomica, and gelsemium. Many conventionally trained medical doctors seem annoyed or baffled when the subject of homeopathy comes up. But in practice, many homeopathic remedies have proven their merits and recent studies support their use.

The oft-repeated principle of homeopathy is that "like cures like." What that means, in practical terms, is that we can prepare a solution that includes an infinitesimally small amount of a substance that *causes* a problem, and then, when the patient takes some of that preparation, it *cures* the problem. Nux vomica, for instance, includes minute amounts of the substance that causes cramps and vomiting. When given to a patient in its highly diluted, homeopathic form, the tonic does just the opposite: It helps relieve cramping and prevent nausea.

Odd? Mysterious? Yes—and trying to explain homeopathic remedies is particularly frustrating if you're a biochemist or an anatomist, because no one has been able to trace the pathways that lead from the substance to the cure. What practicing physicians do know, however, is that these tonics are capable of producing the healing effects that we'd like to see. As a researcher, I would love to have access to a full explanation of the science that can explain these remedies. But in the meantime, as a practicing doctor of integrated medicine, I'm quite happy to use familiar concentrations of these remedies to help ease the pain, discomfort, and illness of patients. There are no side effects; no drawbacks whatsoever to using them; and as long as they produce healing, I'll happily recommend them to anyone who can reap their benefits.

A similar principle applies to another category of healing therapies that I include in this book—natural supplements. We are fortunate to live in a time when there is worldwide exchange of information and data about all kinds of natural healing substances, and many of them are being found outside the laboratories of pharmaceutical companies. We now also have access to many of these natural supplements in many forms.

On the shelves of your local pharmacies, supermarkets, and health food stores, you'll find the now-familiar, standard bottles of multivitamins alongside such newly compounded supplements as glucosamine sulfate (often helpful for arthritis), SAMe (a promising supplement for depression), or CoQ10 (the valuable new heart-helping remedy), to name just a few.

*A note about supplements:* There's sometimes an L form of a supplement, which is used interchangeably with the non-L form. Whether I'm referring to an L form or non-L form, I'm talking about the same supplement.

It may be years, even decades, before mainstream doctors feel comfortable prescribing these supplements—and much more research must be done before we know the full range of their healing powers. But the ones I've reported on in this book are among the most promising, and if there are any questions about using them, I've been careful to note the possible side effects or potential drawbacks in each section.

My personal experience in recommending these supplements to patients has been positive. The ones included here have promising uses for prevention, recovery, and relief of many symptoms and illnesses.

Since I've just described some "categories" of healing therapies, you may wonder why I didn't organize the book that way. There's a simple explanation. I'd like you to be able to get access to the information and advice in this book as quickly and easily as possible, which just isn't possible if you're thinking in terms of categories of healing—or, as they're sometimes called, "modalities."

As you can see from the table of contents, the healing therapies are arranged in A-to-Z order, with nutritional therapies, herbs, supplements, and alternative healing methods side by side. In my own holistic medical practice, I simply don't think in terms of "categories" of healing therapies. It would be short-sighted—and unfair to patients—if I favored herbal remedies over homeopathic remedies for one patient, or decided that an individual should only use supplements while ignoring therapies like exercise or water.

Again, the whole person needs to be considered—and if I'm treating an individual, the pathway to good health for that person may be the sum of all possible avenues of healing. That's why I include information about some of the problems that medical doctors might neglect, such as "leaky gut syndrome" or the importance of detoxification. After all, what "works" for one person might not work for another—but why not consider the *many* possible alternatives that could help?

I want to provide you with the opportunity to become familiar with numerous opportunities for healing that are now within your reach. You'll find herbal remedies alongside homeopathic cures. You'll find sections on fat reduction, food therapies, and juicing next to vitamins, supplements, and specific foods like onion and garlic.

Today, if you're facing a difficult choice or an anxiety-producing situation, the section on mental imagery might tell you about the key therapy that can help you. Tomorrow, if you feel like you're coming down with a cold or experiencing the first signs of flu, it could be the information on echinacea or zinc that you need for information and guidance.

Of course, if you have a health problem or an ongoing condition that concerns you, the first thing you want to do is find all the therapies that might be helpful.

Turn to the "Quick Cure Finder" on page 531 first, and you can find out which of the therapies in this book I personally recommend.

In each section, you'll find out the experiences my patients have had when they used these therapies as recommended. I give you some background on the traditional or historical uses of the therapy, and an overview of the research. (The reference sources can be found at the end of this book.) In addition, I have included specific dosage recommendations and some cautions about possible side effects or negative interactions.

Throughout this book, you'll also find my advice about consulting a medical or naturopathic doctor or specialist before you begin the therapy or while you're using it. I'm fully aware that you may need more than one opinion to help you monitor your health, protect yourself from dangerous interactions, or optimize the benefits of certain natural therapies. I should add, please get medical help or call an experienced and qualified practitioner if you have pain or other symptoms that you don't understand, or if you have any sudden changes in your health.

People, often ask me, "Is this something that you'd use for yourself?"

The answer is yes. Each of these healing therapies in some way supports the healing powers of the body. This book embraces the most effective and sometimes miraculous, nontoxic solutions to healthcare needs that I know. They *do* work as I've described them—not always, not for everyone all the time, but often enough that I readily recommend them to patients, friends, family. Yes, I readily use them myself when necessary. I am always learning more about these and other healing techniques, too, so I constantly review credible scientific studies that evaluate effective uses of holistic methods and medicines.

I realize that you are looking for results. Believe me, I'm on your side. As a naturopathic and homeopathic doctor, I believe the book in your hands is a reliable guide to the best healthcare in the emerging field of integrative medicine.

Yours in good health and vitality,

Mark Stengler ND, CHT, HHP
Doctor of Naturopathy
Homeopathic Doctor

La Jolla, California
*www.thenaturalphysician.com*

# Acknowledgments

I would like to acknowledge Ed Claflin for his help in the conception and development of this book. Also, to Deb Yost for her support in helping me to bring the "good news" of natural medicine to people. Many thanks to Sybil Grace for her editorial help, to Yvette Romero for her expert help with publicity and promotion, and to everyone at Prentice Hall Direct who helped bring this book into being. To my agent, Jeff Herman, for all his help.

My gratitude to Jean Robertson, a mentor of mine, who years ago gave me the sound advice of "Just be yourself."

As always, many thanks to my family and friends.

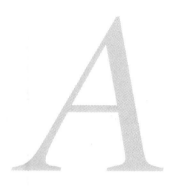

# Acidophilus

· · · · · · · · · · · · · · · · · · · · · · · · · · · · · · · · · · · · · · · · · · · · · · · · · · · · · · · · ·

"Doc, I just don't understand why my digestive system is so messed up. Can you help me?"

The question came from a new patient, Steve, a 19-year-old who had been suffering digestive problems for at least two years.

"Yes, I probably can," I replied. "But let me get some more information from you first."

I was reasonably confident that I *could* help. Most digestive problems, in my experience, improve with specific natural healing therapies.

Some very important background came to light as Steve revealed his past health history. Steve's digestive problems included extreme bloating, gas, loose stools, and abdominal cramps. When we looked at the period when the trouble started—about two years before—Steve realized that it coincided with the start of his acne treatments.

After dealing with acne through his early teenage years, Steve decided when he was seventeen that it was time to take more drastic measures. He requested antibiotic treatments. His doctor prescribed tetracycline, an antibiotic that helps suppress acne flare-ups.

Tetracycline helps combat bacteria that accumulate in the skin oil (sebum), which is overproduced when someone has acne. By destroying bacteria, the antibiotic reduces skin inflammation.

For treatment of acne, antibiotics must be used on a long-term basis. The acne returns when they are stopped. Unfortunately, tetracycline is not a magic bullet.

While it destroys the bacteria that contribute to acne, it also wipes out a number of helpful bacteria, including *Lactobacillus* and *Bifidobacterium.* Sometimes called "friendly flora," these are completely benign organisms that reside in the mouth, digestive tract, respiratory tract, and urinary tract. (In women, these bacteria are also found in the vagina.)

The antibiotic is like a bombshell that indiscriminately destroys allies as well as enemies. When antibiotics are needed for serious bacterial infections, they can be lifesaving—and the benefits of using the bombshell clearly outweigh the drawbacks. But antibiotics are now widely overprescribed for less-than-critical situations—specifically, for conditions such as acne. With prolonged or inappropriate use, they can cause more problems than they solve.

A comprehensive stool analysis proved that my suspicion about Steve's condition was correct. The lab test showed that his "good bacteria" count was very low. The report also indicated that he had an overgrowth of potentially pathogenic "bugs" such as *Candida Albicans* (yeast) and some other organisms that shouldn't be thriving in the digestive tract. Clearly, the shortage of friendly bacteria such as *Lactobacillus* was related to the overgrowth of harmful bacteria.

Once I had the lab report, it was easy enough to help Steve. Plain yogurt that contains "live cultures" has acidophilus and other friendly bacteria. I recommended that Steve eat live-culture yogurt, and I also prescribed an acidophilus supplement known in the natural health industry as a *probiotic* (which simply means "healthful to life").

## THE BACTERIA YOU CAN'T LIVE WITHOUT

It was Dr. Eli Metchnikoff, a colleague of Louis Pasteur's, who did the first, groundbreaking work in the study of *Lactobacilli* and other "good" bacteria. Dr. Metchnikoff was awarded the Nobel Prize in 1908 for discovering that these bacteria played an important role in immunity. Most disease, he surmised, begins in the digestive tract. When the "good" bacteria were not successfully controlling the "bad" ones, Dr. Metchnikoff labeled the condition dysbiosis, which simply means that the bacteria were not living in mutual harmony. His research has led to the understanding we have today of the numerous benefits of the good bacteria and the importance of their role in balancing the "bugs."

It is amazing to realize that acidophilus and the other friendly flora are part of the one hundred trillion bacteria that live together in the human digestive system. Together, these bacteria comprise as much as 4 pounds of our body weight!

This fertile colonization of the human body begins even before birth. An infant enters the world with a preordained measure of both good and potentially harmful bacteria. With the very first breath, a baby inhales bacteria from the environment, bringing those "bugs" into the mouth and mucous membranes. From there the bacteria go on to colonize the rest of the body.

From then on, the balance of bacteria is in a continuous state of adjustment. Breast milk supplies beneficial bacteria, so as long as a child is nursing, he or she has the benefit of an extra boost. Aided by the friendly flora in mother's milk, *acidophilus* and other beneficial bacteria set up their own "territories" where they act to prevent the potentially harmful accumulation of bugs that might attack the body.

## BENIGN BEINGS

In recent years, researchers have come to understand many of the chemical and biological reactions that characterize acidophilus and other beneficial bacteria. Acidophilus produces an acidic environment, which inhibits the reproduction of many harmful bacteria. Acidophilus also produces substances called bacteriocins, which act as natural antibiotics to destroy harmful microorganisms.

Along with other friendly flora, acidophilus also activates the immune system by increasing antibody response in the mucous tissues.

Friendly bacteria also help produce what are known as short-chain fatty acids. These fatty acids are important as they help the regeneration of colon cells. They also have anti-cancer effects.

Acidophilus and the friendly flora of the digestive system help break down foods in the colon, particularly undigested fiber from fruits and vegetables. They help to digest milk sugar and promote regular bowel movements. Acidophilus also works to prevent the growth of *H. Pylori*, a bacteria implicated in many cases of stomach ulcers.

While most physicians know something about these benefits of friendly flora, other rewards are less well recognized. For instance, many physicians are unaware that acidophilus and the good flora help to manufacture vitamins in the body. These include vitamins $B_2$, $B_3$, $B_5$, $B_{12}$, biotin, and vitamin K.

Acidophilus is also important for proper absorption of minerals in the small intestine.

## FOODS ON THE SIDE OF GOOD

Many societies throughout the world have recognized the health benefits of cultured foods that are high in acidophilus. Sauerkraut is one. This traditional German side dish is also taken for ulcers and a variety of digestive problems. Cottage cheese, kefir, and miso are other potential sources.

Yogurt, however, is probably the most convenient source of friendly bacteria. Just make sure to buy organic brands that list live cultures on the label. Flavored yogurt often has a lot of sugar or sweeteners, so I generally recommend the low-fat, plain kind.

In addition to getting more acidophilus from food sources, you can also support the growth of these good bacteria with a type of indigestible carbohydrate called FOS (fructooligosaccharides). Food scientists have learned that FOS not only supports the selective growth of *Lactobacillus acidophilus* and *Bifidobacteria* (another beneficial kind), it also interferes with harmful bacteria.

FOS has other benefits as well, because it inhibits parasites and toxic bacteria from attaching to the digestive tract.

Sources of this unique good bacteria promoter include bananas, barley, garlic, honey, chicory, fruit, wheat, onions, soybeans, and tomatoes. Jerusalem artichoke is particularly high in FOS. The Japanese are so impressed by the health benefits of FOS that they have added it to over 500 food products.

## ADDING TO IMBALANCES

The most common cause of dysbiosis or bacterial imbalance is chronic antibiotic use. But there are other pharmaceutical medications that contribute to dysbiosis. Among the common culprits are pain medications, steroids such as Prednisone, and nonsteroidal antiinflammatories (NSAIDs) such as aspirin and ibuprofen. Another possible contributing factor is low stomach acid, which leads to the buildup of bad bacteria.

As you might suspect, foods play a role in the balance of the microbes in our system. Sugar and alcohol feed the bad bugs. The chlorine in drinking water can contribute to the destruction of acidophilus and the good bacteria. A plant-based diet and cultured foods feed the good bugs.

Chronic stress can also alter flora balance.

## DOSAGE

To determine the levels and balance of bacteria (good and bad), I recommend a comprehensive stool analysis. Specialized labs will do this test. I use the Great Smokies Lab in North Carolina (see resource section for more information).

Some people with a strong dairy allergy cannot tolerate yogurt of any kind, so the best food source—live-culture yogurt—is not appropriate. But supplemental sources of probiotics come in many other forms, including capsule, liquid, or powder. Most of these probiotic formulas need to be refrigerated.

For adults who have a chronic condition, I recommend any product that provides a daily dose of at least two billion viable organisms. For acute infections like diarrhea, I suggest triple that dosage. The best supplements also contain FOS that helps encourage the growth of good flora.

Most probiotic supplements should be taken between meals or 30 minutes after eatin because stomach acid—produced in quantity when you're digesting your food—can destroy acidophilus. Some probiotic supplements are specially coated capsules to prevent the beneficial bacteria being destroyed by stomach acid.

If you've had an antibiotic treatment, I recommend taking a probiotic supplement for at least two months afterward. People who are taking certain medications for chronic illness may need to supplement with acidophilus indefinitely.

Children should use special children's acidophilus supplements. The mixture of probiotics includes a higher percentage of *Bifidobacterium*.

## WHAT ARE THE SIDE EFFECTS?

Side effects are very rare. Some people who have an overgrowth of yeast *(Candida)* may notice some "die off" symptoms in the first few weeks of supplementation. These symptoms include gas, bloating, and diarrhea. A few people have noted that they seem to have poor concentration when they're taking supplements.

As I've noted, people with severe dairy allergies may not be able to tolerate acidophilus in a milk product such as yogurt. They can supplement with a dairy-free probiotic instead.

# ACIDOPHILUS
## Recommendations from the Natural Physician for . . .

### ❧ Cancer Prevention

Probiotics, especially acidophilus, help eliminate or reduce the production of cancer-causing chemicals. They also help to deactivate cancer-promoting enzymes. This is particularly important if you want to lower your risk of colon and breast cancer.

### ❧ Constipation

Acidophilus can be one of the key supplements to use in cases of chronic constipation. One study showed it beneficial for those with constipation who had colitis, irritable bowel syndrome (IBS), and other various disorders. I find it particularly helpful for infants suffering from constipation as a result of antibiotic use.

### ❧ Digestive Health

Acidophilus is my automatic prescription for patients suffering from most digestive disorders. These can include Crohn's disease, ulcerative colitis, irritable bowel syndrome, and ulcers.

I have also prescribed it, quite successfully, for a fairly rare condition called antibiotic-associated colitis. This condition is an acute inflammation of the colon caused by the overgrowth of harmful bacteria, known as *Clostridium difficile*, after the use of antibiotics. Symptoms usually include diarrhea and abdominal pain.

### ❧ Food Allergies

People who suffer from food allergies often have an underlying digestive imbalance. A study looking at a group of children suffering from food allergies showed evidence of *Lactobacillus* and *Bifidobacteria* deficiency.

### ❧ Lactose Intolerance

Acidophilus also helps to produce the milk sugar enzyme lactase. It is well known that 75 percent of adults (except those of northwest European descent) have a deficiency of this enzyme, which means the digestive system cannot break down milk sugar products effectively. This leads to lactose intolerance, indicated by symptoms that include diarrhea, gas, bloating, and bad breath.

### ❧ Leaky Gut Syndrome

This is a very common digestive disorder that involves the "leaking" or malabsorption of undigested food particles. When these particles pass through the intestinal wall, inflammatory chemicals are released. Symptoms of leaky gut syndrome may include abdominal pain, joint pain, fuzzy thinking, gas, weakened immunity, and skin rashes as well as other symptoms. Many conditions ranging from arthritis to irritable bowel syndrome are associated with leaky gut syndrome.

Acidophilus is one of the key supplements used to help heal the damaged intestinal wall so that proper absorption can occur.

### ❧ Traveler's Diarrhea

Numerous studies have shown that acidophilus and other good bacteria are helpful in the prevention and treatment of cases of infectious diarrhea. I recommend my patients take a probiotic supplement preventatively when traveling, especially to other countries.

### ❧ Vaginitis

Acidophilus is commonly used by natural healthcare practitioners for the treatment of

*(continued)*

6

vaginal infections caused by bacteria (*gardnerella*) and yeast. Women generally experience burning, itching, and an odorous discharge with this condition. Vaginitis can often be treated with direct, daily insertion of two acidophilus capsules into the vagina for up to two weeks. At the same time, I recommend that women with vaginitis eat live-culture yogurt and take acidophilus supplements as well. This helps to repopulate the good bacteria and provide an acidic environment that discourages the invading microorganisms.

However, it's important to see a doctor for a diagnosis before using this treatment. Other infectious agents may be contributing to the symptoms—and if so, you may require a different therapy.

# Aconite

"Doctor, is there something natural I can take when I break out into a panic attack?"

Kristina was a new patient, but I was already familiar with her history of chronic anxiety and panic attacks. She was familiar with many of the prescription drugs that she had discussed with other doctors—but she was seeking some form of relief that wouldn't involve the use of pharmaceuticals. I would need to know more about the nature of her anxiety before I made a recommendation.

"Tell me more about what happens to you," I prompted.

"Well, sometimes when I am out in public or before meeting with someone, I get all clammy. My heart starts to race, my body freezes up, and then a wave of fear comes over me—like I'm going to die!"

The natural medicine that instantly came to mind was homeopathic aconite, also known as *Aconitum Napellus*. This remedy covers symptoms such as the kind of anxiety that's accompanied by a tremendous fear of death, which is one of the characteristics of a panic disorder. In fact, aconite is one of the main remedies for phobic states as well as anxiety disorders.

I advised Kristina on how and when she could take aconite. Subsequently, she carried it with her wherever she went. As instructed, when she felt a panic attack coming on—which could happen as frequently as every couple of days—she would take a dose of the remedy.

A few weeks later, at a follow-up visit, Kristina reported that the aconite had helped her calm down. A number of times, it helped prevent a full-blown panic attack with that dreaded fear-of-death feeling.

I had explained to Kristina that aconite was not a cure for her condition, but, as she discovered, it did provide some relief. It also fulfilled her own wish for an effective alternative to the pharmaceutical anti-anxiety medications that had left her with many side effects—including grogginess and what she described as "feeling like a zombie."

There were a number of underlying psychological and biochemical reasons for Kristina's anxiety disorder. The homeopathic remedy would not make those factors go away. What it did, however, is give her relief from the most acute symptoms.

It would be enough if that were the only benefit of aconite. But many homeopathic practitioners have reported other benefits as well. With patients who have suffered from a very violent or traumatic event, such as an earthquake or car accident, practitioners have found that aconite helps relieve some of the symptoms of shock.

## REMEDY VS. HERB

The homeopathic remedy called aconite is different from the herb with the same name. Herbal aconite is sometimes used in Chinese medicine in very small amounts. But a homeopathic remedy contains aconite in an almost infinitesimally dilute form—in such tiny amounts, in fact, that many scientists have been baffled by the healing effects of homeopathy.

In the remedy Kristina received, the amount of aconite was analogous to one drop in a swimming pool filled with water. For such a small concentration to have such a powerful healing effect sounds bizarre—but again and again, homeopathy has produced results that seem to defy explanation.

In brief, the practice of homeopathy is based on the science of "like cures like." For example, a high concentration of aconite would produce results that were just the opposite of what we wanted. One of my colleagues, for instance, took too much of the herb aconite, and was immediately attacked with a number of symptoms that scared the heck out of him—including increased heart rate, elevated blood pressure, sweating, and a feeling of anxiety and of impending doom. We know for a fact that the herb aconite, taken in large doses, is potentially lethal. But in very small concentrations (homeopathic form), it produces symptoms that are precisely the *opposite* of those that my colleague experienced.

That's where "like cures like" comes in—the phrase most commonly used to describe homeopathy. If we know what symptoms are produced by the crude herb, we have guidelines for using the nontoxic homeopathic preparation to *cure* those symptoms. That is to say, a substance that causes symptoms in a healthy person can be used to cure or improve those same symptoms in someone who is ill.

## BEATING THE FLU BUG

Aconite is one of the most common remedies for an acute, infectious disease like the flu—and I've experienced the results firsthand. I vividly recall one rainy, winter's day in Portland, Oregon when I felt the symptoms coming on—first the chills, then weakness in my legs, arms, and finally my whole body. Before long, the fever began.

But there was a weird aspect to this start of the flu. I began to have the sensation that something was *seriously* wrong with my body—and that something terrible was going to happen to me. In other words, the physical sensations were accompanied by mental anxiety along with the onset of a sense of fear.

This was strange. As a trained physician, I was not usually aware of any feelings of fear, even when I became ill. Perhaps this is because I'm generally in good health, and I trusted in my own vitality. This time, however. . . .

So I wondered what was going on—and mentally ran through the usual checklist. Was my blood sugar low? I had recently eaten, so that didn't seem likely.

Was I stressed out and just experiencing a stress reaction that I'd never had before? That, too, seemed improbable since I wasn't in a particularly stressful situation at that time.

It soon dawned on me that the fear was actually one symptom of the onset of the flu. For this particular combination of the symptoms, the most effective cure was likely to be homeopathic aconite.

I knew that if aconite is taken in the first hour of a flu, cold, or other infectious disease, it often stops the illness in its tracks. The first dose had an immediate effect. In less than five minutes, I noticed that I had already started to feel calmer.

I took another dose 30 minutes later. The fever broke. Muscle strength began to return. It was actually a strange experience—to feel the sensations of muscle weakness and achiness begin to dissipate within a matter of minutes.

By the end of the day, I was able to continue my regular routine as if nothing had happened. Thanks to the power of homeopathy—and the remedy aconite—I had beaten the flu bug!

## CHILDREN'S REMEDY

Every home should have a homeopathic remedy kit that includes aconite. It's one of the most common remedies to use for many minor childhood afflictions, including ear infections, sore throat, croup, flu, and fever. For example, a homeopathic doctor is sure to recommend aconite for high fever if the fever comes on suddenly; if the child is crying, restless, and anxious; and if one cheek is pale and the other red.

There are two key characteristics of a condition that requires aconite. First, the symptoms usually come on very quickly. If it's a fever, for instance, the onset can occur in just a matter of minutes, and the temperature spikes quickly. The second characteristic is that the illness often comes after an exposure to the wind, especially the cold, dry wind. For instance, if a child gets an ear infection after being outdoors on a windy, cold day, I would recommend a dose or two of aconite within the first 30 to 60 minutes after the symptoms begin. There's a good chance the treatment will abort the whole infection.

I've seen a child who has been screaming in pain from an ear infection become calmer—to the point of falling asleep—within 10 minutes of being given homeopathic aconite. Best of all, the symptoms do not return. It's times like these when you say "Thank goodness for homeopathy."

## DOSAGE

Dissolve two pellets of the 30C potency (strength) in your mouth every 15 minutes for the relief of shock, anxiety, panic attacks, or an acute infection like the flu or ear infection. If there is no relief of symptoms within one hour, discontinue use and use a different treatment.

Since aconite can contribute significantly to the relief of anxiety, it is one of the main remedies for women during labor who feel absolutely certain they are about to die.

**Note:** Dosage is the same for all age groups.

## WHAT ARE THE SIDE EFFECTS?

As with any homeopathic medicine, side effects are rarely an issue. By taking aconite too frequently, however, you might bring on symptoms of anxiety. Take enough of the remedy to bring symptoms under control, then reduce the dosage or stop taking it.

# Acupressure

Dan, a 41-year-old executive, kept rubbing his neck as he described to me the torment that it was putting him through.

"At work, my neck gets so stiff that I get tension headaches all the time. I see a massage therapist once a week, and that helps. I even have one of those special chairs that help my posture. But if there's anything else you can recommend, I'll do it!"

"You can try acupressure," I suggested. "Let me show you some acupressure points you can press on during the day. This will help to reduce the tension in your muscles and promote relaxation."

To start, I demonstrated by pressing on two points on the back of the neck, known as Gallbladder 20. I showed him how to massage those points with his fingertips. Then I introduced him to "Tai Yang," the points near his temple where gentle pressure would relax the muscles almost instantly.

After that we moved on to Yuyao, a spot located in the middle of the eyebrows.

Then I showed him the spot on his hand where pressure would bring relief. "Push on this mound of flesh that pops up between your thumb and index finger, then squeeze the fingertips together. Tender isn't it?"

In traditional Chinese medicine—as practiced by an acupuncturist—this point is known as Large Intestine 4, I explained. "It helps to relieve pain and discomfort of the face and head."

For the next two weeks, Dan worked on the acupressure points I showed him. Periodically during the day, he would stop work for a couple of minutes and apply pressure to these specific acupressure points. He noticed quite a reduction in his neck discomfort. He never experienced any headaches either.

## KEEPING UP THE PRESSURE

Many people are aware of acupuncture as a treatment to relieve pain. However, acupressure was used long before acupuncture in China, Japan, and India. Actually, it could be said that most every culture used acupressure to some degree. Simply, it was pushing on "tender" spots to relieve local pain and discomfort. Sometimes, it's what we do naturally—pressing on a sore, aching muscle, for instance. But practitioners in acupressure and acupuncture have identified less obvious, specific points of the body that can contribute to pain relief or healing.

Chinese medicine has relied on acupressure for over 4,000 years. Today, it remains a major treatment at Chinese hospitals. Its popularity has been growing steadily throughout the world.

## CHANNELS OF ENERGY

The traditional Chinese system of medicine focuses on the concept that the life-giving energy called "Qi" (pronounced "chee") circulates throughout the body in 12 main channels. Each channel represents a certain organ system—such as kidney, lung, and large intestine. The points that connect to that system are located bilaterally—that is, on both sides of the body. These channels are all interconnected, so they link up to one another.

Along each of the channels, known as meridians, are specific acupressure points that can relieve local pain and inflammation, and also affect pain or tension in other areas of the body. Many of the points can be used to influence the function of internal organs. It is believed that when there is a blockage of Qi circulation in the channels, then disease or illness arises.

To prevent a disease from occurring, or to treat a disease, one must keep the Qi moving. One way to do this is to stimulate the acupressure points where a blockage is occurring. Usually these points are tender to the touch, indicating a blockage. Whether you relieve sore muscles or an internal problem such as digestive upset depends on which points you press. Mental and emotional imbalances can also be helped with acupressure.

## CHEMICAL REACTION?

It is not known exactly how acupressure relieves pain or improves the functioning of internal organs. One theory is that the brain releases certain chemicals that inhibit pain and stimulate the immune system. It is also thought that acupressure relaxes trigger points so muscle tension calms down.

Acupressure may improve blood and lymphatic circulation, as well as improve electrical flow along nerves and between cells. Much research is ongoing in this area, including studies funded by the prestigious National Institutes of Health. Acupressure does work and is a major reason why traditional Chinese medicine is one of the fastest growing medical fields.

While someone trained in acupressure can obtain the best results, there are many easy-to-locate points that you can apply pressure to yourself to alleviate discomfort or improve certain conditions. These points are shown in the illustration on pages 16 and 17.

## ADMINISTERING AN ACUPRESSURE TREATMENT

Here are four easy steps to follow for self-treatment.

1. Make sure you are relaxed. The room should be free of noise. If possible, you should wear light clothing.

2. Locate the desired point to which you are going to apply pressure. Press on the point using your thumb or fingers. The pressure should be direct, yet not cause great discomfort. Some points may be very tender, indicating a blockage.

Start with very light pressure, see how you feel, and adjust the pressure accordingly. Press the acupressure point and hold for 10 to 15 seconds. This can be repeated 5 to 10 times to see if it helps relieve the symptoms.

Chronic conditions will need more treatments to see if the acupressure is working. Some people prefer rubbing or massaging the acupressure points; this is fine to do as well. As the same channel runs on both sides of the body, try to stimulate the points on both sides simultaneously. For example, massaging Gallbladder 20 on both sides of the back of the head helps to relax tense neck muscles. Or, Stomach 36, located four finger widths below the kneecap and one finger width toward the outside of the leg (outside the shin bone on the muscle), can be stimulated simultaneously to improve digestive function.

3. Make sure to breathe while you stimulate the acupressure point. Slow, deep, relaxed breaths are best.

4. Relax in a quiet atmosphere after a treatment and drink a glass of water to help detoxify your body.

## WHAT ARE THE SIDE EFFECTS?

Acupressure is a very safe treatment. Temporary soreness of the acupressure point is common and normal. Acupressure should not be applied to open wounds or areas of extreme swelling or inflammation, such as varicose veins.

There are certain points that should not be stimulated on a pregnant woman because of the risk of miscarriage. It is important that pregnant women avoid the use of Gallbladder 21, Large Intestine 4, and Liver 3. Pregnant women should consult with a practitioner of acupressure before self-treating.

---

# ACUPRESSURE
## RECOMMENDATIONS FROM THE NATURAL PHYSICIAN FOR . . .

### ◌ Allergies

Large Intestine 4, located between the webbing of the thumb and index finger, relieves nasal symptoms and head congestion.

Large Intestine 20, located on the lower, outer corner of each nostril, reduces sneezing and nasal symptoms.

### ◌ Anxiety

Pericardium 6, located two-and-one-half finger widths below the wrist crease in the middle of the forearm (palm side), helps relieve anxiety.

### ◌ Cold and Flu

Large Intestine 4, located between the webbing of the thumb and index finger, relieves head congestion and sinus discomfort. Gently push on this

spot. You want to work this acupressure point on both hands, so after you've treated your left hand, be sure to do the same to the right.

Large Intestine 20, located on the lower, outer corner of each nostril, reduces sneezing and nasal symptoms.

### ◌ Cough

Lung 1, located in the front of the shoulder area, in the space below where the collarbone and shoulder meet, reduces cough.

### ◌ Constipation

Large Intestine 4, located between the webbing of the thumb and index finger, relieves constipation. Gently push on this spot on both hands.

*(continued)*

### ❧ Eyestrain

Stomach 2, located one-half inch below the center of the lower eye ridge (you can feel an indentation), relieves burning, aching, and dry eyes.

Bladder 2, located on the inner edge of the eyebrows beside the bridge of the nose (you can feel an indentation), relieves red and painful eyes.

### ❧ Headache

The following are all helpful. Choose the point or points that provide the most effective relief for you.

- Gallbladder 20, located below the base of the skull, in the space between the two vertical neck muscles.
- Large Intestine 4, located between the webbing of the thumb and index finger. Gently push on this spot on both hands.
- Liver 3, located on top of the foot in the hollow between the big toe and second toe.
- Yuyao, indentation in the middle of the eyebrow (directly straight up from pupil).

### ❧ Indigestion

Stomach 36, located four finger widths below the kneecap and one finger width toward the outside of the leg (outside of shin bone on the muscle), improves digestive function.

Conception Vessel 6, located two finger widths below the navel, relieves abdominal pain, gas, and other digestive problems.

### ❧ Muscle Pain

Find the points that are most tender in the sore muscle and gently press on them and release, or massage these points.

### ❧ Nausea

Apply pressure on Pericardium 6, which is located two-and-one-half finger widths below the wrist crease in the middle of the inside of your forearm. This point works so well for nausea that special wrist bands can be bought that stimulate this point. They are used for any kind of nausea, including morning sickness and motion sickness.

Conception Vessel 6, located two finger widths below the navel, relieves nausea and abdominal symptoms. It is also effective for motion sickness.

### ❧ Neck Pain

Gallbladder 21, located on the highest point of the shoulder (trapezius muscle), relieves stiff neck and shoulder tension. Feel for a tender spot.

Gallbladder 20, located below the base of the skull, in the space between the two vertical neck muscles, relieves stiff neck and neck pain.

Large Intestine 4, located between the webbing of the thumb and index finger, reduces neck and head discomfort. Gently push on this spot on both hands.

### ❧ Sinusitis

The following two points relieve sinus pain and promote drainage:

- Large Intestine 20, located on the lower, outer corner of each nostril
- Large Intestine 4, located between the webbing of the thumb and index finger

# Acupressure Point Location Chart
## (Front)

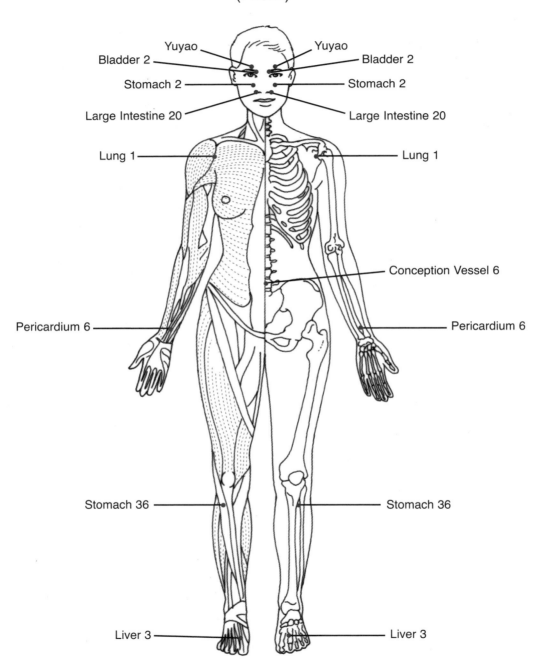

Yuyao

Yuyao

Bladder 2

Bladder 2

Stomach 2

Stomach 2

Large Intestine 20

Large Intestine 20

Lung 1

Lung 1

Conception Vessel 6

Pericardium 6

Pericardium 6

Stomach 36

Stomach 36

Liver 3

Liver 3

# (BACK)

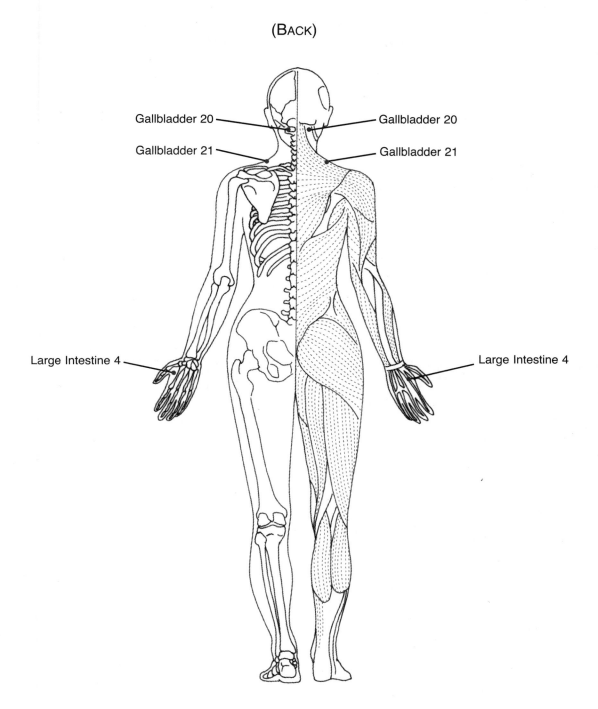

Gallbladder 20

Gallbladder 21

Large Intestine 4

Gallbladder 20

Gallbladder 21

Large Intestine 4

# Aloe

There are over 300 different types of aloe plants in the world, but aloe vera (also called aloe barbadensis) is the one that people are usually talking about when they mention "aloe." Aloe vera is one of the most popular all-round herbs, because it does so much for the skin: It soothes and smoothes the skin, and reduces healing time, if you have any kind of sunburn.

If you have applied aloe vera gel soon after getting a sunburn, you were likely very impressed by how effectively it healed the burn and prevented blisters. In fact, it's so kind to the skin that it's included in many cosmetic products.

But aloe also has medicinal properties when you take it internally. You can take the juice to heal digestive ailments such as ulcers and inflammatory bowel disease (IBD). In addition, it's been known to help heal arthritis, diabetes, and constipation.

The medicinal aloe that's used as a skin gel comes from a different part of the plant from the aloe that's taken internally. The gel comes from the center part of the leaves. That part of the plant is also the source of aloe vera concentrate, a type of aloe vera gel with the water removed. The concentrate, like the gel, is used topically.

To get the aloe vera juice that is usually taken internally, herbalists remove the latex (which has a bitter taste) and dilute the gel with water. But there's also a product called aloe vera latex, aloe bitter latex, or drug aloe. This is derived from the rind—the lining just underneath the leaf surface—and it's bitter tasting. Bitter latex acts as a powerful laxative.

## THE ROLES OF ALOE

Aloe grows in most of the warm, sunny climates of the world. As far back as 550 B.C., Egyptians were already using aloe to treat certain skin conditions, according to written sources.

Elsewhere in the world, similar discoveries were made. The Zulu of southern Africa use it to heal wounds, as do the Chinese. In Ayurvedic medicine the bitter latex, taken internally, is one of the medicines that's used to expel worms.

The plant is also well known for its properties as a laxative. European colonists to Africa, praising the laxative properties, brought some samples back to Europe, where its popularity soon spread. It was also brought to North America from Europe. In fact, if you asked a nineteenth-century pharmacist anywhere in the western world to recommend some kind of laxative, he would almost certainly have named aloe.

The plant contains many different compounds that account for its diverse medicinal properties. A group of compounds known as anthraquinones, found in the rind part of the leaf, make up the bitter latex and account for its powerful laxative effects.

Another active ingredient is the polysaccharide (long sugar chain) known as acemannan. This compound has been shown to stimulate the immune system. It has strong antiviral effects and is being further investigated in the hope that it will be effective with HIV and cancer.

Aloe also contains prostaglandins and fatty acids (including gamma linolenic acid). These compounds are thought to give aloe some of its wound-healing and antiinflammatory powers.

Also, many different vitamins are found in aloe including vitamins C, E, $B_1$, $B_2$, $B_6$, folic acid, choline, and beta carotene. Aloe is also a source of many minerals including zinc, which is well known for its wound-healing properties as well. Aloe also contains 20 different amino acids that are known to help with tissue repair.

Scientists still don't know exactly how aloe heals the skin so effectively, though parts of the puzzle are beginning to fit together. It has been shown to stimulate the cells that grow collagen, the protein substance that binds skin together. The polysaccharides are thought to have an antiinflammatory effect on the skin. The gel that reduces pain contains salicylic acid, the same component that's active in aspirin, so that might account for some of its pain-quelling property. That substance also inhibits many different bacteria and fungus from growing on the skin.

# DOSAGE

## ❧ Gel

The gel can be applied liberally to the skin. You can cut open an aloe leaf and squeeze the gel onto your skin. Any health food store, pharmacy, and most grocery stores carry aloe gel products. Look for one that contains a high concentration of aloe gel (80 percent or higher).

## ❧ Juice

There is not much literature on the proper dosage of juice, which is taken internally. I recommend that people start at 1 teaspoon daily and work up to 6 teaspoons a day. It is recommended to not consume more than 1 quart daily. People with HIV/AIDS use approximately 800 to 1,600 milligrams per day of acemannan, the active antiviral agent in aloe.

### ✺ *Bitter aloe latex*

This substance, taken internally, is such a powerful laxative that you really need to have the guidance of a doctor when you're taking it. Even with this caution, you should keep the daily dosage under 300 milligrams, and stop using it after a few days.

## WHAT ARE THE SIDE EFFECTS?

On rare occasions, people have reported allergic skin reactions to aloe vera gel, though I've never seen this side effect. If you do notice your skin reddening or getting itchy, just stop using the gel. For some people it can worsen dry skin.

Too much of the juice, taken internally, may cause diarrhea. Long-term use of bitter aloe latex is highly inadvisable. It can cause diarrhea and the loss of minerals such as potassium—and for this reason, it's not readily available to consumers. Using it frequently can lead to a condition known as "lazy colon," whereby the lower part of your intestinal tract more or less goes on strike and relies on the laxative effect of the aloe.

Pregnant women and children under the age of 13 should not use the bitter aloe latex at all. Also, don't ever use this aloe compound if you have intestinal obstruction.

---

## ALOE
### RECOMMENDATIONS FROM THE NATURAL PHYSICAN FOR . . .

#### ✺ *Asthma*

Aloe vera extract can help treat asthma, but needs to be taken for 6 months or more before you can tell whether it's effective. My information about this is all secondhand, however. I have never used aloe vera to treat patients with this condition, and I have not met anyone with asthma who has tried the extract as a cure.

#### ✺ *Burns and Wound Healing*

On most of the occasions when I'm recommending aloe vera gel, it's for burns. Either kitchen burns or sunburn are equally well treated with this topical remedy, so it makes sense to have some gel in your kitchen near the stove and also in your beach bag for the shore. It seems to make a dramatic difference in tissue healing.

*(continued)*

### ❧ Canker Sores

One study found a special form of acemannan gel—derived from aloe vera—to be more effective than a conventional medication (Orabase) in speeding the healing of canker sores. In a study of 31 children with canker sores, researchers got good results with nearly four out of five. Improvements usually began on the second day of treatment. (While I have not yet recommended aloe for this purpose, the studies are convincing, and I intend to try it myself if I get canker sores.)

### ❧ Diabetes

Researchers in Thailand investigated the effects of aloe on 77 people who had just been diagnosed with diabetes mellitus (Type 2). People in the study received either 1 tablespoon of aloe vera juice or 1 tablespoon of an inactive substance that looked and tasted just like the medicine. After taking their doses twice daily for 42 days, people taking the aloe vera juice had significantly lower blood sugar levels than those who got the "fake" medicine (placebo). In addition, the treated patients had lower triglyceride levels, which meant their blood was in better condition and they were less likely to have strokes or heart attacks. My feeling is that more studies need to be done, but I would certainly consider that this study opens the door to future possibilities.

### ❧ Psoriasis

This condition can be challenging to treat with either conventional or natural methods. One study showed that a 0.5 percent aloe vera cream used for 4 weeks was significantly effective in relieving psoriasis lesions. The aloe cream helped cure four out of five people who used it, whereas the improvement rate was only about 6 percent among those who used the inactive placebo.

Psoriasis lesions tend to be very dry and flaky. I assume aloe's emollient and antiinflammatory effects were the reason why it was so helpful in this study. In my experience, not all psoriasis patients find aloe helpful—but a surprising number do.

### ❧ Ulcers and Inflammatory Bowel Disease

Aloe juice has become popular as an ulcer treatment in the past few years. One of aloe's constituents, known as emodin, may actually destroy the bacteria *H. Pylori*, which is implicated in causing stomach ulcers.

Anecdotally, many people have told me that it helped relieve their longstanding ulcer symptoms. At first I was skeptical but I have had many people report this benefit to me. Also, aloe juice is gaining popularity for inflammatory conditions of the digestive tract such as Crohn's disease and ulcerative colitis.

### ❧ Viral Infections and AIDS

The antiviral component, acemannan, also has a virus-fighting effect against measles, influenza, and herpes simplex viruses. The injection of acemannan was shown in one study to be very effective against feline leukemia virus: 71 percent of the cats were alive after 12 weeks in what is usually a fatal disease.

Acemannan is showing some promise when used in combination with AZT in the treatment of AIDS. The combination may allow a person with AIDS to use lower dosages of AZT, which would reduce the risk of toxicity and side effects. Studies using acemannan by itself for the treatment of AIDS have been inconclusive.

# Amino Acids

Amino acids are the building blocks of protein and are essential for life. Almost every structure in the body requires amino acids—including enzymes, hormones, muscle, skin, nails, and connective tissue.

When you eat food containing protein, your body acquires a resupply when amino acids are broken down by the digestive system and then absorbed into the bloodstream. Your body will use the amino acids wherever they are most needed.

If you have a deficiency of one or more amino acids due to your diet, digestive problems, or a genetic predisposition, then you may benefit from taking amino acid supplements. Also, certain illnesses have been shown to improve dramatically with specific amino acid therapy.

There are a number of classic examples of amino acids that help fight disease. Lysine inhibits the herpes virus, while arginine can help to heal burns. Tryptophan reduces depression and anxiety; histidine alleviates allergies; and taurine is effective for helping to prevent heart failure. While these are perhaps the best-known medical uses of amino acids, there are hundreds of other conditions for which the supplements can be helpful.

Amino acids are integral to the whole chain-of-execution process that begins with the "commands" that are given out by DNA, the critical genetic material within your cells. Through activation of amino acids, your body manufactures, or replaces, tissues and organs. So your health is determined, at least in part, by how efficiently amino acids are utilized in the body. Disease can arise when there is a deficiency of amino acids or when they are connected improperly (such as in genetic defects).

There are approximately 20 amino acids that compose more than 50,000 different protein structures in the body. Enzymes, vitamins, and minerals are required for the metabolic pathways that convert amino acids into specific body structures, which include not only whole organs like your stomach, heart, or nerves but also the delicate, transient items like hormones and enzymes. The demand for certain amino acids increases when we are under stress, exposed to environmental toxins, afflicted with disease, and other factors.

## THE BIG NINE

There are nine "essential amino acids." These must be ingested, as your body cannot manufacture them. The essential amino acids are phenylalanine, tryptophan, methionine, lysine, leucine, isoleucine, valine, histidine, and threonine.

If your gut bacteria, or flora, are healthy, they help synthesize these essential amino acids—and you need them! To put it bluntly, we'd die without these essential amino acids. But if these essential amino acids are available, your body can manufacture nonessential amino acids, as long as certain vitamins (such as $B_6$), minerals (e.g., magnesium), and enzymes are available for these metabolic reactions to occur. Examples of nonessential amino acids include tyrosine, taurine, cysteine, arginine, ornithine, glutamic acid, glutamine, proline, and glycine.

## FOOD SOURCES

Amino acids are found in protein-containing foods such as meat, eggs, milk, and fish (animal products), and nuts, seeds, soy, corn, and other grains (plant sources). Animal proteins are called "complete" because they contain all the essential amino acids. But even vegetarians can get all the essential amino acids by carefully combining selected plant foods during a 24- to 48-hour period. Spirulina contains all the essential amino acids. Soy comes close to being a complete plant protein. Strict vegetarians can combine whole grains and legumes to achieve all the essential amino acids; for example, by eating peanut butter on whole grain bread or having brown rice with beans.

## AMINO ACID THERAPY

The use of amino acid therapy is an emerging field in nutritional medicine. Amino acids are available as supplements. The most common are called "free-form" amino acids. "Free form" refers to the fact that the amino acids have been "freed" from their protein chain from foods like soy or molasses.

Different amino acids have a variety of different effects. Some amino acids act directly as neurotransmitters. For example, GABA has an inhibitory or calming effect on the body. Other amino acids are precursors that the body converts into neurotransmitters. For example, tryptophan is converted into the serotonin, a neurotransmitter that prevents depression.

## Conditions for Which Amino Acids May Be Helpful

Here are some commonly used amino acids and the conditions for which they are used.

| Amino Acid | Usage |
| --- | --- |
| Arginine | High cholesterol, congestive heart failure, angina, impotence, wound healing, low sperm count |
| GABA | Anxiety, depression, seizures, hypertension, hyperactivity |
| Glutamine | Wound healing, inflammatory bowel disease, leaky gut syndrome |
| Lysine | Herpes, osteoporosis (For more recommendations, see LYSINE, page 316.) |
| Phenylalanine | Pain, weight loss |
| Tryptophan | Depression, anxiety, insomnia, migraine headaches, PMS |
| Tyrosine | Depression, hypothyroidism |

The form known as "branched chain" amino acids is a group of three essential amino acids known as L-leucine, L-isoleucine, and L-valine. The branched chain amino acids are important for muscle growth and wound healing. They are different in that they are metabolized in the muscle instead of the liver.

## DOSAGE

Amino acids can be purchased individually or as blended formulas. These are generally taken for nonspecific reasons—such as to recover from strenuous exercise or for general immune support. Single amino acids are used for therapeutic reasons. For instance, lysine is used specifically for the treatment of herpes.

Amino acids come in different forms. The form best utilized in the body is the "L" form, as opposed to the "D" or "DL" form. The exception to this is DL-methionine or DL-phenylalanine. (The FDA prohibits the sale of "D" or "DL" except for the two exceptions noted.)

Amino acids are available in powder, capsule, or liquid format. The typical dose is 500 milligrams one to three times daily or as recommended by your healthcare practitioner. In some cases, much higher dosages are required for therapeutic results. (An example is the amino acid arginine, which is used in as high a dosage as 8,000 milligrams daily for the treatment of heart failure.)

It usually takes at least a few weeks for results to be noticed, but in some cases, improvement can be felt within several minutes. For example, I have had patients tell me their energy or mood improves within 30 minutes of taking amino acids on an empty stomach. As with any supplement, generally, the longer you have had the condition for which you are using the amino acid (or combination of amino acids), the longer it will take to feel some improvement.

Amino acids are best taken on an empty stomach to maximize their absorption. When taken with food, the amino acids compete with each other for absorption.

I usually advise people to work with a nutritional doctor before they begin amino acid therapy. Lab testing of blood (plasma) or urine can help identify deficiencies or imbalances of the amino acids and then specific therapies can be implemented.

## WHAT ARE THE SIDE EFFECTS?

Digestive upset (diarrhea, constipation, or flatulence) are the most common side effects but are not experienced by most users.

If you have phenylketonuria (a genetic condition), you should not take phenylalanine (DLPA). Do not take phenylalanine, tyrosine, or tryptophan if you are taking a class of antidepressants known as MAO inhibitors or high blood pressure medications. Persons with liver or kidney disease should not take amino acids unless instructed to do so by their doctor. If you're caring for someone who has a mental illness—or if you have a history of mental illness—be sure to seek the guidance of a doctor before you use amino acid therapy. Avoid the use of arginine if you have herpes.

Pregnant women should not take amino acids unless instructed to do so by their doctor.

# Antioxidants

• • • • • • • • • • • • • • • • • • • • • • • • • • • • • • • • • • • • • • • • • • • • • • • • • • • • • • • • • • • • • •

The term "antioxidant" has become a buzzword in the media. Anyone who listens to the radio, watches TV, or reads a magazine or newspaper has heard the term.

But what are antioxidants and what do they do? When I hear people talking about antioxidants, they usually say something like "antioxidants prevent or slow down the aging process" or "they prevent cancer." These people are on the right track.

To understand what antioxidants are, let's first discuss the term "free radical." A free radical is an unstable molecule that is missing an electron (charged particle). It is very reactive and potentially damaging to the tissues and organs of the body.

A free radical seeks out another molecule to pair up with to gain another electron. It will steal an electron from another molecule, which in the process creates another free radical.

Free radicals are a natural byproduct of energy production, what biochemists call oxidation. Hence, the term antioxidant means "against oxidation."

## LIFE WITH RADICALS

It is impossible to avoid free radicals. When cells "burn" oxygen as fuel to produce energy, free radicals are one of the byproducts of this life-sustaining metabolic process. Research has shown that free radicals are implicated in most diseases, including arthritis, cancer, cataracts, fatigue, heart disease, Parkinson's disease, and even the aging process.

Our bodies produce certain antioxidants to fight against this continuous onslaught. Other antioxidants are found naturally in foods, including vitamins, minerals, and phytonutrients. Therefore, we can consume valuable antioxidants found in foods that help to quench free radicals. Also, we can avoid foods that produce free radicals, such as fast foods, which are loaded with unhealthy fats such as hydrogenated oils.

In general, it's a great idea to avoid hydrogenated oils (found in margarine, vegetable cooking oils, packaged foods) and saturated fats (found in red meat and dairy products) that lead to the production of free radicals.

In addition to getting a diet that favors antioxidants, we can take antioxidant supplements to ensure adequate levels.

Why all the fuss about using antioxidant supplements? Well, antioxidants are mainly found in plants. How many people are eating seven or more servings of fruits and vegetables a day? The government promotes five servings a day, but seven to ten is what one should consume for optimal health and to prevent diseases like cancer. According to studies, not too many people come close to having three servings on a regular basis.

# POLLUTION PROBLEMS

There are sound reasons why antioxidant supplements have been in the news so much. As pollution has increased, so has the burden of body stress created by free radicals. Industrial pollution, which contaminates our water, air, and food, has contributed to increased exposure to free radicals and to an increased need for antioxidants.

Radiation from the sun also produces free radicals. Too much exposure to solar rays leads to a much higher free radical load than our body's antioxidant systems can handle. As a result, conditions such as skin cancer, wrinkles, and cataracts develop. As the ozone layer becomes more depleted, the intensity of solar radiation and free radical damage increases.

Unhealthy lifestyle habits such as smoking and drinking alcohol also contribute to free radical damage. Of course, these are controllable factors.

Even high-performance athletes are prone to excessive free radical damage from intensive training. Marathon runners and triathletes are prime examples. It is well known that after exhaustive training and competitive events, many of these athletes become sick with infections or chronic fatigue. High levels of free radicals are to blame for many of these illnesses. Antioxidant supplements can go a long way to protect these athletes.

Certain diseases, such as diabetes, lead to an increased production of free radicals.

Another problem area is digestive health. The result of poor digestion and malabsorption of food is the development of metabolic toxins, and thus free radicals.

Pharmaceutical medications can and often do increase free radical formation, causing damage to the liver and kidneys. I recommend that people who take medications should increase their intake of antioxidants to prevent such side effects.

Paradoxically, free radicals also have a good side. Immune cells use free radicals to destroy bacteria, viruses, and other invading microbes. As a matter of fact, our immune system uses free radicals to kill cancer cells.

Free radicals are also used as messengers in the body. They help to regulate blood pressure and serve other important functions. So the real key is to have a balance between the amount of free radicals and an ample amount of antioxidants to control them.

## SHIELDING THE GENETIC CODE

One of the most important functions of antioxidants is to protect the genetic code of our cells, known as DNA. This is important because DNA controls all the cellular activities that goes on in the body. One of the more fundamental roles of DNA includes cell division.

According to one leading theory, cancer begins when there's oxidative damage of DNA, which then leads to the uncontrolled division of cells—in other words, tumor formation. This theory would help explain, for instance, why smokers are much more prone to lung cancer than nonsmokers. If we inhale cigarette smoke—or any kind of smoke, for that matter—it damages the DNA in the lungs.

But even without such a clear violation of our defenses, scientists estimate that each human cell's DNA receives thousands of "oxidative hits" a day. So antioxidants are critical to our survival, and they need all the help they can get from the enzymes in cells that help protect cell DNA from oxidation.

## DOSAGE

The recommended dosage for antioxidants varies depending on the health of a person. For example, the dosage of the antioxidant for vitamins E and C would be much higher for a person with heart disease than a person who does not have heart disease. I have listed the general daily dosage of the antioxidants in Table 1. These are dosages for a person who wants to take antioxidants for optimal health and for disease prevention.

It is most important to get a full spectrum of antioxidants on a regular basis rather than just to take a few of the antioxidants at higher dosages. Remember, they all work together as a team. I find too many people focusing on one or a few of the antioxidants because of some advertisement they read from a supplement company. Getting the most out of antioxidants can be done through a balanced diet, a full-spectrum multivitamin, or a full-spectrum antioxidant complex supplement. The exception to this rule is when someone has a specific condition, and needs much higher dosages of a single antioxidant.

## WHAT ARE THE SIDE EFFECTS?

Side effects are not a problem with normal dosages. High dosages of fat-soluble vitamins like vitamin A can cause side effects, especially if one has liver or kidney disease.

# SPECIFIC RECOMMENDATIONS FOR SPECIFIC PEOPLE

In addition to a full-spectrum multivitamin, I recommend the following antioxidants so that the daily total (taking into account what is in the multivitamin) equals the recommended dosage.

## ∾ *Athletes*

These supplements are recommended to help athletes recover more quickly from training. Studies have shown that vitamins C and E help to reduce muscle soreness after physical activity.

> Vitamin C—1,000 milligrams
>
> Vitamin E—400 IU to 800 IU
>
> Coenzyme Q10—50 to 100 milligrams
>
> L-carnitine—250 to 500 milligrams
>
> Lipoic acid—100 milligrams

## ∾ *Arthritis Patients*

Oxidative damage leads to the destruction of joint tissue such as cartilage. These antioxidants have been shown to prevent or slow down this degeneration.

> Lipoic acid—100 milligrams
>
> Vitamin C—1,000 to 3,000 milligrams
>
> Vitamin E—400 to 800 IU
>
> Selenium—200 micrograms
>
> Grape seed extract or Pycnogenol—50 to 150 milligrams

## ∾ *Cancer Patients*

I recommend the following for those who have a strong genetic susceptibility to cancer or for those who want a more aggressive prevention protocol.

> Lipoic acid—100 milligrams
>
> Vitamin E—400 to 800 IU
>
> Tocotrienols—100 milligrams

Coenzyme Q10—100 to 300 milligrams

Turmeric extract—900 to 1,800 milligrams of curcumin

Mixed carotenoid complex—25,000 IU

## ∾ Detoxification Patients

People in detoxification programs benefit from antioxidants. The process of detoxification itself creates free radicals that need to be detoxified with antioxidants.

Vitamin C—500 to 1,000 milligrams

Vitamin E—400 IU

Lipoic acid—100 milligrams

Milk thistle (85% silymarin)—450 milligrams

Mixed carotenoid complex—25,000 IU

Selenium—200 micrograms

Green tea—2 to 5 cups daily

## ∾ Diabetes

People with diabetes have many extra nutritional needs. The following antioxidants are very important.

Vitamin E—800 IU

Lipoic acid—100 to 600 milligrams

Vitamin C—1,000 to 3,000 milligrams

Coenzyme Q10—100 milligrams

## ∾ High Cholesterol and Heart Disease

High cholesterol levels by themselves are not the problem when it comes to heart disease. It is when cholesterol, especially LDL cholesterol that becomes oxidized, that an inflammatory response by the immune system leads to plaque buildup in the arteries. These antioxidants are important to prevent this oxidation of cholesterol.

Vitamin E—400 to 800 IU

Tocotrienols—100 to 400 milligrams

Vitamin C—500 to 1,000 milligrams

Coenzyme Q10—100 milligrams

Grape seed extract or Pycnogenol—50 to 100 milligrams

Green tea—1 to 3 cups daily

## ❧ Smokers

Smoking is a sure way to deplete the body's antioxidants. Supplementing antioxidants can help reduce, but not eliminate, some of the damaging effects. When smokers take antioxidants, the first thing they usually notice is an increase in energy. This is probably because the antioxidants are helping the body detoxify these poisonous chemicals, which frees up energy production of the cells.

Vitamin C—1,000 to 2,000 milligrams

Lipoic acid—100 milligrams

Coenzyme Q10—100 milligrams

Vitamin A—1,500 to 5,000 IU

Selenium—200 micrograms

Tocotrienols—100 milligrams

Mixed carotenoid complex— 25,000 IU

Green tea—1 to 3 cups daily

## Recommended Foods

Many fruits and vegetables are high in antioxidants, and the more you can get in your diet, the better. Here are some of the stars.

- Grapes, strawberries, cherries, and blueberries all contain phytonutrients known as flavonoids that have potent antioxidant activity.

- Red wine and red grape juice have also been shown to have the flavonoids that are protective against heart disease.

- Citrus fruit—including oranges, lemons, and limes—all contain flavonoids.

- Carrots contain the carotenoids that help prevent cancer. These carotenoids are also found in orange and yellow types of squash.

- Cruciferous vegetables including broccoli, cauliflower, cabbage, Brussels sprouts, and kale contain various antioxidants. (They also have cancer-preventing phytonutrients such as indoles and sulforaphane.)

- Garlic and onions have antioxidants that help prevent cancer and heart disease.

- Tomatoes are rich in the antioxidant lycopene that helps to prevent prostate cancer.

- Tea contains polyphenols, potent antioxidants that protect humans against cancer and heart disease. Both green tea and black tea have polyphenols (green tea has the higher concentration).

## TABLE 1
## SOURCES OF ANTIOXIDANTS

There are many vitamins, minerals, and phytonutrients that are known for their antioxidant activity. The list below will help you find some of the more popular antioxidants and some of the conditions they can help prevent or control. (For more about some of these antioxidants, see other sections.)

| Substance | Indicated Use | Dosage |
|---|---|---|
| *Nutritional Supplements* | | |
| Vitamin A | Cancer, immune deficiency, respiratory tract infections, vision | 1,500 to 5,000 IU |
| Vitamin C | Arthritis, cancer, heart disease, skin conditions, common cold, heart disease, diabetes, hypertension, liver disease | 500 to 3,000 milligrams |
| Vitamin E | Arthritis, cancer, heart disease, Alzheimer's disease, smokers | 400 to 800 IU |
| Selenium | Cancer, heart disease, viral infections, HIV | 200 to 400 micrograms |
| Carotenoids | Cancer, vision, skin health | Mixed carotenoid complex 25,000 IU |
| Lipoic Acid | Arthritis, cataracts, stroke, heart disease, liver disease, diabetes, AIDS, Alzheimer's disease, Parkinson's disease, radiation exposure | 50 to 300 milligrams |
| Grape Seed Extract (Pycnogenol) | Varicose veins, heart disease | 50 to 150 milligrams |
| Coenzyme Q10 | Heart disease, chronic fatigue, hypertension, cancer, gum disease | 50 to 300 milligrams |
| Lutein | Vision problems (cataracts, macular degeneration) | 6 milligrams daily |
| Lycopene | Prostate cancer | 30 milligrams daily |
| *Herbal Supplements* | | |
| Ginkgo | Alzheimer's disease, age-related memory loss, circulatory problems, asthma | 120 to 240 milligrams of a 24% standardized extract |
| Milk Thistle | Cancer, liver disease | 450 milligrams of a 85% silymarin standardized extract |
| Turmeric | Cancer, liver disease | 900 to 1,800 milligrams of curcumin |

# Apis

· · · · · · · · · · · · · · · · · · · · · · · · · · · · · · · · · · · · · · · · · · · · · · · · · · · · · · · · · · · · · · ·

"Veronica has just been diagnosed with rheumatoid arthritis in her hands. The pain and stiffness keep her from writing at times," said Veronica's mother who had brought her to my office.

"What does the pain feel like?" I asked Veronica, who was only 10 years old.

"It feels like it's burning, and sometimes stinging," she replied.

I put Veronica on a special diet for six weeks. Unfortunately, it did not seem to help as I had expected. I prescribed the homeopathic remedy apis when she came for her next visit. This remedy is indicated in cases of arthritis where there is burning and stinging pain.

Two weeks later, Veronica's mother called me to report that "Veronica's pain is gone."

"That's excellent," I replied. "Veronica needs to keep taking the apis; we need more time to make sure it has a lasting effect."

I kept Veronica on homeopathic treatment for another three months. The last time I talked to Veronica's mother was four years after we started treatment. Veronica's arthritis had not returned.

## THE BUZZ ABOUT APIS

Apis is a remedy that is derived from the honeybee—the stinger as well as the whole bee. Think of the symptoms that a bee sting causes such as stinging, burning, swelling, and itching. These are all the symptoms for which apis is beneficial. So a homeopathic doctor may recommend it for bee stings, allergic reactions including hives, arthritis, urinary tract infections, kidney disease, herpes, sore throat, and ovarian pain.

Apis is indicated when symptoms include a lack of thirst, a negative response to heat, and a positive response to cold applications.

# APIS

## RECOMMENDATIONS FROM THE NATURAL PHYSICIAN FOR . . .

### ❧ Allergic Reactions

Allergic reactions that cause hives or burning and stinging pains that move around the body can be improved quickly with apis. Apis also improves other symptoms of allergic reaction such as swelling of the throat and eyes. These could be allergic reactions to food or to drugs.

**Note:** Seek emergency medical treatment for allergic reactions, especially if you start to have trouble catching your breath.

### ❧ Arthritis

If you have swollen joints that burn or sting—and if your joints feel better after applying cold compresses—then the condition can probably be alleviated with apis.

### ❧ Bee Stings

Apis quickly relieves the pain of a bee sting. This is proof of the homeopathic principle that "like cures like." Take it as soon as possible after getting stung to prevent swelling and other symptoms from getting severe. It is a remedy that should be in your home first-aid kit.

### ❧ Herpes

Apis is a common remedy for herpes infections. Herpes of the mouth—cold sores that sting and burn and that have a vesicle formation—improves quickly with apis. This also applies to the acute treatment of genital herpes.

### ❧ Kidney Disease

Apis is used in acute kidney disease such as glomerulonephritis or nephritic syndrome where there is protein loss in the urine and edema of the body.

### ❧ Meningitis

Symptoms include a stiff neck, high fever, and dilated pupils. Homeopathic apis is most effective in patients whose symptoms are made worse when heat is applied. This remedy can be used in conjunction with conventional treatment.

### ❧ Ovarian Pain

Apis is specific for right-sided ovarian cysts where there is burning and stinging pain. It not only reduces the pain, but also stimulates dissolving of the cysts.

### ❧ Shingles

Apis is one of the primary homeopathic medicines for shingles, especially when there is stinging or burning. Apis helps to relieve the pain and heal the shingles.

### ❧ Sore Throat

Apis is very effective for relieving a sore and swollen throat, especially when the sore throat has specific characteristics. Those characteristics include a burning pain (that feels better when you have a cold drink) and a bright red, swollen uvula (the flap of tissue in the middle of the mouth).

### ❧ Toxemia in Pregnancy

Apis is a good remedy for toxemia in pregnancy where there is protein in the urine, high blood pressure, and lots of body swelling.

### ❧ Urinary Tract Infections

Urinary tract infections can be helped by apis. This is particularly true for bladder infections that cause scalding pain during urination. If you have a right-sided kidney infection, it's another indication that this remedy will probably work well.

## DOSAGE

For acute conditions such as a bee sting or allergic reaction, I recommend taking the homeopathic formulation with a 30C potency every 15 minutes for two doses. Then wait and see if the remedy is helping. The other option is to take one dose of a higher potency such as a 200C.

For skin rashes, sore throats, and other conditions that are not so acute, I recommend taking a 6C, 12C, or 30C potency twice daily for three to five days, or as needed for continued improvement.

## WHAT ARE THE SIDE EFFECTS?

Side effects are not an issue with apis. It either helps or there is no effect at all. It is also safe to use for children.

# Arnica

If I had to choose only one homeopathic medicine for doctors to use in their practice, it would be arnica *(Arnica montana)*.

Even the staunchest skeptic is likely to be swayed by observing what this homeopathic remedy can do. I doubt that any other medicine exists that can so demonstrably and effectively relieve the effects of physical trauma. I have prescribed arnica for many relatives as well as patients—and almost without exception, they have described the results as "miraculous!"

Not long ago, my sister phoned and, with a great deal of concern in her voice, asked whether I could do anything for my four-year-old nephew. Over the sound of his wailing, she told me how he'd been running through the house, tripped, and banged his head, very hard, on a table. He already had a big goose egg over one eye.

Usually, when people call for advice, I like to ask questions and take time to think about what I am going to recommend—but in this case, it was such a common childhood accident, I only needed to know whether he was fully conscious. Just the background wailing answered that question.

I told my sister to give him a dose of arnica from her homeopathic first-aid kit and to call me back in 15 minutes.

My sister called back and her first words were "It's incredible!"

The wailing had stopped.

"I can't believe it," my sister continued. "I gave him the arnica and within a minute or two I could actually see the bruise decreasing in size. Is that possible?"

"Yes," I replied. "I've seen the same thing myself."

Many times, in fact.

## NATURE'S ANSWER TO TRAUMA

Always helpful when someone is recovering from a physical trauma—such as a fall, blow to the body, sprain, or surgery—arnica is most useful whenever there's any kind of bruising. It not only helps prevent the bruise from developing, it also eases the ache or soreness.

## CONCUSSION

It's a shame that every emergency room does not use homeopathic arnica. This is especially true in cases of concussions. Although there are many medicines that can relieve pain, I can't think of any that help speed the recovery from a concussion—a condition where the brain is actually bruised. Arnica plays a crucial role with an injury of this kind. It's helpful when there's any kind of head trauma or concussion, whether the result of a car accident, collision, or fall.

Arnica does not only relieve pain, however; it can also help a person refocus when he or she is acting or feeling disoriented. Arnica helps to reduce the swelling of the brain that occurs with a serious head trauma, which is precisely why I strongly recommend it for every first-aid kit. Keep some on hand in your home, office, and car for emergency situations. It can come in handy.

## MUSCLE RECUPERATION

Arnica can come to the rescue when your muscles feel sore from overexertion. I vividly remember the aftermath of one workout when—after a long hiatus—I'd gone to the gym and did a number of weight-lifting exercises for my chest and arms.

The next day, I could barely lift my briefcase without groaning. My muscles felt like they'd been hammered with a baseball bat.

Physician, heal thyself! After a couple doses of arnica, the soreness greatly improved, and by the afternoon of the same day, I scarcely felt a trace of the pain that I had experienced earlier. It was a lesson, of course, that I needed to get back in shape more gradually. But even the most consistent athlete is likely to experience occasional strains, sprains, and traumatic body-blows. Whatever the sport or cause of the discomfort, arnica can come to the rescue. In fact, I know of many a world-class athlete who keeps a supply of arnica ready to use at a moment's notice.

## DOSAGE

A potency of 30C is common, but you can take whatever potency you have on hand. Dissolve two pellets of arnica in your mouth every 15 minutes for the relief of physical trauma. Two to three doses should be sufficient.

**Note:** Dosage is the same for all age groups.

## WHAT ARE THE SIDE EFFECTS?

While there are few side effects, it is best not to use arnica on a regular basis as your response to the remedy may diminish. For instance, I wouldn't advise using it after every workout if you regularly exercise. Instead, take it for more serious injuries or traumatic accidents when it is greatly needed.

Arnica does not interfere with painkillers or other pharmaceutical medicines that may be prescribed for an injury.

*One warning, however:* Do not mistake the herbal form of arnica for homeopathic arnica. The herbal form of arnica (available in creams and tincture) is applied topically to unbroken skin to relieve muscle soreness. The herbal form should not to be taken internally.

# Arsenicum Album

Homeopathy is one of the most fascinating and effective healing therapies. Although it is one of the more difficult therapies to learn, it is one of the most rewarding. Interestingly, tens of thousands of medical doctors (and hundreds of thousands of other practitioners) around the world use homeopathic medicine on a routine basis in their practice.

Millions of people benefit from homeopathy. In Germany, approximately 40 percent of all medical doctors prescribe homeopathic remedies or refer to practitioners who do. According to Dana Ullman, coauthor of *Everybody's Guide to Homeopathic Medicines,* over 70,000 registered homeopaths practice in India.

Another country with a strong homeopathic following is Britain, which is home to the Royal London Homeopathic Hospital. Also, the Royal Family has been under homeopathic care since 1930. In France, more than 6,000 physicians practice homeopathy and over 18,000 pharmacies sell homeopathic remedies.

Homeopathy is one of the fastest growing retail lines in the North American health-food industry. Hollywood celebrities such as Lindsey Wagner and Jane Seymour openly endorse homeopathy and relate the benefits they have received from homeopathic treatment.

There are still many doctors, however, who are resistant to homeopathy in North America. Their minds could be changed by seeing the beneficial effect of a remedy like arsenicum.

Even though the root word suggests "arsenic," this homeopathic medicine has none of the harmful effects that are commonly associated with the poison called arsenic. Homeopathic physicians in Europe and the U.S. have been prescribing arsenicum to patients for more than two centuries without a single case of poisoning.

## DRAMATIC PHYSICAL RELIEF

My patient's wife called me one night at around midnight. Her husband was suffering from food poisoning. He was lying on the floor near the bathroom, in agony, having bouts of vomiting and diarrhea. Understandably, he wanted to be close to the toilet.

When I hear of these two symptoms occurring together—vomiting and diarrhea—I prescribe arsenicum as the homeopathic remedy. Things settled down after my patient took a dose of arsenicum. His diarrhea improved, as well as the vomiting, and he was able to get some much needed sleep that night.

I recommend arsenicum when physical symptoms include chills, with worsening of symptoms between 12 A.M. and 2 A.M., burning pains relieved by heat, and thirst for frequent sips of water.

I frequently prescribe arsenicum for anxiety, asthma, diarrhea, food poisoning, and allergies, although it can be used for many other conditions.

## DRAMATIC PSYCHOLOGICAL RELIEF

Arsenicum is not only helpful for physical symptoms, but for psychological states as well.

Jolene was a patient who responded well to arsenicum. She suffered from a lot of anxiety and worry, had a hard time relaxing, and was constantly on the move. She worried about many things, but particularly her own health. No doctor was able to find anything wrong with her, but for years she went from doctor to doctor to get reassurance that nothing was medically wrong. Jolene would wash her hands several times a day, especially after shaking hands with someone because she had a fear of germs from touching things or people. Her health concerns and general anxiety caused insomnia.

After talking with Jolene, I prescribed arsenicum. She was very concerned about taking the remedy, for fear of side effects, so I had her take her first dose in my office. This seemed to alleviate some of her concern.

As time passed, Jolene's insomnia gradually improved. Four months later, she reported that she felt calmer in general and had less anxiety. While her anxiety and fears are still a problem, Jolene is able to function more effectively, and, even more important, she has better peace of mind.

Arsenicum is a great remedy for those who are fastidious and feel the need to be in control of things at all times.

## DOSAGE

Dissolve two pellets of the 30C potency (strength) in your mouth every 15 to 30 minutes for the relief of acute symptoms, such as diarrhea or anxiety. If there is no improvement of symptoms within one or two hours, discontinue and use a different treatment. For chronic conditions, treatment should be prescribed and monitored by a homeopathic practitioner.

**Note:** The same dosage is effective for people of all ages.

## WHAT ARE THE SIDE EFFECTS?

As with any homeopathic medicine, side effects are not much of an issue. If you take arsenicum too frequently though, it could aggravate the symptoms you are treating, or bring on other symptoms common to the remedy—such as anxiety or insomnia.

Try arsenicum for a few days. If your symptoms improve, take it for another week and then stop. If your symptoms return, take it as needed to relieve the symptoms. If your symptoms get worse, or if you are not sure if it is the right remedy, stop using it and see a homeopathic practitioner.

---

## ARSENICUM ALBUM
### RECOMMENDATIONS FROM THE NATURAL PHYSICIAN FOR . . .

**∾ Allergies**

Arsenicum is one of the best hay fever remedies. It is especially indicated for symptoms of burning, watery eyes, and clear nasal discharge or dripping that leaves the upper lip red and excoriated. It is also a good remedy for people with multiple chemical sensitivities.

**∾ Anxiety**

Many patients with anxiety have benefited from treatment with arsenicum. People whose general fears and phobias interfere with their lives may require this remedy. These people are often perfectionists who need to have things exactly to their liking. A key symptom is waking up with anxiety or panic attacks between 12 A.M.

*(continued)*

and 2 A.M. These people also tend to be restless and have a hard time relaxing because of their anxiety and fears.

### Asthma

Arsenicum is the most common remedy to treat and prevent worsening of asthmatic attacks. I recommend taking it when the very first symptoms of asthma appear. If it does not help immediately (within a few minutes), then a pharmaceutical bronchodilator should be used. It can also be taken in conjunction with a bronchodilator for quicker relief of symptoms.

**Warning:** Do not discontinue the use of your bronchodilator without your doctor's guidance.

### Cancer

Arsenicum is one of the chief remedies used by homeopaths for the complementary treatment of cancer. Many homeopathic doctors have observed cases where burning pains that can accompany certain cancers are alleviated with arsenicum, even when painkilling medications were of no benefit.

### Diarrhea

Arsenicum is used for acute cases of diarrhea, especially when the stools are watery and burning. It is also a great remedy for cases of chronic diarrhea as found in colitis. The diarrhea is often worse from anxiety, cold drinks, and eating fruit. If arsenicum is the right remedy, relief is noticed after taking only a dose or two.

Acute diarrhea is the leading cause of childhood mortality worldwide. This occurs mainly in third-world countries where poor sanitation, malnutrition, and poor medical care are commonplace.

Oral rehydration treatment can prevent death from dehydration, but does not reduce the duration of individual episodes. A randomized double-blind clinical trial comparing homeopathic medicine with placebo in the treatment of acute childhood diarrhea was conducted in Leon, Nicaragua, in July 1991. Eighty-one children aged 6 months to 5 years of age were included in the study. An individualized homeopathic medicine (some received arsenicum) was prescribed for each child and daily follow-up was performed for 5 days. Standard treatment with oral rehydration treatment was also given. The children receiving homeopathic treatment had a statistically significant decrease in duration of diarrhea.

Homeopathic remedies cost only a fraction of what drugs cost. They have no toxicity and are effective against bacteria, viruses, and parasites that cause diarrhea. Antibiotics, on the other hand, treat only bacterial-caused diarrhea.

### Flu

People get different symptoms, even with the same strain of flu virus. The symptoms depend in part on how your body reacts to the infection. Arsenicum is helpful for the flu bug that hits and gives you a double whammy of diarrhea and vomiting at the same time. Chills and restlessness are also characteristic of the flu that requires this remedy.

### Ulcer

Ulcers and gastritis (inflammation of the stomach) can be helped by arsenicum, especially when the stomach pains are made better by drinking milk. This is the second most common remedy for ulcers after nux vomica.

# Ashwagandha

In the ancient tradition of Ayurvedic medicine—as practiced in India for thousands of years—the herb ashwagandha *(Withania somnifera)* has been used to treat conditions such as fatigue, chronic disease, impotence, and waning memory. Now, in twenty-first-century United States, this well-respected herb has a new and even brighter reputation as a much-needed stress reliever.

Sometimes referred to as "Indian Ginseng," "Winter Cherry," or "Withania," ashwagandha herb has many similarities to Chinese ginseng. In Ayurvedic medicine, it may be used to treat a number of other diseases besides those already mentioned—including asthma, bronchitis, psoriasis, arthritis, and infertility. Ayurvedic doctors prescribe it in very specific ways that are suited to certain constitutional types. It's often given with the so-called "warming herbs," such as ginger, to increase its tonic effect.

Ashwagandha root differs from Chinese ginseng in having a mild sedative action. This makes it well suited for the Type A person—that is, someone who's always "on the go" at such a high rate that he or she may be headed for burnout.

## MULTITONIC

Research shows that this herb is an excellent adaptogen that helps the body cope with physical and mental stress. Studies show that ashwagandha can help people who have exhaustion from chronic stress, weakened immunity (for instance, if they have cancer), and as a tonic for chronic diseases, especially inflammatory disorders.

This herb also has overall benefits for many body systems. Ashwagandha is unique in acting as a tonic to the nervous system, but also has sedative and antiepileptic effects. It mobilizes different components of the immune system to fight invading microbes and has a modulating or balancing effect if you have inflammation.

A number of animal and laboratory studies have shown this herb has antitumor activity. Ashwagandha has also been shown to have antioxidant activity, so it's helpful in protecting brain cells (which could explain why it helps to prevent memory loss). It also stimulates red blood cell production. Ashwagandha is also said to be a rich source of iron, so it's a potential choice for the treatment of iron-deficiency anemia.

Animal studies have shown that it increases thyroid hormone levels.

Over 35 chemical constituents have been identified, extracted, and isolated in this plant. These include some groups of chemicals such as alkaloids, steroidal lactones, saponins, and withanolides.

Ashwagandha has been used in only a few human studies—far outweighed by the number of animal or test-tube studies that have been done. However, it has remained popular and highly valued through thousands of years of use in Ayurvedic medicine. This is a classic case of an herb that has often been used for successful treatments yet never "proven" by modern scientific research. In my opinion, ashwagandha should be used when indicated. I am sure there will be continued scientific research that will eventually shed light on the reasons why this wonderful plant has proven so helpful to so many people.

## DOSAGE

The standard adult dosage is 1,000 to 3,000 milligrams daily of the root.

## WHAT ARE THE SIDE EFFECTS?

No side effects or toxicity have been reported with ashwagandha.

---

## ASHWAGANDHA
### RECOMMENDATIONS FROM THE NATURAL PHYSICIAN FOR . . .

**∾ Aging**

For one full year, 3,000 milligrams of purified ashwagandha powder or placebo was given to 101 normal healthy male volunteers, all between the ages of 50 and 59. The herb had some physical effects that slowed the effects of aging for all the men in the study. All men showed significantly increased hemoglobin and red blood cell count. Improvements in nail calcium and cholesterol were also noted. In addition, nearly 72 percent of the men reported improvement in sexual performance.

**∾ Anemia and Slow Growth**

Ashwagandha has been shown in two human studies and several animal studies to increase

*(continued)*

---

43

hemoglobin, red blood cell count, and serum iron levels. In a scientific trial that continued for 60 days, 58 healthy children between the ages of 8 and 12 were given milk that was treated with fortified ashwagandha (2,000 milligrams a day). The herb improved the health factors that contribute to growth—leading to a significant increase in hemoglobin and albumin. Researchers concluded that ashwagandha can be a growth promoter in children—and they also noted that these children were less likely to have anemia.

### ❧ Arthritis

Ashwagandha is used in Ayurvedic herbal formulas for the treatment of arthritis and conditions involving inflammation. In a double-blind, placebo-controlled study, 42 people with osteoarthritis were given a formula containing ashwagandha (along with the herbs boswellia, turmeric, and zinc) for three months. Their health was compared with a control group that received a placebo.

The herbal formula significantly reduced the severity of pain and the degree of disability. There were no significant changes in the control of inflammation, however. For this reason, ashwagandha is mainly used in formulas where inflammation-controlling substances are also part of the mix.

### ❧ Fatigue

Ashwagandha has been historically used for the treatment of chronic fatigue, especially a patient who shows signs of nervous exhaustion.

### ❧ Memory Problems

Some holistic practitioners recommend ashwagandha for its benefit to the brain. It helps improve the ability to reason and solve problems as well as improve memory. Practitioners of Ayurvedic medicine, who are familiar with these outcomes, often recommend it for patients who are starting to experience memory loss. Studies on rats have shown that it improves cognitive function.

### ❧ Stress

Ashwagandha appears to help the body cope with the effects of stress more effectively. I am sure that ashwagandha will become as popular as the ginsengs in helping to deal with this all-too-common problem.

# Astragalus

Jerry had been undergoing chemotherapy for cancer, and he fully understood the ramifications of continued treatment. In addition to side effects such as nausea, chemotherapy contributes to a breakdown of the immune system.

Without question, Jerry was going to continue chemotherapy treatments to control and, hopefully, eradicate the cancer. But at the same time, he wondered what he could do to help protect his immune system while the treatments continued.

I had been down this road many times before, so I was prepared for the question of what Jerry should take to help tolerate the ravages of chemotherapy. As I explained to him, it's especially important to make sure the concentrations of good immune cells, known as white blood cells, don't fall too low. If those immune cells are deficient, serious secondary infections can set in.

"My recommendation is astragalus root," I told him.

This Chinese herb *(Astragalus membranaceus)* is one of the best long-term immune tonics. It is commonly used in China, Japan, and—now—some North American hospitals to protect people against the side effects of chemotherapy treatments.

Acting on my suggestion, Jerry immediately began taking the recommended dose. He reported that his cancer doctors were surprised at how well he tolerated his chemotherapy treatments over the next few months.

After the round of treatments, when his cancer appeared to be in remission, Jerry approached me once again.

"Should I stop taking it?"

My answer was immediate. "No way!"

In fact, I recommended some other detoxifying and immune-building supplements to reinforce and enhance the benefits of the astragalus root. "You need to continue to build your immune system," I reminded him. We mapped out a supplement regimen that would continue for more than a year—both to buttress his immune system and help prevent a reoccurrence of cancer.

## CHINESE TREASURE

Having been trained in Oriental medicine, I have a tremendous respect for the healing powers of Chinese herbs. Among the most treasured of these herbs is astragalus, also known as Huang Qi.

Roughly translated, Huang Qi means yellow energy. The suffusion of energy is suggested by the yellow color of the root, which grows wild in northern China, Taiwan, Mongolia, Japan, and Korea. (In recent years, astragalus has also been grown commercially in North America.) As with many Asian herbs, astragalus has been used for its medicinal properties for over one thousand years.

In traditional Chinese medicine, herbalists and Asian doctors prescribe astragalus to help prevent colds and upper respiratory tract infections. It's effective with people who are susceptible to asthma. It's also known as a remedy for poor appetite, weak digestion, and diabetes.

Practitioners of traditional Chinese medicine sometimes recommend astragalus for organ prolapse—that is, conditions like prolapsed uterus or hemorrhoids. In addition, it acts as a natural diuretic, helping to excrete excess fluids and relieve conditions such as edema. Astragalus is also known to heal ulcerations of the skin and help with the underlying cause of weak muscles (due to poor digestion).

As with most Chinese herbs, astragalus is generally used in a formula that's made up of a blend of herbs, and it's a perfectly good addition to soup or rice. In fact, in China, it's not uncommon to use astragalus root as a standard ingredient in cooking.

## ACTIVE CONSTITUENTS

There is not a whole lot known about the exact constituents of astragalus that boost the immune system. Large, sugarlike molecules known as polysaccharides probably help to stimulate the "good" immune cells. Astragalus also contains substances called saponins, which have a similar immunity-enhancing effect.

## IMMUNE TONIC

Astragalus is one of the best herbs in the world for enhancing the protective effects of the immune system. How does it actually work? Similar to echinacea, astragalus increases the levels of certain immune cells that fight viruses and other microbial intruders. This includes macrophages, which are analogous to a Pac-man that swims around and eats tasty microbes.

Natural killer cells are also activated. These fearless warriors attack and destroy cancer cells and viruses. This is important considering cancer cells develop in our bodies on a daily basis and are kept in check by our immune system.

Astragalus also stimulates the secretion of a powerful antiviral chemical known as interferon, which prevents viruses from replicating. One eye-opening study looked at 28 people over a 2-month period and their levels of interferon. Compared with controls, those receiving astragalus had a significant increase in the production of interferon. In addition, the interferon levels remained elevated for 2 months after astragalus supplementation ended.

What I find interesting is that, for many years now, medical researchers have been trying to use synthetic versions of interferon for immune system enhancement. People with diseases like cancer and hepatitis C are commonly given interferon, but many are forced to discontinue using it because it produces so many side effects. I would suggest that it's time for researchers to focus on finding the active constituents in herbs like astragalus that stimulate the production of the body's own natural interferon, instead of trying to artificially duplicate it. More conventional studies using the whole herb would be even better.

In addition, it's been shown that astragalus has a supportive effect on bone marrow, the core of the bones where white blood cells mature. Animal studies have shown that astragalus increases the army of white blood cells that are needed to fight invading microbes.

Finally, astragalus boosts the levels of antibodies in the body. Antibodies bind foreign invaders and signal the immune system to destroy the most common intruders—bacteria, viruses, fungi, and other microbes.

## DOSAGE

Typical adult dosage for the tincture form is 20 to 30 drops three times daily. If you're taking it in capsule form, the recommended dose is 1,000 milligrams, three times daily.

In traditional Chinese medicine, between 8 to 15 grams of the root are decocted—that is, boiled in water to extract the crucial ingredients that support and enhance the immune system.

## WHAT ARE THE SIDE EFFECTS?

Very high dosages may cause indigestion. In traditional Chinese medicine, astragalus is not prescribed by itself or in high dosages in formulas when a patient has certain kinds of fevers. Otherwise, it is considered a safe herb to use at all times.

# ASTRAGALUS
## RECOMMENDATIONS FROM THE NATURAL PHYSICIAN FOR . . .

### ∾ Cancer

Astragalus is often a key herb in both Chinese and Western herbal formulas for immune support for people with cancer because it enhances the activity of immune cells such as macrophages and natural killer cells that are known to destroy cancer cells.

In one interesting study at the University of Texas Medical Center in Houston, researchers found that astragalus enhanced or restored the function of white blood cells that were taken from people with cancer. In fact, some of the damaged cells were so much improved that they became more active than normal cells taken from people who were cancer free.

As I've mentioned, though, astragalus is rarely administered as a solo cure—and this presents a challenge when we try to figure out what the herb does by itself. Historically, the herb is just one of a blend of Chinese herbs that, together, stimulate immunity. In my own experience, these traditional blends are the most effective. Nonetheless, I have seen patients improve when they only took astragalus, and some studies do find that it's effective by itself.

More commonly, astragalus is used the way Jerry used it—to reduce the side effects of chemotherapy drugs. In Chinese and Japanese oncology hospitals, doctors often rely upon astragalus to reduce the potentially damaging effects of chemotherapy by helping bone marrow produce more white blood cells.

Also, astragalus appears to have a protective effect on the liver. In one study, astragalus helped protect the liver against the toxin carbon tetrachloride.

### ∾ Common Cold and Upper Respiratory Tract Infections

Astragalus is an excellent herb if you're prone to frequent colds and upper respiratory tract infections like bronchitis. One Chinese study looked at 1,000 people with lowered immunity and found they experienced fewer colds, with less-severe symptoms, when they took astragalus either in the form of a nasal spray or a tablet. Reviewing studies like this makes me realize that an herb like astragalus can save a person a lot of time from missed work and family time. It has also been shown to be effective in the treatment of chronic bronchitis.

### ∾ Digestion

Astragalus is known to be a digestive tonic in Chinese medicine. While I have never seen it used by itself for the treatment of digestive disorders, it is an integral component of traditional Chinese digestive formulas.

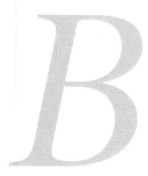

# Bach Flower Remedies

"I get very uptight and restless when I fly," said Tina. "Can you recommend something to calm me down? I'm taking a four-hour flight tomorrow, and I don't want to take sleep medication."

"I can recommend the Bach Flower Rescue Remedy," I said. "I'm confident that it will calm you down and help you relax on the plane."

This homeopathic combination of different flower and plant extracts is well known in the natural health field for its ability to calm people (and even pets) during emotional situations.

A few weeks later, Tina reported that regular doses of the Rescue Remedy kept her calm during the flight.

I have found the Rescue Remedy also works well to prevent jet lag. I add 10 drops to a bottle of water and sip it during the flight. Many friends and patients have reported that it works well for them, too.

## GIFTS FROM THE GARDEN

In the early 1900s, Dr. Edward Bach developed what he called "the Bach Flower Remedies" from flower and plant extracts. His focus was to find a gentle system of medicine that released emotional blockages and restored emotional and physical health to the patient.

Dr. Bach developed 38 different remedies, each addressing a different emotional state. These gentle extracts have been remarkably effective in promoting emotional healing.

If you are having problems with emotional issues that do not seem to be getting resolved, Bach flower remedies are worth trying. Many patients tell me they have a synergistic effect with their counseling. Others tell me the remedies have helped them break through emotional issues that counseling could not help. I do not recommend Bach flower remedies as a substitute for counseling—but, in my experience, they work well when they're used as supplemental therapy to effective counseling.

These remedies can also help relieve physical ailments. For example, people suffering from stress-induced digestive problems notice a lessening of their symptoms when using the Bach flower stress-related remedies.

## DOSAGE

Bach flower remedies come in liquid solutions. The typical dosage is 5 to 15 drops as needed for relief of emotional stress. For long-term use, the remedies are usually taken two to three times daily. For best effect, I recommend you wait at least 10 minutes after eating before taking the remedies.

Many practitioners combine different Bach flower remedies to address multiple issues that patients may be facing. For example, a widow may be given sweet chestnut for feelings of despair combined with the flower remedy heather, which is used for feelings of loneliness.

## WHAT ARE THE SIDE EFFECTS?

As with other homeopathic preparations, side effects are not really an issue. The most important aspect of the remedies is to pick the one remedy (or the group of remedies) that best addresses the underlying emotional imbalance.

## SELECTING BACH FLOWER REMEDIES

Pick the Bach flower remedy from Table 2 that best matches your emotional symptoms. If more than one of the remedies matches your symptoms, then combine 5 drops of each remedy in a glass of water. The longer you've had an emotional imbalance, the longer you'll need to take the Bach flower remedies. Health food stores and some pharmacies carry Bach flower remedies.

## TABLE 2

| Flower Remedy | Emotional Theme | Flower Remedy | Emotional Theme |
|---|---|---|---|
| Agrimony | Suppressed grief | Mustard | Unexplainable sadness that comes and goes |
| Aspen | Fear and anxiety | Oak | Struggling against the odds and not giving up |
| Beech | Critical and intolerant | | |
| Centaury | Weak-willed and seeks praise of others | Olive | Mental and physical exhaustion |
| Cerato | Lack of confidence | Pine | Unsatisfaction |
| Cherry Plum | Fear of losing control | Red Chestnut | Overly fearful for others |
| Chestnut Bud | Repeating old patterns | Rock Rose | States of terror, such as nightmares |
| Chicory | Controlling others | | |
| Clematis | Lack of motivation and concentration | Rock Water | People too strict with themselves |
| Crab Apple | Poor self-image | Scleranthus | Indecisive |
| Elm | Feeling of inadequacy, overwhelmed | Star of Bethlehem | Emotional trauma |
| | | Sweet Chestnut | Despair |
| Gentian | Self-doubt and discouragement | Vervain | Argumentative |
| | | Vine | Strong-willed to the point of dictatorial |
| Gorse | Hopelessness | | |
| Heather | Loneliness | Walnut | Emotional adjustments |
| Holly | Negative feelings | Water Violet | Independent |
| Honeysuckle | Dwelling in the past | White Chestnut | Persistent worry |
| Hornbeam | Fatigue of mind and body | Wild Oat | Unfulfilled ambitions |
| Impatiens | Impatience | Wild Rose | Indifferent |
| Larch | Lack of self-confidence | Willow | Bitterness |
| Mimulus | Fear | | |

# B-Complex Vitamins

B-complex vitamins include $B_1$ (thiamin), $B_2$ (riboflavin), $B_3$ (niacin), $B_5$ (pantothenic acid), $B_6$ (pyridoxine), $B_{12}$ (cobalamin), folic acid, and biotin.

I often refer to these B vitamins as the stress or energy vitamins. However, they do far more than just combat stress and improve energy levels. B vitamins are also effective in preventing certain types of birth defects, cancer, and heart disease, among other conditions.

A patient of mine brought her 75-year-old mother, Dolly, to see me.

"My mother's memory is deteriorating," Theresa told me. "Her doctor said she has age-related memory impairment. It's really bad now. She can't remember where she leaves things and has trouble remembering people's names."

"Did he suggest any course of treatment?" I asked.

"He said there wasn't much he could offer. It's just normal aging."

When I ordered a test to check Dolly's $B_{12}$ and folic acid levels, I discovered that her $B_{12}$ level was very low. I had Dolly use a supplement of sublingual $B_{12}$ (2 milligrams daily) that also included folic acid. I also recommended an herbal formula that stimulated stomach acid and improved digestive function, as I knew Dolly was probably not getting adequate vitamin absorption from her foods.

Two months later, Dolly returned to my office with her daughter.

"I noticed a great improvement in my mother's memory!" Theresa exclaimed excitedly.

I had Dolly continue the $B_{12}$ folic acid supplement for another 6 months, and then was able to reduce the dosage in half as a maintenance dosage.

## RATING: B MINUS

Many people in our society are deficient in one or more of the B vitamins. There are a variety of reasons for this. In a general sense, many of us do not get enough of the B vitamins because we eat refined grains. We lose a high degree of B vitamins when the outer shell of grain kernels is milled.

Another reason is that many of us have a lifestyle that promotes the excretion of B vitamins; for example, we drink coffee and alcohol. In addition, certain medications (birth-control pills, seizure and ulcer medications, and steroid medications, to name a few) can also lead to specific B-vitamin deficiencies. Mental stress and physical activity also lead to a greater need for the B's.

B vitamins are best taken together, hence the term "B complex." Taking one of the B vitamins by itself for long periods of time may lead to an imbalance in other B vitamins.

There are certain conditions, though, for which high single doses of one or more of the B vitamins are required for therapeutic effects. For example, high dosages of $B_6$ are needed to relieve the symptoms of carpal tunnel syndrome or morning sickness.

Another common example is niacin, which is used in very high dosages for the treatment of high cholesterol levels. Like vitamin C, the B vitamins are all water-soluble. This means they do not need to be taken with meals to be absorbed (unlike fat-soluble vitamins such as A, D, K, and E, which require fat and bile to be absorbed). Also, water-soluble vitamins are more sensitive to the environment as they are more easily lost during cooking and storage.

## DOSAGE

B-complex vitamins come in two standard dosages—50 milligrams and 100 milligrams. I recommend 50 milligrams as the daily dosage for most patients because the majority of people I see are already taking a multivitamin, which has B vitamins in it. Therapeutic dosages of individual B vitamins are given in specific profiles for each that follow.

$B_{12}$ and folic acid are also available in sublingual (under the tongue) form, which gets absorbed directly into the bloodstream from the mouth. This is good for people who have absorption problems. Also, B vitamins are available in liquid form and by injection.

## WHAT ARE THE SIDE EFFECTS?

There are few potential side effects from B vitamins, but some people do get nausea and skin flushing, which is associated with vitamin $B_3$ (niacin).

I have had a few patients who cannot tolerate any amounts of supplemental B vitamins. In these cases, an underlying metabolism problem in the liver is often the root cause. This may be helped with a detoxification program and by using food-based vitamins. Specific B vitamin recommendations follow.

## THE B-COMPLEX ROSTER

### ❧ Vitamin $B_1$ (Thiamin)

Alcoholics are at the biggest risk of having a $B_1$ deficiency. Alcohol use, over time, reduces the absorption of $B_1$ through the intestines—and $B_1$ is needed for alcohol metabolism. A deficiency of $B_1$ due to alcoholism can lead to permanent memory impairment, problems with eye movement, and a condition known as Wenicke's encephalopathy, where psychosis or brain damage can occur.

People with epilepsy who use the seizure medication Dilantin are prone to $B_1$ deficiency, as are people with diabetes, Crohn's disease, and several neurological diseases. In addition, antibiotics are known to deplete thiamin.

Good sources of thiamin are whole wheat products, soy, brown rice, peanuts, sunflower seeds, and milk. Therapeutic dosages range from 50 to 8,000 milligrams daily.

### ❧ Vitamin $B_2$ (Riboflavin)

Vitamin $B_2$ has become popular for the prevention of migraine headaches. One of the theories about migraine headaches is that they are caused by insufficient energy production within brain cells. Riboflavin is an integral factor in cell energy production. Preliminary studies have shown the benefits of riboflavin. One study compared the effects of riboflavin (400 milligrams) and a placebo in 55 patients with migraine headaches. Riboflavin was found to reduce the frequency and duration of the headaches.

Several antibiotics and drugs that treat migraines, such as Imipramine, can lead to a $B_2$ deficiency.

Symptoms of a riboflavin deficiency can include cracks in the corners of the mouth, inflammation of the tongue (glossitis), visual problems, and seborrheic dermatitis.

Good sources of riboflavin are organ meats, eggs, whole grains, green leafy vegetables, and almonds. A therapeutic dosage is up to 400 milligrams for the prevention of migraine headaches.

## ～ Vitamin B₃ (Niacin)

Niacin plays a role in many different functions in the body. It remains one of the cheapest and most effective cholesterol-lowering substances that we know about. It lowers all those blood markers that should be low, such as total cholesterol, LDL (the so-called "bad cholesterol"), lipoprotein A, triglycerides (fats in the blood), and fibrinogen. At the same time, niacin also increases HDL (the so-called "good cholesterol"), which transports cholesterol away from the blood vessels to the liver.

One of the side effects of this vitamin, as I've mentioned, is what's called the "niacin flush." I had a patient who came to me for natural treatment to reduce his high cholesterol markers. His blood test showed elevations of most of the cholesterol markers, and his protective HDL was too low. He was started at a beginning dose of 1,500 milligrams of niacin that was to be increased over time. He had a reaction to the niacin. He became hot and clammy, his skin turned red, and he experienced nausea. He said he felt as if he was having hot flashes.

I prescribed, instead, a nonflushing form of niacin called Inositol Hexaniacinate. (European physicians have used this form of niacin for decades.) He started with a dosage of 2,500 milligrams daily and never had any reactions. Over the next six months, his cholesterol returned to the normal range.

Good sources of niacin are organ meats, peanuts, poultry, milk, eggs, legumes, and whole-grain products. A therapeutic dosage is from 500 to 3,000 milligrams.

I advise against using time-released niacin, which can be toxic to the liver.

## ～ B₅ (Pantothenic acid)

I call B₅ the adrenal vitamin. The adrenal glands need pantothenic acid to produce stress hormones. Therefore, when people are under chronic stress, whether it be physical or mental, B₅ supports the adrenal glands in producing adequate levels of stress hormones such as cortisol. This enables the body to handle stress successfully.

Other conditions are alleviated with vitamin B₅. People with fatigue notice a difference when they take pantothenic acid. Vitamin B₅ is also commonly prescribed for allergies. A number of my patients reported that B₅ was of great benefit in reducing their allergy symptoms.

A different form of pantothenic acid called pantethine has proven to be effective in lowering total cholesterol, LDL, and triglyceride levels while increasing the good HDL. This supplement can also benefit people with diabetes who have elevated triglyceride levels.

Good sources of vitamin $B_5$ are chicken, fish, eggs, organ meats, whole grains, avocados, and cauliflower. A therapeutic dosage is from 500 to 1,500 milligrams daily of pantothenic acid, or 900 milligrams of pantethine. (**Note:** Many nutritional adrenal support formulas contain pantothenic acid in combination with other adrenal support supplements such as vitamin C, ginseng, and adrenal glandular.)

## ❧ *Vitamin $B_6$ (Pyridoxine)*

Vitamin $B_6$ has a multitude of uses. It is intricately involved in amino acid metabolism. A deficiency in $B_6$ can lead to weakness, confusion, depression, and skin conditions like eczema. Drugs that can cause a $B_6$ deficiency include birth-control pills and antibiotics. Smoking contributes to $B_6$ deficiency as well. It has been shown to be effective for alleviating PMS.

Vitamin $B_6$ is also important in reducing the risk of cardiovascular disease. Along with $B_{12}$, trimethylglycine, and folic acid, $B_6$ helps to lower a toxic component of protein metabolism called homocysteine. This metabolite is a causative factor in approximately 10 percent of heart attacks.

Another condition that $B_6$ can alleviate is carpal tunnel syndrome. This painful condition involves compression of the main nerve in the wrist from swelling and inflammation as a result of repetitive work (such as typing or carpentry). Carpal tunnel syndrome can also flare up in pregnancy due to fluid retention.

There are many other conditions that are alleviated with $B_6$—including depression, asthma, water retention, diabetes, epilepsy, and morning sickness. I have also treated patients who were suffering from kidney stones. Vitamin $B_6$, along with magnesium, helps to prevent the buildup of the most common type of kidney stones—those composed of calcium oxalate.

Good sources of vitamin $B_6$ are meats, poultry, fish, eggs, walnuts, peanuts, bananas, and whole-grain foods. A therapeutic dosage is 50 to 200 milligrams. (**Note:** Too much $B_6$ supplementation can lead to nerve toxicity. Symptoms may include tingling and changes in coordination. This may happen with dosages above 200 milligrams. Most reported cases occur in people who have taken dosages of above 500 milligrams for a prolonged period of time.)

### ❧ *Folic Acid*

Folic acid is important for the brain. It can be helpful for those who suffer from depression and poor memory, especially the elderly.

One of the most important functions of folic acid is to prevent neural tube defects in newborns (the incomplete development of the spinal cord and/or the brain) as well as cleft palate. The majority of these defects can be prevented with daily folic-acid supplementation of 400 to 800 micrograms. Taking the folic acid before conception gives the best results. It can reduce the risk of a neural tube defect by 60 percent if taken one month prior to conception and during the first trimester.

As I mentioned earlier, folic acid is important for preventing the buildup of homocysteine, thus reducing the risk of heart disease in genetically susceptible individuals. In addition, maintaining lower homocysteine levels also helps in preventing osteoporosis.

As with $B_{12}$, folic acid is required for cell division.

Folic-acid deficiency competes with iron for the most common vitamin deficiency in the world. A deficiency of folic acid can lead to anemia, gingivitis, depression, memory problems, and many other symptoms. Drugs that can lead to a deficiency of folic acid include barbiturates, corticosteroids, estrogen, chemotherapy medications such as methotrexate, birth-control pills, antacid medications, and many others.

Folic acid is found in high concentrations in green leafy vegetables such as spinach, chard, and kale. Other sources are asparagus, organ meats, orange juice, and whole-grain foods. A therapeutic dosage is 400 to 2,000 micrograms.

### ❧ $B_{12}$

Vitamin $B_{12}$ works in tandem with folic acid for many biochemical processes such as cell division and formation of the myelin sheath (the covering of nerve cells).

Many vitamin users refer to $B_{12}$ as the energy vitamin. I have seen many patients with fatigue experience tremendous boosts of energy after receiving $B_{12}$ injections. Other conditions that are alleviated by taking supplemental $B_{12}$ include asthma, depression, multiple sclerosis, shingles, and chronic fatigue.

$B_{12}$ is one of the critical nutrients to lower homocysteine, a substance that increases the risk of heart disease.

Drugs known to deplete $B_{12}$ stores in the body include birth-control pills, stomach acid blockers, antibiotics, and some seizure medications.

A deficiency of $B_{12}$ will result in anemia. In addition, the nervous system is quite dependent on adequate levels of $B_{12}$. Memory loss is a symptom, especially in the elderly. As a matter of fact, physicians have reported cases of suspected Alzheimer's disease that actually turned out to be $B_{12}$ deficiencies, which were improved with $B_{12}$ supplements.

Other signs of $B_{12}$ deficiency include a beefy, red tongue and diarrhea. Blood and urine tests can be done to evaluate the levels of $B_{12}$ in the body.

Vegetarians may require $B_{12}$ supplementation as animal foods contain the highest quantities. They can take whole-food supplements such as spirulina and chlorella, which contain $B_{12}$, or a B-complex supplement can be taken on a regular basis.

Other food sources of vitamin $B_{12}$ are liver, eggs, fish, cheese, milk, meat, dark green leafy vegetables, asparagus, organ meats, orange juice, and whole-grain foods. A therapeutic dosage is 400 to 2,000 micrograms.

## ❧ Biotin

Biotin is a B vitamin known for its benefit to nails and hair. It is manufactured by *bifidobacterium bifidus,* a group of friendly bacteria that reside in the intestines. Therefore, a suspected biotin deficiency in an infant or adult should also be treated with probiotic supplements containing these helpful and necessary bacteria. As the bifidus bacteria in the intestines manufacture biotin, it is logical that antibiotics can deplete body stores of biotin.

Biotin is also helpful for cradle cap, also known as seborrheic dermatitis. Yellow scales that may be greasy or dry form on the scalp of an infant or adult. Many cases of infant cradle cap have been reported to respond to biotin supplementation. Of course, you must check with your pediatrician before giving any supplement to your baby.

Studies have shown that biotin supplementation can be helpful for improving blood-sugar control in both Type 1 and Type 2 diabetes.

Good sources of biotin are brewer's yeast, liver and other organ meats, milk, cheese, soybean, eggs, cauliflower, mushrooms, and whole-wheat products. A therapeutic dosage to strengthen nails and hair in adults is 1,000 to 3,000 micrograms daily. For cradle cap, a breast-feeding mother can take 6,000 micrograms daily or the infant can be given 200 to 300 micrograms daily.

# Bee Pollen

I can usually figure out a way to help my patients when they complain of allergy problems. There are many good remedies for hayfever symptoms—the sinus pressure, headache, fatigue, runny nose, sneezing, and itchy nose that seriously impinge on your quality of life. But one spring, when I had exactly those symptoms myself, I found it impossible to come up with natural treatments that were any help at all. I was just plain miserable—and, I'll admit, more than a little humbled by the fact that I couldn't heal myself.

Of all the remedies that I'd considered for myself, however, there was still one that I hadn't tried. Some colleagues, and even a number of patients, had told me that bee pollen products had helped them to relieve or cure their allergies.

Up to that point, I'd had no reason to use or recommend bee pollen. On the other hand, I'd never been so taxed for ideas. I wasn't having any success at all with the homeopathic and nutritional supplements that normally worked so well. So why shouldn't I test bee pollen on myself?

I began to take bee pollen capsules. The product I used was harvested from a bee farm in Peace River, Alberta.

Typically, people are advised to take 2 to 4 capsules daily of bee pollen for a therapeutic effect. Being an aggressive supplement taker, I started at 8 capsules daily. On the first day of use, I did not notice any change in symptoms, but by the sixth day, most of my hayfever symptoms had disappeared.

Ecstatic with the results, I was still fearful that my symptoms would come back, so I stayed on a regimen of 8 capsules per day, which is about double the dose that's usually recommended. (Bee pollen is nontoxic, so I knew I was perfectly safe taking the higher dosage.) When I remained allergy-free, I decided to try a reduced dose, and within three weeks I was down to 4 capsules per day. Still, no symptoms—so in another week, I reduced my dosage to 2 capsules daily.

I stayed on the 2-capsules-a-day schedule for another two months, then stopped taking the bee pollen. I knew there was a risk of the symptoms returning because I'm in an area (San Diego) where there are different types of pollens all year round. But the hayfever was gone for good.

## THE BUZZ ABOUT POLLEN

Produced by flowering plants, pollen clings to bees as they go about their business of gathering nectar. It's sometimes referred to as Nature's Superfood because it includes a wide spectrum of nutrients, from vitamins A and C to the B-complex vitamins and amino acids. Among the other nutrients are carotenoids, calcium, magnesium, copper, iron, potassium, and flavonoids such as rutin and quercitin—all of which are believed to give bee pollen a large part of its anti-allergy effect. In addition, it contains those hard-to-get trace minerals such as silicon, molybdenum, boron, and sulfur. It also contains life-sustaining enzymes and plant hormone structures known as sterols, which are thought to have hormone-balancing effects.

Bee pollen is used to treat or prevent many different conditions, from arthritis and allergies to depression and fatigue. Many people who are active in sports rely upon bee pollen to increase their energy and endurance. It is said to have benefits for the reproductive system as well.

## DOSAGE

The typical adult dosage for chronic health conditions is 2 capsules daily (equivalent to 500 to 1,000 milligrams). For the relief of acute symptoms, higher dosages of 4 to 8 capsules or more may be used, as long as there are none of the side effects mentioned below.

## WHAT ARE THE SIDE EFFECTS?

The most talked-about concern is that people who are allergic to bee stings should not use bee pollen. Experts state the bee pollen allergies are quite rare—but they do occur, and in some cases can be quite severe. If you've ever had an allergic reaction to bee stings, avoid bee pollen completely.

A small percentage of users may also experience digestive upset.

Even if you've never had an allergic reaction to bee stings, I'd advise that you test a very small amount of bee pollen—just to make sure—before you take a whole capsule. Open one capsule and place a small amount of the powder on your tongue. If you have any allergic symptoms at all—such as wheezing or a rash—don't take any more.

Some bee pollen products are tainted with contaminants from air pollution (pesticides, herbicides) and environmental chemicals (heavy metals). Therefore, I advise that you only use a product from a company that uses a quality bee pollen source and tests their product to make absolutely sure it is not contaminated.

# BEE POLLEN
## RECOMMENDATIONS FROM THE NATURAL PHYSICIAN FOR . . .

### ◌ *Allergies*

It is thought that the pollens in bee pollen have a desensitizing effect on the immune system. In other words, you may be allergic to certain pollens that are in very small concentrations in the pollen that bees have collected. When you take bee pollen, your immune system starts to become desensitized to the point where you can tolerate more of these pollens, with less allergic reaction. Essentially the bee pollen has a homeopathic effect.

### ◌ *Arthritis*

After one lecture, I met a 64-year-old man who appeared healthy and full of vitality. Ten years before, he said, he had visited a naturopathic doctor for treatment of rheumatoid arthritis. By the time he went to see that doctor, his arthritis was so bad that he couldn't even walk. He was in a wheelchair.

As he told his story, his wife stood beside him nodding her head in agreement.

"When did you get better?" I asked, since his condition had obviously improved.

He told me his doctor had given him a bottle of bee pollen and specified a daily dose. The man was told to return to the clinic in two weeks.

In those two weeks, he recalled, his symptoms improved so much that he was able to walk into the doctor's office on his own.

Needless to say, I had just met a great believer in bee pollen. Since then I have paid more attention to this remedy and have met a number of people who have had success with it. While the effects are not so dramatic for everyone with arthritis, bee pollen is used by natural healthcare practitioners around the world to help alleviate arthritis symptoms.

### ◌ *Energy Boost*

Bee pollen is a popular supplement among many athletes, who report that it helps them train hard and recover quickly. Many athletes report that it helps increase stamina.

### ◌ *Immune Support*

Bee pollen is reported to help strengthen the immune system. People susceptible to reoccurring colds and respiratory tract infections may be helped.

Since bee pollen is so high in nutrients, you might want to take it if you're detoxifying. When you detoxify, you reduce the intake of foods that normally keep your immune system in good working order.

# Bilberry

· · · · · · · · · · · · · · · · · · · · · · · · · · · · · · · · · · · · · · · · · · · · · · · · · · ·

"The eye doctor says my eyes are going bad. I guess it's just part of aging," said 72-year-old Maureen.

"Oh, a lot of things get blamed on aging," I said. "Tell me more about your eyes."

"Well, I can't read as well as I used to," Maureen continued. "But what really bothers me is that my doctor said I am developing bad cataracts. He said if they get worse over the next year or two I will need cataract surgery, and I don't want surgery of any kind!"

"Let me take a look," I said.

While examining Maureen's eyes through my ophthalmoscope, I could see clouding in the lenses of each. But I didn't think surgery was called for—and told her that.

"Compared to a lot of people your age, your eyes look pretty good. If we get you on a good, comprehensive protocol now we should be able to halt any further progression of the cataracts."

"What is it that can help me?" asked Maureen.

"Lots of good things," I said. "You need to increase the fruits and vegetables in your diet, and take some antioxidant supplements. One of the main supplements you need to take on a regular basis is bilberry."

Fortunately, it was easy to convince Maureen to try this herb. She had already heard about it from a friend, and was wondering about its effectiveness. What I told her confirmed her assumption that it would be helpful.

Ten months later, Maureen had her eyes examined by an ophthalmologist. She was told that her cataracts had not worsened at all, and, if anything, had slightly improved. There was no doubt in my mind that bilberry extract was benefiting Maureen.

## TRIED AND TRUE BLUE

Bilberry *(Vaccinium myrtillus)*, European blueberry, is one of the more popular herbs in Europe and North America. Millions of Europeans are fond of bilberry jam, and many eat the berries. Thousands rely on it for its medicinal benefit for the eyes and as a tonic to the circulatory system.

Bilberry fruit has been used medicinally since the Middle Ages; historically, for the treatment of scurvy. (Bilberries are high in vitamin C and flavonoids.) Bilberry leaves and the fruit are also known to have an astringent effect. This is why it was and still is used today for diarrhea and urinary tract infections. It is also used medicinally for diabetes, varicose veins, and other circulation-related conditions.

The German Commission E, the government-backed medical board in Germany that helps regulate herbal medicine, lists bilberry as a treatment for acute diarrhea, and mild inflammation of the mucous membranes of the mouth and throat. Modern interest in bilberry was sparked during World War II when British Royal Air Force pilots reported that consuming bilberry jam improved their nighttime vision and accuracy on bombing missions. Almost 20 years later, scientists began studies on bilberry and its benefit for the eyes.

## A POTENT SPECIAL PIGMENT

Researchers have concluded that potent antioxidants called anthocyanosides are responsible for many of the healing properties of bilberry. This antioxidant effect reduces cellular damage and breakdown. As a result, anthocyanosides improve circulation through the smallest areas of circulation—through the capillaries.

Bilberry actually strengthens the capillary walls, thus preventing easy bruising, bleeding, varicose veins, and poor circulation. In addition, improved circulation allows valuable nutrients to flow efficiently to specialized structures such as the retina of the eye. This is why visual problems such as cataracts, macular degeneration, and poor night vision can be prevented and treated with bilberry.

The special pigment in bilberries also has a natural antiinflammatory effect, making it potentially useful for conditions such as rheumatoid arthritis.

## DOSAGE

For most adults, I recommend a standardized extract containing 25 percent anthocyanosides, at 160 milligrams twice daily. For adults with more severe problems, the dosage may be increased to 160 milligrams three times daily. For example, for a case of inflamed varicose veins (phlebitis), a dosage of 480 milligrams daily should be taken for a week or longer until the inflammation calms down, and then 320 milligrams can be taken as a maintenance dosage. Most of my patients notice improvement with 320 milligrams and take bilberry on a long-term basis.

Bilberry is most commonly taken in capsule form. It is also available as a tincture and in tablet form as well. As I mentioned, people in Europe use bilberry as a fruit the way we use its cousin, the blueberry, but it takes a lot of fruit to equal one capsule: You'd have to eat three bowls of bilberries to equal what is found in 320 milligrams of a standardized extract!

My guess is that blueberries have very similar properties to bilberry. Studies have shown that blueberries are also high in antioxidants.

Incidentally, these same types of antioxidants are found in red grapes, which have been shown to reduce the risk of heart disease. (Both red wine and red grape juice, containing these antioxidants, are often recommended.)

## WHAT ARE THE SIDE EFFECTS?

There is no known toxicity with bilberry. It does have a blood-thinning effect, however. Therefore, if you are on blood-thinning medication, let your doctor know that you are taking bilberry. This may require your doctor to prescribe a lower dosage of the pharmaceutical blood thinner you are taking.

---

# BILBERRY
## RECOMMENDATIONS FROM THE NATURAL PHYSICIAN FOR . . .

### ∾ Cataracts

Cataract surgery is very common in the United States. Oxidative damage from sunlight exposure is the leading cause of cataracts. Bilberry and its antioxidant properties are well recommended for those with cataracts.

Of course, it makes more sense to take it on a preventative basis or in the early stages of cataract development rather than waiting until the onset of cataracts. I also recommend antioxidants such as vitamins A, C, E, selenium, carotenoids, zinc, and a few others to be taken for the treatment of cataracts as well as bilberry for a more aggressive treatment.

The power of bilberry and vitamin E in preventing the progression of cataracts was shown in a randomized, double-blind, placebo-controlled study. This high-quality study found that the combination of bilberry (360 milligrams) and vitamin E (100 milligrams) daily for four months prevented the progression of cataracts in 97 percent of 50 people with mild senile cataracts. As an added bonus, no side effects were reported. This study is encouraging as it demonstrates that a lot of people with early-stage cataracts could avoid surgery with safe supplements such as bilberry and vitamin E.

*(continued)*

### ❧ Diarrhea

European doctors recommend bilberry for the treatment of acute diarrhea, although I have never used it for this. It is said to have an astringent effect on the mucous membranes, thus relieving diarrhea. The German Commission E recommends it for "nonspecific, acute diarrhea."

### ❧ Eyestrain

Many of my patients report eyestrain and headaches from working on their computers all day long. Most people notice their eyes feel much better after they take bilberry. Patients tell me their vision improves, their eyes get less tired and bloodshot, and they are less prone to headaches. Bilberry is quite helpful for anyone who has to spend long hours in front of a computer screen. (But for anyone who has to sit in front of a computer many hours a day, I also recommend the new flat computer screens—which emit less radiation—and advise taking regular breaks.)

### ❧ Glaucoma

Glaucoma is a disease that causes pressure to build up in the tissues of the eye. This is the result of fluid not being able to drain properly out of the eye chambers.

Glaucoma is a serious condition and is the second leading cause of blindness after macular degeneration. Bilberry may have a protective effect against glaucoma by improving the strength of the eye tissues. Although I have not seen any studies supporting this, many holistic physicians recommend bilberry for this condition.

### ❧ Hemorrhoids

Bilberry strengthens the capillary walls, thus preventing the buildup of fluid in the blood vessels and surrounding tissues. In addition, it promotes circulation through the blood vessels.

These actions make bilberry effective for the prevention and treatment of hemorrhoids.

I was impressed by a study that examined 51 pregnant women who took bilberry extract. Bilberry significantly improved the pain, burning, and itching associated with their hemorrhoids. After reading this study, I now consider bilberry for the prevention and treatment of hemorrhoids and varicose veins in pregnant patients.

### ❧ Macular Degeneration

The macula is the portion of the retina in the back of the eye responsible for fine vision. Degeneration of the macula leads to a slow or sudden loss of central vision. Macular degeneration is the leading cause of blindness in people 55 years and older.

There are two types of macular degeneration—dry and wet. There is hemorrhaging of blood vessels in the wet type. Bilberry treatment is most indicated for the dry type, which is more common. Free radical damage from smoking and sunlight appears to be the underlying cause of macular degeneration. Risk factors also include hypertension and atherosclerosis. Bilberry's antioxidant effect may offer protection against macular degeneration.

A protocol of antioxidants (such as lutein, zinc, carotenoids, vitamins C and A, and grape seed), along with bilberry and ginkgo extract is what I routinely recommend to people with this condition.

### ❧ Night Vision

Research has shown that bilberry improves energy production in the eye, critical to good night vision. Bilberry extract demonstrated significant improvements in pilots' speed-adaptation ability to light changes. While one study has challenged this assumption, we know that

(continued)

bilberry has been helpful for people in the past. Since it's nontoxic, there's no reason why you shouldn't try it for a while to find out whether it improves your night vision.

### ❧ *Varicose Veins*

Many of my female patients over the age of 40 want natural treatments for varicose veins. Bilberry improves circulation, so it's certainly one of the better herbs to use. In the same study where researchers studied the ability of bilberry supplements to reduce hemorrhoid symptoms in pregnant women, doctors saw that it improved varicose veins as well.

My patients who use bilberry for varicose veins report that it noticeably improves the appearance of their veins and prevents them from getting worse. Bilberry works nicely in combination with the herb horse chestnut and grape seed (or pycnogenol) extract for varicose veins.

# Black Cohosh

"I have a hot flash every hour of the day; it's driving me crazy! The doctors I have seen all recommend hormones. I assume there is something else you can recommend?"

Kristy, a 50-year-old patient of mine, was going through the transition of menopause and wanted nothing to do with the standard prescription of synthetic hormones.

I asked whether she had heard of the herb black cohosh.

"Well, yes," said Kristy, "but does it actually work? Remember, I am having hot flashes all day long, I need something strong!"

"I don't think you will be disappointed."

I talked to Kristy two weeks later, and she said her hot flashes had decreased to a frequency of about three a day. Then I followed up again, about six weeks after she began treatment. Kristy reported she no longer had any hot flashes at all. As an added bonus, she also had less depression and insomnia—two problems that had started when she began menopause.

These are the kinds of results I have come to expect from black cohosh. As you will read, this menopause-specific herb is effective in other areas as well.

# A CLOSER LOOK

Black cohosh (*Cimifuga racemosa)* is also known as "black snakeroot" because of its black roots—the part of the plant that's used for medicinal purposes. This member of the buttercup family grows wild in the eastern forests of the United States. Other similar species grow in China, Japan, Korea, and Siberia. Commercial black cohosh farms in Europe now supply much of the raw materials for the North American herbal industry.

Native American Indians—particularly the Iroquois and Cherokees—used black cohosh for many different reasons including menstrual cramps, childbirth, arthritis and sore muscles, coughs and upper respiratory tract complaints, and snakebites. It was also used by "eclectic medical doctors," as practitioners of herbal medicine were called in the 1800s and early 1900s. Naturopathic doctors also used it later on in the early 1900s for headaches, heart conditions, and as a digestive tonic. Black cohosh is also known as "bugbane," since the strong smell of the flowers works as a natural insect repellant.

Black cohosh was imported to Germany in the early 1900s. Since the 1940s, German research has heavily influenced the various uses and scientific validation of black cohosh. Today, black cohosh is the most popular herbal treatment for the symptomatic relief of menopausal symptoms. It can be found everywhere—in health food stores, pharmacies, grocery stores, and even on the Internet.

# ACTIVE INGREDIENTS

Most of the studies done on black cohosh have used an extract containing 2.5% triterpene glycosides that include the markers actein and cimicifugoside. Researchers disagree on exactly how black cohosh relieves menopausal symptoms. There is some literature that supports the idea that taking black cohosh lowers the hormone LH (lutenizing hormone).

During menopause, estrogen and progesterone levels drop, while the pituitary gland increases levels of the hormone LH. The rise in LH is believed to be one of the causes of menopausal symptoms. The inhibition of LH release by the pituitary gland is a leading factor in the relief of menopausal symptoms. Some researchers also feel that estrogen-balancing chemicals in black cohosh—known as "phytoestrogens"—may act to relieve menopausal symptoms as well.

## DOSAGE

Black cohosh supplements are available in capsule, tablet, and tincture form. The tea form is also available, though it's not commonly used.

As a standard dosage, I recommend a black cohosh extract standardized to 2.5% triterpene glycosides. The typical dosage used in studies for the relief of menopausal symptoms was 80 milligrams of the tablet or 80 drops of tincture. Most women notice improvement within four weeks of starting supplementation.

For severe menopausal symptoms or for women who do not see improvement at 80 milligrams, I recommend using 160 milligrams daily. In time, usually after 6 months or longer, the daily dosage may be reduced to 80 milligrams. A similar dosage can be used for other conditions such as fibromyalgia or arthritis.

## LENGTH OF USE

The duration of menopausal symptoms varies from woman to woman. I have had women tell me they have been having hot flashes and other menopausal symptoms for over 5 years.

How long can you take black cohosh? Many books quote the German Commission E, which states that black cohosh should not be used for more than six months. The Commission's recommendation appears to be based on the fact that no studies have yet shown whether side effects occur with long-term use. However, it is important to note that there is no information showing that long-term use is detrimental.

Historically, black cohosh has been used for long periods of time without problems. I have to disagree with the Commission E on this one. I and other experts in the field of herbal medicine find no problem with prescribing black cohosh on a long-term basis. It is no doubt safer than long-term hormone replacement therapy.

## WHAT ARE THE SIDE EFFECTS?

Though side effects are uncommon, a small percentage of users get digestive upset. This may be corrected by taking black cohosh with food.

Clinical studies involving more than 1,700 patients over a 3- to 6-month period showed excellent tolerance of black cohosh. Using higher dosages than I recommend may result in headaches and dizziness. Black cohosh should not be used during pregnancy and while breast-feeding.

## CANCER SAFETY ISSUES

Studies have shown that black cohosh is safe to use by women with a history of breast or uterine cancer. For example, one study showed that black cohosh does not have the same effects that estrogen does—that is, the breast cancer cells whose growth is dependent on estrogen were *not* stimulated by black cohosh. As a matter of fact, just the opposite; black cohosh inhibited the cancer cells from proliferating.

This study underscores the point I emphasize about the hormonal effects of black cohosh. It alters the levels of hormones already present in the body, as well as hormone cell receptors, instead of supplying actual hormones as in hormone replacement therapy.

## BLACK COHOSH
### RECOMMENDATIONS FROM THE NATURAL PHYSICIAN FOR . . .

#### ❧ *Arthritis and Fibromyalgia*

Black cohosh has a natural antiinflammatory effect. This makes it helpful in reducing pain, stiffness, and soreness associated with all types of arthritis. Arthritis pains are also a common symptom associated with menopause. Hormonal changes can result in circulation and immune system imbalances that may lead to joint inflammation.

It is also one of the better herbs to use in cases of fibromyalgia. In this condition, muscle pain is more of a problem, as opposed to joint pain. Black cohosh has a muscle-relaxing effect and reduces some of the soreness that people with fibromyalgia invariably suffer from. Women ages 25 to 45 are most commonly afflicted with fibromyalgia.

I have found a strong connection between hormone imbalance and fibromyalgia. I believe black cohosh's hormone-balancing qualities are one of the main reasons it helps improve fibromyalgia.

#### ❧ *Anxiety and Depression*

Black cohosh is effective for anxiety and depression that is associated with menopause. In the study I cited earlier, 85 percent of the 629 menopausal women who were given black cohosh extract had improvement in their anxiety and irritability, and almost 83 percent had improvement in their depression, with 46 percent no longer having any symptoms of depression.

Another study showed that black cohosh relieved anxiety and depression more effectively in menopausal women than the anti-anxiety drug diazepam. That is remarkable considering that diazepam is a powerful sedative drug. But the connection makes sense, because hormone imbalance leads to chemical imbalance in the brain's neurotransmitters (messengers). By balancing the ratios of the hormones estrogen and progesterone with black cohosh, you can indirectly balance the brain's chemicals and relieve symptoms such as anxiety and depression.

*(continued)*

### ∾ Menopausal Symptoms

Black cohosh is one of the best natural therapies a woman can use to relieve menopausal symptoms. All the clinical studies on black cohosh that I have seen relate to its benefit for menopausal women. The vast majority of the studies have been done in Germany and the results are impressive to say the least.

In a study of 629 menopausal women who used black cohosh extract for 6 to 8 weeks, 80 percent noticed improvements within the first 4 weeks of use. These are very impressive results, considering that hormone replacement can take 4 to 8 weeks to begin to relieve menopausal symptoms. Symptoms that were noticeably improved included nervousness and irritability, hot flashes, headache, insomnia, vertigo, heart palpitations, ringing in the ears, and insomnia.

Another interesting double-blind study followed 80 menopausal women for 12 weeks. Women were given black cohosh, synthetic estrogen, or a placebo. Women who were given the black cohosh had the best results in relieving menopausal symptoms including reduced anxiety and decreased hot flashes. This study is quite powerful as it proves the effectiveness of black cohosh over estrogen replacement.

Women who still have their ovaries may be able to switch from estrogen replacement therapy to black cohosh extract. I have done this with several women by slowly reducing their hormone replacement while starting them on black cohosh extract or a menopausal formula containing black cohosh. Researchers have studied women who were making the transition from hormones to black cohosh. For example, one study involved 50 women who were taking hormone replacement to relieve menopausal symptoms. Out of the 50 women, 28 were able to make the switch to black cohosh without being given additional hormones.

My patients tell me they feel better both physically and mentally when they switch from synthetic hormones to natural therapies like black cohosh extract. Psychologically, they feel safer getting off hormones that have a reputation for causing cancer and other diseases.

Keep in mind that black cohosh has not been shown to reduce the risk of osteoporosis or heart disease. These factors need to be addressed on an individual basis. It is also helpful for menstrual cramps and may be included in PMS formulas.

### ∾ Menstrual Cramps and PMS

Black cohosh helps to reduce menstrual cramps by relaxing the smooth muscles of the uterus. While it does not have so strong of an antispasmodic effect as the herb cramp bark, it can help relieve the cramping associated with premenstrual syndrome and dysmenorrhea (painful menses).

# Boswellia

In the news some time ago was a well-known basketball player who had been diagnosed with a rare kidney disease. He was forced to stop playing, at least temporarily, while he waited to find whether he was a candidate for a kidney transplant. With the tragic news of this player's health problems, the spotlight turned on the long-term use (some would say abuse) of antiinflammatory medications. These medications are given, as a matter of course, to many professional athletes. But other people take them, too, and in so doing they may run the risk of kidney, liver, and gastrointestinal problems.

For anyone who has been taking antiinflammatory pharmaceuticals, herbs such as boswellia *(Boswellia serrata)* offer an effective and much safer natural alternative.

My own knowledge of traditional herbal remedies, such as this one, comes from the experience of healing remedies that date back many generations. Boswellia is one of these valuable herbs that originates in Ayurvedic medicine. It is often used to treat inflammatory conditions like rheumatoid arthritis, osteoarthritis, and cervical spondylitis. It also has been used in traditional Ayurvedic medicine for diarrhea, chronic lung disorders, menstrual disorders, and skin problems.

Though the use of boswellia was initiated in India, today it is commonly prescribed in the West, particularly Europe and now North America.

Boswellia serrata—a branching tree found in India, Northern Africa, and the Middle East—is a close relative of frankincense *(Boswellia carteri)*, which contains similar compounds. When the bark of the Boswellia tree is stripped away, the trunk yields a milky gum resin. Constituents found in this resin include oils and triterpenic acids.

The boswellic acids are among those triterpenic acids, and most of the antiinflammatory properties are thought to come from the boswellic acids. When you're looking for boswellia on the shelf, you want an herbal product that is "standardized to boswellic acids."

It is believed that the boswellic acids interfere with leukotriene synthesis. That could explain why it brings some relief. Leukotrienes are hormonelike compounds that cause pain and inflammation.

## DOSAGE

I recommend 1,200 to 1,500 milligrams of a standardized extract containing 60–65% boswellic acids taken two to three times daily.

# WHAT ARE THE SIDE EFFECTS?

Boswellia appears to be very safe. Animal studies have shown no toxicity problems. It is known to occasionally cause mild digestive upset. Safety for pregnant and nursing women has not been established, so until testing is done, I'd advise pregnant women to avoid taking it.

## BOSWELLIA
### RECOMMENDATIONS FROM THE NATURAL PHYSICIAN FOR . . .

### ๛ *Arthritis*

Boswellia has been traditionally used for both rheumatoid arthritis and osteoarthritis. But there are many other kinds of arthritis as well, and boswellia is now quite popular in the natural healthcare field as a natural antiinflammatory for all the different types.

One researcher who reviewed 11 German clinical studies found that boswellia had been beneficial for 260 people who did not respond well to conventional treatments. Researchers found that standardized boswellia extract significantly reduced swelling and pain and usually reduced morning stiffness for people with rheumatoid arthritis.

Even more impressive was that some people were able to reduce their intake of NSAIDs (nonsteroidal antiinflammatories). The dosage used in most studies was 1,200 to 1,500 milligrams of extract in capsules that were taken two to three times daily—so people were getting a total of 3,600 to 4,500 milligrams of extract each day.

It is important to note that NSAIDs, the pharmaceutical medicines most often taken for arthritis, help to relieve pain and inflammation, but may actually accelerate cartilage degeneration. Boswellia does not cause this cartilage degradation. It actually reduces the breakdown of cartilage building blocks known as glycosaminoglycans.

More research needs to be done before we'll know whether boswellia slows down or halts the underlying disease process that's associated with arthritis. But we do know that boswellia works very well when combined with glucosamine sulfate and MSM for the treatment of osteoarthritis.

### ๛ *Injuries*

Boswellia, along with other natural products with natural antiinflammatory properties (such as bromelain, MSM, and vitamin E), should be considered for the prevention and treatment of athletic injuries and other kinds of muscle and joint problems.

### ๛ *Ulcerative Colitis*

Boswellia is useful in alleviating the inflammation associated with inflammatory bowel disease (IBD). In a 6-week study involving 42 people who had ulcerative colitis symptoms, researchers found that boswellia extract was just as effective as the high-powered pharmaceutical drug sulfasalazine in producing remission.

# Bromelain

• • • • • • • • • • • • • • • • • • • • • • • • • • • • • • • • •

"Mark, you should see the bruise I have on my shoulder. It's massive!"

For my friend Les, such bruises came with the territory. He was in the midst of hockey playoffs. Bruises like this had happened before and they would surely happen again—as long as he stuck with the sport.

"Do you still have any bromelain left?" I asked, reminding him of the remedy I'd given him just a week before.

"Oh yeah, I still have some left."

I have noticed that many people completely forget that they have supplements on hand that may be precisely what they need.

"How about taking two tablets every couple of hours?" I suggested.

It was no more than two days later that Les returned to tell me that the bruising—along with the shoulder pain—had improved remarkably.

I wasn't surprised. It was the kind of results I'd come to expect from bromelain.

## PLUNDERING THE PINEAPPLE

Bromelain is actually a group of protein enzymes derived from the pineapple plant, whose healing powers were described in the medical literature as

## Maxing Your Antibiotics

Bromelain is used in many countries to increase the absorption and utilization of antibiotics.

In one study, 53 hospitalized patients were given bromelain in various combinations with appropriate antibiotic medications. Their conditions included a wide range of health problems, including pneumonia, bronchitis, skin staphylococcus infection, thrombophlebitis, cellulitis, pyelonephritis (kidney infection), and abscesses of the rectum. Twenty-three of the patients had been on antibiotic therapy without success. Bromelain was administered four times a day along with antibiotics or by itself.

To compare, a control group of 56 patients was treated with antibiotics alone.

Of the 23 patients who had been unsuccessfully treated with antibiotics, 22 responded favorably to the combined treatment. The rate of improvement was across-the-board, for every type of disease, when patients were given the combination of bromelain and antibiotics.

For doctors involved in the study, it was an eye-opener. Many had not realized that bromelain was able to potentiate the effects of antibiotics in this way.

I hope we'll see larger-scale studies in the near future. Such promising results suggest that people may be able to take lower doses of antibiotics if they simultaneously take bromelain. (Many doctors are eager to reduce the rampant overuse of antibiotics, which is leading to ominous new strains of resistant bacteria.)

Those with weak or compromised immune systems could be the greatest beneficiaries of combination treatments with bromelain and antibiotics. Infants, seniors, and AIDS patients are particularly good candidates for the combined therapies.

**73**

far back as 1876. Though the active enzymes are found in the fruit as well as the stem, commercial products are made exclusively from the stem.

Bromelain is used for many purposes—as a digestive aid, natural blood thinner, antiinflammatory, mucus-thinning agent, immune system enhancer, and for skin healing. It also helps improve the absorption of certain supplements (such as glucosamine) and drug medications such as antibiotics.

One of bromelain's unique actions is to reduce inflammation in people who have conditions such as arthritis or heart disease. It can also help control the inflammatory process after an injury. It breaks down blood clots at the site of an injury, so swelling is reduced and, at the same time, there's increased circulation to the site of injury or inflammation. Bromelain also helps control some of the body's naturally produced chemicals that tend to increase an inflammatory reaction after an injury.

## DOSAGE

The dosage of bromelain is designated in two different ways with regard to supplements. One is milk-clotting units (M.C.U.) and the other is gelatin-dissolving units (G.D.U.). Look for products that are standardized to 2,000 M.C.U. per 1,000 milligrams, or 1,200 G.D.U per 1,000 milligrams. Most people require a dosage of 500 milligrams three times daily between meals.

## WHAT ARE THE SIDE EFFECTS?

Side effects are rare with bromelain. However, allergic reactions can occur in sensitive individuals. Increased heart rate and palpitations have been observed in some people at dosages near 2,000 milligrams. Those on blood-thinning medications should check with their doctor first before using bromelain.

---

### BROMELAIN
#### RECOMMENDATIONS FROM THE NATURAL PHYSICIAN FOR . . .

**❧ Arthritis**

Bromelain is a popular component of natural arthritis formulas. It is helpful for both osteoarthritis and rheumatoid arthritis.

One study found that the supplementation of bromelain enabled people with rheumatoid arthritis to reduce their corticosteroid medications. In addition, patients noticed significant

*(continued)*

---

improvements in joint mobility and also noticed less swelling. This study is encouraging because many people suffer side effects from corticosteroid therapy—and the less medicine they have to use, the better. If bromelain supplementation can reduce the amount of steroids needed, the risk of serious side effects decreases as well.

My experience is that most people with arthritis can maintain a good quality of life if they take the opportunity to try bromelain and other natural treatments.

### ❧ Burns

A specially prepared bromelain cream has been shown to eliminate burn debris and speed up the healing of burned skin.

### ❧ Cancer

Various studies have looked at a link between bromelain treatments and cancer deterrence or recovery. In one study, 12 patients with ovarian and breast tumors were given 600 milligrams of bromelain daily for at least 6 months. (Some treatments continued for several years.) Resolution of cancerous masses and a decrease in metastasis was reported.

Bromelain in doses of over 1,000 milligrams daily have been given in combination with chemotherapy drugs such as 5-FU and vincristine, with some reports of tumor regression.

Although I do not rate bromelain as one of the more potent anti-cancer herbs, it is worthy of more study. For those who are using chemotherapy to fight cancer, the addition of bromelain offers the promise of making the therapy more effective.

### ❧ Cardiovascular Disease

Holistic practitioners have expressed a great deal of interest in using bromelain for treatment and prevention of cardiovascular disease. We know that bromelain helps break down fibrinous plaques in the arteries, allowing for more efficient circulation. In theory, at least, this is a sure way to help prevent strokes.

When we take routine tests to determine whether people are at risk of cardiovascular disease, fibrin is one of the markers that we're beginning to look at routinely. (In other words, a lot of fibrin in the blood is one indicator that stroke could be somewhere on the horizon.) The fact that bromelain can help "break down" this fibrin is significant. In one study, bromelain administered at a dosage of 400 to 1,000 milligrams per day to 14 patients with angina (chest pain) resulted in the disappearance of symptoms in all patients within 4 to 90 days.

Bromelain also has the potential to break down plaque, the fatty deposits that impair blood flow through the arteries. The enzyme has been shown to dissolve arteriosclerotic plaque in rabbit heart arteries. While more studies need to be done, I've talked to many practitioners who notice that their heart patients do better on bromelain.

### ❧ Digestive Problems

Bromelain has long been used as a digestive aid in the breakdown of protein, and there are now many "digestive-enzyme formulas" that routinely include bromelain as one of the key ingredients. Either bromelain alone or the enzyme formulas can be helpful for people who have digestive conditions such as colitis or irritable bowel syndrome (IBS). In addition, we know that incomplete protein breakdown is implicated in immune reactions that lead to inflammatory conditions such as arthritis.

### ❧ Injuries

Bromelain's most well-known use is in the treatment of injuries, and it definitely helps to reduce pain and swelling if you have bruises. In one early clinical trial, doctors gave bromelain to 74 boxers who regularly suffered bruising on the face, lips,

(continued)

ears, chest, and arms. When bromelain was given four times a day, all signs of bruising disappeared by the fourth day among 58 of the boxers.

A control group, comprised of 72 boxers, were given a placebo—a look-alike capsule made up of inert substances. In that group, 62 of the boxers needed 7 to 14 days before the bruises cleared up. (Only 10 were free from signs of bruising after 4 days.)

### ∿ Respiratory Mucus

Bromelain thins mucus. If you have bronchitis and another kind of respiratory-tract condition, you'll probably discover that dosing with bromelain will help you expel the mucus more easily. For similar reasons, taking bromelain has been shown to improve cases of sinusitis.

### ∿ Surgery Recovery

Bromelain is a valuable supplement in helping people recover more quickly from surgery.

In one study, patients who were given bromelain supplements two to four days before surgery were able to recover from pain and inflammation more quickly than those who didn't take the enzyme. The bromelain-takers took an average of 1.5 days to be pain free, compared with an average of 3.5 days for those who went without it. Without bromelain, it took an average of 6.9 days for inflammation to go down, but only about 2 days for those who had bromelain supplements.

In my opinion, supplements such as bromelain should be routinely given to those recovering from surgery. Just think of all the days of suffering patients could avoid!

### ∿ Thrombophlebitis

In studies, bromelain has been proven very effective in the treatment of vein clots, as thrombophlebitis is commonly called.

### ∿ Varicose Veins

Bromelain has value in the treatment of varicose veins. I do not rate it so effective as horse chestnut and some of the other herbs, but it certainly helps.

# Burdock

"This cleansing formula contains burdock root. I have never heard of it before. What does it do, Dr. Stengler?" asked Wendy, a patient of mine.

"Burdock is a great herb to help a person detoxify," I replied. "In your case, I think it will help with your chronic eczema. If we get your digestion working better and liver filtering toxins more efficiently, then your skin should also improve. Burdock works to do all these things."

Burdock *(Arctium Lappa)* is an amazing herb to use for detoxification. It supports the liver, our primary organ of detoxification. It also supports kidney detoxification and destroys impurities of the blood such as harmful bacteria and yeast. An underrated aspect of detoxification is lymphatic drainage, which Burdock also enhances. Burdock seeds act as a natural diuretic to flush out water-soluble toxins.

## BURDOCK BASICS

Burdock exemplifies an important class of herbal medicines called "alteratives." An alterative herb improves general health by balancing and tonifying body functions. Alteratives improve nutritional status through improved digestion and elimination. They are sometimes referred to as "blood purifiers" as they help cleanse the liver and blood. They often are rich in minerals, phytonutrients, and other nutrients that stimulate metabolism and healing.

They are also referred to as "tonics," as they tonify and optimize different organ systems of the body. They also help indirectly with energy production by improving the body's overall level of health. Alteratives generally have low potential for toxicity and can be used on a long-term basis.

Burdock is native to Asia and Europe, and is grown in North America. North American herbalists and naturopathic doctors mainly use the roots for their medicinal properties, but the leaves and fruits are also used. A related species, common burdock *(Arctium minus)*, can also be effective.

Burdock root contains many different constituents including inulin, phytosterols, polyacetylenes, arctic acid, volatile acids, tannins, vitamin A, iron, calcium, sodium, and other minerals. It is said to be "cooling" in terms of its effect on body temperature.

Burdock is an excellent herb for skin disorders such as acne, eczema, psoriasis, and rashes. Its hormone-balancing qualities are useful for the treatment of premenstrual syndrome and relieving menopausal symptoms. It is also used for diabetes, arthritis, and gout. This herb will improve digestion and help detoxify the lymphatic system. In addition, burdock will tonify the urinary system and help treat fevers and sore throats.

It has often been included in herbal cancer formulas as well.

## DOSAGE

I recommend that adults take 20 to 30 drops (0.5 milligram) or 300 to 500 milligrams of the capsule form two to three times daily with meals.

# WHAT ARE THE SIDE EFFECTS?

Burdock is very safe; however, there are a few caveats. Those who have chronic diarrhea should start with a low dosage at first, as burdock stimulates the digestive organs. In some people, prolonged use of burdock seed can cause urinary tract irritation. Burdock should not be taken during pregnancy.

## BURDOCK
### RECOMMENDATIONS FROM THE NATURAL PHYSICIAN FOR . . .

**∾ Acne and Skin Conditions**

Burdock is my favorite herb for the treatment of acne—with vitex and milk thistle not too far behind. I have seen dramatic effects from the use of burdock in the past to improve low- to moderate-grade acne. I find it consistently helps my patients.

It works well because it treats all the root problems of acne: hormonal imbalance, poor digestion, inefficient liver activity, intestinal and skin bacteria and yeast overgrowth, and general toxicity.

Improvements are usually noticed within four to six weeks of consistent use, although teenagers may need to take it longer before they see results.

It is also a favorite for the treatment of eczema.

Along with sarsaparilla, burdock is one of the best herbs for psoriasis. For an aggressive treatment of psoriasis, I'd recommend taking both burdock and sarsaparilla together.

**∾ Cancer**

Burdock is often a component of western herbal formulas targeted toward cancer. While cancer can be a complex disease, many researchers detect a connection between cancer and "toxicity" in the body.

Burdock improves detoxification and supports the immune system. In addition, its hormone-balancing properties may be beneficial for hormone-dependent cancers. (Research on natural therapies and cancer is limited.)

**∾ Constipation**

Bowel movements are easier when the liver and gallbladder secrete more bile. This is why it is a good idea to take burdock with meals to help improve digestion and elimination.

**∾ Diabetes**

Animal studies have shown that burdock improves glucose tolerance. This is attributed to the inulin—the substance that makes up between 20 percent and 40 percent of the root.

**∾ Fever and Infection**

Burdock is "cooling." The seeds are known to be especially effective in helping to reduce fever. It is also used for sore throats and mouth sores.

**∾ Indigestion**

As a bitter herb, burdock stimulates most of the digestive organs to work more effectively. Over time, this herb can help strengthen weak digestive organs and improve digestion.

(continued)

## ❧ PMS and Menopause

The liver works to metabolize all the hormones in the body. The better the liver is working, the better the overall hormone balance. PMS is caused by a hormone imbalance, which burdock helps to correct. Also, as a "cooling" herb, it helps reduce hot flashes.

## ❧ Urinary Tract Infections

Burdock is used to help support kidney function, and for the treatment of chronic urinary tract infections.

# Butcher's Broom

"These dang hemorrhoids are killing me. I can't sit or lie down. And there is no way I am getting the rubber band treatment or surgery like my friends have had!"

Jim, a 65-year-old retired farmer, was living with the classic problem of a twentieth-century average person—the excruciating and embarrassing pain of hemorrhoids. In his case, we were able to relieve his rectal symptoms without drugs or surgery. One of the main components of his treatment was a capsule extract of butcher's broom.

Untold numbers of people have hemorrhoids—and a quick tour of pharmacy shelves will quickly reveal how many products are available. But whether you take those products or have conventional treatments, the "cure" usually isn't lasting. Fortunately, nature has provided remedies that shrink hemorrhoid tissue and without side effects.

One such herb is butcher's broom *(Rusculus aculeatus)*. Coming from an evergreen bush that's a member of the lily family—native to the Mediterranean and northwest Europe—the herbal preparation is actually made from the rhizome that grows along the ground.

## A GOOD VENOTONIC

Butcher's broom has a long and noble history as the chosen preparation for hemorrhoids and varicose veins. Long ago, its bundled branches were made into brooms that were used by butchers—hence the name. But these days the herbal preparation comes in various bottled and packaged forms that suggest neither butcher shop nor busy sweeper.

The active constituents in butcher's broom are believed to be ruscogenins. They work to treat hemorrhoids by constricting blood vessels and reduce inflammation in the hemorrhoidal tissue.

Butcher's broom is a classic example of what is called a venotonic, which simply means that it improves the tone of the venous wall. If you have hemorrhoids, the veins have become weakened because of swelling and abrasion. So a venotonic is exactly what you need for treatment.

## DOSAGE

I recommend a standardized extract that gives you a total dosage of 100 milligrams of ruscogenins daily. Creams that contain butcher's broom extract are widely available in Europe, but you can find ointments at some stores in the United States.

## WHAT ARE THE SIDE EFFECTS?

There are no known side effects for butcher's broom.

---

## BUTCHER'S BROOM
### RECOMMENDATIONS FROM THE NATURAL PHYSICIAN FOR . . .

### ❧ Hemorrhoids

Butcher's broom can be used for treatment of an acute hemorrhoid condition or on a long-term basis to keep hemorrhoid tissue from becoming engorged and inflamed.

In studies, researchers have usually given butcher's broom combined with flavonoids and vitamin C—which is the formula I recommend for maximum healing benefits.

### ❧ Varicose Veins

Butcher's broom is a venotonic, so it can also be used for varicose veins.

A study was done of 40 people with chronic venous insufficiency. They had various symptoms—such as varicose veins in the legs, edema (swelling caused by buildup of fluids), itching, and leg cramps—that indicated poor venous blood flow. Those taking the butcher's broom extract in combination with a flavonoid improved significantly without side effects.

---

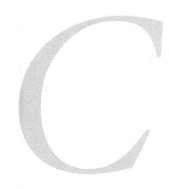

# Calcium

All the milk ads say you need calcium from cow's milk for strong bones and healthy teeth. True enough. Calcium is essential for strong bones—as long as you're getting many other minerals as well—and it's certainly beneficial for teeth. But there are more food sources of calcium than milk, and many of them are actually *better* than milk.

But let's look at the mineral itself before we get to sources.

Calcium is required by every cell of your body for a multitude of different actions. This is the mineral that helps your muscles contract, keeps your nerves lively, facilitates cell division, and helps arrange for the release of neurotransmitters, the chemical signals that scoot between nerve cells. Among its other valuable services, calcium helps your heart beat, your blood clot, and your hormones stay active. It's a factor in enzyme reactions and sperm motility.

So important is calcium, that it makes up almost 2 percent of your body weight, more than any other mineral. No question about it—for good health and vitality, you have to consume and absorb enough calcium on a regular basis.

## SOME NOTABLE DEFICIENCIES

We have an epidemic of calcium deficiency in North America. Only 10 percent of adults get the recommended amount of calcium each day. Our kids aren't getting enough, either. Approximately 70 percent of teenage boys and 95 percent of girls get less than the minimum amounts recommended in standard nutrition guidelines. Of course, this deficiency is particularly alarming among the teenage girl population,

*If you are lactose intolerant or have other kinds of problems with dairy products, here are some alternative food sources that can help you meet your daily requirements of calcium.*

| Food Source and Serving Size | Calcium (in milligrams) |
| --- | --- |
| Sardines (3 ounces) | 375 |
| Collard greens (1 cup) | 355 |
| Calcium-enriched rice milk (1 cup) | 300 |
| Calcium-enriched soy milk (1 cup) | 300 |
| Sesame seeds (1/2 cup) | 250 |
| Broccoli (1 cup) | 180 |
| Almonds (2 ounces) | 150 |
| Kale (1 cup) | 150 |
| Salmon (3 ounces, canned) | 150 |

since females are particularly susceptible to bone loss, and postmenopausal women are much more likely to have fragile bones if they don't get enough calcium in their earlier years.

As for postmenopausal women, they too seem oblivious to the risks of underconsumption of calcium. Most American women get 600 milligrams of calcium daily, which is far below the 1,200 milligrams per day that's recommended by the National Academy of Sciences. Is it any wonder that approximately one out of every three postmenopausal women will develop osteoporosis? This dreaded condition accounts for over 1.5 million fractures each year.

Now comes the question that nutritionists and doctors haggle over all the time: Given that we need more calcium, what are the best sources?

Most conventional doctors will immediately say cow's milk. It's true, milk does contain calcium. One 8-ounce serving of skim milk contains 302 milligrams. So, at least theoretically, a postmenopausal woman could meet her calcium requirement with just four glasses of milk every day.

But that's not quite the whole story.

First of all, some people simply don't tolerate cow's milk very well. If you lack the enzyme lactase—as many of us do—it's difficult to digest milk sugar (lactose), and you're likely to have symptoms of gas, bloating, nausea, abdominal cramps, and diarrhea. According to *The Merck Manual*—the "bible" of health statistics—75 percent of adults have some degree of lactase deficiency. For those of northwest European descent, lactase deficiency is much lower, around 20 percent, but that's a small proportion of the world's population. At the other extreme, 100 percent of Chinese have lactase deficiency, so all Chinese are lactose intolerant to some extent. Seventy-five percent of African Americans have lactase deficiency, as do a high percentage of those from Mediterranean descent.

Another problem is that cow's milk and the products derived from cow's milk tend to create excess mucus. I have seen many patients with chronic sinusitis and upper respiratory tract problems (including chronic bronchitis and asthma) who improve as soon as they go on a dairy-free diet. The same is often true of children who have reoccurring ear infections, since those conditions just get worse when the children have too much mucus.

Some researchers suspect a link between cow's milk and hardening of the arteries, while others suspect that consumption of cow's milk may be a factor in autoimmune diseases such as lupus and rheumatoid arthritis. Cow's milk is also known to be a common cause of iron deficiency anemia because it can create the conditions for internal bleeding. (Anemia is a possibility any time there's excessive blood loss.)

For children who get more than 24 ounces of whole cow's milk daily after the first year of life, there's an additional risk of iron deficiency because milk has little iron, may replace foods with higher iron content, and may cause occult (hidden) gastrointestinal bleeding.

Studies have also shown that cow's milk is a major cause of chronic constipation in children.

## ARE YOU LOSING CALCIUM?

While milk isn't quite the calcium hero that it's made out to be, some other common foods are worse villains than we recognize.

There are a number of foods, beverages, and habits that can cause you to lose calcium. It has been proven that caffeine (coffee and soda), alcohol, and sugar all promote the urinary excretion of calcium. Also, you lose more calcium if you have a diet that's high in animal protein. Smoking causes calcium loss, too. It's also been shown that hormonal imbalances and poor digestive function can contribute to a calcium deficiency.

You should also be aware of the dietary factors that *improve* the absorption of calcium. Vitamin D, vitamin C, and the mineral magnesium are among the nutrients that help your cells absorb and use calcium.

## DOSAGE

The National Academy of Sciences recommends the following for daily calcium intakes. These doses apply to males as well as females. In my view, you should be getting at least these amounts—and for most people, more is better. I especially feel that children 8 years and younger should be getting closer to 1,000 milligrams daily of calcium.

6 months or younger—210 milligrams

7 months to 12 months—270 milligrams

1 to 3 years—500 milligrams

4 to 8 years—800 milligrams

9 to 18 years—1,300 milligrams

19 to 50 years—1,000 milligrams

51 years or older—1,200 milligrams

For a calcium supplement, I recommend calcium citrate or calcium citrate-malate. Studies show that these are the forms best absorbed by the body.

I'm sometimes asked about taking TUMS® as a supplement. It does contain a form of calcium carbonate, so my reply is an absolute "no." The carbonate form is not so well absorbed and it buffers stomach acid—that is, gets in the way of the stomach acid that's needed for calcium absorption. If calcium carbonate is used, then higher amounts are required due to the decreased absorbtion.

Make sure to use a reputable brand, as some calcium supplements have been found to be contaminated with lead. Avoid dolomite and bone meal: These calcium supplies are poorly absorbed, and some sources have a history of lead contamination.

I recommend most adults and children take 500 to 1,000 milligrams daily of a good-quality calcium supplement. You'll probably need at least this much added to whatever calcium is in your diet, because dietary deficiencies are so common. Make sure to take a high-potency multivitamin that contains other vitamins and minerals needed to absorb and utilize calcium effectively.

Also, use calcium supplements that contain magnesium, as this mineral is very important in helping your body absorb and use as much of the calcium as possible. Magnesium should be taken at half or equal to the amount of calcium each day. If you take a magnesium supplement that's separate from the calcium supplement, you'll find it in many acceptable forms—as magnesium citrate, chelate, or glycinate aspartate, fumarate, malate, and succinate. You'll need 500 to 600 milligrams daily of magnesium—though I'd advise taking 1,000 milligrams or more if you have osteoporosis.

Calcium supplements are best absorbed if you take them with food. Your body releases hydrochloric acid when you eat, which helps with the absorption process.

## WHAT ARE THE SIDE EFFECTS?

At one time, doctors thought high calcium intake could raise your risk of kidney stones—but studies have shown this isn't so, especially in the case of calcium citrate. Any dosage below 2,000 milligrams is safe. People who have been diagnosed with thyroid problems—in particular, hyperparathyroidism—should not supplement calcium unless under a doctor's supervision. You'll also need to follow a doctor's guidance if you have kidney disease.

Calcium does interfere with iron and zinc absorption. If high levels of iron and zinc are required, then take them at different times of the day, away from calcium. For example, if you're taking iron for anemia, take a separate iron supplement, and make sure it's a couple hours before or after you take your calcium.

# CALCIUM
## RECOMMENDATIONS FROM THE NATURAL PHYSICIAN FOR . . .

### ᴏᴡ *Colon Cancer*

Colon cancer ranks number two, after lung cancer, among fatal cancers. Many human and animal studies show that you'll have a decreased risk of colon cancer if you take more calcium. Researchers still don't know the best dose for achieving this protective effect, but meanwhile, you can't go wrong by getting more calcium in your diet.

### ᴏᴡ *Circulatory Problems and Heart Disease*

By taking calcium supplements, you'll excrete more saturated fat, which is a dietary factor that contributes significantly to heart disease. At the same time, you'll *decrease* the absorption of cholesterol, thus lowering blood cholesterol

levels. Because calcium has both a fat-removing and cholesterol-lowering effect, it may reduce your risk of stroke and heart attack.

### ᴏᴡ *Growing Pains*

I have found that almost 90 percent of all cases of growing pains in children are related to a deficiency of calcium, magnesium, vitamin D, or all three. Unfortunately, many family doctors still do not recognize this solution to what can be an excruciating problem for a child.

### ᴏᴡ *High Blood Pressure*

Calcium should definitely be one of the supplements prescribed for high blood pressure. It is

*(continued)*

theorized that calcium helps relax the muscle cells that line your blood vessel walls, thus decreasing pressure inside the arteries. I find it works very well in combination with magnesium, potassium, vitamin C, and coenzyme Q10.

### ❧ Muscle Cramps and Spasms

Calcium deficiency is often the underlying problem when people have muscle problems. Again, it works well in combination with magnesium and potassium. I've found that chronic muscle spasms often disappear after people take calcium and magnesium supplements for a week or two.

### ❧ Osteoporosis

Calcium is constantly flowing in and out of bones. Bone density decreases when we're not supplying enough absorbable calcium to make up for daily losses. Studies have shown that calcium supplementation slows down bone loss.

*The New England Journal of Medicine* reported that postmenopausal women who added 1,000 milligrams of calcium to their normal daily diets experienced a 43-percent reduction in bone loss when compared with women who weren't getting the supplements.

### ❧ PMS

Along with magnesium and vitamin $B_6$, calcium supplementation has been shown to help alleviate premenstrual syndrome. It takes one to two cycles of supplementation for significant reductions in PMS symptoms.

### ❧ Pregnancy

Calcium appears to reduce the risk of pregnancy-induced high blood pressure. It also lowers the risk of a pregnancy-related condition called preeclampsia—higher blood pressure combined with increased water retention and more loss of protein in the urine. I recommend calcium to pregnant women to prevent these two conditions and also to prevent the muscle cramps and spasms that frequently occur during pregnancy.

# Cantharis

One night I got a call from a relative of mine. Her husband, Darrel, had been burned in an accident at work, and he was in serious pain.

Darrel worked at an oil compressor station, and he had received steam burns on his thigh when one of the pipes broke. The pain was excruciating.

This all occurred in the dead of winter, where the temperature was about minus 4 degrees below Fahrenheit. Though he was in severe pain, Darrel managed to pull off his jeans before he got into his truck and raced to the hospital some 20 miles away. So it happened that around 7 o'clock on a bitter winter's evening, a man came running into the emergency room of an Alberta hospital, clad only in his underwear.

Darrel was given some cream for second-degree burns, along with a shot of morphine. He took home some pain medication as well as antibiotics to prevent a secondary bacterial infection. His wife had picked him up from the hospital.

When I received the call from Darrel's wife, many hours had passed since his release from the hospital, but the pain-relieving medications weren't helping.

I recommended that he take homeopathic cantharis that was in their homeopathic first-aid kit. Thirty minutes later, I called again to find out how he was faring. He reported a dramatic reduction in pain. A short time after my call, I later learned, he fell asleep and slept soundly for the rest of the night.

The next day, when Darrel saw the doctors at the emergency room, they asked how he'd coped with the pain overnight. He pulled out his bottle of cantharis and said, "I quit using the pain medication because it was not helping. Instead, I have been using this. I really do not feel much pain at all!"

The attending doctors looked at him in disbelief. They had no idea what cantharis was.

## A BEETLE BONUS

In my view, many burn victims could be spared a lot of pain and agony if emergency-room doctors knew a lot more about homeopathic remedies such as cantharis.

The cantharis preparation comes from the blister beetle, sometimes called the Spanish fly. The beetle contains a chemical called cantharadin, which can raise blisters and cause severe inflammation on human skin. Based on the homeopathic premise that "like cures like," this is the perfect substance to use in a homeopathic dilution to heal burns. It's very effective with second-degree burns—the kind that raise blisters on the skin. It also helps relieve pain and promote healing if you have a third-degree burn, the most severe kind.

Homeopaths tell of cases of hospitalized patients with the severest of burns who have gotten relief from cantharis. Other homeopathic remedies to consider include arsenicum and urtica urens.

Cantharis is also one of the best remedies for urinary tract infections, especially bladder infections.

## DOSAGE

Cantharis is generally used for severe acute burns and bladder infections, so I recommend using the highest dose possible. I typically use a 200C potency or higher. Most health food stores and pharmacies carry the 30C potency as the highest strength. This too can work; it just needs to be taken more often, such as two to four times daily. If it helps, but wears off, then contact a homeopathic practitioner for a stronger potency.

## WHAT ARE THE SIDE EFFECTS?

I have never seen any side effects with cantharis. If it doesn't help, it does nothing at all, in which case you should simply try a different remedy.

---

## CANTHARIS
### RECOMMENDATIONS FROM THE NATURAL PHYSICIAN FOR . . .

**❧ Burns**

While cantharis is most helpful for the type of burns that raise blisters, I have also found it helpful for severe sunburns. I found myself recommending it just a few days before my wedding, when one of my "best men" got a nasty-looking sunburn. (I didn't make him feel any better by commenting that he resembled a baked salmon—but it was true, his whole upper body was bright pink.) So he got a high dose of cantharis (and also aloe vera gel) just to get him to the church on time. Surprisingly, he had no blistering or peeling, and none of the typical sunburn pain!

For burns that cover a large area of the body, one homeopath recommended dissolving two pellets of cantharis in a bottle of purified water.

Spray the solution over the burn areas as needed during the day.

**❧ Urinary Tract Infections**

Cantharis is very effective in the first stages of a urinary tract infection, especially if you've experienced a burning sensation while urinating. One source describes this as "Each drop passes as if scalding water."

Cantharis is prescribed if blood accompanies the stream of urine, which often happens with bladder infections, or if there's dribbling as a result of the infection. Cantharis can be combined with antibiotics to speed recovery and reduce urinary pain, especially if the infection has spread to the kidneys.

# Carotenoids

"As you can tell, I'm a sun worshipper. So I already know you're going to recommend sunscreen," said Barb, a 35-year-old fitness trainer. She assured me that she already did that—and she was also trying to limit the time she spent in the sun. "But besides that . . . ?"

"Antioxidants are what I recommend," I answered. "A diet rich in fruits and vegetables is your best choice. There are also many antioxidants in the multivitamin that you are taking. But I also recommend a mixed carotenoid complex. The carotenoids act as antioxidants to protect the skin and help absorb the sun's ultraviolet rays."

"My multivitamin contains beta carotene. Is that one of the carotenoids?" asked Barb.

"Yes it is." But I also wanted her to know that she might need more than that. "Most multivitamins do not contain a mixed carotenoid complex," I noted. "There are several carotenoids besides beta carotene. As a matter of fact, it appears that getting a combination of them are more important than taking any single one by itself."

Researchers estimate that over 700 different carotenoids exist in nature. Fruits and vegetables are rich in carotenoids, especially ones with bright colors such as red, yellow, orange, purple, and dark green.

## WHAT ARE CAROTENOIDS?

Carotenoids are actually fat-soluble pigments that are responsible for the brilliant colors in the full spectrum of the fruit and vegetable rainbow. Apart from their colorful contribution, they are also responsible for protecting the plant from oxidants formed during photosynthesis.

Beta carotene is the most well-known carotenoid but not necessarily the most potent. Other important carotenoids that have been the focus of recent research include alpha carotene, cryptoxanthin, lutein, lycopene, and zeaxanthin.

Some of the carotenoids are converted into vitamin A, but many are not. Essentially, nature has intended for us to get a mix of carotenoids.

In general, the brighter the food, the greater the carotenoid concentration. For example, a pale orange carrot contains less beta carotene than a dark orange carrot. General sources include carrots, pumpkins, squash, sweet potatoes, broccoli, peas, collard greens, kale, peppers (all colors), spinach, apricots, cantaloupe, papaya, peaches, tangerines, tomatoes, watermelon, and cherries.

Most supplements use a mixed carotenoid complex from the sea algae *Dunaliella salina* from the waters of Australia.

## A FULL SPECTRUM OF HELP

As a whole, the carotenoids are protective against a variety of cancers and cardiovascular disease. They also enhance the immune system and act as antioxidants.

Specific carotenoids are known to benefit specific organs of the body. For example, the carotenoids lutein and zeaxanthin (found in high concentration in spinach and dark green leafy vegetables) appear to be important in protecting against macular degeneration. Lycopene is carotenoid found in high concentration in tomatoes and appears to be protective against prostate cancer.

Carotenoids are important for proper lung function as they suppress free radicals from air pollution. A study of 528 people ages 65 to 85 years old found that persons with high blood levels of beta carotene, lycopene, and alpha carotene had significantly better lung function than those with low levels of these nutrients.

Studies have shown that carotenoids help to prevent the damaging effects of the sun's ultraviolet rays on the skin. A recent study showed that 25 milligrams of a natural carotenoid complex protected against sunburn after eight weeks of supplementation. (However, the combination of carotenoids and vitamin E worked better to provide protection after four weeks of use.)

## DOSAGE

I recommend taking one capsule of a mixed carotenoid complex. A typical soft gel carotenoid complex will contain a mixture similar to the following:

Beta carotene—25,000 IU

Lycopene—5,000 micrograms

Alpha carotene—492 micrograms

Cryptoxanthin—115 micrograms

Zeaxanthin—98 micrograms

Lutein—74 micrograms

Specific conditions require higher dosages of the individual carotenoids.

It is important to note that zinc, vitamin C, and thyroid hormone are required for the conversion of carotenoids to vitamin A.

Note that carotenoids are helpful in preventing many health problems, especially for the conditions listed below.

## WHAT ARE THE SIDE EFFECTS?

The carotenoids are nontoxic. A yellowish discoloration of the skin (carotenemia) can result from taking too high a dosage. The discoloration goes away when the dosage is reduced.

## CAROTENOIDS
### RECOMMENDATIONS FROM THE NATURAL PHYSICIAN FOR . . .

### ◌ Cancer

It has been well documented through population studies that carotenoid-rich diets are protective against a variety of cancers. Specifically, the carotenoid lycopene seems to have powerful preventive effect, especially in guarding men against prostate cancer.

Interestingly, lycopene is the most abundant carotenoid in the prostate gland. Researchers feel that lycopene is better absorbed from tomato sauce as opposed to raw tomatoes.

A 6-year Harvard study of 48,000 male physicians found that men who consumed tomato-rich foods (tomatoes, tomato sauce, and pizza) at least ten times a week, had a 35 percent decreased risk of prostate cancer as compared with those men who had less than a serving-and-a-half of those high-lycopene servings every week.

Men have asked me whether it makes sense to use lycopene as a supplement for prostate cancer. One study has been done. In this study researchers looked at 30 men with localized prostate cancer who were scheduled to undergo surgical removal of the prostate. For three weeks prior to surgery, the participants were randomly assigned 30 milligrams of lycopene supplement or a placebo—that is, a sugar pill that resembled the real supplement. After the men underwent surgery, follow-up examinations showed that the treated group had smaller tumors than the group of men who received the placebos. Also, the PSA value had declined in those taking lycopene. PSA is a "marker" that is used to help doctors determine the presence of prostate cancer, so a decline in PSA was considered an excellent indicator that the lycopene was having a beneficial effect.

A recent study showed that high-lutein diets were associated with a 17 percent decrease in colon cancer risk, and young people with a diet high in lutein had a 34 percent lower risk of colon cancer.

*(continued)*

Many studies have shown a protective effect of beta carotene, especially in early-stage cancers of the mouth and esophagus—though studies have shown the protection is not powerful enough to help prevent lung cancer in smokers.

Overall, for cancer prevention it makes sense to eat a diet rich in carotenoids. If supplements are used, then mixed carotenoid supplements make the most sense to me. Higher dosages of lycopene—30 milligrams daily—are a good idea for men with prostate cancer.

### ❧ Cardiovascular Disease

Carotenoids also appear to be important for the prevention of cardiovascular disease. This may be due to their protective effect, since they help to prevent the oxidation of cholesterol.

One study showed that eating a diet rich in carotenoids may reduce the risk of angina. Researchers found that people with the highest levels of alpha carotene, beta carotene, and beta cryptoxanthin were on average 50 percent less likely to develop angina.

### ❧ Macular Degeneration

This condition is the leading cause of blindness in the United States. The macula—the part of the retina responsible for visual acuity—deteriorates. Population studies show that the risk of developing age-related macular degeneration is significantly reduced in people whose diet is rich in fruits and vegetables containing beta carotene.

Lutein and zeaxanthin are two carotenoids that appear to be even more important. These carotenoids are found in dark green vegetables such as spinach, kale, and collard greens. They function in the macula to absorb light and protect our eyes against light's damaging effects.

A survey of 876 elderly individuals showed that those whose intake of these two carotenoids was high, were 56 percent less likely to develop age-related macular degeneration.

# Cayenne

Spicy food lovers crave it, people with pain need it, and those with heart disease swear by it.

Also known as red hot pepper or chili pepper, cayenne *(Capsicum annum)* is actually the dried form of a ripened berry. This medicinal food has a history that goes back thousands of years. Chili pepper was used for many kinds of healing in South America and the West Indies. It was Christopher Columbus who brought cayenne to Italy from the West Indies—and before long, it was one of the more popular European spices. Western herbalists use cayenne for the treatment of asthma, poor circulation, respiratory tract infections, sore throats, digestive disturbances, toothaches, fevers, and heart disease. It's also used as a "synergist" in some herbal formulas—that is, an added ingredient that enhances the effects of the other herbs in the formula.

Cayenne is such a potent spice that it may seem contradictory to use it for pain relief. But many holistic practitioners as well as conventional medical doctors recommend the topical use of cayenne to relieve joint and muscle pain. The active ingredient—capsaicin—blocks the neurotransmitter substance P, so that the nerves to the skin and spinal cord do not receive any "pain signals." This is also the chemical that gives cayenne its hot taste.

When cayenne is first applied, you may feel a burning, stinging sensation as substance P actually increases for a short time. But as you use cayenne for a longer time, the sensations diminish as substance P activity decreases.

Some people, including myself, have stomach irritation when we eat cayenne or take a cayenne supplement. But I've found that this reaction isn't universal—it all depends on the person. Whatever your reaction, however, there's no evidence that chili peppers damage the intestinal tract. On the contrary, one study has shown that capsaicin actually inhibits the growth of the bacteria *H. Pylori,* which is implicated in many cases of stomach ulcers.

Cayenne has also been praised as a natural ingredient that improves circulation. Many herbalists and supplement companies claim that cayenne helps to "clean out" the arteries and reverse the effects of atherosclerosis. More studies must be done before we can be sure of these effects, but I do believe cayenne benefits the heart and cardiovascular system based on the feedback I get from patients. It's also known to be a great source of antioxidants such as vitamins A and C, and phytochemicals that protect against cellular damage. Some laboratory studies have also shown that cayenne reduces cholesterol levels and acts as a natural blood thinner.

Cayenne is used by many herbalists and naturopathic doctors in formulas for sore throats, upper respiratory tract infections, and sinusitis. It helps to reduce congestion and inflammation of these areas.

# DOSAGE

### ∾ *Topical use*

The cream should be an 0.025–0.075% capsaicin extract. Apply the cream two to four times daily.

∽ *Internal use:*

Take a 500-milligram capsule or 15 drops of tincture two to three times daily with meals.

## WHAT ARE THE SIDE EFFECTS?

Some people do experience digestive upset from taking cayenne internally. The cream form, which is applied to the skin only, has been shown to be very safe in clinical studies—though some people may initially experience a burning sensation that goes away after three or four days. *One caution about the topical treatments, however:* The cream should not be applied on open skin or near the eyes.

Cayenne probably has blood-thinning properties, so you should let your physician know you're taking the drops or capsules if you happen to be on blood-thinning medications.

## CAYENNE
### RECOMMENDATIONS FROM THE NATURAL PHYSICIAN FOR . . .

∽ *Arthritis*

Studies have shown capsaicin cream effective for osteoarthritis. Keep in mind, however, that this approach alleviates the pain, not the underlying cartilage deterioration. Supplements such as glucosamine sulfate, SAMe, and antioxidants (selenium, vitamin C, alpha lipoic acid) help to regenerate cartilage tissue and should also be used simultaneously.

Rheumatoid arthritis can also be helped with capsaicin cream.

∽ *Diabetic Neuropathy*

Diabetic neuropathy is the nerve damage related to a diabetic condition, and it's characterized by pain and abnormal sensations in the legs and feet. In studies, researchers have found that capsaicin is effective in relieving this kind of pain.

When researchers tried the cream with 49 patients who had moderate to severe diabetic neuropathy, it was found that 90 percent of the people who took capsaicin had pain reduction by the eighth week of use. Remember, capsaicin is the active ingredient in cayenne.

Other studies have confirmed this benefit as well—so cayenne is a simple, nontoxic way to relieve nerve pain if you have severe diabetic neuropathy. To make the treatment even better, I recommend adding alpha lipoic acid, vitamin $B_{12}$, and gingko biloba, which work internally to reverse this painful condition.

∽ *Heart Disease*

Cayenne has been shown to reduce the risk of heart disease by reducing cholesterol and triglyceride levels. Despite the lack of studies

*(continued)*

about this effect, hundreds of people have testified to the tremendous benefits they have experienced from supplementing with cayenne.

As a natural blood thinner, cayenne helps promote optimal circulation through the arteries of the body and heart. It is theorized that cayenne improves circulation through the coronary arteries. It is a great herb to include in herbal cardiovascular formulas.

### ℘ Psoriasis

This painful and itchy skin condition is one of the most stubborn conditions to treat because flare-ups can occur almost any time. The best long-term treatments involve herbs, supplements, and therapies that will help balance the internal environment. However, topical treatments with capsaicin have also proven effective.

For difficult cases, capsaicin is a treatment to consider.

### ℘ Shingles

The pain from shingles can be excruciating. I've had patients who couldn't even lie on their side on the examining table because the pain was so bad. Yet these "worst cases" are, fortunately, the very ones who are likely to benefit the most from treatment with cayenne.

When tested in controlled studies, capsaicin has relieved shingles pain in about 50 percent of users. I usually like to combine this treatment with other therapies, including vitamin $B_{12}$ injections, acupuncture, and homeopathic remedies. Capsaicin cream can be used to help relieve pain while these other natural therapies are working internally for a long-term cure.

### ℘ Surgery Recovery

Surgery can be traumatizing enough, but when you have additional nerve pain after surgery, life can be pretty miserable. Fortunately, capsaicin cream has proven helpful for people who have had nerve trauma and lasting pain after surgery.

Several studies support this recommendation. In a study of 23 patients who had mastectomies for breast cancer, researchers found that a cream with 0.075% capsaicin significantly reduced pain levels. These types of pain studies are encouraging because, so often, physicians don't know how to treat postsurgical nerve pain except with more surgery or with pharmaceutical pain medications, many of which have side effects. (Other natural treatments that work well include acupuncture and homeopathic remedies such as hypericum.)

# Chamomile

You'll routinely be offered chamomile tea in many restaurants and homes in Germany. It's an herb with a pleasant taste—so tasty, in fact, that even hard-core coffee-lovers can be found drinking it from time to time. If you ever need a tonic, too, to help anyone in the family overcome stomach upset, chamomile *(Recutita matricaria)* is the one to choose.

Much of chamomile's medicinal effects are targeted toward the digestive tract and nervous system. It's a synergistic combination, since the state of your nervous system is quite likely to dictate the health of your digestive system. In a world where high stress predominates, chamomile offers welcomed relief to "jangled nerves."

Chamomile has a rich history of use around the world. Ancient Egyptians, Greeks, and Indian healers relied on chamomile for its healing properties. It's a leading treatment for digestive conditions in many parts of Africa. It's officially considered a drug rather than an herb in many parts of the world—notably in Belgium, France, and the United Kingdom.

It comes in many forms. You'll easily find chamomile tea in the supermarket. The tinctures and capsules are in many health food stores and pharmacies. Chamomile is even used as an ingredient in shampoos. (It brings out blonde highlights, as well as acting as a cleanser.) Widely used as a homeopathic remedy, it's also a popular essential oil that's much valued for its aroma.

## A CHOICE OF TEAS

Two species of chamomile are used medicinally. German chamomile, also known as *Matricaria chamomilla* or *Matricaria recutita,* is the species of chamomile that has been most frequently used in research. This is the variety I recommend for patients. There's also a Roman chamomile, but I prefer the German. According to my sources in the health food industry, German chamomile is not contaminated by pesticides and other chemicals that are frequently found in Roman chamomile products.

Researchers have identified two major classes of active constituents in chamomile. Essential oils in the herb appear to have potent antiinflammatory and antispasmodic effects. This accounts for the many beneficial ways it soothes the gastrointestinal tract by relieving spasms, preventing gas, and even helping to ward off ulcers.

Chamomile also enhances antiviral and antibacterial activity, promoting the proliferation of substances that help fight off infection.

Because of its antiinflammatory properties, chamomile is also used topically for the treatment of skin disorders such as eczema. Even pets can benefit from this herb. I recall the time when my wife's cat had a very painful-looking patch of ulcerated skin on its belly—an area where a patch of hair was missing. The vet wanted to prescribe antibiotics and a topical cortisone cream. Instead, we used a treatment of fresh cool chamomile tea applied topically to the wound a few times each day. Within a week this raw-looking flesh wound had healed up nicely.

Another group of important compounds in chamomile is the flavonoids. Flavonoids promote an anti-anxiety effect. Scientists have shown that they do this by binding to special receptor sites in the brain, helping to induce a state of relaxation. Flavonoids also add to the antiinflammatory effects of chamomile.

# DOSAGE

### ❧ Tea

Chamomile works best, I've found, when you brew fresh tea. When the chamomile flowers are freshly steeped in boiling water, the essential oils form a high concentration. Also, just taking the time to make a fresh cup of chamomile tea is therapeutic. It's a way of saying, with your actions, "My health is important so I will take the time to make a health-promoting cup of tea."

I recommend steeping 1/2 to 1 teaspoon of dried chamomile flowers in a cup of freshly boiled water. Just one fresh cup helps to relieve digestive cramps and flatulence—and reduces anxiety, too—and you can have several cups during the course of the day.

Traditionally, mothers gave their infants a teaspoonful of freshly made chamomile tea to help relieve colic. I recommend it—but make sure the teaspoonful of tea is room temperature or cooler before giving it to a baby.

### ❧ Tincture

I recommend 10 to 30 drops (0.5 milliter) of the tincture form. For best results, add this tincture to 1/2 cup warm water. The tincture and the warm liquid combine to help relieve spasms in the digestive tract.

Infants also respond well to this mixture, but you only need to mix a few drops of chamomile tincture in the warm water.

### ❧ Capsule

You can get chamomile capsules, but often the capsulized herb is combined with other herbs to create a formula. I recommend that adults take 250 to 500 milligrams in the capsule form three to four times daily.

### ❧ *Creams*

Chamomile is used in creams and salves for various skin conditions such as rashes. Apply as directed on the container.

## WHAT ARE THE SIDE EFFECTS?

A number of herbalists have suggested that people should avoid use of chamomile if you're allergic to plants in the ragweed family, but I haven't seen any clinical evidence to support this view.

The warning signs would be reactions like an outbreak of hives, difficult breathing, or digestive upset. Of course, you should stop taking chamomile if you have any of these reactions. But millions of people use chamomile each year, and I haven't seen any reports of these adverse reactions.

---

## CHAMOMILE
### RECOMMENDATIONS FROM THE NATURAL PHYSICIAN FOR . . .

### ❧ *Colic*

Chamomile can be a godsend for parents whose child is suffering from colic. While experts do not agree on the cause of colic, it is clear that many cases are related to abdominal pain from the buildup of intestinal gas. Chamomile with its antispasmodic action can relieve colic in short order.

To prevent a flare-up of colic, administer 1/2 to 1 full teaspoon of cooled-down chamomile tea every 10 minutes or so until the infant stops fussing or crying. Quite often, parents will comment that after taking the chamomile the infant will pass gas, then settles down.

An even better way to use chamomile for colic is by giving the child the homeopathic form. Mix a pellet in water, and when it's completely dissolved, give the child 1/2 teaspoonful.

Herbal combinations can be very effective, too. In one study, 69 infants who were prone to colic were given a variety of different teas. Of those who got an herbal tea consisting of chamomile, vervain, licorice, fennel, and lemon balm for seven days, 57 percent had fewer colic symptoms.

Whether you're giving the child herbal or homeopathic forms of chamomile, be sure to treat the underlying cause as well. If the infant is still breast-feeding, the mother should avoid eating chocolate, peanuts, cow's milk, and spicy foods. Some children have an adverse reaction to cow's milk-based formulas and even soy formulas.

### ❧ *Earache*

While the herbal form of chamomile can be used to treat mild cases of childhood earaches,

*(continued)*

---

I consider the homeopathic form to be almost a wonder remedy. If the child is very irritable and holds one ear in pain, I would give the homeopathic cure. Chamomilla, the homeopathic form, is particularly recommended if one cheek is red while the other is pale, and the earache is so acute that nothing will settle down the child.

I remember one child who was brought into my clinic screaming and kicking from the intense ear pain. Examining the child's ear, I could see that she had a middle ear infection. The parents were at their wits end—but they didn't want to treat their daughter with antibiotics.

Five minutes after I gave the girl one dose of chamomilla, she was asleep in the mother's arms. When I saw the child the next day, the parents told me the child had slept through the night and was back to her regular self. I have seen dozens of cases like this, and so have other colleagues who practice homeopathy.

### Flatulence

To help relieve flatulence, many people combine this herb with other digestive tonics such as fennel, peppermint, and ginger.

### Irritable Bowel Syndrome (IBS)

IBS is a condition characterized by abdominal pain, flatulence, constipation, and/or diarrhea. In many cases, this all-too-common condition is in many cases correlated with high stress levels. Many stress-reduction techniques are helpful—including exercise, prayer, and counseling. But along with those strategies, I recommend chamomile to help relax the nervous system.

When you're more relaxed, digestive organs work more efficiently. In addition, the antispasmodic effect of chamomile provides pain relief for anyone with IBS.

I recall working with Michael, a 34-year-old mechanic, who had a fairly typical case of IBS. His worst symptom was the buildup of gas, which often caused great abdominal pain. In addition to testing Michael for food sensitivities, I recommended he drink a cup of chamomile tea with each meal.

Michael reported a dramatic improvement within two weeks. His condition greatly improved over time—only flaring up when he ate too much fast-food. Even when he had a flare-up, however, the chamomile helped alleviate most of the discomfort.

### Insomnia

Chamomile is one of the herbs to consider using before you go to bed if you occasionally have a problem with insomnia. I find this herb also works well in a combination formula with herbs such as valerian, oatstraw, skullcap, and passionflower.

### Menstrual Cramps

Chamomile can be used to relieve the pain of menstrual cramps, particularly when combined with herbs such as cramp bark.

If you are experiencing menstrual cramps, I recommend placing a hot water bottle over the lower abdomen and taking chamomile every 15 minutes.

In its homeopathic form, chamomilla is also quite effective for menstrual cramps. My wife, Angela—who is also a natural doctor—once suffered from cramps so badly that she had to lie down. I came to see her between patients one day and found her lying on a table in one of the exam rooms. She said she felt like she was going to die.

I immediately gave her a dose of chamomilla, and within 10 minutes the pains greatly sub-

(continued)

sided. An hour later, she was back seeing patients with me.

Angela later told me that after taking the remedy, she passed a huge clot, which was likely causing most of her discomfort.

### ❧ Skin

The use of chamomile in natural skin products continues to become more popular. Its antiinflammatory effect makes it valuable for rashes of all types. European practitioners recommend that it be added to baths for skin ailments.

One study found chamomile to be effective in speeding up the healing of skin abrasions after tattoos were surgically removed with abrasive materials.

### ❧ Stress

The nerve-relaxing properties of chamomile make it a popular herb for anxiety. Although not so strong as the nerve-soothing herbs kava root or valerian, it does work well for mild cases of anxiety. It's often included in herbal formulas, particularly for people whose muscles get very tight and tense from stress.

### ❧ Teething

Homeopathic chamomilla is the number-one remedy for children who have discomfort and pain from teething. Not only does it provide relief from the pain, chamomilla also helps alleviate the diarrhea that can accompany teething. (Homeopathic doctors look for a green stool color to determine whether chamomilla is the remedy of choice.)

You can give a child chamomilla in the usual homeopathic form or in the form of teething tablets. Herbal teas or tinctures also help, but I've found they don't work so well as the homeopathic form.

### ❧ Ulcers

Chamomile has a rich herbal history of use in the treatment of ulcers. One of its key components, azulene, is believed to promote healing in the mucus layer of the stomach. Animal studies have demonstrated the anti-ulcer effects of chamomile.

One old-time naturopathic doctor taught me a treatment that I have frequently given to my patients. First, I have the patient drink a half cup of chamomile tea, then lie down on her back. Fifteen minutes later, the patient drinks another half cup and lies on her left side. After 15 minutes and another half cup of chamomile tea, the patient shifts to her stomach. A final dose, and she lies on her right side for the last 15 minutes.

As the doctor had indicated, having someone shift positions in this way allows the chamomile to settle in different areas of the stomach, and 15 minutes is enough time to let the healing properties go to work on the contacted tissue.

The highly regarded German medical doctor and herbalist Rudolph Weiss states in his book *Herbal Medicine* that "Chamomile does not merely give symptomatic relief in these cases [of ulcers], but directly effects a cure. . . ." But he also notes that large doses of chamomile tea or tincture need to be given for prolonged periods of time for complete healing to occur.

I would recommend at least two months of continuous use.

# Chromium

"Mark, I have been following the exercise program you recommended and have been doing pretty well on my diet. But there is one little problem—well, it's actually a big problem. I can't stop eating those sweets. I crave them all day long!"

Susan, a 33-year-old mother of three, had made it her goal to lose 20 pounds of "leftover pregnancy weight." But this craving for sweets—certainly a common problem—was making it impossible.

"Let's have you take some chromium to help with your blood-sugar regulation," I suggested. "Maybe you crave sweets because your body wants to compensate for low blood-sugar levels."

Any kind of sweets—whether chocolate, candy, or soda—gives you an instant "blood sugar fix." Unfortunately, those foods also cause blood sugar irregularity and cause insulin levels to rise, leading to fat storage. (Insulin is the hormone produced by your body that helps open the gates of your cells to blood sugar and, therefore, fat storage.)

When Susan heard that chromium would help reduce sweet cravings, her response was predictable: "Great, I would like to get started on it right away!"

She reported four weeks later that her sweet cravings were much improved. Chromium was "doing the trick," to use her phrase.

## TRACE-MINERAL POWER

Chromium is a trace mineral, meaning that our bodies only require very small "trace" amounts. While we need many milligrams of some vitamins and minerals, a trace mineral like chromium is fine if it comes in microgram dosages—that is, one-thousandth of the other requirements.

Chromium facilitates the uptake of glucose (blood sugar) into the cells so that it can be "burned" for energy. Admittedly, the hormone insulin is the substance that's mainly responsible for transporting glucose into the cells—but chromium teams up nicely with the hormone to carry out the delivery function.

Without insulin, serious disease such as Type 1 diabetes can occur. Commonly called juvenile-onset diabetes, this type occurs when the pancreas does not secrete enough insulin. People with Type 1 diabetes need regular injections of insulin so that their cells can get a sorely needed, steady supply of glucose.

Type 2 diabetes (adult onset or noninsulin dependent) usually occurs later in life and has a different type of pathology. This is not a disease where there is a lack of insulin; rather, it occurs when the cells are insensitive to insulin. If the insulin doesn't unlock the door of the cell, glucose can't get in. It's like a taxicab pulling up to the door—but the passengers can't get out and go in the building.

Chromium—and another trace mineral called vanadium—both have the keys to help get the doors unlocked. By enhancing the action of insulin, the trace minerals help glucose penetrate the cells.

But apart from playing a role as a "glucose tolerance factor"—as it's sometimes called—chromium is good for a variety of other applications. We are learning more about a condition called "Syndrome X," which occurs when people have an inherited problem—they can't metabolize carbohydrates (including sugar) very effectively. If someone has high blood-sugar levels because of Syndrome X, that person is going to have increased levels of the hormone insulin—and if you have elevated insulin levels, you're prone to many health problems including obesity, high blood pressure, fatigue, and heart disease, to name a few. Minerals like chromium are a godsend for people with Syndrome X, as it optimizes the cells' ability to metabolize carbohydrates.

Chromium is found in whole grains. Deficiencies are quite common, because most of the grains found in processed or packaged food are highly refined and just don't have enough chromium content. Meat and brewer's yeast are also rich sources of chromium.

# DOSAGE

If you have no blood sugar or weight problems and want to take an extra chromium supplement just to see how you feel, I recommend 200 micrograms daily. Many multivitamins now contain this amount. But if you're supplementing with chromium specifically for weight, you should generally take 400 to 600 micrograms daily.

If you have diabetes or blood-sugar problems (for example, hypoglycemia), the recommended dose is between 400 and 1,000 micrograms daily. But anyone taking these dosages should have their blood sugar and medications monitored by a doctor.

Chromium picolinate is the type that has been most widely researched in reliable studies. It works hand-in-hand with the trace mineral vanadium to help regulate blood sugar.

## WHAT ARE THE SIDE EFFECTS?

Dosages at 1,000 micrograms and lower appear to be very safe and nontoxic. If you're taking drugs for diabetes, however, the addition of chromium can affect your need for pharmaceutical medication. Often, diabetic pharmaceutical medications (insulin or Type 2 diabetic drugs) need to be reduced or the blood-sugar levels can get too low. That's why it's essential for anyone with diabetes to discuss their plans with a doctor before starting a supplement program with chromium.

# CHROMIUM
## RECOMMENDATIONS FROM THE NATURAL PHYSICIAN FOR...

### ∾ Cholesterol and Triglycerides

Chromium has been shown to lower total cholesterol and triglycerides by about 10 percent in people with Type 2 diabetes and also those who do not have diabetes. Both of these effects help to lower your risk of heart disease. It also increases the good cholesterol HDL. While the improvements are not dramatic, it makes sense to include chromium for improved heart health.

### ∾ Diabetes and Hypoglycemia

Anyone with diabetes or hypoglycemia should definitely be supplementing with chromium. The fact that chromium makes the cells more sensitive to insulin has been borne out by studies done with people who had Type 2 diabetes. Often, those who have Type 2 diabetes have a chromium deficiency, which appears to make them more susceptible to the condition.

In one study, for instance, researchers examined 29 overweight individuals who also had a family history of diabetes. Using the usual methods of controlled experiment, some of the patients received 1,000 micrograms (1 milligram) of chromium daily, while others received a placebo. After four months, the patients were tested again, and researchers found that the chromium-takers had a 40 percent reduction in insulin resistance. The same improvement was maintained at the end of eight months. This study suggests the need for people who have a strong family history of diabetes to begin chromium supplementation on a preventative basis, especially if they are overweight.

On the heels of research like this, the arguments for taking chromium are compelling. The trace mineral is nontoxic—so why not try this natural therapy (along with lifestyle changes) if it can help prevent this disease?

*(continued)*

When I had first started my practice many years ago, I saw a patient who was showing the early warning signs of diabetic retinopathy, an eye disease—potentially leading to blindness—that's directly related to high blood-sugar levels. From the patient's description, I realized that his diet varied enormously from day to day—yet it seemed like he would benefit from chromium supplementation, so I started him on 400 micrograms a day. Six months later he told me that the medical doctor whom he'd been seeing could no longer find any evidence of retinopathy. The physician simply recommended that my patient continue to do whatever he had been doing. Such a reversal of the condition was rare, his doctor noted.

I find that hypoglycemia also responds well to chromium supplementation. One small study of eight females with hypoglycemia found that their condition was alleviated when they took 200 micrograms for three months.

### ❧ Weight Loss

Human studies have shown that chromium supplementation at doses of 200 to 400 micrograms can help people lose weight and increase lean muscle mass. Larger studies need to be done—but, in the meantime, I've seen this type of regimen help about 50 percent of the patients I've treated with similar amounts of supplementation. Remember that it may take a couple of months before the beneficial effects start to show.

The supplements work best when the doses are combined with a steady, good diet and regular exercise.

# Coenzyme Q10

Several pictures come to mind when someone mentions the supplement coenzyme Q10 (also referred to as CoQ10). One is that of the heart. I see this big, red pumping muscle contracting and relaxing. Inside the heart cells are tiny explosions where energy is being created. Within these cells I see the spark plug. The spark plug is CoQ10.

Without coenzyme Q10, heart cells could not produce energy, known as ATP. Though the heart is the most famous center of operations for CoQ10, it's found in other body cells as well—and in all of them, it's important for energy production.

But the heart suffers most when there's a lack of CoQ10. It beats slowly. Its contractions are wimpy. Its rhythm goes awry. When a heart doesn't have enough CoQ10 for proper electrical conduction, it suffers as it starves—and, of course, the whole circulatory system pays the price.

Fortunately, when new CoQ10 comes on the scene, recovery can be noticeable and rapid. As CoQ10 saturates the heart cells, life returns; the heart resumes its strong, regular series of rhythmical contractions; tissues fill with more oxygen as blood flow improves; and energy abounds.

## BETTER VESSELS

Not only does CoQ10 improve heart cells, it also renovates the highways and byways of all our blood vessel walls. Subjected to constant pounding from the surge of blood flowing through them, our arteries and veins can get damaged over time as the pressure builds. As those blood vessels absorb some of the coenzyme Q10 that's circulating through the body, the walls relax and blood pressure drops. Blood flow hits an optimum level—not too fast and not too slow, but just right to deliver oxygen and nutrients to the tissues.

The blood vessel walls are safer when blood pressure is lower—hence, the premium that we place on "normal blood pressure." As pressure rises, so does the risk of heart attack or stroke.

## A UBIQUITOUS SUBSTANCE

With so many benefits for the body, in so many places, it's appropriate that CoQ10 should also be known by the medical term ubiquinone. A ubiquitous substance, found in all the cells of the body, coenzyme Q10 was originally discovered in 1957 by scientists from the Merck pharmaceutical company. They used the number 10 in reference to its biochemical structure (ten isoprenoid units on its side chain), but apart from assigning the name that stuck, they didn't do much to explore its properties.

The Japanese began testing CoQ10 on humans in 1963, and by 1976 it was "placed on the formulary" (that is, accepted as a medicine) for Japanese hospitals.

### Fuel for the Athletic Set

Though exercise is certainly healthful, committed athletes get so much of it that their bodies produce what are known as metabolic byproducts, including free radicals. These are runaway substances that, left unchecked, can cause rapid cell aging.

By taking low levels of antioxidants such as CoQ10, the body counteracts some of the effects of these free radicals. Athletes can become more resistant to fatigue and immune-system breakdown. Therefore, anyone who is involved in rigorous physical activity would do well to supplement at least a minimal amount of CoQ10.

In 1978, Peter Mitchell was awarded the Nobel Peace Prize for his studies of energy production in the human body, which led to hypotheses on how CoQ10 works and how it relates to heart disease.

From that time on, hundreds of studies on CoQ10 have been done in Japan, the U.S., and other countries. (So much of the research has been done by Dr. K. Folkers of the University of Texas that he is often referred to as the "father of coenzyme Q10.") By the mid 1990s coenzyme Q10 was widely accepted in the health food industry as a popular supplement to help improve heart health. Unfortunately, even today, there are many cardiologists who do not recommend CoQ10.

CoQ10 is found in high amounts in meat and fish. Nuts are also a source as are some vegetables like broccoli and spinach. The body manufactures CoQ10 from the amino acid tyrosine. This synthesis requires the action of vitamins C, $B_2$, $B_6$, $B_{12}$, folic acid, niacin, and pantothenic acid. Another important function of CoQ10 is that it works to recycle vitamin E.

# DOSAGE

If your health is good but you just want to take coenzyme Q10 for prevention, I'd recommend 25 to 100 milligrams daily. It does make sense to supplement with CoQ10, whatever the state of your health, as cardiovascular disease can sneak up on just about anyone (it's the leading cause of death in the U.S.) and CoQ10 is one of the best antioxidants for the entire cardiovascular network.

If you have cardiovascular disease or any other serious illness (such as cancer), you should take between 300 and 450 milligrams daily.

CoQ10 is available in different forms. You can get soft gel capsules, sublingual tablets, and powder-filled capsules. Coenzyme Q10 creams are now available, as well, to help prevent aging of the skin.

A few human studies have shown that certain brands of soft gel capsules have two to three times the bioavailability as the dry-powder form of capsules. CoQ10 is both water- and fat-soluble in its gel form, which means it's much more effectively absorbed into the bloodstream. If you take the gel form, you only need to take half to one-third as much as you would with the powdered form to get the same recommended dose.

CoQ10 is best taken with meals.

# WHAT ARE THE SIDE EFFECTS?

Coenzyme Q10 is very safe, but we don't know about its effects on pregnant or lactating women, or higher dosages on young children. Until it has been tested, I would not recommend it to these groups unless a patient has an urgent medical problem, such as a heart condition, that warrants its use (and then, only with the supervision of a doctor).

CoQ10 may interfere with the action of the blood-thinning drug Coumadin. If you're taking that pharmaceutical, let your doctor know that you plan on supplementing with CoQ10 so that your blood-clotting ability can be closely monitored. Personally, I have never seen a bad interaction between Coumadin and CoQ10, but some problems have been reported in the medical literature.

## COENZYME Q10
### RECOMMENDATIONS FROM THE NATURAL PHYSICIAN FOR . . .

#### ❧ Angina
If you have this symptom of heart disease, it actually feels like your heart is being squeezed, or you experience the sensation of a great pressure in the chest. Angina is almost always caused by a lack of oxygen to the heart muscle. Because the arteries are partially blocked by plaque—a buildup related to high cholesterol—your heart isn't getting enough blood flow to provide oxygen to the heart muscle. Spasm of the coronary arteries can also lead to angina.

Several studies have shown CoQ10 to be effective for this condition. Pharmaceutical medications are useful for treating acute episodes of angina, but CoQ10 is the supplement of choice for prevention of future attacks. I have had outstanding results in patients who have had a history of angina. Sometimes I recommend CoQ10 by itself while, for other patients, I favor combining it

with magnesium, hawthorn berry extract, and cactus extract (*Cereus grandiflorus*).

#### ❧ Arrhythmia
People who have this condition say they have the sensation that their heart is missing a beat. Coenzyme Q10 has a stabilizing effect on the electrical conductivity of the heart, so it helps to prevent arrhythmia. Studies have shown it to be effective in nearly one-quarter of cases where people are having a particular kind of arrhythmia related to premature ventricular contractions.

Magnesium, L-carnitine, and potassium supplements are also indicated for arrhythmias.

#### ❧ Atherosclerosis
When cholesterol and other fatty substances go through an oxidation process in the arteries, they begin to damage blood vessel walls. As a result, plaque builds up as your immune system

*(continued)*

reacts to what's going on inside the blood vessel. If this process continues undeterred, it can lead to the blocked condition commonly called "hardening of the arteries" or atherosclerosis. But that process can be slowed or stopped if you make dietary changes and use coenzyme Q10 to inhibit the oxidation of cholesterol and other fatty substances in the body.

### ❧ Cancer

Researchers have discovered that anything we do to bolster the immune system can also help fight cancer, and we know that CoQ10 is required as a nutrient for a healthy immune system. Many holistic doctors recommend CoQ10 in high dosages (300 milligrams or higher) along with other therapies in the treatment of cancer. Five cases of metastatic breast cancer have been documented in which there was complete reversal of metastasis with high doses of CoQ10 (390 milligrams). Obviously, there needs to be more studies done on CoQ10 and cancer. It does make sense though to at least use it as a complementary therapy when treating cancer.

### ❧ Cardiomyopathy

This is a disease of the heart that results in a reduced heart contraction force. Cardiomyopathy may be caused by a variety of factors, including viral infections, nutritional deficiencies, and autoimmune reactions. The progression of this disease can lead to congestive heart failure, where the heart refuses to pump. (If the heart isn't jump-started again, congestive heart failure can be fatal.)

One study looked at 34 people with severe cardiomyopathy who were given 100 milligrams of CoQ10 daily. Eighty-two percent of the people showed improvement—as measured by heart tests—after the therapy. Their 2-year survival rate was 62 percent, compared with a second group of people who only had conventional therapy. (Of the latter group, the 2-year survival rate was only 25 percent.)

### ❧ Congestive Heart Failure

If you have this condition, the heart simply "gives out" as a pump, and your system is deprived of blood. Shortness of breath, fatigue, and water retention in the lungs and lower legs are common symptoms of this disease. Dr. Sinatra, a cardiologist and author of the *Coenzyme Q10 Phenomenon*, has found that higher dosages of CoQ10 can have dramatic, lifesaving benefits for people with congestive heart failure. Several studies support the use of CoQ10 for this serious condition.

### ❧ Diabetes

People with diabetes have been found to have low levels of CoQ10. Theoretically, they have a higher need for this natural substance because the disease increases the need for antioxidants. I recommend that people with diabetes should take CoQ10 as part of an antioxidant regimen.

### ❧ Drug Damage

Several drugs deplete the body of CoQ10. Adriamycin, a chemotherapy drug used for various types of cancer, can cause irreversible heart damage and possible heart failure. Coenzyme Q10 works as an antioxidant to protect the heart from the damaging effects of this chemotherapy agent. One study of children with cancer who were being treated with Adriamycin showed that CoQ10 had a protective effect when they were given 200 milligrams daily.

Beta blockers are a class of drugs that deplete CoQ10 as well. These medications are commonly used for conditions like high blood pressure and arrhythmia. Interestingly, beta blockers can lead to congestive heart failure in people, though it isn't known whether the heart

*(continued)*

failure is a side effect of the beta blocker or is caused by depletion of CoQ10. While more research needs to be done in this area, it seems prudent to take CoQ10 as a preventative supplement if you're taking a beta blocker.

Millions of North Americans take cholesterol-lowering drugs, and many of these drugs have well-reported side effects. CoQ10 is a very important supplement if you're taking a class of cholesterol-lowering drugs known as HMG CoA reductase inhibitors such as Mevacor, Pravachol, and Zocor. These drugs work by inhibiting the enzyme HMG CoA reductase that is required by the liver to manufacture cholesterol. This same enzyme is also involved in the synthesis of CoQ10. If you are taking a a lot of this class of medicine, it can lead to tissue depletion. For anyone taking these kinds of drugs, I recommend an additional dose of 100 to 200 milligrams of CoQ10. (I also recommend other liver-protective substances such as alpha lipoic acid and milk thistle.)

Some psychoactive drugs, including tricyclic antidepressants and phenothiazines, also deplete CoQ10 levels. Some heart conditions such as arrhythmias, congestive heart failure, and heart attacks have been associated with the use of these medications. Taking CoQ10 will help you protect yourself against the cardiac toxicity of these drugs.

### ❧ Male Infertility

Coenzyme Q10 has been shown to improve the fertility potential of sperm. This may occur because CoQ10 is an energizing substance that could literally help the sperm to swim more rapidly or more strongly. It is also likely that CoQ10 protects the sperm from the damaging effects of free radicals.

CoQ10 is well worth trying for low sperm counts or poor motility. When I recommend it, I often suggest other supplements as well, including the amino acid arginine, and vitamins $B_{12}$, C, E, zinc, and L-carnitine.

### ❧ Mitral Valve Prolapse

Mitral valve prolapse means that one of the heart valves is not closing properly as your heart contracts and expands. CoQ10 may help this condition.

### ❧ Muscular Dystrophy

This refers to a group of genetic diseases characterized by progressive muscle weakness. Most of us have become familiar with this disease through the annual Jerry Lewis telethons. Dr. Folkers has shown in two small studies that CoQ10 improved physical performance in people with this disease. He recommends people with muscular dystrophy supplement with CoQ10 indefinitely, as it has been proven safe and it improves quality of life. CoQ10 is well worth trying, and I would recommend L-carnitine as well.

### ❧ Periodontal Disease

Several studies have shown that CoQ10 improves the health of the gums—a significant finding, since more than 30 million Americans suffer from gum disease. In theory, CoQ10 improves oxygenation of the gum tissues and also has a supportive effect on the immune system. So it not only helps the gums heal, it also helps to suppress the bacteria that lead to gum inflammation and erosion.

CoQ10 is definitely worth trying if you have chronic bleeding gums due to gingivitis. I recommend taking the supplement for several months before your dentist makes an assessment of progress.

CoQ10 is now available in special toothpastes for people with gum disease.

*(continued)*

**❧ Skin Health**

I have noticed that skin creams containing CoQ10 have come onto the market. Although I was skeptical at first, there is research showing that creams containing antioxidants such as CoQ10 and vitamin C do, indeed, help to pro-tect the skin. It could be that these products help the rehydration of the skin, giving it a more youthful appearance.

CoQ10 also helps protect the skin against the ultraviolet radiation from the sun.

# Cranberry

The medical community scoffed for decades at the notion that cranberry juice could clear up urinary tract infections. It was widely regarded as nothing more than a folk remedy.

Yet there's a rich history behind this tart berry *(Vaccinium macrocarpon),* and many people have reported medicinal benefits. Although I like to see scientific studies, the many stories of its healing power added up to strong empirical evidence. Now the research has caught up with the folk history. A number of studies in the last decade have shown that cranberry is quite effective for the prevention and relief of urinary tract infections.

Cranberry has long been used for medicinal purposes by Europeans as well as Native American Indians. It won acceptance as a cure for urinary tract infections—but beyond that, it was used to deal with gallbladder attacks, liver and stomach problems, and for the prevention of scurvy. (Both vitamin C and flavonoids, which are contained in cranberry, help to prevent scurvy.)

Today, cranberry juice and supplements are used by millions around the world—and the medical community has become more accepting. In the past few years, many more conventional physicians have been recommending cranberry for their patients.

The fruit called cranberry comes from the vine of a plant that belongs to the same genus *(Vaccinium)* as bilberry and blueberry. It grows in North America in marshlike conditions, such as the famous "cranberry bogs" of Cape Cod, Massachusetts and southern New Jersey.

I mainly recommend cranberry for the prevention and treatment of urinary tract and prostate infections. Research has shown that cranberry inhibits growth of the bacteria *E. coli,* which is the culprit most commonly associated with urinary tract infections. As a food source, cranberry provides ample vitamin C and flavonoids for people who need higher amounts for conditions such as varicose veins and cataracts.

## DOSAGE

### ✺ *Juice*

It is important to drink the unsweetened form of cranberry juice. "Regular" cranberry juice—the kind that appears on most supermarket shelves—is sweetened with sugar that suppresses the immune system and feeds harmful bacteria.

For anyone dealing with urinary tract infections, I recommend 8 ounces of unsweetened cranberry juice four to five times daily. If the tart taste is too much for you, dilute the juice with water. For long-term use and prevention of urinary tract infections, I recommend having one or two 8-ounce glasses of unsweetened cranberry juice daily.

### ✺ *Capsules and Tablets*

If you take cranberry in capsule form, the dosage varies depending on the potency of the product. In the past, the capsules had such a low concentration of cranberry that you'd have to take eight capsules or more to get the same therapeutic effect as four 8-ounce glasses of the juice. Currently, the standardized capsules and tablets have higher concentrations. You can take three to four capsules or tablets daily to achieve therapeutic benefit.

## WHAT ARE THE SIDE EFFECTS?

There are no reported side effects. However, I would recommend anyone with diabetes to check with his or her doctor first before using cranberry juice on a long-term basis. The naturally occurring fruit sugars could cause blood-sugar problems. But if you have diabetes, you might be able to avoid spiking blood-sugar levels by taking cranberry juice with your meals.

# CRANBERRY
## RECOMMENDATIONS FROM THE NATURAL PHYSICIAN FOR . . .

### ∿ Prostate Infections

Known as prostatitis, prostate infections are more common in men who have an enlarged prostate gland—a condition that occurs in about half of all men over the age of 50. *E. coli* is the most common bacteria associated with prostate infections.

An enlarged prostate pinches on the urethra (urinary tube), causing a slowdown or backup of urine flow. As a result, bacteria and other microbes are more likely to grow in the urethra, leading to infection. Cranberry can help prevent this problem.

### ∿ Urinary Tract Infections

It was generally believed up until the last decade that cranberry juice prevents urinary tract infections by lowering the pH of urine. A lower pH makes for an inhospitable environment for bacteria like *E. coli*.

But studies done in the 1990s demonstrated that phytochemicals in cranberry—known as proanthocyandins—prevent bacteria from attaching to the bladder wall and urinary tract. Researchers also discovered that the sugar molecule fructose helped prevent a certain strain of *E. coli* from adhering to the urinary tract cells. Finally, a 1998 study in *The New England Journal of Medicine* demonstrated that cranberry prevents the fimbriae (analogous to arms and hands of bacteria) from attaching to the urinary tract walls. In research, cranberry's cousin blueberry was found to have a similar action.

I recommend cranberry juice or cranberry extract in supplemental form be used by people who have been taking prescription antibiotics for a urinary tract infection—especially if they have any kind of kidney infection. This simultaneous use optimizes the chances of a quick recovery.

A 1994 study in *The Journal of the American Medical Association* found that regular consumption of cranberry juice significantly reduced the frequency of bacteria and pus in the urine of elderly women. In this 6-month study, the 153 women drank less than one pint of cranberry juice every day—with the usual "control group" drinking a placebo drink that had a similar flavor to cranberry. Improvements were noticed in the cranberry drinkers within 4 to 8 weeks.

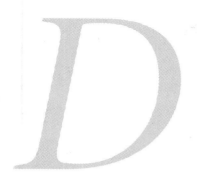

# Dandelion

· · · · · · · · · · · · · · · · · · · · · · · · · · · · · · · · · · · · · · · · · · · · · · · · · · · · · · · ·

One person's weed is another's healing herb. The same dandelion *(Taraxacum officinalis)* that so many homeowners set out to pull, eradicate, or destroy has a rich history of medicinal use in Europe, China, Japan, and Russia. Even in the U.S., this herb has been used for detoxification for more than a century.

Dandelion root is revered for its ability to tonify the liver. The leaves have a natural diuretic effect—that is, they'll help remove excess water from the body. In addition, the whole plant is a nutritious and healing food. You can use the leaves in salads or in teas. The roots can be roasted and used as a coffee substitute, while the flowers have gone into a variety of alcoholic beverages, including dandelion wine and the after-dinner liqueur schnapps.

## WEEDING OUT THE GOOD STUFF

Dandelion is a rich source of minerals such as magnesium, potassium, manganese, copper, phosphorous, sodium, iron, and silicon. The leaves are also rich in vitamin A. According to Dr. Bernard Jensen, author of *Foods That Heal,* "Dandelion greens have more vitamin A than almost any other vegetable."

Other nutrients found in dandelion include the B-complex vitamins as well as vitamin C, vitamin D, vitamin K, and calcium. Choline, a relative of the B-vitamin family is also found in relatively high amounts in dandelion. This nutrient is important for preventing and treating a fatty liver, and it also serves as an aid in bile production.

**113**

The chemical constituents of dandelion lend additional healing properties. One of the more important chemicals, taraxacin, which has a bitter taste, is thought to stimulate the digestive organs. It plays a role in prompting the liver and gallbladder to release bile. Improved bile flow is important, because it helps the liver to detoxify (that is, get rid of toxic chemicals) more effectively.

Dandelion also contains two hormone-balancing constituents: taraxerol and taraxasterol. It's one of the premier herbs recommended for hormone-related conditions like PMS.

Pectin is also found in dandelion. This is a type of fiber that helps to relieve constipation and reduce cholesterol levels. It also binds with toxins, which helps get rid of them. (The toxic substances that bind with pectin pass more readily through your digestive system.) Finally, dandelion contains a type of resin that helps in eliminating lung congestion, so it's a helpful remedy for coughs.

Dandelion ranks alongside milk thistle as the most frequently recommended herbs to help patients who need liver detoxification. Doctors who use natural healing methods are often concerned with the overall condition of the liver because it performs so many functions. Among other things, it detoxifies the chemicals and pollutants that get into our body, produces bile to help digest fats, stores and helps to regulate blood sugar, and metabolizes hormones. As one expert noted, the liver performs over 5,000 different enzymatic reactions every second. It's no wonder so many conditions can be helped by improving liver health. Just by treating the liver, we can sometimes resolve numerous conditions, ranging from physical problems such as indigestion and hepatitis to the emotional imbalances that contribute to irritability and depression.

# DOSAGE

Dandelion root is most often taken in the capsule form. A typical adult dose is a 250- to 500-milligram capsule taken three times a day with meals. Since the dosage may vary depending on the strength of the extract, I recommend that you follow the directions on the label.

If you're taking the tincture form, 20 to 30 drops with each meal is an average dose.

You can have dandelion leaf tea any time you need the benefits of its diuretic effect, as it will help you get rid of excess water and reduce bloating. Use one heaping tablespoon of dandelion leaves per cup of water. If you pick local dandelion to make a tea or add the leaves to your salad, be sure you're getting the plant from an area that has not been sprayed with herbicides.

Dandelion leaf is also available in both capsule and tincture form.

## WHAT ARE THE SIDE EFFECTS?

While the dandelion plant is not toxic, some people get loose stools because it increases bile flow in the body. Therefore, it's not advisable to take capsules, tincture, or tea if you have diarrhea.

Some people are allergic to dandelion. Don't take it if you get an inflammation—contact dermatitis—when the leaves touch yours skin. Dandelion should not be used if you have bile duct obstruction, acute gallbladder inflammation (cholecystitis), or intestinal blockage. Also don't take dandelion to relieve gallstones unless you have been given a dosage that's prescribed by a knowledgeable herbal practitioner.

The German Commission E states that dandelion is a safe herb for women to use during pregnancy or while breast-feeding.

---

## DANDELION
### RECOMMENDATIONS FROM THE NATURAL PHYSICIAN FOR . . .

**≫ Constipation, Flatulence, and Indigestion**

Poor bile flow can lead to chronic constipation. If you have enough fiber in your diet and consume plenty of water but still have constipation problems, then it is a sign that the liver needs some work. Your bowels move more easily with some dandelion to increase the bile flow. Unlike pharmaceutical laxatives—which should only be used for a short time—you can take dandelion root in any of its forms for a few months and then gradually discontinue it. Once the liver and gallbladder are "tuned up," the bowels should move on their own without continual use of the herbal remedy.

Indigestion or flatulence might be caused by insufficient stomach acid or bile production. If you're having these problems, dandelion is helpful because it stimulates natural actions and secretions of the digestive organs. Taken with meals, over time, it helps "retrain" the digestive organs so they'll function more effectively.

Dandelion is especially helpful if you have any problems digesting fats. When that's the case, it's usually because bile flow is insufficient.

**≫ Diabetes**

Dandelion root can be helpful for the long-term treatment of diabetes. It contains inulin, which

*(continued)*

---

**115**

is known to help balance blood-sugar levels. When you improve liver health by taking an herb like dandelion, you're assisting one of the organs that's most essential for blood-sugar regulation.

### ⚘ Edema

I have had several elderly patients come to see me for the treatment of edema in their lower legs and ankles. That's the swelling or bloating that's caused by fluids in the extremities. Dandelion leaf extract works very nicely without side effects to substantially reduce this swelling.

I have determined in some cases that water retention is due to a weak heart. If the heart doesn't contract forcefully, water can back up in the tissues, which is a common symptom of congestive heart failure. Conventional medical tests such as an EKG (electrocardiogram) and ultrasound can reveal whether you have symptoms of congestive heart failure. To treat the heart weakness along with the edema, I not only recommend dandelion but also add herbs like hawthorn berry and nutrients like CoQ10 and L-carnitine.

I commonly recommend dandelion leaf for edema that occurs with pregnancy, when many women experience swelling of the hands and ankles. Dandelion leaf extract will usually help reduce some of the bloating. One of the benefits of dandelion leaf as a diuretic is that it does not cause the loss of potassium. (Potassium loss is a common side effect of some pharmaceutical medications that are prescribed for relief of edema.)

### ⚘ Gout

Dandelion has traditionally been used for the treatment of gout because it helps lower the levels of uric acid—and excess uric acid is often responsible for this problem. From my own observations, dandelion doesn't have dramatic effects in the short term, but it can be helpful on a long-term basis. (Cherries and celery seed extract are also excellent for relieving gout.)

### ⚘ Hepatitis

A valuable herb when it comes to liver problems, dandelion has been shown to improve liver function and alleviate the symptoms of liver toxicity. So it's well-suited as a treatment for hepatitis. If you are taking medication for hepatitis, you should continue to follow your doctor's advice, but dandelion can help improve bile flow so that there is no back up of bile in the ducts. Most herbal liver formulas contain dandelion root as one of the main herbs.

### ⚘ High Blood Pressure

I almost always recommend dandelion leaf in the treatment of high blood pressure. It acts as a natural diuretic so that blood volume is reduced, which has the effect of relieving high blood pressure.

Prescription blood-pressure medications, which are mostly diuretics, work on the same premise. But I prefer dandelion leaves over medication because of the way some pharmaceuticals cause potassium depletion.

An ideal herbal formula for high blood pressure includes dandelion leaf, hawthorn berry, viscum, and valerian. I've found that this combination is successful in a high percentage of cases, and many patients are able to reduce their pharmaceutical medications. At the same time, I always emphasize the importance of keeping your doctor informed if you have high blood pressure—and you should never discontinue a blood-pressure medication without the approval of your doctor.

(continued)

### Loss of Appetite

Dandelion root, like many other bitter herbs, can help restore your appetite. Just a daily cup of dandelion tea may be enough to improve appetite if you haven't been feeling hungry.

### PMS, Menopause, and Hormone Balancing

Dandelion root is excellent for conditions related to hormone balance. The liver has to metabolize hormones, so you may develop a hormone imbalance if this organ is not working effectively.

In Chinese and naturopathic herbal medicine and in many other natural healing systems, optimizing liver health is considered very important if you want to treat conditions such as PMS, irregular menstrual cycles, or the symptoms associated with menopause.

In addition to helping out the liver, dandelion has two chemical constituents—taraxerol and taraxasterol—that help balance hormones as well.

### Weight Loss

If you take dandelion leaf tea or extract, you'll encourage the excretion of water, which leads to weight loss. It's not an easy weight-loss route, however, because it just reduces fluids without affecting the underlying causes of being overweight.

# D-glucarate

I had a conversation not long ago with Dr. Thom Slaga, a well-known researcher at the prestigious American Cancer Research Center in Denver, Colorado. We were discussing his ongoing studies of a naturally occurring nutrient called glucaric acid.

Dr. Slaga piqued my interest with his explanation. Glucaric acid, he said, is a potent phytonutrient (plant nutrient) that helps the body detoxify toxic substances. This amazing phytonutrient, he went on to say, seemed to prevent certain types of cancers in animals. It was soon to become available as a supplement, in a form known as calcium d-glucarate, often referred to as d-glucarate.

I was struck at once by the possibility that d-glucarate might offer tremendous benefits for my patients. If this supplement stood up to scientific scrutiny, it was just what I was looking for. I had been intrigued about the new frontier in natural medicine—the role of phytonutrients and whole-food extracts—and here was a supplement that represented the latest discovery in that frontier.

## TOMORROW'S BREAKTHROUGH TODAY

I would expect that we will all be hearing a lot more about this breakthrough supplement in the coming years. As a medical advisor for the health food industry, I am sometimes privy to leading-edge research, years before it becomes public knowledge. Often, new supplements are slow to be accepted. But I expect calcium d-glucarate will prove to be one of the most important nutritional supplements on the market.

The phytonutrient occurs naturally in fruits and vegetables such as apples, broccoli, alfalfa, cherries, and grapefruit. In this naturally occurring form, it's known as glucaric acid. When it's made into a supplement, calcium is added to help improve absorption.

Most people don't eat enough fruits and vegetables to get therapeutic amounts of phytonutrients like glucaric acid. That's where the supplement comes in handy. We would have to eat seven to ten servings of fruits and vegetables a day for cancer prevention, according to current recommendations. Living in a world where fast-food is the norm, most people struggle to get two servings a day. By taking glucaric acid in supplemental form—as d-glucarate—we can take a step toward cancer prevention by making up some of that daily deficit.

## LIVER SUPPORT

D-glucarate helps the liver metabolize or "burn up" some dangerous toxins, preventing these chemicals from causing harm. The toxins include carcinogens—that is, cancer-causing agents—as well as certain hormones. In the liver, d-glucarate helps the toxins turn into a water-soluble form, after which, they can be excreted in urine.

When toxins enter the body, they go through two main detoxification phases in the liver. Phase one breaks down the compound and turns it into what's called an intermediate form, which is less toxic. Then the less-toxic form enters phase two, where it becomes water soluble. If either one of these phases doesn't work correctly, the toxic substances continue to circulate in the body, causing damage. Eventually, these toxins get stored in tissues such as the brain, bone, or fat—or they build up inside other organs.

D-glucarate is important in the process because it helps carry out phase-two detoxification efficiently. But it does more than remove cancer-causing chemicals. In addition, d-glucarate helps metabolize hormones and many other potentially harmful substances.

## HORMONE BALANCER

While healthy levels of hormones help the body function properly, excessive amounts of certain hormones can cause serious problems. Studies have shown that unhealthy levels of hormones like estrogen, progesterone, testosterone, and other hormones can cause cancer. For example, excess levels of estrogen and some estrogen-related compounds have been associated with breast, uterine, ovarian, and prostate cancers. Calcium d-glucarate has been shown to inhibit the incidence of breast tumors in animals. In one study, supplementing 2 percent of the animals' diets with d-glucarate produced dramatic results, among them:

- A 50-percent inhibition of beta glucoronidase. This is an enzyme that, by reversing the beneficial breakdown of hormones, allows risky amounts of hormones to build up in the body.

- A 23-percent reduction in the levels of estradiol. Estradiol is one of the estrogens known to promote breast and uterine cancers, so the reduction of estradiol is the equivalent of a reduced risk of cancer. (It also reduces the levels of toxic estrogen metabolites.)

- A fourfold reduction in the numbers of tumors.

## GETTING BALANCE BACK

It's quite common for people to suffer from hormone imbalances, so all of us can benefit from eating foods that contain d-glucarate as well as taking the supplemental form. I particularly recommend supplements for women who have a family history of breast cancer. Women who have had breast cancer, or are currently being treated, can also use this supplement, because it may help correct the underlying hormonal imbalance that is likely one of the root causes of the cancer. I also recommend it for women who are using birth control pills. I commonly use it in combination with the phytonutrient indole 3 carbinol.

Women and men on hormone-replacement programs would do well to take d-glucarate on a preventative basis to prevent the toxic buildup of these hormones. Men with an enlarged prostate or with those trying to prevent or treat prostate cancer should be on this supplement. We now know that testosterone and estrogen imbalances are implicated in this hormone-sensitive gland.

In addition to its cancer-preventive properties, d-glucarate is generally effective in detoxification—that is, removing many different harmful compounds from the body. It makes a lot of sense for those on any type of detoxification program to get this nutrient into their body at therapeutic levels.

## DOSAGE

Toxicity studies have shown d-glucarate to be very safe. I generally recommend patients take 400 milligrams daily as a preventative dosage and up to 2,000 milligrams if they're on a detoxification program. Studies as high as 10,000 milligrams a day have been done with calcium d-glucarate with no side effects reported.

I usually recommend the capsule, which is most readily available and is convenient to use. But you can also get d-glucarate in tablets and in powdered drinks.

The supplement does not require a prescription. You can purchase it at health food stores, pharmacies, and some grocery stores.

# DHEA

My suspicions were confirmed by the test.

Bob, a 51-year-old businessperson, had come to me complaining of a profound feeling of burnout. As a result, I'd sent out for a saliva DHEA hormone test. It showed that his DHEA levels were very low for his age.

"You have the DHEA levels of a 70-year-old," I told him. "That helps to explain why you feel burned out. It also helps to explain why your libido is so low."

"What can we do to get it back to normal?" Bob asked.

"Anything you can do to cut down on stress will help," I answered. "The way you perceive stress is important, too."

We discussed some of the approaches he could take to help alter his approach to stressful situations and control his response. Then we moved on to the subject of nutrition and herbal supplements.

"I want you to start taking fifty milligrams of DHEA daily," I said. "Your levels are so low that you need the supplementation."

Bob felt a surge in his energy levels over the next two months. Also, he reported that his wife was pleasantly surprised to find his sex drive had been renewed.

He was also surprised that a single supplement could make such a difference. Though he had been to several physicians before seeing me, he said that I was the first to request the DHEA hormone test that showed what the problem was.

# FROM THE ADRENALS

Dehydroepiandrosterone (DHEA) is a steroid hormone that is mainly secreted by the adrenal glands, which are located on top of both kidneys. It was first identified in 1934 and since then over 5,000 research studies have been completed on it.

In the past decade, some enthusiastic researchers have referred to it as a "fountain of youth" and an "anti-aging" hormone. That's based upon the way DHEA levels decline as we age. They tend to peak in people when they reach the age of 30. After that, there's a general decline until, by age 70, DHEA levels are about 20 percent of those of a young adult. Since it seems to be associated with youthful energy, appearance, and immunity, DHEA has many applications.

DHEA is the most abundant steroid hormone in the body. It serves as a precursor to other hormones such as testosterone, androstenedione, and estrogen. It also has many direct effects on the body. For example, population studies show that higher DHEA levels are associated with the prevention of heart disease and cancer. It has a profound benefit to the immune system and is thought to be an important factor in autoimmune conditions.

DHEA is found in very high concentrations in the brain and is thought to play an important role in memory and cognitive function. Depression may be related to low levels of DHEA. Doctors are increasingly recommending hormones like DHEA for the treatment of chronic inflammatory conditions such as arthritis.

**121**

Hormone specialists also recommend it as part of a comprehensive treatment for osteoporosis. It may also benefit women suffering from menopausal hot flashes.

DHEA supplementation appears to protect against bone loss (osteopenia). It also improves cognitive function in people who are taking prednisone, the hormone that's most often prescribed by medical doctors to help prevent bone loss.

## DOSAGE

The dosage for DHEA should be determined by a doctor well-versed in natural hormone replacement. Although blood tests for DHEA can be done, I have my adult patients undergo a salivary hormone test instead, because I have found that measurement of blood levels is usually not so accurate.

The starting dose I recommend is based on the levels determined by the saliva test. For many of my patients who have low levels of DHEA, I recommend a starting dose of 20 to 50 milligrams of DHEA daily. I then monitor their levels and observe their subjective symptoms to find the right dosage for them.

People with conditions such as lupus may require 200 milligrams or more daily. I do not recommend that people routinely take a DHEA supplement without knowing what their levels are. DHEA is often used in conjunction with its precursor, a hormone known as pregnenelone.

DHEA is available over the counter in capsule form. It is also commonly used by doctors in the sublingual, microionized capsule, and transdermal forms.

## WHAT ARE THE SIDE EFFECTS?

Even though DHEA is available over the counter, this hormone—as with any hormone—should be used with caution. One of the first side effects that typically occurs is an acne breakout, especially on the back.

Too high a dosage of DHEA can cause masculine effects in women, such as facial hair growth. This is reversible when the dose is lowered.

The long-term effects of DHEA supplementation are unknown at this time. It is unclear whether it will cause problems for people who have hormone-dependent cancers such as breast and prostate cancers. Until we know the possible side effects for people with those conditions, I would not advise taking DHEA.

Women who are pregnant or breast-feeding should not take DHEA unless instructed to do so by a physician under special circumstances.

# DHEA
## Recommendations from the Natural Physician for . . .

### ❧ Allergies

Some people with chronic allergies, especially multiple chemical sensitivity, notice reversal of their condition after taking a DHEA supplement.

### ❧ Cancer

Preliminary research has shown that DHEA may be protective against cancers such as breast cancer, but more research is needed. However, DHEA appears to be important for a healthy functioning immune system.

### ❧ Circulatory Health and Heart Disease

DHEA may have a protective effect against heart disease. The Massachusetts Male Aging Study looked at the relationship between heart disease and levels of DHEA. The study included men between the ages of 40 and 70. There was an inverse relationship found between the levels of DHEA and heart disease.

### ❧ Chronic Fatigue Syndrome

I have had some patients with chronic fatigue syndrome respond quite dramatically to DHEA supplementation. In all cases the patients had tested low in DHEA before therapy was started.

### ❧ Dementia

Stress hormones such as cortisol and DHEA appear to play a role in dementia and diseases such as Alzheimer's. More research needs to be done in this area but DHEA appears to have a beneficial effect on aging brain function.

### ❧ Diabetes

DHEA may be a key supplement for those with diabetes. Benefits have been shown in animal studies. Many holistic doctors report benefits with patients who have diabetes. It helps to prevent infections, build immunity, and improve wound healing.

### ❧ HIV

A longitudinal study showed a relationship between low serum DHEA levels in HIV-infected men and a more rapid progression to AIDS. Since there is currently no cure for HIV, we must use all possible means to help people with this condition, including hormones such as DHEA.

### ❧ Impotence

I have found DHEA to be helpful for some men with impotence, which may be because DHEA is converted to testosterone. Researchers from the University of Vienna who tracked the results of DHEA replacement therapy in a group of 40 men found that the hormone was helpful for impotence (erectile dysfunction). The men—who were all between the ages of 41 and 69—were given DHEA supplements or inactive placebos over a 24-week period.

All of the men in the study had been experiencing early loss of erection, which made them unable to complete intercourse. The study showed that the men who took DHEA—as opposed to the placebo—had improved sexual response in a number of areas. They reported improved erectile function, orgasmic function, sexual desire, intercourse satisfaction, and overall satisfaction.

*(continued)*

### ❧ Inflammatory Bowel Disease (IBD)

Researchers evaluated DHEA and cortisol levels in patients with ulcerative colitis and Crohn's disease. DHEA was found to be much lower in IBD patients than in a group of healthy people.

Although treatment with a corticosteroid such as prednisone can inhibit adrenal hormone production, these DHEA deficiencies were found even in patients who had not been subjected to previous treatment with corticosteroids. Researchers also found that as DHEA-S levels rose and cortisol levels dropped, the patients who were being monitored showed fewer signs of inflammation.

### ❧ Lupus

I have found DHEA supplementation to be helpful for some female patients who have lupus. Many other doctors of natural medicine report similar experiences. I find it to be a good alternative to prednisone therapy, especially when combined with other naturopathic therapies such as homeopathy and nutrition.

In one study, some women with systemic lupus erythematosus were given 200 milligrams of DHEA daily, and others were given a placebo. Those given DHEA had better improvement as rated by the patients and physicians, while there were more flare-ups of the disease in the group that was given the placebo. Those taking DHEA were also able to reduce their dosage of prednisone while those taking the placebo had to slightly increase their dosage.

### ❧ Menopause

DHEA decreases (as do estrogen, progesterone, and testosterone) in women going through menopause. DHEA can be helpful in increasing libido, reducing hot flashes, and protecting against bone loss. In rare cases it may help relieve vaginal dryness and thinning of vaginal tissue.

### ❧ Osteoporosis

DHEA should be considered as part of an aggressive treatment protocol for those who have osteoporosis, as it appears to prevent bone loss.

### ❧ Prednisone Tapering

DHEA is an excellent hormone to use to help people lower their dosage or discontinue using the drug prednisone. Long-term prednisone use can damage the immune system, liver, kidneys, and cause osteoporosis. Making the transition from prednisone to DHEA must be done under the guidance of a knowledgeable physician.

# E

# Echinacea

It's not unusual to get calls at my office from patients wondering what to do about the cold or flu that just hit them. My first thought is: What natural supplements can they get quickly, right off the shelf?

Well, just about anyone can find echinacea (pronounced eck-in-ay'-sha) at a nearby store. It's one of the five top-selling herbs in North America. In fact, it's a worldwide best-seller, as herbalists and doctors in Europe have been prescribing echinacea for decades. Carrying the popular name of purple coneflower (so-called because of its beautiful, purple, daisy-like petals), echinacea is renowned as an herb that enhances the immune system. It's commonly used to treat a number of conditions from flu and the common cold to a range of other infectious diseases.

## THE SNAKEBITE CONNECTION

Native Americans of the Plains are believed to be the first to use echinacea. As today, it was a remedy for colds, coughs, and sore throats, but also toothaches, battle wounds, and even rattlesnake bites.

During the latter part of the 1800s, Plains settlers adopted the purple coneflower as a common remedy; and by the 1920s, echinacea was being sold as a commercial product and prescribed by the many physicians who were comfortable with herbal medicines.

Dr. H.C.F. Meyer of Pawnee, Nebraska was a keen commercial promoter. Adding his own recommendations to what he had learned from Native Americans,

Dr. Meyer sold echinacea as a "cure all" for various ailments. His reputation was considerably enhanced by the claim that he had successfully treated 613 cases of rattlesnake poisoning. One doctor gave the following candid account of Dr. Meyer's own, personal echinacea experiment:

"With the courage of his convictions upon him, he injected the venom of the crotalus (rattlesnake) into the first finger of his left hand; the swelling was rapid and in six hours up to the elbow. At this time he took a dose of the remedy, bathed the part thoroughly, and laid down to pleasant dreams. On awakening in four hours, the pain and swelling were gone."

## INFECTION FIGHTER TO THE RESCUE

I can't say I have had any patients come to me for the natural treatment of rattlesnake bites. (If I did, I would quickly hurry them off to a hospital emergency room for a dose of up-to-date antivenom.) But it's interesting to note that echinacea does have the special property of preventing the spread of infectious substances to tissues.

Echinacea as a healing remedy was introduced to Europe during the 1930s. Since then the preponderance of scientific research on echinacea has been done in Western Europe, especially Germany, where the government plays an active role in funding natural medicine research. But Canadian and American researchers have recently made similar strides in echinacea research, with clinical studies and bio-chemical analysis of the healing herb.

Over 400 studies to date have looked at the pharmacology and clinical uses of echinacea. Not all studies have shown efficacy of the herb, but most of the research indicates that echinacea helps reinforce the immune system.

Echinacea is consistently one of the best-selling herbs in North America and Europe. Over 10 million units are sold annually in Germany alone.

Though there are nine species of echinacea, *Echinacea purpurea* and *Echinacea angustifolia* are the two most often used commercially. Most clinical studies are done with these species, especially *purpurea*.

## TONGUE-TINGLING CHEMICALS

Scientists have not reached a consensus about the active ingredients in echinacea. Though researchers acknowledge the herb has many immune-boosting properties as well as antiinflammatory and antimicrobial effects, they're not sure what chemicals or combination of chemicals are responsible.

It's known, however, that echinacea contains caffeic acid derivatives such as cichoric acid and polysaccharides. The plant also has compounds known as alkylamides that are thought to be important. (Alkylamides are the substances that make your tongue tingle and go numb if you take a hefty dose of straight echinacea.)

Some of these compounds are water-soluble and some are alcohol-soluble. When tinctures, pills, or tablets are being created from echinacea, the manufacturer must go through an elaborate process to extract the compounds. Recent research done at the University of British Columbia in conjunction with the University of Alberta has shown that the ratio of the actives in echinacea is important for optimal immune response. So in other words, not only is it important to have active constituents in echinacea products, but to also have them in a specific ratio or blend.

## A Boon in Pregnancy

Pregnant women have to be careful about anything they eat, which includes supplements, so I'm often asked whether echinacea is safe to use during pregnancy. My answer is yes. Echinacea has a long history of use by herbalists and naturopathic doctors for the treatment of acute infections during pregnancy. If a pregnant woman has a cold, flu, or urinary tract infection, I would not hesitate to recommend echinacea. Side effects or problems with the pregnancy or health of the baby have not been reported. In fact, my wife used echinacea during her entire first pregnancy with no adverse effects.

A study by the Hospital for Sick Children in Toronto, in conjunction with the Canadian Naturopathic College, has confirmed the safety of echinacea use during pregnancy. A group of 206 women who used echinacea during pregnancy for upper respiratory tract infections were analyzed along with a control group of 198 pregnant women who had upper respiratory tract infections but never used echinacea. The researchers found no association with the use of echinacea and birth defects. There were also no differences in the rate of live births or spontaneous abortions between the two groups.

## AROUSING IMMUNE CELLS

Echinacea doesn't work like the pharmaceutical antibiotics that "kill" microbes like bacteria. Instead, echinacea arouses the immune cells that patrol and defend the body against these invaders. It increases the number and activity of disease-fighting white blood cells, and it activates antiviral chemicals such as interferon. Echinacea can even activate the immune cells that fight tumors. In addition, research has shown that the chemicals in echinacea have the power to inhibit an enzyme released by bacteria, called hyaluronidase. Bacteria normally produce this enzyme to penetrate into human tissue. Echinacea prevents this from happening.

Researchers in a German study found clear evidence that echinacea helps to promote good immune cells, called phagocytes. One group of people were given 30 drops of echinacea three times daily for five days, while people in the control group were given a placebo. The level of phagocytes was measured at the beginning and throughout the study. At day three, the phagocyte activity of those taking echinacea increased by 40 percent. By the fifth day, phagocyte activity had increased 120 percent. When people stopped taking echinacea, immune-cell activity dropped off sharply. After three days, there was no difference in immune-cell activity between the group taking echinacea and the control group.

Leading researchers now feel that echinacea may actually be more of an immune-modulating herb, meaning it has a balancing effect on the immune system. As research continues, this may mean that echinacea may be more valuable than just boosting immune function.

## VIRUS SLAYERS

While there are a host of modern antibiotics for killing bacteria, modern medicine has a limited arsenal of weapons to defeat viral infections. This presents a problem for the many doctors who rely on conventional pharmaceuticals in their medical practice. Over 65 million people in the U.S. each year "catch" the common cold, while another 108 million get the flu—and these are just two of the infectious diseases caused by viruses. Others include genital herpes, which affects an estimated 45 million people, as well as hepatitis C, which afflicts 170 million people in the world. Even a simple viral infection like a viral sore throat poses a challenge for any doctor who relies exclusively on antibiotics and other conventional prescription medications.

Echinacea, like some other immune-enhancing herbs, has a direct antiviral effect. Even better, it seems to summon all the resources of the immune system to help destroy viral invaders.

It also works well in combination with other antiviral plants and herbs. I like to prescribe echinacea in a formula called the "virus cocktail," which is comprised of echinacea, lomatium, astragalus, reishi, and licorice root. The synergistic blend of these herbs tends to be more effective than any one herb by itself.

## BACTERIA AND FUNGUS

Since echinacea enhances the action of your immune cells, it is also effective against bacterial, fungal, and yeast infections. This is especially helpful if you're fighting a bacterial infection, because many bacteria are now resistant to antibiotics (because they're overprescribed by doctors for things like viral infections). If needed, there is no problem using echinacea in combination with antibiotics. As a matter of fact, I find when people are on antibiotics for a bacterial infection and use echinacea simultaneously, they recover more quickly.

### Benefits for Athletes

Sports medicine specialists studied the effect of echinacea on men who participated in triathlons—those grueling events that involve long-distance swimming, running, and cycling. It is well known that triathletes are at an increased risk for infection because they train so exhaustively for each event. Among the participants of the study, some took a placebo, others were given a mineral supplement (43 milligrams of magnesium), while a third group took 8 milliliters of *Echinacea purpurea* daily. All three groups of athletes took the supplements for 28 days before a triathlon.

During training, one-quarter to one-third of the athletes taking a placebo or mineral supplement ended up getting colds. (Those taking magnesium missed 13 days of training, while those in the placebo group missed a total of 24 days.) None of those who were taking echinacea showed any cold symptoms, and none missed any training days.

At least one study—which included 4,190 patients—confirmed this observation. Researchers divided the patients into two groups and gave about half of them an antibacterial formula that included echinacea (along with two other herbs—thuja and baptisia). Along with that formula, the patients received antibiotics that were chosen by the doctors. For comparison, the rest of the patients received only antibiotics, with no herbal formula.

The results showed the effectiveness of taking herbal antibacterial agents along with antibiotics. In the group that got an echinacea-based formula plus an antibiotic, people were cured significantly faster and there was a lower incidence of recurring infection than in the group of people who just got an antibiotic. Also, the symptoms of "sore throat" and "difficulty in swallowing" were improved much more efficiently in the first group than in the second group.

# DOSAGE

Echinacea is generally available as a tincture, capsule, tablet, or cream in the U.S. It's also possible to take it in the form of an injection, though this method is mainly used in Germany.

Glycerine (alcohol-free) tinctures are available. These are good for kids, who especially enjoy the berry-flavored varieties.

### ❧ Tincture

I recommend 20 to 60 drops of the tincture every two to three hours for acute infections or twice daily for long-term use.

### ❧ Capsule

I recommend 500 to 1,000 milligrams every two to three hours for acute infections or twice daily for long-term use.

**Note:** High-potency, quality echinacea products are standardized to contain active ingredients such as alkylamides, cichoric acid, and polysaccharides.

Some controversy surrounds the length of time one can use echinacea. Many authors state that echinacea should not be used on a long-term basis. However, there are no studies showing that long-term use is harmful or that echinacea loses its effectiveness.

I generally recommend patients use echinacea for acute infections until they are completely over the illness. For those who are very susceptible to infections, especially during the winter, and do not want to change their lifestyle, echinacea can be used on a long-term basis (although it is not so effective as improving diet, reducing stress, and exercising). Long-term use of echinacea throughout the winter season is common in European countries.

# WHAT ARE THE SIDE EFFECTS?

There has been no reported toxicity with echinacea, but two patients of mine have had allergic reactions, with some throat swelling after they started taking echinacea. Such a reaction has the potential of being life threatening. In both cases, I recommended that my patients avoid using echinacea and switch to other immune-enhancing herbs instead.

There have been some concerns about echinacea affecting fertility. An animal study that appeared in 1999 suggested that echinacea might adversely affect fertility—but, in my view, the research was seriously flawed. Researchers directly exposed hamster eggs to echinacea extract and concluded that at high concentrations echinacea impaired or prevented the sperms' ability to penetrate the eggs.

The flaw of the study is that echinacea is broken down in the digestive system to various components, each of which is highly diluted. Putting echinacea directly on sperm or hamster eggs does not replicate what happens in real life. Perhaps there will be further studies that give us a better idea of echinacea's effects on fertility, but this one isn't worth taking seriously.

# ECHINACEA
## RECOMMENDATIONS FROM THE NATURAL PHYSICIAN FOR . . .

### ∾ Autoimmune Conditions

There's some controversy about prescribing echinacea to patients who have autoimmune diseases—that is, conditions that become worse when the immune system is overactive. The German Commission E, the government-backed medical board in Germany that helps regulate herbal medicine, recommends that echinacea should not be used in those who have tuberculosis, leukosis, collagenosis, multiple sclerosis, AIDS and HIV, lupus, rheumatoid arthritis, and other autoimmune conditions. The assumption is that echinacea will worsen the hypersensitivity of the immune system, causing a flare-up of problems.

While I often agree with many of the Commission E recommendations, many physicians point out that there have not been any studies showing that echinacea is harmful for autoimmune conditions. I have not seen or read any reports where a patient with one of these conditions was made worse from using echinacea, despite the fact that millions of people take it every year.

That said, echinacea would not be my first choice for a condition like multiple sclerosis, rheumatoid arthritis, or other autoimmune diseases. But when my patients with these conditions have an acute infection, such as a cold or urinary tract infection, I do recommend echinacea and other immune-enhancing herbs to fight off the infection. Usually these herbs are helpful; in any case, they don't seem to aggravate the autoimmune disease.

Interestingly, German physicians commonly use echinacea as a topical cream to relieve rheumatoid arthritis symptoms. These same doctors also frequently recommend echinacea be taken internally for its natural antiinflammatory effects. Furthermore, newer research is showing that many autoimmune conditions are due to the immune system reacting to infectious agents, and cross reacting with the body's own tissue at the same time. In theory, this would make echinacea helpful for these conditions. More studies are needed to tell us exactly what effect—both good or bad—echinacea has

*(continued)*

for people with inflammatory or autoimmune conditions.

## ∾ Common Cold

I have found that echinacea can help prevent the common cold as well as reduce the symptoms and shorten the duration—but results differ. Some people respond almost miraculously, while others get no benefits at all. Overall, though, echinacea is more effective than over-the-counter medicines, which only help to reduce some of the symptoms of a cold and do nothing to assist the immune system or battle the infection.

One clinical study looked at the effectiveness of *Echinacea purpurea* for 120 patients who had the initial symptoms of the common cold, with "acute, uncomplicated upper airways infection." When these patients took 20 drops of echinacea every two hours for the first day—and thereafter three times daily—they fared much better than another group that took a placebo. At the end of the 10-day study, patients were questioned about the intensity of their illness and the time it took them to improve. The time to improvement was significantly shorter. In the echinacea group, people averaged four days to recover, while those in the placebo group took an average of eight days to recover.

## ∾ Flu

Yes, there are a few antiviral drugs that can help treat the flu. However, the clinical data on these drugs does not impress me very much. The most commonly prescribed drug, amantadine, isn't at all effective in the first two or three days. This is a real drawback because most people experience their worst symptoms during the first 72 hours of a flu attack.

Fortunately, my clinical experience has shown that herbs like echinacea can often help with symptoms the first 24 hours. This is sup-

ported by research—but the research also suggests that the size of the dose is an important factor. In a study of 180 men and women between the ages of 18 and 60, researchers compared three different groups. The first group took a placebo. The second got 90 drops of *Echinacea purpurea* every day, which is the equivalent of a 450-milligram dose, while the third group received double that, or 900 milligrams daily. Symptoms of all participants were evaluated after three to four days and again after eight to ten days. The results showed that 90 drops of tincture had little effect, but the people who took 180 drops were significantly better off, with less-severe symptoms that lasted for a shorter time.

## ∾ Skin Conditions

In North America, echinacea has not quite caught on as a topical treatment for skin conditions. But many European makers of skin products are including the herbal ingredient.

A review of 4,958 clinical cases focused on the effectiveness of echinacea ointment. The main researcher in the study concluded that the ointment was highly effective for many skin conditions. These included 1,453 patients with wounds, 900 with varicose ulcers, 629 with eczema, 26 with burns, 222 with herpes simplex, and 212 with inflammatory skin problems. More than 90 percent positive results occurred when the ointment was used to treat burns, wounds, and herpes.

## ∾ Vaginitis

Reoccurring vaginal yeast infections can be quite troublesome for women. One German study looked at 203 women with this condition. Of the 60 women taking echinacea (while the rest took a placebo or other medicines), only 10 had recurrences of yeast infections.

# Enzymes

. . . . . . . . . . . . . . . . . . . . . . . . . . . . . . . . . . . . . . . . . . . . . . . . . . . . . . . . . . .

"I travel a lot on business," said Jeremy, a 35 year old in the software business. "I wish I could eat good food all the time—but it's just impossible."

Dependent on restaurant food, often obliged to eat with customers, at the mercy of in-flight meals, Jeremy was having increasing problems with his colitis.

"I know what will help a lot," I replied. "Enzymes!"

When taken with meals, enzymes help with digestion. I recommended that Jeremy always have a bottle with him wherever he traveled, just to prevent flare-ups.

In addition, I recommended a number of other herbs to take in combination with the enzymes. Last of all, "I still want you to follow the diet recommendations we talked about."

From that point on, Jeremy started taking the enzymes with every meal, whether or not he was in-flight, on the road, or eating hotel food. Not only would these enzymes help to repair his digestive tract, they would also help increase the supply of enzymes produced by his own body.

Enzymes are protein molecules found in every cell in humans, animals, and plants. As you read this sentence, millions of enzymatic reactions are occurring, regulating all the chemical reactions that occur in your body.

Enzymes perform many life-sustaining functions. Some, known as digestive enzymes, help break down food so the nutrients can be absorbed from the digestive tract into the bloodstream. Others, called metabolic enzymes, are involved in energy production, detoxification, immunity, and many other important activities.

All the vitamins and minerals found in food, or taken as supplements, require the action of enzymes to make them active. Those nutrients also boost enzyme activity, since these molecules require what are called cofactors—magnesium and other minerals—to help them function. In addition, coenzymes such as B vitamins or coenzyme Q10 are needed to activate the enzyme. Working together, the enzymes, cofactors, and coenzymes sustain the energy creation that sustains every one of our living cells.

There is no doubt that a healthy body requires a rich supply of enzymes. Though many supplement programs focus on our vitamin and mineral requirements, we may see more interest in enzyme therapies in the future. An increasing number of nutrition-oriented doctors are beginning to make enzymes a central focus of healing therapies.

## BEST SOURCES

There are several ways our bodies get life-sustaining enzymes. Some are manufactured by our body organs. Our saliva glands, stomach, and liver all produce enzymes—and the pancreas is the major factory.

Raw foods are another important source because plants produce enzymes to sustain their own metabolic activities. Raw fruits and vegetables provide many of the nutrients we need to help replace our enzymes, but they do have to be raw. You don't get the same boost from these foods when they're cooked, because the enzymes in food are destroyed when temperatures hit 140 degrees Fahrenheit.

Besides getting enzymes from raw fruits, vegetables, herbs, and seeds, you can also get a good supply from juices. It's best to drink juice that's as freshly made as possible if you want to get the highest amount of vitamins, minerals, phytonutrients, and enzymes from that source.

Other food sources of enzymes include fermented foods such as yogurt, kefir, sauerkraut, miso, tempeh, and natto (fermented, cooked soybeans). You can also get good, healthy doses from wheatgrass, alfalfa, algae (chlorella, spirulina), and raw honey.

You can also take supplements for a boost. The three main forms of supplements provide plant, microbial, and animal enzymes. Research has shown that the body uses these enzymes for different activities such as digestion and other metabolic functions. Another category of supplements—whole-food supplements—may contain some live enzymes, though not in such high concentrations as enzyme supplements.

## THE DEPLETION EFFECTS

Enzyme deficiency may be a major factor in chronic disease. Since our cells can't possibly function without enzymes, it's reasonable to conclude that any deficiency could contribute to health problems. So if you're not getting enough enzymes from your diet—particularly if you don't eat enough raw fruit and vegetables—it's reasonable to make sure you take supplements.

Studies have shown that the average American eats approximately two servings of fruits and vegetables daily. This is a far cry from the government-recommended five to seven servings or the seven to ten servings advocated by most nutritional experts. Even when we do eat these foods, we're usually getting them after they've been cooked, when the enzymes have been destroyed by frying, boiling, steaming, baking, or microwaving.

Enzymes are also destroyed by pesticides, herbicides, food preservatives, additives, colorings, and flavor enhancers. They're also depleted by other substances, such as smoke and other air pollutants, excessive sun (UV rays), and medications. Illness also depletes enzymes; in addition, they can be diminished by the free radicals produced during normal cell activity or by the physical demands of increased activity.

Enzymes are critical to good digestion, so you may need to get additional enzymes to improve digestion. While your body produces many different enzymes to assist in the assimilation of food (see Table 3), you might need to take enzyme supplements to help these internally-created enzymes break down food more efficiently. This can be very helpful for people with digestive conditions such as IBS, Crohn's disease, or other inflammatory bowel disorders.

Also, people with food sensitivities and general digestive weakness (gas, bloating, diarrhea) can benefit from enzyme supplementation. Keep in mind that a lot of chronic illnesses are caused at least in part by the malabsorption of food and nutrients, which creates toxic byproducts that get into the bloodstream. Therefore, supplements such as enzymes can indirectly help conditions such as arthritis, cancer, fatigue, and allergies.

# TYPES OF SUPPLEMENTAL ENZYMES

As mentioned, there are three main types of enzymes that you can purchase commercially.

### ᴄᴡ *Plant Enzymes*

The two best examples are bromelain from pineapple and papain from papaya. Both of these supplements can be taken with meals to help with the digestion of protein. If you take either of them—especially bromelain—on an empty stomach, they help to prevent inflammation. These enzymes assist with the breakdown of protein, but not other foodstuffs such as carbohydrates and fats.

## TABLE 3
## WHERE FROM AND WHAT FOR?

Enzymes are produced in many different parts of the digestive system, and they perform a wide variety of functions in the breakdown of food. Here's an overview of some of the most important and what they do.

| Enzyme(s)/Source of Production | Location of Activity/Action |
| --- | --- |
| Amylase (ptyalin)/Saliva glands | Mouth/Breaks down carbohydrates |
| Gastric lipase/Stomach | Stomach/Breaks down fats |
| Renin/Stomach | Stomach/Breaks down milk protein |
| Pepsin/Stomach | Stomach/Breaks down protein |
| Proteolytic/Pancreas | Small intestine/Breaks down protein |
| Amylolytic/Pancreas | Small intestine/Breaks down carbohydrates |
| Lipolytic/Pancreas | Small intestine/Breaks down fats |
| Peptidases/Small intestine | Small intestine/Breaks down protein |
| Amylolytic/Small intestine | Small intestine/Breaks down sugars |
| Lipase/Small Intestine | Small intestine/Breaks down fats |

### ✑ Microbial Enzymes (Fungal Enzymes)

This group of enzymes has a much broader scope of use—especially for digestion—than the plant enzymes. All the microbial enzymes are derived from the fermentation of fungus. Though some people in the health industry commonly refer to microbial-derived fungal enzymes as plant enzymes, they actually come exclusively from fungi rather than other types of plants. The fungi are fermented in a specific way to produce a full spectrum of enzymes.

The two most common types of fungi are *Aspergillus oryzae* and *Aspergillus niger,* which are grown on a base of wheat or rice bran that's been enhanced with other substances that encourage good enzyme growth. Extracted from the fungi, the enzymes then go through a purification and separation process. They're dried, concentrated, and analyzed by a quality-control technician.

European doctors give microbial-derived enzymes by injection, using the intravenous form in the treatment of disease. I often recommend the supplement form of microbial-derived enzymes because of their potency, purity, and stability.

I've found that full-spectrum fungal enzyme formulations are extremely helpful to people who need to improve their digestion. They can also help with tissue repair from injuries.

### ❧ Animal Enzymes.

These are derived from animal organs. Typically, pancreatic enzymes are derived from pig or sheep pancreas, while bile enzymes and salts are derived from ox gallbladder. Some of these formulations seem to be unstable—which means they quickly break down (and therefore lose their effectiveness) when they're exposed to stomach acid.

To get around this problem, the extracts are made into tablets with a special coating (enteric coating) to avoid being destroyed by stomach acid. Many researchers state that even with the enteric coating, many of the enzymes are still destroyed by stomach acid.

The other concern I have with animal enzymes is the issue of purity. Seeing as the extracts are ground up pancreatic tissue, can the consumer be guaranteed that all

## A Wrap-up of Commercial Enzymes

Most of the following enzymes can be purchased individually. More commonly, they're part of multi-enzyme formulas.

- **Alpha galactosidase** The best known of these alpha glactosidase products has the brand name Beano®. The enzyme helps break down the carbohydrates that cause gas formation from eating beans. It is also found in full-spectrum microbial-derived enzymes.

- **Amylase** Breaks down carbohydrates. *Sources:* plant, microbial, animal.

- **Bromelain** Breaks down protein and has natural antiinflammatory effect. (See BROMELAIN). *Source:* plant (pineapple stem or fruit).

- **Cellulase** Breaks down fiber. *Source:* microbial.

- **Chymotripsin** Breaks down protein and reduces inflammation. *Source:* animal.

- **Invertase** Breaks down carbohydrates, especially sugar. *Source:* microbial.

- **Lactase** Breaks down milk sugar (lactose). Found in milk products (LactAid®) as well. *Source:* microbial.

- **Lipase** Breaks down fats. *Sources:* microbial, animal.

- **Maltase** Breaks down carbohydrates, specifically maltose. *Source:* microbial.

- **Pancreatin** Breaks down proteins, fats, and carbohydrates. *Source:* animal (derived from cow or hog pancreas).

- **Papain** Breaks down proteins and has a natural antiinflammatory action. *Source:* plant (papaya).

- **Pepsin** Breaks down protein. *Source:* animal.

- **Phytase** Breaks down phytic acid of plants. *Source:* microbial.

- **Sucrase** Breaks down the sugars sucrose and maltose. *Source:* microbial.

- **Trypsin** Breaks down protein and has natural antiinflammatory effect. *Source:* animal.

contaminants are removed, including things such as viruses? I have not seen this issue fully addressed by manufacturers. However, many people do get therapeutic benefits from pancreatic extracts—and studies show they work.

Given the choice among plant, microbial, and animal enzymes, however, I generally choose microbial- (fungal) derived enzymes.

## DOSAGE

Different measurements are used for enzymes. Microbial-derived enzymes have different units of measurement than animal- and plant-derived enzymes.

When enzymes are taken as a digestive aid, the typical dosage is one to two capsules with each meal. Some people may need to take three capsules with each meal for a better digestive effect.

The dosage for plant enzymes is the same, but you don't want to take them with meals if you're using them for their antiinflammatory effect or to heal wounds. Instead, take them between meals.

Enzymes should be kept away from heat and moisture when they're in storage. They should also not be exposed to light. Make sure the lid to the enzyme supplement container is closed tightly.

Individual enzymes can be taken between meals for specialized therapeutic effects. For example, proteolytic enzymes—such as bromelain or protease—help to reduce inflammation and heal injuries and wounds when used in higher concentrations between meals. Practitioners use lipase enzymes to help metabolize triglycerides. Follow the directions on the container.

I mainly recommend the use of microbial-derived enzymes derived from *Aspergillus oryzae*, as do many health professionals. They are a very concentrated source of enzymes and appear to be more stable than animal enzymes. If you do use animal-derived pancreatic enzymes, then make sure they are enteric coated.

## WHAT ARE THE SIDE EFFECTS?

Side effects are not common with enzymes. However, a small percentage of people get gas and bloating when they first start taking them. These initial symptoms are often the result of the digestive system "rebalancing" itself as yeast and undesirable bacteria are killed from the changes in the digestive flora. Less often, it could be a sensitivity reaction, in which case the symptoms will not go away.

Those with active ulcers or a history of ulcers should avoid the use of protein (protease) enzymes as they can further irritate an ulcerated stomach. If you suffer from ulcers and also need digestive support, you can obtain digestive enzyme formulas that are made without protein enzymes.

Persons with blood-clotting disorders, those on blood-thinning medications, and people about to undergo surgery should avoid the use of protein (protease) enzymes as they can thin the blood, especially when taken between meals. You might be able to use digestive enzyme formulas that contain proteolytic enzymes, as long as you take them with your meals—but be sure to consult with your doctor first.

If you're allergic to pork, avoid porcine- (pork) derived animal enzymes.

People always ask if they can take microbial (fungal-derived) enzymes if they have *candida* (yeast overgrowth). I have not seen a problem in these cases. The enzymes come from yeast, but in the end-product of the whole extraction process, no yeast are left in the formulation.

# ENZYMES
## RECOMMENDATIONS FROM THE NATURAL PHYSICIAN FOR . . .

### ᴧ *Arthritis*

Poor digestion is one of the major factors associated with the development of arthritis. Enzymes help to reduce the toxic load in the body and improve the absorption of nutrients. This is especially important for people who have rheumatoid arthritis. Proteolytic enzymes like bromelain help to reduce inflammation. (For more information, see Bromelain, page 73.)

### ᴧ *Autoimmune Conditions*

If you improve the absorption of foods, it means you're getting more and better nutrition, and that helps anyone who has an autoimmune condition. There's a well-established connection between poor intestinal absorption (leaky gut syndrome) and autoimmune diseases.

Inflammatory chemicals are released in the body when the immune system reacts to poorly digested proteins.

### ᴧ *Cancer*

Proteolytic enzymes are used by holistic cancer specialists to help break down cancer cells. Also, full-spectrum enzymes enhance digestion, which helps to improve the nutritional status of the body and makes for a healthier immune system.

Many cancer clinics in Europe and now the United States use enzyme therapy as a complementary therapy in the treatment of most types of cancers. Dr. Nicholas Gonzales, a medical doctor who practices in New York City, has raised quite a few eyebrows in the medical community with his successful natural treatment of cancer. The results of his clinical trial showed

*(continued)*

**139**

that a treatment protocol consisting of diet, nutritional supplements (which included mega doses of animal-derived pancreatic enzymes), and detoxification was significantly more successful than conventional therapy (chemotherapy) for inoperable pancreatic cancer. For example, his patients had an 81-percent survival rate after one year as compared with a 25-percent average survival rate for those undergoing conventional treatment for the same cancer. Currently, a large-scale study of Dr. Gonzales's enzyme treatment of advanced pancreatic cancer is about to get underway and is being funded by the National Institutes of Health's National Center for Complementary and Alternative Medicine, with collaboration from the National Cancer Institute.

### Colic

One technique that can help improve colic is to add full-spectrum microbial-derived enzymes to the baby's formula. Just by adding one enzyme you help to predigest the proteins and other foodstuffs in the formula so that they can be more easily digested. Breast-feeding mothers can take enzymes with meals so that the food they eat is broken down better—but consult with your doctor first. Taking enzymes makes it less likely that food allergens will be passed through breast milk.

### Digestive Disorders

This is a huge category of conditions that really includes pretty much every digestive disorder. Simple indigestion, flatulence, and chronic diarrhea can be helped with enzyme supplementation.

Those with Crohn's disease, irritable bowel syndrome, and ulcerative colitis should definitely consider supplementing with enzymes to help get their condition under control. Enzymes are helpful to prevent indigestion when eating a large meal or food that is hard to digest. (My occasional pizza binges are accompanied with enzymes.)

### Food Sensitivities

Supplements that improve digestion can help improve or eradicate food sensitivities. While avoiding the foods that may be causing a food-sensitivity reaction, you can also help the condition by taking enzymes.

### Injuries

Proteolytic enzymes have long been used for the treatment of injuries, particularly athletic injuries. They help decrease inflammation and swelling, and stimulate immune activity in the repair of the injury. Bromelain is the most well-known proteolytic enzyme for these kinds of treatments. Microbial-derived protease is also effective.

### Skin Rashes

Chronic skin rashes can be the result of poor intestinal health. The irritation from toxic metabolites of poor digestion can cause inflammation of the skin. Along with dietary improvement, enzymes help to decrease this toxic load and, over time, can improve various skin conditions.

### Viral Infections

A number of people have told me that they took proteolytic enzymes (microbial-derived) on an empty stomach to help fight viral infections such as the common cold and flu. Advocates of this type of therapy say that the enzymes help to break down the protein coat (capsid) that surrounds the virus. Though I'm not aware of any studies that validate this use, many popular European pharmaceutical products include a combination of proteolytic enzymes and "cold drugs" together in a formula.

# Evening Primrose Oil

Few supplements are as confusing to people as the essential fatty acids (EFAs)—probably because "fatty" has such a sinister connotation. But the "essential fatty acids" are not at all synonymous with weight gain or poor health or any of the other things that "fatty" seems to imply. Rather, they're essential to life itself.

The human body doesn't "manufacture" EFAs, so we either have to attain them from our diet or through supplementation. They're what we need to help build the basic structure of our cells and also to help those cells function as they should. They're also the essence of what's good about evening primrose oil (*Oenothera biennis*).

Evening primrose oil—commonly referred to as EPO—is an essential fatty acid supplement comprised of oil that's extracted from the seeds of evening primrose. For a number of years, an increasing number of holistic doctors have been recommending it for treatment of women who have PMS symptoms and cyclical breast pain. It's also recommended for eczema, diabetic neuropathy (the nerve damage experienced by some people who have diabetes), and arthritis pain.

Evening primrose oil is high in the group of essential fatty acids known as omega-6. It's not hard to get omega-6 fatty acids from other food sources, because it's in red meat and most vegetable oils such as safflower and sunflower. But evening primrose oil does have one other very special constituent, which is the main reason why so many people can benefit from it. This constituent is known as gamma linolenic acid (GLA). In fact, evening primrose seeds yield between 7 and 10 percent GLA. (Other plant sources of GLA include borage and black currant seed.)

GLA is an essential fatty acid that is required for proper brain development and function. Infants receive GLA from breast milk. As GLA is metabolized in the body, it's transformed into other chemical substances (metabolites) that help control inflammation, prevent blood clots, reduce some kinds of muscle cramping, and balance hormones. Some people actually need a direct source of GLA to help prevent nerve damage from diabetes or conditions such as eczema. Therefore, they benefit from a direct source like EPO.

# DOSAGE

The amount of evening primrose oil that should be used depends on your weight and, of course, the condition you're treating. The most important aspect of evening primrose is the amount of GLA that is contained in each dose. Evening primrose oil capsules usually come in 500-milligram sizes—and from that, you should be getting about 50 milligrams of GLA.

There's also an oil form, which is usually more cost effective. Adults with specific conditions such as eczema and PMS can benefit from 150 to 400 milligrams of GLA daily, which means taking between 1,500 and 3,000 milligrams of evening primrose oil. (For some diseases, such as neuropathy, higher doses are needed.)

The optimum doses for children are between 50 and 200 milligrams of GLA, or 500 to 2,000 milligrams of evening primrose oil capsules.

For those taking evening primrose oil on a preventative basis, I recommend 500 to 1,500 milligrams daily in combination with an omega-3 oil such as flaxseed, hemp, or fish oil. Most people are deficient in omega-3 fatty acids, so it is important to take evening primrose with omega-3 fatty acid-rich foods or supplements.

As with other fats, evening primrose is best taken with meals. It is wise to make sure you are taking some extra vitamin E each day (400 IU), because it helps maximize the benefits of the fatty acids. In fact, many of the oil blends contain vitamin E, which helps prevent the oils from becoming rancid.

I also recommend taking a multivitamin if you're taking evening primrose oil. You need a variety of different vitamins and minerals for essential fatty acid metabolism. Vitamin C, vitamin $B_6$, magnesium, zinc, and biotin are among the important nutrients needed for optimum metabolism.

# WHAT ARE THE SIDE EFFECTS?

A few people experience digestive upset and headaches when they take evening primrose oil, especially if they don't take it with meals. These side effects usually go away when the dosage is reduced. (Before reducing the dosage, however, try taking evening primrose oil with meals.)

My biggest concern with EPO is that it needs to be balanced with dosages of omega-3 fatty acids. Long-term solo use of EPO, without simultaneous doses of omega-3's, may set the stage for disease or worsen existing conditions. I have patients come into my office saying that they have been taking evening primrose oil because they heard or read that it is good for their nails, hair, menopause symptoms, and many other things. In some cases it has worsened their problem because they were not simultaneously taking omega-3's and creating an essential fatty acid imbalance.

Natural physicians are particularly concerned that people may worsen existing diseases like heart disease, arthritis, and cancer with unbalanced EPO supplementation. Using evening primrose oil in the short term (a few months) is unlikely to cause any kind of harm—but, still, I always recommend taking EPO in a blend with omega-3 fatty acids such as fish oil, flax oil, or hemp oil.

# PRIMROSE OIL
## RECOMMENDATIONS FROM THE NATURAL PHYSICIAN FOR . . .

### ❧ Arthritis

For most people who have rheumatoid arthritis, I've seen best results from oil blends that contain omega-3 fatty acids and some GLA. Flaxseed or fish oil supplementation seems to do the most good.

### ❧ Attention Deficit Disorder (ADD) and Attention Deficient Hyperactivity Disorder (ADHD)

I usually recommend the fatty acid DHA for children who have attention deficit problems. However, some children need extra amounts of GLA to help this condition—and for them, I'll specify an oil blend containing DHA and GLA. Fortunately, we now have blood tests that can measure the levels and ratios of the essential fatty acids, and based on these, we can develop specific fatty-acid formulas that are best for each individual.

### ❧ Diabetes

Neuropathy is a common complication that affects 30 percent of people with diabetes. Often the first signs of this condition are "pins and nee-

dles" feelings in the feet and hands. In several studies it has been shown that nutritional therapies are beneficial, especially evening primrose oil. People with diabetes often have problems converting linoleic acid into GLA, and a deficiency of GLA leads to circulation problems, so insufficient oxygen reaches the nerves. Evening primrose can be a big help because it's a direct source of GLA.

Researchers in one study looked at the effects of GLA on 84 people who had Type 2 (adult-onset) diabetes. All participants had neuropathy symptoms such as tingling, burning, weakness, and impaired reflexes. They were given either 12 capsules of evening primrose oil containing 480 milligrams of GLA or a placebo capsule with no active ingredients. During the following year, the patients in the study met with their doctors every three months for evaluations. The researchers used 16 different ways to measure neurological damage or improvement. Among the people who took evening primrose oil, there were greater positive changes in all 16 measurements.

Studies like this show the value of evening primrose oil and GLA for people with diabetic neuropathy. My feeling is that even better

*(continued)*

results would be attained with an oil blend of omega-3 and omega-6 fatty acids. Better yet, you may be able to prevent a condition like diabetic neuropathy by taking these oils well before symptoms of neuropathy ever show up. I recommend combining the essential fatty acids with supplements like ginkgo, bilberry, alpha lipoic acid, vitamins E and B$_{12}$, and folic acid. This is a very powerful, comprehensive, nutritional approach for diabetic neuropathy.

### ∿ Eczema

Children with eczema tend to have an inherited problem of converting linoleic acid into GLA. Studies have shown that their mothers also have a history of eczema and have low levels of GLA in their breast milk. They also have higher levels of linoleic acid, signifying a conversion problem.

Studies show that internal use of evening primrose oil provides relief from itching but can take up to four months of continuous use to be fully effective. Again, I would recommend it be taken in an oil blend with fish or flax oil.

Adults with eczema can also benefit from evening primrose oil. A study of 52 adults with eczema found that evening primrose oil was very effective in reducing skin redness and damage.

### ∿ PMS and Cyclical Breast Tenderness

Evening primrose oil can be helpful as part of a comprehensive nutritional approach for treating premenstrual syndrome (PMS). It helps reduce symptoms of irritability and depression, and it can also help prevent fluid retention. Some women find that it takes care of monthly breast tenderness and pain—but it may take four months or more of supplementation before evening primrose oil begins to be really effective.

British doctors use evening primrose oil as a first choice treatment for cyclical breast pain and fibrocystic breast syndrome. For these conditions, I recommend a combination of evening primrose oil, omega-3 fatty acids, vitamin E, and the herb vitex.

# Exercise

"I'm a mess," said Cheryl, a 31-year-old mother of three. "I've gained a lot of weight, I'm tired all the time, and I'm depressed."

"You used to be fit and energetic," I said. "What's happened?"

"Since I had the baby, I've just been falling apart," Cheryl replied.

As I was taking a comprehensive history, I began to suspect that a large part of Cheryl's health problems stemmed from a single source.

"You're doing lots of good things," I told her. "Your diet is good; you have a positive attitude toward your family, and you're actively involved in a women's group to help reduce your stress. However, you're not taking time out to exercise."

There were a lot of other things I could have done to help her, such as homeopathic and herbal treatment. But I knew that until we got her moving with some simple exercise, we were not going to get the results that Cheryl needed and deserved.

"Cheryl, what type of exercise did you enjoy doing in the past?" I asked.

"I used to like walking and swimming," she answered.

"Are you willing to start back on one of those two exercise programs?" I asked.

"I'll do the walking," she replied, "but I don't want to go swimming at this point. I'm embarrassed by the 30 extra pounds I put on over the last five years."

So walking became the mantra. She started doing 10 minutes every other day for the first two weeks. Then she increased the time to 15 minutes, five times a week.

Three months later, Cheryl was doing 30 minutes of brisk walking five times a week. She had lost 10 pounds, was feeling more energetic, and her depression had greatly improved. After just three months, she knew she still had a way to go—but now she had the confidence and motivation to continue. I was certain she could take her health to a higher level.

As an added bonus, she had seen her relationship with her family improve, too. She was less irritable with her kids and husband—partly because she felt better about herself, psychologically, and also because her vitality and energy were on the rise.

## THE BENEFITS OF MOVING AND SHAKING

I wrote this section after coming back from a 3-mile run. I felt great—and knew why. Every time anyone does exercise like this, there's a surge in endorphins and enkephalins—the body chemicals that make you feel good. I was highly motivated to discuss this major component of health and vitality.

Exercise is essentially some form of movement. This ranges from walking to jogging, from biking to playing tennis, to dancing and Tai Chi, and all the other forms of movement you can think of.

Many people think of a gym when they hear the word "exercise." For some people this brings up images of large muscular men or women grunting and groaning as they lift weights. They equate "exercise" with painful exertion.

My goal here is to get you motivated to exercise and then to select exercises that excite you. I also want you to realize the benefits of exercise and what it can do for you physically and mentally. In addition, I want to give you a sense of what *kind* of exercise you may want to be doing.

# GETTING STARTED

The first step to a successful exercise program is to get motivated. Think of the health improvements you can get by exercising. Also, think how the quality of your life will improve when you lose weight, gain muscle, and have an abundance of energy.

With more exercise, many areas of your life can improve, including relationships and work. Exercise is also an effective way to increase sex drive and libido naturally in men and women.

Next, think about what will happen if you don't exercise. See yourself as out of shape, having less energy, and your body "falling apart." It's not a pleasant sight. Make up your mind right now that you will begin to figure out and implement an exercise program immediately. Feel good about it and get excited.

I think it's a mistake to select an exercise that you don't really like. For example, a friend invites you to go jogging, so you go, but you really have no interest in jogging. You would rather go swimming. If you pick an exercise that you don't have an interest in, you are not likely to stick with it. For an exercise program to be worthwhile, you have to stick with it over the long term. Studies show that if you abruptly stop exercising, you lose within a couple of weeks most of the benefits that you gained.

Besides motivation, compliance is everything when it comes to getting the benefits of exercise and sticking to an exercise program long term. By choosing one or two forms of exercise that you really enjoy, you increase your chances of sticking with it. Exercise should be something to which you look forward. It's something from which you can gain energy.

# CHOOSING THE MIX

When choosing your exercise program, focus on aerobic work first. By this I mean walking, jogging, biking, swimming, tennis, dancing—any activity that keeps you constantly moving.

By contrast, there is also anaerobic exercise—such as weightlifting—but it's secondary. For example, weightlifting can improve muscular strength, muscle mass, and bone density. It is also good for the heart and cardiovascular system. However, I recommend beginning with an aerobic exercise program, and then adding an anaerobic exercise like weightlifting.

A combination of cardiovascular training like walking or swimming (or many others) plus some form of resistance training like weights is best. This works all the systems of the body.

Don't feel you have to engage in vigorous physical activity to get the benefits of exercise. A study of over 72,000 female nurses found that women who walk briskly five or more hours a week cut their risk of heart attack by 50 percent.

## FREQUENCY AND LENGTH OF EXERCISE

The frequency and length of exercise depends on your current level of health. Your doctor and a fitness trainer can best determine this. In general, moderately healthy people should start with 10 to 15 minutes of aerobic exercise three times a week and work up from there.

Over time, the length of the exercise period can be increased to 30 to 45 minutes, and the frequency should be four to six times a week. If you experience muscle soreness, and it does not seem to be going away, then cut down the frequency and length of your exercise. If you're starting a weightlifting program, be sure to work with a personal trainer.

If you want some guidance in starting an exercise program, I recommend *Weight Training for Dummies* by Liz Neporent and Suzanne Schlosberg and *The Aerobics Program for Total Well Being: Exercise, Diet, Emotional Balance* by Kenneth H. Cooper.

## WHAT ARE THE SIDE EFFECTS?

Initially, muscle soreness will be the most common side effect as your body becomes accustomed to the exercise. This soreness will become less of a problem after the first three weeks. Proper form is required for weightlifting; otherwise, injuries can occur. In addition, proper warm-up and post-exercise stretching are important to prevent soreness and injuries.

## EXERCISE
### RECOMMENDATIONS FROM THE NATURAL PHYSICIAN FOR . . .

**∾ Anxiety and Depression**
Exercise reduces the effects of stress on the body and should be an important part of a treatment program for anyone with these conditions. It also stimulates the release of chemicals in the brain that are important for mood.

*(continued)*

A study reported in the *Journal of Epidemiology* showed that those who participated in exercise, sports, and physical activity experienced a decrease in depression, anxiety, and malaise.

### ☙ Arthritis

The right kind of exercise can be helpful for the different forms of arthritis. For example, swimming is a good choice of exercise for someone with rheumatoid arthritis or osteoarthritis as it is gentle on the joints. Exercises performed improperly, such as running on a hard surface or using an improper weightlifting technique, can aggravate arthritis.

### ☙ Detoxification

Regular exercise is helpful for anyone in a detoxification program. It promotes increased circulation and lymphatic drainage. It also causes sweating, and thus stimulates detoxification.

### ☙ Diabetes

Exercise increases insulin activity, reduces total cholesterol and triglycerides, and increases the good HDL cholesterol in those who have diabetes. It stimulates blood flow that is more easily impeded in someone with this condition. However, anyone who has diabetes should be monitored by his or her doctor, and follow an exercise program under medical supervision.

### ☙ Fatigue

By expending energy, you can actually increase your energy and vitality level. This is the paradox of exercise, which works well to increase energy levels when done within the parameters of a person's exercise limits. On the other hand, over-exercise can lead to fatigue.

### ☙ Heart Disease

It is a well-known fact that exercise reduces the risk of most cardiovascular diseases. Part of this effect comes from the lowering of cholesterol and triglycerides, and the increase in good HDL cholesterol. It also helps to reduce the effects of stress, another big risk factor for heart disease. Exercise also strengthens the heart muscle. However, anyone who has heart disease should be monitored by his or her doctor, and follow an exercise program under medical supervision.

### ☙ Hot Flashes

Regular exercise has been shown to reduce the number of hot flashes that women experience during menopause.

### ☙ Immunity

Exercise done in moderation strengthens the immune system. For example, breast-cancer risk is reduced in women who exercise. But it's important to note that overtraining, as seen sometimes in marathon runners or triathletes, for example, can lead to suppression of the immune system. Again, balanced exercise is the key.

### ☙ Osteoporosis

It is undisputed that weight-bearing exercise stimulates the growth of bone cells and thus increases bone density. Actually, swimming and some other forms of less weight-bearing exercise have also proven to be effective. This is why exercise is so important to prevent and help treat osteoporosis.

### ☙ PMS

Regular exercise is quite helpful for women who consistently suffer from premenstrual syndrome.

### ☙ Stress

Exercise is one of the most effective techniques to alleviate the effects of stress on the body and mind.

**148**

# *F*

# Fat Reduction

. . . . . . . . . . . . . . . . . . . . . . . . . . . . . . . . . . . . . . . . . . . . . . . . . . . . . . . . . . . . . . . . .

"I have tried many different diets over the years. With some of them, I improved for a period of time, but the weight keeps coming back. I don't know why my body wants to carry around this extra 30 pounds."

Betty's words were an echo of the words I'd heard many times from many other patients. A 32-year-old housewife with two children, she was very familiar with a number of books and weight-loss programs—and she had tried more than one. Nothing, so far, had worked for her, but she still believed there was a "simple secret" to losing fat and lowering her weight.

"My secret for helping people lose weight? It's simply to treat the cause of the weight problem."

My answer obviously puzzled her. "And what's the cause of my weight problem?" Betty asked.

"That's what we need to find out today," I answered. "I believe there are seven main causes of weight problems. One is genetics. Some people just are genetically programmed to store more fat. However, they can overcome this with a strong program.

"Two is diet. You need to have a diet or nutritional program that is compatible with your metabolism.

"Three is exercise. It is very important to burn that fat and speed up your metabolism. The trick is finding an exercise program that you enjoy, and getting the maximum benefit without having to kill yourself with endless hours of workouts.

"Four is hormone balance. Over 50 percent of all women have hormonal imbalances. In addition, blood-sugar balance is connected to the hormone insulin, and is very important. Blood sugar that goes up and down stimulates the release of insulin, which causes fat storage. If your hormones are out of whack, your metabolism is messed up.

"Five is toxicity. If you are full of toxins, your enzyme systems cannot work properly. As a result, your body stores fat and retains water. Detoxification is often important for people with weight problems.

"Six is nutritional deficiencies. They can interfere with your metabolism.

"Seven is the emotional and spiritual component. Suppressed or unresolved issues in these areas can be a major contributor to weight problems. For example, I talk to patients all the time who overeat or eat junk food because they're filling a void for their loneliness, depression, or some other emotion."

"Sounds pretty comprehensive," said Betty.

"Yes, it is. People with weight problems have a problem in one or more of these areas. From your health history and the metabolic testing, I can pinpoint exactly why you have the problem and then together we can correct it. This will not only help you lose weight in a safe manner, but you'll keep it off for good."

Betty's response was optimistic. But even when she declared "I feel very hopeful about this," I could sense that her optimism was tinged with reservations. After all, this wasn't the first time she'd tried.

But by the next year, she no longer had hesitations about the program. She lost 25 pounds. Her total cholesterol dropped 20 points, and her blood-sugar levels balanced out. She also knew that it wasn't a passing phase of dieting or weight loss. She had no problem keeping the weight off—and her optimism was sustained by a new sense of vitality and self-esteem.

## THE SEVEN CAUSES OF WEIGHT PROBLEMS

Think of being overweight as a symptom of an underlying imbalance. When you identify why you have the weight problem, you can shed those extra pounds more quickly and with less effort.

Trying a fad diet is a "shot in the dark," as is the latest "breakthrough" weight-loss supplement or drug. The simple fact is that most of the "breakthrough" dieting or weight-loss programs are not sustainable in the long term, and some are downright dangerous.

I've found that it's quite feasible for you, on your own, to go through the seven causes of weight problems. If you do an honest evaluation of the cause or causes, you can make your own analysis of why you are having difficulty losing weight and keeping it off. Whether you're male or female, young or old, your weight problem is certain to relate, in some way, to one or more of these seven causes. But it's up to you to decide *which* of these are more pertinent than the others.

## 1. GENETICS

You may come from a family that tends to have weight problems. Quite often, when a number of people in the same family are overweight, it's easy to conclude that "it's in the genes."

But is it?

Except in rare cases, the notion that you are genetically "doomed" for fat accumulation just isn't true. What we really are talking about is genetic tendencies or genetic predisposition. Everyone comes into the world with some distinct, genetic predispositions, and it's true that people can have a genetic makeup that makes them more prone to having weight problems. If you already have a predisposition toward being overweight, and you're in a family where people consume a lot of high-calorie foods—well, between genetics and lifestyle, you are, indeed, in a situation that makes weight gain a near certainty. However, you can overcome or reduce your fat-storage tendency by focusing more on the other six causes. It just takes a little more work.

## 2. DIET

The biggest problem with general weight-loss diets is that they put everyone on the same regimen. Any diet that does this is destined to fail for a certain percentage of people.

Everyone is biochemically unique and responds differently to different foods. Food preferences are as unique as taste in clothes. But you may "wear" one diet a lot better than you do another one. Some people do better on a vegetarian diet, while others do worse. Others do fine on a diet that focuses more on protein foods. Also, I have seen some people do well on a diet that's custom-designed for a specific blood type.

Deciding *which* diet is for you may be a process of trial and error unless you see a physician. However, I have found some successful diet guidelines that will help you turn on your body's fat burners.

### ∾ *Watch Your Sugar Intake*

The average American consumes 125 pounds of sugar a year. It is no wonder this country has a weight problem. Consumption of refined carbohydrates, which are essentially simple sugars, leads to a condition known as insulin resistance.

Your body responds to simple sugars by releasing insulin, which transports blood sugar (glucose) into the cells. The rapid release of sugar into the bloodstream results in insulin "spikes"—so called because if you charted your blood glucose during the day, you'd see times when insulin spiked upward on the chart. This response helps get glucose into the cells, but when you have those sudden spikes of insulin, it has the effect of causing fat storage.

But there's another response, as well, that occurs over time. If you consume a diet of refined sugars for very long, the cells' response to insulin becomes sluggish, leading to the condition known as insulin resistance. When glucose isn't transported into the cells so efficiently—because of this insulin resistance—the body stores it as fat.

Refined carbohydrates that you should try to avoid or minimize include pastas, white rice, non–whole-wheat grain products such as white bread, and most bakery items. You'll also want to avoid sugars such as white and brown sugar, corn syrup dextrose, fruit juices, and maple syrup. Of course, candies and chocolate bars fall into the "unwanted" category.

These are probably foods that you eat at nearly every meal, so you may be wondering what's left. As a rule of thumb, I'd advise that you stick to what nature has provided by eating whole foods such as fresh vegetables. Based on the same principle, whole-grain pastas and breads are better to eat because the grain is unrefined, and brown rice is better than white rice. These foods have fiber—among other good nutrients—and the fiber helps slow the release of sugar into the bloodstream.

But there's another fact to remember about refined carbohydrates. They can actually be consumed in moderation if you also eat high-fiber foods like vegetables, whole grains, and legumes. The reason for this is that each food has what is called a glycemic index. The glycemic index is a rating of how high glucose levels rise after a food is consumed. The higher the glycemic rating, the faster the glucose enters the bloodstream, and the greater the insulin response.

Glucose has a rating of 100. Lentils have a rating of 30, while a bagel has a rating of 72. So if you were to have a bagel along with a salad, your blood-sugar elevation would not be nearly so high.

People always ask about fruit juice, which is concentrated sugar. Fruit juice can be consumed in moderation as long as you don't drink it on an empty stomach and you have it with foods that will slow the sugar absorption. For example, drinking fruit juice along with fish and salad would have much less effect on fat storage than drinking fruit juice by itself.

The best way to avoid refined sugars is to prepare meals yourself or eat with a discriminating eye when you eat out.

One ray of hope: The herb stevia is excellent to use as a sweetener. It's actually sweeter than sugar and does not adversely affect blood-sugar levels, even in people with diabetes. It can be purchased as a liquid or powder at health food stores and some grocery stores.

## ॐ *Watch Which Fats You Eat*

The wrong types of fats worsen insulin resistance and contribute to fat deposits. Avoid saturated fats—those found in red meat and dairy products. They not only worsen your weight problem, but also increase your risk of heart disease and certain cancers.

Avoid fake fats, too. These synthetic fats include trans fatty acids as found in fried foods, margarine, and products containing partially hydrogenated oils (such as cookies and crackers). Instead, focus on healthy omega-3 fats that are highly concentrated in cold-water fish such as salmon, mackerel, and herring. Omega-3's are also found in flaxseeds, flaxseed oil, and walnuts.

Stay away from oils that are rich in omega-6, such as sunflower, corn, soy, and most other cooking oils. Use heart-healthy and fat-friendly extra-virgin olive oil instead.

## ॐ *Balance Your Carbohydrates, Proteins, and Fats*

The ratio of carbohydrates, proteins, and fats is important in a successful program of fat reduction. Many weight-loss books advocate certain proportions among these three components of the diet. In general I find that a lot of people lose weight more efficiently on a diet that emphasizes a little more protein and less carbohydrates and fats. A major reason this works is because people consume less refined carbohydrates when they focus on getting more protein. Also, protein does not cause blood-sugar spikes and thus does not generally cause fat deposition.

The trick is to eat high-quality proteins such as fresh fish, nuts, seeds, and relatively high-protein plant foods such as soy and corn. Other good animal sources include organic eggs and poultry.

I find that a good diet for fat reduction has approximately 40 to 50 percent carbohydrates, 30 percent fat (mainly "good fats" such as omega-3's), and 20 to 30 percent protein. Don't stress yourself by trying to calculate the percentages of calories that fall into each category for each meal. Instead, simply make sure you include a good protein, a complex carbohydrate, and a good fiber source in each meal.

Find what proportions of carbohydrates, proteins, and fats are optimum for you and adjust the percentages accordingly. In general, you will attain a percentage close to what I recommend, and will turn on the fat burners while shutting down the fat storers.

## ∾ Counting Calories Isn't Necessary

Calories are a factor in fat reduction. The higher the number of calories from food, the more energy you must expend burning them off. With my system, counting calories becomes obsolete. The real issue is focusing on quality foods in moderate portions.

If you focus on quality foods and the right ratio of the different types of foods, the calorie count will remain at a level where you can lose weight.

## ∾ Eat Smaller Meals

Eating smaller, more regular meals throughout the day helps to quell the appetite and level the blood sugar. This is a long-term strategy for fat reduction.

## ∾ Do Not Skip Meals

I would say 30 percent of all my weight-loss patients tell me on our initial visit they skip breakfast. Never skip a meal. This is a signal to the body to conserve energy and store fat.

If time is an issue, prepare breakfast the night before or make yourself a protein shake by combining 1 scoop of soy or whey protein powder with soy or rice milk and 1 to 2 tablespoons of ground-up flaxseeds. Add some blueberries or another fruit that you like.

This takes a whopping two minutes and supplies you with protein, carbohydrates, good essential fatty acids, and fiber. It will help to level out your blood sugar and prevent fat storage. It will also increase your energy and mental sharpness as opposed to being tired and mentally dull from skipping breakfast.

## ∾ Harness the Power of Plant Foods

Don't forget the power of plant foods when you're on a fat-reduction diet. Vegetables and some fruits are excellent sources of fiber, which helps to bind fat from foods and expel it in the stool.

Fiber also helps to slow the release of sugar from foods into the bloodstream. This is especially true of soluble fiber—found in oat bran, dried beans, peas, rice bran, barley, and apple skin.

Plant foods are also excellent sources of phytonutrients that aid the body in many ways, including the process of "burning fat"—that is, fat metabolism.

You can get the full spectrum of amino acids from the combination of various plant foods. They are also very important for detoxification. That's significant because proper detoxification removes toxins that cause fat storage and water retention.

## ∾ Watch Your Water Intake

Drinking an adequate amount of water is critical for weight loss. Dehydration, even at a marginal level, actually causes the body to store water, and water retention is a large factor in weight gain. In addition, water is essential for detoxification.

You should drink at least six to eight 8-ounce glasses of water daily (48 to 64 ounces). Also, avoid those substances that cause dehydration such as caffeine (coffee), salt, and alcohol.

## ∾ Identify Your Food Sensitivities

One of the ways I expedite the weight-loss process for my patients is to identify their food sensitivities. Different people are sensitive to different foods. Food sensitivities cause water retention and make metabolism and detoxification more sluggish.

Many of my patients who have had food-sensitivity testing report that they lost extra weight by avoiding the foods to which they are sensitive. (See FOOD-SENSITIVITY THERAPY, page 189.)

# 3. EXERCISE

Without question, exercise is a cornerstone of any fat-reduction and weight-loss program, but it may be a challenge to find an exercise program you like so that you will stick with it long term. Fat reduction will also be fastest if you do aerobic exercise such as walking, jogging, swimming, biking, or dancing, because you burn fat more efficiently.

Weightlifting isn't such an efficient fat burner, but it does increase your body's metabolism—and a combination of the aerobic activities along with some weightlifting (called "anaerobic") is ideal.

Sports such as racquetball or tennis are excellent, too.

How often should you exercise and for how long? That depends on your current level of health. Your doctor and a fitness trainer can best determine the optimum periods.

In general, moderately healthy people should start with 10 to 15 minutes of aerobic exercise three times weekly and work up from there. Ideally, the time of exercise should be 30 to 45 minutes (or longer) and the frequency should be four to six times a week. If you're just starting a weightlifting program, work with a personal trainer who can help you begin at a reasonable level without risk of injury. You can always build up to higher weights or more repetitions over time.

## 4. HORMONE BALANCE

Hormones are powerful chemicals that control your body's metabolism. One of the most important in the fat-reduction equation is the thyroid gland. It is well known that if thyroid hormone is low, cell metabolism slows down and weight gain is a pretty sure thing.

Many physicians, including myself, believe that hypothyroid (low thyroid function) is epidemic in our society, especially among women over the age of 25. Unfortunately, blood tests often do not pick up borderline cases of low thyroid.

The best diagnostic procedure is to have a thyroid panel done by your doctor (including the tests called "free T3" and "TSH"). Saliva thyroid hormone tests have recently become available. Also, take your temperature each morning at the same time for five days straight. Temperature is an indication of thyroid function, and if the temperature reading is consistently below 98.2 degrees Fahrenheit, then you have a sluggish thyroid.

If you do have low thyroid, I recommend you find a holistic doctor for natural thyroid support. I don't favor conventional thyroid hormone replacement (with the medication Synthroid) because it weakens the thyroid. Over time, patients on Synthroid need to take increasingly higher dosages to equal results.

Estrogen and progesterone balance is also very important for weight loss. Many women have too much estrogen relative to progesterone, a condition referred to as "estrogen dominance." I find that synthetic estrogen and progesterone lead to water retention and hinder thyroid function.

Testosterone and growth-hormone deficiency can also lead to fat deposition, especially in men. Women given synthetic hormone replacement for menopause almost always start to gain weight and increase water retention. The birth-control pill has similar effects.

(For more about natural hormone-balancing options, see BLACK COHOSH, VITEX, and NATURAL PROGESTERONE.)

The last issue of hormone balance is the concept of insulin resistance, which I described earlier. The consumption of refined carbohydrates leads to insulin spikes that promote fat storage. Over time, the cell insulin receptors become less sensitive to insulin so the body stores the glucose as fat.

Another condition known as "Syndrome X" also comes into play. This refers to a cluster of conditions. Insulin resistance is part of the equation, but added to that are two of the following—high cholesterol, high triglycerides, or high blood pressure, or obesity. (The "apple shape" figure is a general sign of Syndrome x— that is, with excess fat around the belly, hips, and thighs.) Researchers feel that anyone who has Syndrome X is only one step away from developing diabetes.

## 5. TOXICITY

Toxins—such as pesticides, herbicides, and other chemicals—that get into the body from the environment wreak havoc on your body's enzyme systems. Toxins known as heavy metals, such as mercury and lead, are particularly dangerous and can suppress thyroid function. They also impair the detoxification process and lead to water and fat accumulation.

Toxins that accumulate as the result of poor digestion are also a problem. For a thorough detoxification program, I generally advise people to work with a holistic doctor who can help you identify the toxins that may be stored in your body and then work with you to help eliminate them. But if you follow a good diet, exercise, and take nutritional supplements, you are already enhancing the detoxification process.

## 6. NUTRITIONAL DEFICIENCIES

Nutritional deficiencies are widespread in a society like ours, because we consume monumental quantities of refined and synthetic foods. Many different vitamins and minerals are involved with fat metabolism in one way or another.

Specifically, I find that chromium, vanadium, and alpha lipoic acid are of particular help in regulating blood-sugar levels, and thus preventing fat storage. Dosages of 400 micrograms of chromium picolinate or chelate, 100 micrograms of elemental vanadium, and 100 to 200 milligrams of alpha lipoic acid are useful.

Zinc and magnesium are required for proper insulin function. A dosage of 30 milligrams daily is good for zinc, and a dosage of 500 milligrams is good for magnesium.

Beyond that, a high-potency multivitamin is helpful as an insurance policy for nutritional support.

An essential fatty acid source such as ground-up flaxseeds, or flaxseed or fish oil is recommended to help metabolize fats and for proper insulin function.

Nutritional deficiencies cause cravings for sweets and fatty foods, which translate into fat gain.

# 7. EMOTIONAL AND SPIRITUAL FACTORS

Many people have weight problems because of past emotional traumas. As a result, they use food to help dampen, reduce, or control emotional pain. I often see this problem in people who have been divorced or been through difficult relationships. People who have suffered physical and sexual abuse often have eating disorders, too—and one manifestation of that could be excessive weight gain because of bingeing or alternate bingeing-and-starving.

Is this an issue for you?

One way to answer that question is to consider whether eating is actually something that compels you. Though you might use food this way—to make yourself feel temporarily "good"—the reality of what it does for you is probably quite different. The excessive food consumption makes you gain weight, which actually decreases your energy levels and vitality. Far from feeling better about yourself, you're more likely to feel reduced self-esteem.

If this is an issue for you, it must become the first thing you address. Work with a counselor or religious leader to overcome the emotional and spiritual traumas that are the underlying cause of your weight problem and unhappiness.

Are you looking for a miraculous weight-loss product you can take without changing your eating habits or doing exercise? I have not yet found such a product—at least, one with no side effects—and I seriously doubt that it exists.

However, you can use certain products that may aid in fat reduction as part of the comprehensive program outlined in this section. These products fall into two broad categories that are worth considering: nutritional supplements and natural stimulants. While I do not recommend the stimulants, I discuss them in this section because they are so popular.

# NUTRITIONAL SUPPLEMENTS

Many nutritional supplements on the market are described as weight-loss products, even when there are few good studies to back up their use. There are a number of products that may be promising, but, as I've noted below, some have only been tested in animals.

### ∾ *Conjugated Linoleic Acid (CLA)*

Promoted as a weight-loss promoter, antioxidant, cancer fighter, and immune system enhancer, conjugated linoleic acid (CLA) is found in red meat. It helps glucose get into muscle cells more effectively, thus preventing glucose from being converted into fat. It also helps fats enter the cell membranes of muscle and connective tissue, where the fat is burned for fuel. Most of the claims about this substance are based on animal studies, but human studies exist. *Dosage:* 1,000 mg three times a day with meals.

### ∾ *Chitosan*

Chitosan is a product that is derived from chitin, which is found in the exterior skeletons or shells of shrimp, crabs, and other shellfish. When taken with meals, chitosan binds fats so that they are not absorbed. It is not a source of calories since it is not digestible.

Some human clinical data exists to support its benefit. *Dosage:* 500 to 1,000 mg at the beginning of each meal.

### ∾ *Hydroxycitric Acid (HCA)*

This extract is derived from the rind of Garcinia cambogia, a fruit grown in Southeast Asia. Laboratory and animal research has shown it helps with weight loss by reducing the conversion of carbohydrates into stored fat. It has been shown to suppress appetite in animals, and seems to have no side effects. Whether it will prove effective in human studies remains to be seen. *Dosage:* 500 mg three times daily before meals.

### ∾ *Pyruvate*

This is an altered form of the sugar molecule. In human and animal studies, pyruvate seems to aid in weight loss when people combine it with a low-fat diet. That doesn't imply, however, that you can take pyruvate on its own—without other dietary alterations—and expect to reverse weight gain. *Dosage:* 6 to 30 grams daily.

# NATURAL STIMULANTS: BE WARY

Many weight-loss stimulants are popular, but I don't recommend them. These "natural stimulants," as their name suggests, actually stimulate the nervous system and help prompt the release of adrenaline. That hormone, produced by the adrenal gland, promotes the burning of fat for fuel.

**The drawback of these products is that they may have serious side effects.** People may have a variety of reactions to these stimulants, such as anxiety, insomnia, chronic fatigue, heart abnormalities, and elevated blood pressure. If you already have one of these conditions, the addition of natural stimulants can make the symptoms more severe.

I am also concerned about their effect on the thyroid and adrenal glands. I advise people never to take natural stimulants for long periods of time. When the thyroid and adrenal glands are overstimulated, they don't function so well (call it "wearing out")—and when their function is inhibited, other health problems can arise.

# CAFFEINE

Good old caffeine is a stimulant that increases the metabolic rate and may curb appetite. As many people have discovered, too much caffeine may cause anxiety, insomnia, heart palpitations, elevated blood pressure, and trembling. Caffeine also increases urinary frequency and can lead to hyperactivity.

### ∾ *Ephedra (Ma Huang)*

This herb has been valued for its medicinal properties in traditional Chinese medicine for thousands of years. In traditional Chinese herbal therapy, it is used for colds, bronchitis, asthma, sinusitis, upper respiratory tract infections, and for its diuretic properties. It is known for its ability to relax the bronchial muscles.

Ephedra contains ephedrine and pseudoephedrine, two nerve stimulants that act like the pharmaceutical epinephrine. In traditional Chinese medicine, ephedra was always used in a combination with other herbs and always in very small amounts. When combined with herbs like licorice root, doctors of Chinese medicine found that ephedra's toxicity was reduced.

Here in the West, it is used more like a drug—taken by itself, and sometimes in high concentrations. There is no doubt that people lose weight by taking ephedra preparations, as it stimulates fat metabolism. But at what long-term costs?

**160**

The problem is, anyone taking ephedra in the "straight" form—without the benefit of other combinations of herbs—may as well be taking amphetamines. For someone with severe obesity who is contemplating surgery, it might make sense to be treated with ephedra by an experienced practitioner—and it certainly is an alternative to more dangerous pharmaceutical medications. But it can have extensive and serious side effects ranging from increased blood pressure and heart rate to anxiety, insomnia, and increased urination.

I would never recommend ephedra to someone with preexisting heart conditions (especially arrhythmias), thyroid disease, and diabetes. It should also never be taken along with pharmaceutical antidepressants or medications for high blood pressure (hypertension).

### ∾ *Guarana* (**Paullina Cupana**)

Guarana seeds were originally used as a medicine by indigenous peoples of the Amazon forest to treat diarrhea, reduce hunger, and relieve arthritis. It contains guaranine, which is a stimulant that is very similar in its structure and effects to caffeine. People use it as an alternative to ephedra and caffeine supplements. It is thought to have fewer side effects than other natural stimulants.

# Ferrum Phosphoricum

Ferrum phosphoricum, abbreviated as ferrum phos, is an important homeopathic remedy for treating anemia and fevers. This remedy is a combination of the minerals iron and phosphate.

Iron is an integral component of red blood cells, helping to bind oxygen so that it can be stored in the cells. Iron is in the food we eat, and a certain amount is added when you cook with cast-iron pots and pans.

The homeopathic form of iron—ferrum phos—is what I recommend to improve the cellular uptake of iron. It's just what you'll need, for instance, if you have iron-deficiency anemia.

A number of health and lifestyle factors can contribute to this type of anemia. Some women suffer from iron-deficiency anemia because of heavy blood loss during their menstrual cycle. Bleeding from injuries is another possible cause. You also have to be alert to the possibility of anemia if you're on a strict vegetarian diet and have digestive and absorption problems. Plant foods are low in iron, and the iron in plant foods cannot be absorbed so well as the iron that comes from meat.

Ferrum phos does not actually supply the body with doses of iron; rather, it works to increase the absorption of iron from the foods we eat. More important, it helps to increase the uptake of iron by our red blood cells. Even if you take high doses of iron supplements to offset low-iron blood, the supplements don't help if the iron cannot be incorporated into your red blood cells and, from there, get carried to other iron-starved tissues.

When Rebecca came to me for treatment of iron-deficiency anemia, she already recognized that an irregular and very heavy menstrual cycle might be contributing to her constant feeling of tiredness. I noticed at once that she had large black "shiners" under her eyes, which is a symptom of iron deficiency.

For the previous three months, she had been taking large doses of iron supplements (120 milligrams daily) as her doctor had recommended—but during that time, her anemia had not improved. Subsequently, the doctor had used injections—and these may have been somewhat more effective, but Rebecca reported the injections were also very painful.

There was more. Because of Rebecca's heavy monthly blood flow, her doctor had prescribed birth-control pills, hoping that the pills would help regulate her menstrual cycles. But Rebecca had experienced severe nausea and headaches and had finally refused to use the pill any more. Furthermore, the benefits were slight. After two months of supplements, injections, and birth-control pills, her blood tests showed only slight improvement.

After talking with Rebecca, I had her stop the injections and began her on a treatment that focused on the use of ferrum phos along with a multivitamin that had a relatively small amount of iron in it. I reasoned that Rebecca's cells were, obviously, not assimilating the iron effectively. Instead of trying to force more iron into her body, I wanted to make changes at the cellular level that would help improve the way her cells utilized and incorporated the iron.

There was another reason to recommend ferrum phos as soon as possible. In women like Rebecca who have iron-deficiency anemia associated with heavy menstrual bleeding, a cycle develops, leading to worsening conditions. The anemia actually promotes even heavier menstrual bleeding. So I knew that until we got the anemia under control, it would be difficult—if not impossible—to get the bleeding under control.

Rebecca took the ferrum phos diligently. Within three weeks her bleeding became lighter and within six weeks her menstrual cycle became regular again. Blood tests showed a 50 percent improvement in her red blood cell levels and ferritin levels (storage levels of iron). The dark eye shiners disappeared and her skin color improved. Rebecca's improvement continued over the next three months until her iron and red blood cells were back to normal.

## DOSAGE

For the treatment of iron-deficiency anemia I recommend ferrum phos 3x or 6x to be taken three times daily. For a more aggressive treatment of anemia, you can also take the herb yellow dock, which contains small amounts of iron and enhances the digestive absorption of iron.

For the treatment of acute illnesses, I recommend the 30C potency or higher. Take the ferrum phos as needed until you feel the relief of symptoms. (However, lower potencies of 3x and 6x also work well for some acute illnesses.)

## WHAT ARE THE SIDE EFFECTS?

I have never seen any side effects with ferrum phos supplementation. It is a homeopathic remedy, so there's no danger of iron toxicity, even with children.

---

## FERRUM PHOS
### RECOMMENDATIONS FROM THE NATURAL PHYSICIAN FOR . . .

#### ∾ *Anemia*
I would not hesitate to give ferrum phos supplementation on a long-term basis for severe anemia. I also recommend it during pregnancy to help women maintain normal iron levels.

#### ∾ *Bleeding*
Ferrum phos is a good remedy to any kind of bleeding, especially nosebleeds and minor cuts. You can crush the tablets of ferrum phos and apply the powder directly to scrapes and cuts.

*(continued)*

### ☙ Earache

Ferrum phos is one of the more common remedies used for childhood ear infections. Homeopathic physicians are most likely to prescribe it if the child's face is flushed and the child has a fever of 102 degrees Fahrenheit or higher.

I also notice whether the child acts sick. Oddly enough, ferrum phos is most effective as a earache remedy for a child who does not even seem to be sick but continues to play around and act as if nothing were wrong.

I also examine the child to find out whether the right ear tends to be more painful than the left. If so, again, it's an indication that ferrum phos may be the most effective earache remedy.

### ☙ Fever

Ferrum phos is also an excellent remedy to help control fevers, especially in younger children. It helps to calm down a fever—unlike fever-reducing pharmaceutical medications that tend to suppress the fever rather than reduce it. Because fever helps to stimulate the immune system, it should be reduced rather than being totally suppressed or eliminated.

### ☙ Sore Throat and Tonsillitis

Both of these conditions can be helped with ferrum phos remedy. It is especially useful when the throat and face appear bright red and the patient has a powerful thirst for cold drinks.

# Feverfew

Feverfew *(Tanacetum parthenium)* is known among herbal enthusiasts as the "migraine headache herb," and there are enough clinical studies to confirm that the leaf of this plant does help to prevent migraines. While herbalists have used feverfew to prevent and treat migraine headaches for centuries, it also has a rich history for the treatment of menstrual cramps, as a pain reliever during labor, and as a remedy that can help reduce fever. It has also helped treat arthritis, toothaches, and respiratory tract conditions such as asthma and bronchitis. Today, most people and practitioners use feverfew for migraine headaches and, to a lesser extent, for arthritis.

Feverfew grows up to three feet tall and is native to different parts of Europe. It is also grown commercially in North America.

Scientists aren't sure why feverfew can help prevent migraine headaches, but they do have theories. It's thought that the herb helps reduce the clumping of specialized cells in blood that form blood clots—the cells called platelets. Researchers believe that platelet aggregation leads to the release of inflammatory chemicals, which alters the way blood circulates through the brain. When platelets begin to aggregate in an abnormal way, the process is thought to cause biochemical imbalances with the neurotransmitter serotonin, and these imbalances, in turn, lead to migraine headaches. Feverfew seems to help prevent this chain reaction.

Also, feverfew contains significant amounts of the hormone melatonin. Low levels of melatonin have been held as a potential cause of migraine headaches.

Another theory about feverfew relates to a substance called parthenolide. Though it's just one constituent found in feverfew, some researchers consider parthenolide to be important in preventing migraines. However, more research needs to be done before anyone can be certain of the precise therapeutic effects of parthenolides.

Feverfew also inhibits arthritis and other inflammatory conditions. In all probability, this occurs because feverfew prevents the release of immune cells that cause problems when they reach a body joint and begin to cause inflammation. So the action of feverfew helps prevent joint and tissue destruction.

## DOSAGE

I recommend the capsule form to patients. Look for a standardized extract that contains 0.3 to 0.7% parthenolides. Make sure the product also contains a base of the whole herb, since we don't know, for sure, which constituents of feverfew are the active components.

For the treatment of acute migraines, take 300 milligrams every 30 minutes to a maximum of four doses daily. If you get improvement, continue on an as-needed basis without exceeding the four-a-day dosages.

While feverfew might help relieve acute migraine in some people, in my own experience I've found that it's a better preventive than treatment of migraines. The preventive dose that I recommend is 300 to 400 milligrams of the standardized capsule, taken daily. If you still get migraines, don't give up on the feverfew. You may need to take it for up to three months before it really begins to work as a preventive.

The tincture form can also be used. I recommend 30 drops per dose.

Though some people make a tea of feverfew, I've found that the tea doesn't contain the active ingredients that you need for best results.

As far as I know, you can also chew on feverfew leaves (although I have yet to meet someone who has done this.)

Be aware that feverfew can take up to three months of use to be effective in preventing migraines.

# WHAT ARE THE SIDE EFFECTS?

A very small percentage of feverfew users may experience digestive upset. Since this herb has some blood-thinning properties, you should check with your healthcare professional if you are already on blood-thinning medication or if you're taking migraine medication.

Also, if you're a woman who's pregnant or breast-feeding, be sure you're under the guidance of a knowledgeable practitioner before you start taking feverfew.

If you are one of the few people who decides to chew the leaves, do so with caution as mouth ulcers may occur.

---

## FEVERFEW
### RECOMMENDATIONS FROM THE NATURAL PHYSICIAN FOR . . .

**∾ Arthritis**

Feverfew can help relieve the pain of osteoarthritis and rheumatoid arthritis. Do not expect immediate pain relief, however, as it takes time for the antiinflammatory action to kick in. I prefer to use feverfew in formulations that contain other natural antiinflammatory supplements such as MSM, boswellia, turmeric, and bromelain. (If you're suffering from osteoarthritis, then glucosamine sulfate is a must, whether or not you also take feverfew.)

**∾ Migraine Headaches**

Some prescription medications can effectively relieve migraine headaches, but there's always the potential of drug toxicity and side effects, which don't occur with feverfew. I typically recommend feverfew along with other natural therapies such as treating food sensitivities, spinal manipulation, hormone balancing, stress reduction, and detoxi-fication. These other therapies address the underlying causes of many migraines—and if one or more is successful, you might be able to stop taking feverfew. Otherwise, as one study has

shown, the migraines may recur as soon as the herbal treatments are discontinued.

The effectiveness of feverfew is supported by some good clinical data. A 1998 study looked at 59 people who suffered migraine headaches. For the first four months of the study, subjects took a daily, regulated dose of feverfew in capsule form. (As usual in such studies, there was a con-trol group for comparison.) Researchers found that daily treatment with feverfew lead to a 24 percent reduction in the number and severity of migraine headaches. Also, symptoms of nausea and vomiting were improved. No side effects were reported from feverfew. It was interesting to note that 47 percent of the people in the study had already tried conventional migraine drugs without any improvement in the severity or frequency of migraines.

**∾ Pain**

Feverfew can be used in the treatment of many other types of pain. Some practitioners and herbalists prescribe it for toothaches, muscle injury, and other, similar types of trauma.

# Fiber

Want to look healthy on the *outside?*

Then you have to look healthy on the *inside.*

That's one of the fundamental premises of natural healing traditions. Of all the substances that help make your insides look healthy, the best is surely fiber. Fiber not only keeps your digestive tract healthy, it also helps create good health and vitality through detoxification.

Hippocrates, the "father of medicine," acknowledged the health benefits of fiber in the fifth century B.C. Some 2,400 years later, an American entrepreneur by the name of Sylvester W. Graham picked up the cause, expounded heartily on the benefits of roughage in the diet, and created the company that produced the eponymous Graham cracker.

However, it was not until the 1960s that researchers seriously studied the role of fiber in the diet. Interest was piqued by studies showing that the native Africans who subsisted on a very high fiber diet had a very low incidence of colon cancer, diverticulosis, gallstones, hemorrhoids, appendicitis, diabetes, and some forms of heart disease. Researchers concluded that there was a clear connection between consumption of high fiber and overall digestive good health.

## BULKING UP FOR GOOD HEALTH

Also referred to as "roughage," fiber is the indigestible portion of plants that forms the bulk of stool. The human body does not secrete enzymes that break down fiber, and the roughage doesn't provide any calories, vitamins, minerals. But having that undigestible matter in the digestive system is actually a benefit. As the fiber moves through, it acts like a broom, sweeping out the garbage and toxins that accumulate in our digestive tract. Without this cleansing effect we could not survive, as infection in our digestive tract would be rampant.

Fiber also helps control blood-sugar levels by slowing the rate at which the intestines release blood sugar into the bloodstream. Even though it doesn't provide any nutrients directly to the body, certain types of fiber feed the friendly bacteria that live in your intestinal tract, helping to speed digestion and preventing unfriendly microbes from causing infection.

## Benefits Galore

Fiber has many important, proven health benefits. Here are the top ten.

1. Decreases appetite and gives a feeling of satiety without increasing body fat or weight. This leads to weight loss.
2. Reduces fat absorption.
3. Reduces cholesterol.
4. Improves blood-sugar regulation.
5. Promotes bowel regularity.
6. Reduces the risk of certain types of cancer.
7. Binds and eliminates toxins.
8. Promotes healthy intestinal bacteria.
9. Promotes hormone balance.
10. Increases your intake of phytonutrients (many of which are found in the fiber portion of plants).

For vegetarians, getting enough fiber is usually no problem. If you're eating a lot of vegetables, fruits, legumes, nuts, seeds, and whole grains, you'll be getting a full spectrum of various types of fiber. Studies have shown that many vegetarians have a lower risk of many chronic conditions such as heart disease and many types of cancers, compared with the general population.

For the average American who is *not* a vegetarian, fiber intake is usually far below what it should be. Most of us eat a dismal 11 to 20 grams of fiber daily—and I'm sure there are many teenagers or college students living on fast-food, soda, and coffee who get as little as 5 grams of fiber daily. Yet, for optimal health and for the prevention of many diseases, we should all be getting 40 to 50 grams daily.

## A DOUBLE REQUIREMENT

There are two main types of fiber that are distinguished by the way they react to water. "Insoluble fiber" is the kind that cannot dissolve in water—and this is the kind that "bulks up" in the intestine and acts like a broom, sweeping undigested or undigestible matter out of your colon. Insoluble fiber includes cellulose, the indigestible portion of plants. This type of fiber is found in the leaves of plants, in the peels and skins of fruits and vegetables, and in the coverings of whole grains.

Both wheat bran and psyllium seed are two excellent sources of insoluble fiber. While it does not dissolve in water, it does bind to water, which helps to bulk up the stool and prevent diarrhea. Insoluble fiber protects against diseases such as diverticulitis, irritable bowel syndrome, and possibly colon cancer.

The second category is "soluble fiber," the kind that dissolves in water. As soluble fiber passes through the digestive tract, it binds together bile acids and cholesterol, so they pass through without being reabsorbed. Oat bran, perhaps the best-known form of soluble fiber, has been shown to reduce cholesterol. But it's not the only beneficial source of soluble fiber. You can get similar benefits from dried beans, peas, rice bran, and barley.

One particular form of soluble fiber known as pectin is found in the outer skin and rind of fruits and vegetables. The skin of an apple contains 15 percent pectin, while an onion skin contains 12 percent. Pectin, like other forms of soluble fiber, lowers cholesterol levels by preventing the reabsorption of cholesterol in the gut.

Mucilages—found in the inner layer of nuts, seeds, grains, and legumes—is yet another kind of soluble fiber. Guar gum, the most common mucilage, is used as a thickening agent and stabilizer in commercial products such as salad dressing, ice cream, and skin creams. As with pectin, mucilage forms a gel in the digestive tract and slows the rate of blood-sugar digestion and absorption. This helps in the regulation of blood-sugar levels.

Flaxseeds contain a high amount of both soluble and insoluble fibers. One-quarter cup of flaxseeds contains 20 grams of fiber. The water-soluble mucilage in flaxseeds is very soothing and healing to the digestive tract, helps to feed the good bacteria, and also has a natural laxative effect. Also a rich source of omega-3 fatty acids, flaxseeds contain hormone-balancing and cancer-protecting lignans.

## EDIBLE GOOD HEALTH

There are many sources of dietary fiber, but, as you can see from Table 4, there is a wide variability in the content of fiber in servings of different foods. To get a good mix of soluble and insoluble fiber in your daily diet, here are some foods to consider.

## FIBER SUPPLEMENTS

Many people benefit from taking fiber supplements. They may be helpful to you if you suffer from constipation, hemorrhoids, or digestive conditions such as irritable bowel syndrome (IBS), Crohn's disease, or ulcerative colitis.

When patients have these conditions, I generally recommend that they first try to increase their dietary intake of fiber before taking supplements. But when you just can't get enough fiber from your daily diet, supplements are extremely helpful.

Psyllium husks are often used because they absorb a lot of water and bulk up the stool, which improves elimination. Another good supplement is wheat bran, which is also a good insoluble source of fiber (but not helpful if you have a wheat sensitivity or allergy).

## TABLE 4

| | Insoluble Fiber (grams) | Serving Size | Total Fiber (grams) | Soluble Fiber (grams) |
|---|---|---|---|---|
| *Fruits* | | | | |
| Apples | 2.6 | 1 | 3.0 | 0.4 |
| Banana | 1.3 | 1 | 1.8 | 0.5 |
| Blueberries | 1.9 | 1/2 cup | 2.1 | 0.2 |
| Blackberries | 4.5 | 1/2 cup | 4.9 | 0.4 |
| Grapes | 0.5 | 10 | 0.5 | trace |
| Grapefruit | 0.3 | 1/2 | 0.1 | 0.4 |
| Honeydew, melon | 0.4 | 1/2 cup | 0.5 | 0.1 |
| Peach | 1.1 | 1 | 1.7 | 0.6 |
| Raisins | 1.4 | 1/4 cup | 1.6 | 0.2 |
| *Vegetables* | | | | |
| Artichoke (fresh, cooked) | 6.4 | 1 medium | 3.5 | 2.9 |
| Beans (black, dry, cooked) | 2.7 | 1/2 cup | 0.1 | 2.8 |
| Broccoli | 1.0 | 1/2 cup | 1.6 | 2.6 |
| Brussel sprouts (frozen, cooked) | 2.8 | 1/2 cup | 0.4 | 3.2 |
| Lentils (dry, cooked) | 2.8 | 1/2 cup | 0.1 | 2.9 |
| Peas (green, canned, or frozen) | 2.8 | 1/2 cup | 0.3 | 3.1 |
| Lettuce | 0.3 | 1/2 cup | 0.2 | 0.5 |
| Spinach (canned, cooked, or raw) | 2.0 | 1/2 cup cooked or canned, 2 cups raw | 0.3 | 2.3 |
| Vegetable soup (canned) | 1.6 | 1 cup | 0.6 | 2.1 |

| | Insoluble Fiber (grams) | Serving Size | Total Fiber (grams) | Soluble Fiber (grams) |
|---|---|---|---|---|
| *Grains* | | | | |
| Bread (white or Italian) | 0.6 | 1 slice | 0.2 | 0.8 |
| Bread, rye | 0.5 | 1 slice | 0.2 | 0.7 |
| Bread, whole wheat | 2.2 | 1 slice | 0.3 | 2.5 |
| Cereal, Total® cornflakes | 0.8 | 1 cup | trace | 0.9 |
| Cereal, Rice Krispies® | 0.4 | 1 cup | 0.1 | 0.5 |
| Cereal, Special K® | 0.7 | 1 cup | 0.1 | 0.8 |
| Cookies, oatmeal | 0.6 | 1 large | 0.3 | 0.9 |
| Cookies, plain sugar | 0.2 | 1 | 0.1 | 0.1 |
| Crackers, Ritz® | 0.2 | 4 | 0.1 | 0.3 |
| Muffin, blueberry | 0.8 | 1 small | 0.2 | 0.6 |
| Oats, whole | 1.6 | 1/2 cup | 0.5 | 1.1 |
| Pancakes | 0.9 | 2 | 0.2 | 0.7 |
| Rice, medium grain | 0.4 | 1/2 cup | trace | 0.3 |
| *Nuts* | | | | |
| Almonds, roasted | 2.5 | 22 whole | 0.1 | 2.4 |
| Peanuts | 2.0 | 30 to 40 whole | 0.1 | 1.9 |
| Walnuts | 1.1 | 14 halves | trace | 1.0 |
| *Legumes* | | | | |
| Beans, black, dry | 2.8 | cooked 1/2 cup | 0.1 | 2.7 |
| Lentils, dry | 2.9 | cooked 1/2 cup | 0.1 | 2.8 |

When you're selecting a supplement, make sure the product doesn't include sugar, artificial sweeteners, or artificial coloring. Any of these added ingredients may cause digestive upset. Whatever supplement you take, be sure to drink lots of water along with it. Otherwise, the supplement can "bulk up" inside your intestinal tract rather than passing readily through it , causing constipation.

## DOSAGE

While adults should get 40 to 50 grams of fiber daily, children need less. For a quick calculation of a child-appropriate dosage, just add five to the age of the child to get the number of grams of fiber the child should be taking. For example, a 10 year old would require 15 grams of fiber daily.

If you haven't been getting sufficient fiber in your diet, and want to work up to the optimum level, you should gradually increase your daily fiber intake. If you suddenly start taking more fiber, you may experience excessive bloating and flatulence—but this is less likely to happen if you raise your intake more slowly.

Whether you're taking supplements or just eating more fiber, make sure to drink plenty of water throughout the day. Try to get six to eight 8-ounce glasses so that the fiber doesn't "plug you up."

It's also helpful to get fiber from a variety of different sources. As you can see in Table 4, there are many common foods you can eat that are good sources of the various fibers. One simple technique is to make sure you are getting one or more fiber-rich foods with each meal. For example, if you can eat whole oat cereal for breakfast, you'll get both soluble and insoluble fiber—about twice as much as you'd get from cornflakes or Special K®.

For lunch or dinner, have some broccoli or a green leafy salad. Whole-grain bread is good with any meal, as it provides plenty of insoluble fiber.

If you still find that your fiber intake is too low, then I highly recommend grinding up flaxseeds each day. You can get as much as 20 grams of fiber from one-quarter cup of ground flaxseeds.

Fiber supplements should be used according to the containers' labels. They are generally available in powder or capsule form. I usually recommend psyllium, with a starting dose of 1 teaspoon or 2 capsules daily along with an 8-ounce glass of water. Over a period of six weeks, you can build up the doses until you're taking the amount of fiber that is necessary for the bowels to move. The maximum is typically 4 teaspoons or 8 capsules of supplemental fiber.

## WHAT ARE THE SIDE EFFECTS?

You can avoid the gas and bloating if you steam or cook vegetables, then gradually switch to more raw vegetables (which have more nutrients and a higher concentration of enzymes) as your body adjusts to the increase in fiber.

Fiber supplements can inhibit the absorption of certain drugs and can "bind up" various minerals, also preventing absorption. This can be avoided, however, if you avoid taking fiber supplements at the same time as medications or vitamin/mineral supplements.

# FIBER
## RECOMMENDATIONS FROM THE NATURAL PHYSICIAN FOR . . .

### ↜ Cancer

One of the benefits of fiber, especially insoluble fiber, is that it binds to cancer-causing substances so that they are excreted out of the body. Epidemiological studies demonstrate that if you have a diet high in saturated fat diets and low in fiber, you increase the risk of many different types of cancer, including colon cancer.

Of course, all these benefits can't be attributed to fiber. Fruits, vegetables, legumes, and whole grains—foods with the most dietary fiber—also contain vitamins, minerals, and phytonutrients, all of which are believed to be responsible for some of the protective effects against cancer. Lignans in flaxseed, for example, are phytonutrients that have a protective effect.

That said, it's evident that a high-fiber diet can be protective against certain kinds of cancer—especially colon cancer. This makes sense to me, as toxins are bound by fiber and removed through the stool. Also, when fiber is acted on by bacteria in the colon, it produces the substance butyric acid, what's known as a "short-chain fatty acid." Butyric acid is the main energy source for the colonic cells, and it's thought to be one of the mechanisms that helps dietary fiber prevent colon cancer.

Hormone-dependent cancers in women—such as breast, uterine, and ovarian cancers—seem to show up more often among women on low-fiber diets. Men on low-fiber diets seem to have a higher rate of testicular cancer.

Women on vegetarian diets have been shown to have up to 50-percent lower levels of free estrogen in their blood than women who eat meat and foods made from animal products. Insoluble fiber helps to bind and excrete excess estrogen. Researchers believe this may be one of the reasons why vegetarian women have lower rates of breast cancer.

### ↜ Cholesterol

Many of the different forms of fiber help to reduce cholesterol levels. Pectin as found in apples and other fruits lower total and LDL cholesterol. Similarly, the water-soluble fiber in oats seems to improve cholesterol levels. It contains a substance called beta glucan, which has been shown to lower cholesterol.

In 1997, the Food and Drug Administration (FDA) allowed oat bran to be registered and promoted as a cholesterol-reducing food. But studies on the effects of oat bran have produced somewhat mixed results. Some oat bran studies have

*(continued)*

been shown to produce very little improvement in cholesterol levels, while others show up to a 21-percent reduction in serum cholesterol. Researchers have found that as little as 18 grams of oat bran fiber favorably affect the total and LDL cholesterol levels in men with mildly elevated cholesterol markers. (In most studies that produced benefits, people ate around 100 grams of oat bran.) Guar gums have also been shown in animal and human studies to lower cholesterol markers. Psyllium has also been shown to lower cholesterol.

The body eliminates cholesterol through bile acids, which are produced by the gallbladder and released into the small intestine. Water-soluble fibers bind to the cholesterol in these bile acids so that they cannot be reabsorbed and are carried out with the stool.

### ✎ Constipation

Fiber bulks up the stool so that gravity and peristalsis (contractions of the smooth muscles of the digestive tract) pull down the stool. Insoluble fiber is most important as it pulls water into the large intestine, and with more liquid, you'll have softer stools and easier elimination.

Soluble fiber also contributes, to a lesser degree, to the weight and water content of the stool. Ground-up flaxseeds as well as vegetables are the best forms of fiber to relieve constipation. (Other major factors contributing to constipation are too little water consumption and not enough exercise.)

If it takes a long time for stool to move through the intestinal tract, there's a higher chance that toxins can be reabsorbed into the bloodstream. The transit time, the length it takes to go from the mouth to the anus, is significantly reduced when you have a high-fiber diet. For example, cultures that consume a high-fiber diet (100 to 170 grams per day) have a transit time of 30 hours. In comparison, the low-fiber American diet (10 to 20 grams per day) have a transit time that exceeds 48 hours.

### ✎ Diabetes and Hypoglycemia

Water-soluble fiber is extremely important if you have diabetes or hypoglycemia. Foods such as oat bran, legumes, nuts, seeds, apples, and most vegetables slow down the release of blood sugar from the intestine to the bloodstream.

In addition, dietary fiber has been shown to increase the cells' sensitivity to insulin, so additional fiber helps balance blood-sugar levels. (I also recommend guar gum for blood-sugar balance.) People with diabetes or hypoglycemia need to consume good portions of fiber with every meal. For someone with diabetes, I recommend 50 grams of fiber a day.

### ✎ Irritable Bowel Syndrome (IBS) and Inflammatory Bowel Disease (IBD)

If you have either of these digestive conditions, it's essential to pay attention to your dietary habits—especially fiber intake. A lack of dietary fiber creates an unhealthy environment in the digestive tract, setting the stage for digestive disease.

Besides helping with elimination, a good supply of insoluble fiber helps to feed the "friendly bacteria" that live in the colon and assist digestion. In fact, if you have IBS or IBD, there's a good chance you have a condition known as dysbiosis or bacteria imbalance, which can be detected by stool analysis.

I find most of my patients with these conditions benefit from increasing dietary sources of fiber, but I generally recommend steamed and cooked sources of vegetables. If you have IBS or IBD, you'll probably want to reduce or avoid wheat and other grain products because they tend to be irritating. Psyllium supplements, for instance, are helpful for some people with these digestive problems, but they can be very irritating to others.

If you want to try ground-up flaxseeds—which are generally well tolerated—start with a low dosage of 1 to 2 teaspoons with one tall glass (8 ounces) of water. If you don't experience discomfort, you can gradually increase the dosage over time.

# Fish Oil

Gary's father had died at the age of 54. "It was a heart attack," Gary told me.

Now 44 himself, Gary almost felt as if he were living on borrowed time. He could hear the clock ticking.

"Gary, most cases of heart attacks can be prevented," I assured him. I also let him know he was doing the right thing—showing some concern about his heart health before anything happened. Most people, sad to say, wait until they've had a heart attack before taking the measures that they could and should have taken years before.

True, there are inherited factors that make some people more susceptible than others to heart attack—specifically, homocysteine and cholesterol levels just seem to be higher in some people than in others. But most heart attacks are due to diet and lifestyle factors.

Gary had done enough reading to be aware of that. It was one reason he wanted to get started on an aggressive program to keep his heart as healthy as possible.

Among the strategies we discussed were stress reduction, exercise, a series of lab tests, and, of course, diet and supplements. I emphasized the importance of omega-3 fatty acids found in fish, especially cold-water fish such as salmon, mackerel, herring, and sardines. Above all, I recommended fish-oil supplements, such as salmon oil, to optimize the amount of these heart-healthy fatty acids. As part of a total strategy for heart health, the steady intake of fish oil could, potentially, add decades to his life expectancy.

## OIL WELL

Among the essential fatty acids that we need to live, omega-3's are very important. It's one of those fats that your body can't manufacture on its own, so it needs to come from food sources or supplements.

While omega-3 is also found in flaxseed and flaxseed oil, the kind that you get from fish and fish oil has some unique properties that are not present in these other foods. The fish and fish oils are a direct source of two long-chain fatty acids known as EPA (eicosapentanoic acid) and DHA (docosahexanoic acid), and both are very important for heart health.

**175**

Another reason doctors are confident about the benefits of fish oil is pragmatic. The vast majority of studies on essential fatty acids have been done on fish oils. There are sound reasons to believe that oils such as flaxseed oil may be nearly as effective, but to date, they haven't been studied so much. It is the fish oils that have been studied and shown to be effective.

Fish became more popular as a "healthy heart" food when researchers studied the "Mediterranean diet"—that is, the diet of many cultures around the Mediterranean during the 1960s in Crete, parts of Greece, and southern Italy. (There, as in many other cultures, the "American diet" has crept in, raising the rate of heart disease and other chronic diseases). In the classic Mediterranean diet, people had many plant foods (vegetables, legumes, fruit, bread, pasta, nuts), lots of olive oil, and low to moderate amounts of fish, poultry, meat, dairy, eggs, and wine.

Nutritionists believe the consumption of fish was one of the key benefits of this diet, which resulted in a much lower incidence of obesity, heart disease, diabetes, and cancer. A 4-year study of the Mediterranean diet found that people could reduce their risk of heart attack by as much as 70 percent.

## SEA RATIONS

In a more direct study of fish consumption, a team of researchers who looked at mortality data from 36 countries confirmed that life expectancy is longer in those countries where people get a lot of fish in their daily diet. Men and women who eat more fish have a lower risk of early death from all kinds of illnesses, particularly stroke and heart disease.

Essential fatty acids form a group of hormone-like messengers known as prostaglandins. The omega-3 fatty acids as found in fish oil—helped along by the EPA and DHA in the fish—tend to decrease inflammation, thin the blood, and balance the immune system.

In the immune system, EPA appears to be particularly important for its anti-inflammatory effects, so it's helpful to people who have arthritis. DHA is critical for the proper development and function of the brain because your brain cells need it to transmit electrical impulses efficiently. It's not surprising, therefore, that a DHA deficiency can lead to memory, behavior, and learning problems.

Some studies have also indicated that supplementing infant formula with DHA can improve children's IQ. Interestingly, it's also important for mood regulation, and studies have shown that a deficiency can contribute to depression.

The DHA found in fish oil also appears to calm down hyperactive children. It's also required for proper retinal development for infants.

## DOSAGE

Fish oil capsules generally are available in 500- to 1,000-milligram doses. When purchasing the capsules, pay particular attention to the amounts of EPA and DHA stated on the labels. You want fish oils that contain about 18 percent EPA and 12 percent DHA: in other words, totalling about 30 percent of the omega-3 fatty acids found in these fish oils. (Some of the newly developed, high-potency fish oils now contain even higher concentrations of EPA and DHA.)

For preventative purposes, I recommend that people eat foods high in DHA and EPA such as cold-water fish. (Eggs also contain DHA.)

If your health is generally good, I'd advise taking 2,000 milligrams of a daily fish-oil supplement such as salmon oil. But if you're susceptible to specific diseases such as arthritis, high blood pressure, and other conditions, I'd advise getting a higher dose—as much as 6,000 to 10,000 milligrams per day. However, you'll probably want to check with your health practitioner to find out an optimal dose for your condition, since the supplement can be costly.

If you're taking the concentrated fish-oil capsules that have higher concentrations of EPA and DHA, I recommend salmon oil or tuna oil capsules that have been tested for heavy metal contamination and rancidity. I am also a big fan of the oil blends that contain a combination of essential fatty acids such as DHA, EPA, and GLA. An ideal formula also has vitamin E in it. If not, take vitamin E *with* the fish oil to prevent the oil from going rancid.

Fish-oil capsules should be stored in the refrigerator once they are opened. Don't leave the container standing in bright light or keep it in a warm room.

## WHAT ARE THE SIDE EFFECTS?

Some people who take fish oil experience digestive upset including burping—which can be disconcerting because you may burp a "fishy" smell. But you probably won't have that problem if you take the capsules with meals.

Also, some companies make specially designed capsules that ensure the oil makes it into the small intestine before breaking down. Such claims are advertised so you might want to try their capsules to see whether their product alleviates the problem of burping or "fish breath."

Since fish oils also have a blood-thinning effect, check with your doctor if you are taking any blood-thinning medications.

You may have an increase in LDL cholesterol while supplementing fish oil. If a blood test shows your cholesterol count is on the rise, you can take a garlic supplement to help neutralize this potential effect of the fish oil.

Although people have relatively few and minor problems with the side effects of fish oil, there's a risk that the capsules can contain rancid oil. It's easy to check, however. Just cut open the end of a capsule. If the fish oil has gone rancid, you can easily smell the strong odor. You're better off getting a fresh bottle with new capsules.

Finally, check the label of any brand you buy to make sure the product was tested for contaminants such as heavy metals.

# FISH OIL
## RECOMMENDATIONS FROM THE NATURAL PHYSICIAN FOR . . .

### ☙ ADD and ADHD

Many school-age children have been diagnosed with Attention Deficit Disorder (ADD) or Attention Deficit Hyperactivity Disorder (ADHD), and their problems are sometimes related to nutritional imbalances. (Excess sugars and some additives in junk food have particularly been blamed.)

Essential fatty acids such as DHA are critically important for proper brain function, but—well, how many children do you know who eat fresh cold-water fish three times a week? When children aren't getting enough DHA and they're loading up on saturated fat, trans fatty acids, and omega-6 fatty acids from fast-foods, the inevitable result is a fatty-acid imbalance.

DHA supplementation has been shown to decrease aggression while a child is under stress. The DHA in fish oil helps to improve the chemi-

cal balance in the brain while giving the general benefits of omega 3 fatty acid supplementation.

I recommend that bottle-fed infants receive omega-3 supplementation, especially DHA, for proper brain and retina development. Breast-fed infants receive these critical essential fatty acids in the breast milk. I suspect that, before long, DHA supplementation will be required in all commercial baby formulas.

### ☙ Arthritis

Numerous studies with fish oil have been done on people with rheumatoid arthritis and the results have been very positive. For aggressive treatment using fish oil, take 6,000 milligrams daily. Some people need doses that are even higher, so talk to your health practitioner about the optimum dose if you have severe rheumatoid arthritis.

If the fish oil is helpful in reducing stiffness and pain, there's a good chance you'll be able to

*(continued)*

178

reduce the dosages of pharmaceuticals. Drug therapy for rheumatoid arthritis focuses on prednisone, methotrexate (also used for chemotherapy), and antiinflammatory medications—all of which can have serious toxicity when used on a long-term basis. With fish oil, on the other hand, there's no toxicity, so it's a far more benign treatment than the classic pharmaceuticals. One study found that many patients were able to go off their antiinflammatory drugs while supplementing fish oil and experienced no relapse in their rheumatoid arthritis. Researchers found that the fish oil had a balancing effect on the entire immune system.

It is recommended, as the result of studies, that a minimum daily dose of 3,000 milligrams EPA and DHA is necessary to derive the expected benefits, although I find not all my patients need this high a dosage. Once you start taking fish oil, you can expect to stay on it for at least 12 weeks before it begins to yield benefits. But after that, you can stay on it indefinitely.

Despite the many improvements you can get from fish oil, I do have to say it should be part of a total program when you're treating rheumatoid arthritis. It's also important to improve your diet and take steps to reduce the toxins in your body. I've seen the quickest results with detoxification programs when they also involved homeopathic remedies. But fish oil is a good long-term therapy for some people, and it can definitely help keep inflammatory conditions under control.

Although not so well studied, essential fatty acids found in fish oil are helpful to decrease the stiffness associated with osteoarthritis, the most common form of arthritis, where the cartilage has degenerated.

## ❧ Asthma

The rate of asthma keeps increasing. Sadly, children's asthma is continuing to rise at an alarm-

ing rate. Environmental pollution and poor dietary habits are largely to blame.

Essential fatty acids in fish and fish oil help to suppress the inflammatory chemicals involved in this disease. Studies show that children who eat oily fish more than once a week have one-third the risk of getting asthma as children who do not eat fish or eat lean fish on a regular basis.

Fish-oil supplements are helpful for both children and adults with asthma. Again, the benefits of fish oil take months before the natural antiinflammatory benefits begin to take hold.

## ❧ Cancer

Omega-3 fatty acids are important for a healthy, well-functioning immune system. If you can get more omega-3 fatty acids in your diet and also take supplements, there's a good chance you can help protect yourself from certain types of cancers.

Animal studies have shown that fish oil can augment certain types of chemotherapy to fight cancer more effectively. Fish oil has also been shown to help treat cachexia, which is the loss of muscle mass and weight in cancer patients.

## ❧ Cardiovascular Disease

With many studies to back up its benefits, fish oil is often recommended as a preventative for heart and circulation problems. Along with the population studies showing that consumption of fish oil slashes the rate of cardiovascular disease, are literally hundreds of studies that support these observations. Fish oils reduce cholesterol and triglyceride levels and also act as a natural blood thinner, which results in the lowering of blood pressure.

## ❧ Chronic Obstructive Pulmonary Disease

Over 17 million Americans suffer from this group of serious breathing disorders that includes asthma, bronchitis, and emphysema. Smoking, as

(continued)

you might expect, is the factor that multiplies your chances of getting any of these diseases. But for smokers as well as nonsmokers, there are some benefits in eating fish as often as possible.

### Crohn's Disease and Ulcerative Colitis

Inflammatory bowel diseases such as Crohn's disease and ulcerative colitis can be helped by fish-oil supplementation.

In one study of ulcerative colitis, people who took fish-oil supplements (high in omega-3's) were able to cut their steroid medications in half. Again, I see fish oil as one component of a total natural-therapy program to address and alleviate these digestive conditions. Other measures include stress reduction, improving digestive capacity, and maintaining a healthful diet.

Herbal medicines and homeopathy are excellent therapies to help turn these conditions around without relying on pharmaceutical drugs that may have many damaging side effects.

### Depression

The brain is 60 percent fat and requires essential fatty acids, especially DHA, to function properly. It has been shown that people deficient in DHA are much more likely to suffer from depression.

Consuming fish on a regular basis is a good way to prevent depression. I recommend concentrated DHA supplements for those already battling depression.

As a side note, I believe it's time that more research is done on nutritional deficiencies to find out how they can cause mental diseases such as depression. I see an increasing number of people using pharmaceutical antidepressants on a long-term basis, without exploring other preventives. As we learn more about genetic susceptibility to depression, we will also discover what nutrients and other therapies can help correct what people have come to call "genetic depression." To date, fish oil is certainly one of the most important of the nutrients we have been able to identify as necessary for healthy brain functioning.

### Eczema

I have found that flaxseeds and flaxseed oil in combination with GLA work well for eczema. It also makes sense to consume cold-water fish rich in omega-3 fatty acids. Fish oil is also another option to treat eczema.

### High Blood Pressure

High blood pressure is one of the biggest risk factors for heart disease and stroke. Numerous studies have shown that fish oil reduces blood pressure. I find fish oil works best as part of a natural program—combined with stress-reduction techniques and a regimen that includes herbs such as hawthorn, minerals such as magnesium and calcium, along with the natural supplement CoQ10.

### High Triglycerides

With fish oil, you can lower high triglyceride levels, which are an independent risk factor for heart disease. As I've mentioned, though, fish oil can increase LDL cholesterol, so you'll want to supplement with garlic to help balance out its effects.

### Insulin Resistance

The inability to metabolize carbohydrates effectively leads to high blood-sugar levels and a corresponding spike of the hormone insulin (the component that helps get the blood sugar into the cells). As a result, many different biochemical reactions can occur, one of which is weight gain.

Clinical studies have shown that omega-3 fatty acids, such as those in fish oil, help improve the body's utilization of insulin. (It's interesting that an essential fatty acid can help *decrease* body fat!) This insulin-balancing effect is also important in relationship to diabetes.

*(continued)*

**180**

### ❧ Kidney Protection

People who receive organ transplants require extensive immune-suppressing drugs. These are needed to keep the body from rejecting the donated organ, but some of the drugs (such as cyclosporine) are so powerful that they can have life-threatening side effects.

In the case of patients who have had kidney transplants, however, it's been shown that they resume normal kidney function more quickly when omega-3–rich fish oil is supplemented. It appears that the fish oil actually protects the kidneys from the damaging effects of the immune-suppressing drugs.

### ❧ Lupus

Two pilot studies have shown fish oil to benefit people with lupus, an autoimmune condition where the immune system attacks its own tissue. For patients with lupus, I suggest eating cold-water fish regularly and supplementing with fish oil. It may take six months to a year before there's any improvement, but sometimes the benefits can be dramatic.

### ❧ Multiple Sclerosis

Dr. Roy Swank, the doctor who developed a natural protocol for multiple sclerosis (MS), recommended fish oil as well as flaxseed oil. In fact, Dr. Swank advocated that patients who have MS should eat fish three times a week or more. He was also a proponent of cod liver oil—one of the popular fish oils—as a daily supplement.

### ❧ Psoriasis

Several studies have shown that 10 to 12 grams of fish oil daily can improve psoriasis. I routinely recommend fish oil and dietary fish as well as other natural therapies to improve this inflammatory condition.

### ❧ Schizophrenia

Some preliminary studies are showing that EPA and DHA may be helpful in the treatment of schizophrenia. More research needs to be done, but I would not be surprised to see these essential fatty acids become accepted as part of the routine treatment for schizophrenia. Dr. Abraham Hoffer of Victoria, Canada has already demonstrated that a knowledgeable practitioner can provide a full-scale treatment of schizophrenia with nutritional therapies.

# Flaxseed

"Dr. Mark, what can I do? My hair is falling out, my nails are peeling, and my skin is flaking because it is so dry!" The plea came from Rachelle, a 23-three-year-old university student.

My first step was to ask her about her usual daily diet and her digestion. She mentioned right away that she had chronic constipation, and wondered whether that could be somehow related to her dry-skin condition.

"Possibly," I replied. But after hearing what she ate on a daily basis, I found another factor that seemed even more important. It appeared that Rachelle had an omega-3 fatty-acid deficiency. Because she didn't enjoy the time and effort of cooking, she was eating about 90 percent of her meals in fast-food restaurants. Also, like many university students, Rachelle liked to eat out so she could socialize with her friends.

Her dry-skin problem could also be caused by low thyroid function—but once I ruled that out, I started Rachelle on flaxseed oil (*Linum usitatissimum* or linseed). Two months later Rachelle was a happier and healthier person. She said the first symptom to improve was the constipation. Instead of having a bowel movement every three days, it was now once daily. Her skin was less dry—and she was no longer losing hair the way she had been. Her nails, though still brittle, were starting to improve. Rachelle also noticed that her memory and concentration were better. (This made sense, as the brain needs a strong supply of essential fatty acids to function optimally.)

Given the success that Rachelle was experiencing, it was simple to make a recommendation at our next appointment. "Keep doing what you're doing," I advised. "Another month or two, and you will feel and look even better. Essential fatty acids take time to work. Sometimes, it's many months before you get the full benefits."

Obviously, this simple supplement had made a profound improvement in Rachelle's life. Ideally, she would have increased her intake of omega-3 fatty acids by eating more foods that were rich in it, such as fish, nuts, and some specific vegetables. Also, cutting down on the fried and fast-foods rich in omega-6 oils and hydrogenated fats would have been a prudent choice as well. But, in reality, Rachelle wasn't about to change her lifestyle. Fortunately, she could get almost the same, optimum results just by taking two teaspoons of flaxseed oil every day.

As Mahatma Gandhi said, "Wherever flaxseed becomes a regular food item among the people, there will be better health."

## CHANGING YOUR OILS

In an ideal diet, there's a balance between two kinds of essential fatty acids: the omega-3's (alpha linolenic) and omega-6's (linoleic). Most of us consume far too many omega-6 fatty acids (from red meat and vegetable oils) and not enough omega-3 fatty acids (from fish, flaxseed, some vegetables). Many experts feel the optimal ratio of omega-6 to omega-3 fatty acids is 4 to 1, while most people are getting these oils in a ratio that's about 20 to 1!

Many diseases are related to essential fatty-acid deficiency. The commercial processing of fats and oils has created an "essential fatty-acid crisis" for industrialized nations. These synthetic, rancid fats not only displace "good fats" in the body, but also have toxic effects on the immune and nervous systems.

More important than the total amount of fats is the *type* of fat we consume. Essential fatty acids such as those found in flaxseed are critical to the optimal health and functioning of all cells in the body, including brain cells. Essential fatty acids improve our cell walls, and this improvement has a direct effect on the functioning of the cells. Essential fatty acids influence the passage of nutrients and information that comes into a cell, and the elimination of toxic waste products. So, healthy cells equal a healthy metabolism and healthy body.

Flaxseed is a powerful disease-fighting food that most people desperately need. It has a history of over 5,000 years of use. Records show that flax was cultivated as a food in ancient Babylon (3000 B.C.). Hippocrates (460–377 B.C.) recommended flax as a food to relieve intestinal discomfort.

## THE GROWTH OF FLAXSEED

For centuries, flax has been a staple of Europeans' diets. No wonder the Latin translation of flax means "useful." There are nearly 100 different species of flax worldwide, and many of its health-yielding properties are now being acknowledged. Almost anywhere you go in North America, you can now find flaxseed breads or you can buy bags of flaxseed in bulk at health food stores.

Flax has a very nutritious profile, containing vitamin A, some of the B's, D, and E, carotene, lecithin, and many minerals. It also contains many different amino acids, the building blocks of protein. While it is not a complete protein source, it combines well with other protein foods, which means it ultimately helps you consolidate more protein in your body.

Well known as an excellent source of omega-3 fatty acids (alpha linolenic acid)—the type of "good fats" in which so many people are deficient—flaxseed oil helps protect against cardiovascular disease, cancer, arthritis, and many other chronic degenerative diseases.

But flaxseed oil has another attribute: an almost perfect balance of omega-3's with other kinds of fatty acids. Flaxseed has approximately 48 to 64 percent omega-3's, 16 to 34 percent omega-6's, and 18 to 22 percent omega-9 fatty acids. This type of fatty acid composition is an excellent fatty-acid balance.

In addition, flaxseed has some very powerful medicinal properties. It's an excellent source of insoluble fiber, which is the kind that helps out the digestive tract by forming the bulk of the stool and absorbing toxins. As an added bonus, flax also contains a second type of fiber, the soluble kind that dissolves in water and is absorbed in the digestive tract. Soluble fiber helps reduce cholesterol levels and regulate blood-sugar levels.

# CONTENTS

One-quarter cup of flax contains approximately 20 grams of total fiber, which is just about half of the recommended daily fiber requirement (doctors suggest 35 to 50 grams daily). Flax also contains mucilage, a gel-like substance that soothes and heals the digestive tract. In addition, flaxseed helps feed the "good bacteria"—the kind that reside in the digestive tract, helping with digestion. It also has a natural laxative effect.

Flaxseed is also one of the top sources of a phytonutrient known as lignans. (Though wheat bran is also known for containing lignans, the amount in flaxseed is about 100 times what it is in wheat bran.) Found in the fiber part of flaxseed, lignans have many benefits, helping to fight cancer, viruses, fungi, and bacteria. Lignans also balance hormones, so it can relieve menopausal hot flashes.

Researchers are particularly interested in the anticancer properties of flax lignans. Research on animals and humans has shown that lignans have a protective effect against hormone-sensitive cancers such as breast, uterine, and prostate cancer. Lignans increase sex-hormone binding globulin (SHBG), which binds estrogen and helps to clear it out of the body. It also appears to block excessive stimulation of testosterone.

Lignans are broken down by the gut flora into two compounds known as enterolactone and enterodiol. These compounds interfere with the cancer-promoting effects of estrogen, especially breast cancer, which is probably a reason why vegetarian women have lower rates of breast cancer than nonvegetarian women. The omega-3 (alpha linolenic acid) has its own immune-enhancing and anticancer properties as well.

# DOSAGE

### ✿ *Flaxseed*

There are various ways to consume flaxseed. If you're dealing with the actual seeds, you need to break the hard outer coating. One way is to grind them in a coffee grinder for about 5 seconds.

The typical adult dose is 1 to 2 tablespoons daily, but there's so much fiber in flaxseed that you may have digestive problems (including excessive flatulence) if you start with that much. If you're not already on a high-fiber diet, or if you're prone to digestive problems, I suggest you start with a quarter tablespoon daily and gradually increase the dosage.

Children can take 1 to 2 teaspoons of ground flax daily, but they, too, may need to start with a lower dose.

Make sure to always drink at least 8 ounces of water when you're taking ground-up flaxseed. The liquid is needed to help move the seeds through the intestinal tract. Alternatively, you can add the ground-up flaxseed to a shake, juice, or a glass of water to help it go down more easily.

Flaxseed is a good addition to salads and granola cereal and can also be used in baking. Try to take the flaxseed as soon as possible after grinding them up, because they start to oxidize as soon as they've been ground. The flaxseed oil starts to turn rancid with oxidation.

You can also let the whole seeds soak in water overnight, then take them the next day. The soaking softens them and makes them more digestible.

### ✿ *Flaxseed Oil*

The adult dosage for flaxseed oil is 1 to 2 tablespoons daily. Children can start at 1 teaspoon daily and the dose can be gradually increased unless the stools get too loose.

Flaxseed oil is also available in gel capsules, which work well if you don't want to taste the flax or take time to grind and/or soak the flaxseed. Unfortunately, the capsules are more expensive. You'll need to take nine to fourteen 1,000-milligram capsules daily if you want to get the equivalent of one tablespoon of flaxseed oil.

When you're storing flaxseed oil, keep it away from light—preferably, in the refrigerator. I recommend buying small bottles of flaxseed, so the oil is always as fresh as possible. Make sure to check the expiration date on the bottle.

Fresh flaxseed oil has a characteristic nutty flavor, and if it goes rancid, you can tell at once by the smell. So as soon as you open a new bottle, give it a sniff to make sure the oil is fresh. Also, you should look for oil that's made from organically grown flaxseed to ensure that it isn't tainted with pesticides.

## WHAT ARE THE SIDE EFFECTS?

People who have gallbladder problems, such as gallstones, may have trouble digesting flaxseed oil. That's because the gallbladder concentrates and releases the bile to help break down oils; if there's not enough bile, digestion is more difficult. This can be resolved if you start with a very small amount of flaxseed oil (1 teaspoon) and build up the dosage over time. Better yet, start by using ground-up flaxseed.

Another possible side effect is constipation if you don't drink enough water when you start taking flaxseed. One patient, for instance, called me with severe abdominal pain after taking a half cup of ground flaxseed; but when I reminded her about taking more water, she recovered. (Having taken that much flaxseed, however, she needed to drink nearly half a gallon of water during the next few hours!)

You should not ingest flaxseed at all if you have bowel obstruction.

A few patients have reported outbreaks of adult acne after starting flaxseed oil—but over time, their skin improved. The outbreaks were probably the effect of the body detoxifying and adjusting to the new balance of essential fatty acids.

The high fiber content of flaxseed may interfere with the absorption of certain medications. If you're taking pharmaceutical doses on a regular basis, be sure to check with your pharmacist about possible interactions.

## FLAXSEED
### RECOMMENDATIONS FROM THE NATURAL PHYSICIAN FOR . . .

೧ *Acne*

Omega-3 fatty acids help reduce skin inflammation and have a balancing effect on the production of sebum, the substance that forms pimples. The results are not immediate, however, and you may have to take flaxseed for several months before you begin to see benefits. However, it is worth taking on a long-term basis to keep acne under control.

Some cases of acne are related to poor elimination. Flaxseed or flaxseed oil help to keep the bowels regular and decrease systemic toxicity.

೧ *Arthritis*

Omega-3 fatty acids as found in flaxseed oil help to keep the inflammatory pathways in the body in balance. It also works to keep joints "lubricated," which makes it especially helpful for osteoarthritis. *(continued)*

It may also help people who have rheumatoid arthritis, but the connection is more indirect. There have been a number of studies using essential fatty acids for rheumatoid arthritis, but the best results have been produced with high doses of fish oil—a direct source of eicosapentanoic acid (EPA), which has antiinflammatory properties. If you take flaxseed, some of the alpha linolenic acid does get converted to EPA, but the amount of conversion varies with each individual—and conversion is further inhibited if you have a deficiency of the mineral zinc.

I recommend more than flaxseed oil for patients who have rheumatoid arthritis. You should also eat cold-water fish such as salmon, mackerel, and herring, and— for more aggressive therapy—supplement with a quality fish oil to further reduce pain and inflammation.

### ✍ Cancer

Flaxseed is an excellent supplement to use for the prevention and treatment of cancer, primarily because of the hormone-balancing and immune-supportive effects of lignans.

Since one out of every eight women is likely to get breast cancer in her lifetime, I recommend flaxseed as a standard preventive for every woman who is concerned about this disease.

In breast cancer research, an increasing number of studies are suggesting that a form of estrogen known as 16 alpha-hydroxyestrone (toxic estrogen) needs to be balanced out with another form called 2-hydroxyestrone to lower the risk of developing cancer. Some plant nutrients can alter this ratio in a positive way, and so can flaxseed.

In one study, researchers compared the health of women who had diets that included flaxseed and, in some cases, wheat bran as well. Researchers found that flaxseed supplementation positively increased the urinary ratio in favor of the "good estrogen" 2-hydroxyestrone,

while wheat bran had no effect. The significance of this study is that serious cancers such as those of the breast, uterus, and cervix may very well be prevented and to some degree treated with flaxseed and possibly flax oil lignan extracts.

The health of the prostate gland in men is also very much associated with essential fatty acid and hormone balance. Flaxseed, with its high lignan content, should be on the dietary list for any men who have enlarged prostates. It's a prostate-cancer preventive, and also useful as part of a comprehensive treatment for prostate cancer.

With its excellent fiber and lignan content, flaxseed has been shown to protect against colon cancer as well.

### ✍ Cholesterol and Heart Disease

You can definitely lower your cholesterol and triglycerides by adding omega-3 fatty acids to your diet—but most of the studies that show the benefits of this therapy have been done with fish and fish oils. However, some research also shows that flaxseed has a similar effect of lowering cholesterol and LDL cholesterol (the "bad" kind).

While I haven't seen flaxseed oil make dramatic improvements in the blood profiles of patients, I think long-term use of flaxseed and flaxseed oil makes sense as part of a comprehensive nutritional approach for the balancing of cholesterol. The high omega-3 fatty acids in flaxseed have natural blood-thinning properties. This helps to prevent strokes and optimizes circulation to the heart and body tissues.

### ✍ Digestive Disorders

What do irritable bowel syndrome (IBS), Crohn's disease, ulcerative colitis, and constipation all have in common? The answer—low fiber intake.

*(continued)*

Not only is flaxseed an excellent way to increase the daily fiber in your diet, it's also a way to get the soothing mucilage that can help heal an inflamed and irritated digestive tract. In addition, flaxseed "feeds" the good bacteria, which are usually deficient in people who have these digestive problems.

In fact, flaxseed oil is a tried-and-true old European treatment for constipation in children and infants. Just a teaspoonful can get the bowels moving in short order.

### Dry Skin

Dry skin, like eczema, is often a sign of essential fatty-acid deficiency—a fact that's acknowledged by most nutrition-oriented doctors. (Low thyroid is another possible contributing factor.)

If I put a patient on an essential fatty-acid supplement, such as flaxseed or flaxseed oil, his or her dry skin starts to improve.

### Eczema

Any kind of omega-3 fatty-acid supplementation, whether it comes from flaxseed or fish oil, can help treat eczema. Often, flaxseed oil alone is not enough. When parents bring their kids with eczema into my office, I always recommend increasing the fish in their diet and check for food sensitivities. When my own son began getting eczema on his cheeks, at the age of about 14 months, we increased the amount of fish in his diet and supplemented with an essential fatty-acid supplement that contained a high percentage of omega-3 fatty acids and some GLA from evening primrose. At the same time, we also cut the cheese and citrus fruit from his diet. Over the next four months, his cheeks cleared up nicely.

It's important to know that essential fatty acids take awhile to "kick in," so be patient and give them at least a few months to work.

### Energy Recovery

Athletes who train hard need extra amounts of essential fatty acids as well as many other nutrients. I recommend supplementing with flaxseed for quicker recovery from workouts. The flaxseed also helps to protect the immune system that can be weakened from exhaustive training.

### Memory Problems

The brain is 60 percent fat—and essential fatty acids are an integral component of this fat. Perhaps the most critical of these essential fatty acids is DHA, which is necessary for memory and learning. Since a certain amount of alpha linolenic acid from flaxseed is converted into DHA, this supplement can be a beneficial memory booster. Also, omega-3 fatty acids have an antiinflammatory effect, which appears to be important for brain health.

### Multiple Sclerosis

Essential fatty acid balance is one of the most important areas to focus on for people with this disease of the nervous system. People with multiple sclerosis may suffer from a multitude of symptoms that range from visual changes to muscle weakness, all related to deterioration of the tissue (the myelin sheath) that covers the nerves.

Dr. Roy Swank, a neurologist from Portland, Oregon, has proven that a diet rich in essential fatty acids and low in saturated fat is key to the successful treatment of multiple sclerosis (MS). Dr. Swank advocates that his patients with MS eat fish and supplement cod liver oil. For MS treatment, many practitioners find that flaxseed works as well as cod liver oil. Both are rich in omega-3 fatty acids.

# Food-Sensitivity Therapy

One of the most misunderstood areas in medicine today is the concept of food allergies. One problem is that people confuse the term "food allergy" with "food sensitivity." Even health practitioners occasionally use the terms interchangeably—but they're quite different.

If you have a food allergy, you'll see some pretty obvious symptoms as soon as you eat the food that's causing the allergy. Those symptoms might be an outbreak of hives, sudden difficulty breathing, or even vomiting. If you get a conventional lab test, it will probably reveal the offending food that's causing an increased immune reaction. Common food allergens, for example, are peanuts and milk, both detectable in a lab test.

But apart from these distinct food allergies, people can experience food sensitivities that involve a whole different set of reactions. Symptoms of food sensitivity may include headache, bloating, cramps, diarrhea, nausea, runny nose, skin rash, mood changes, joint pain, and many other potential symptoms. In children, just the presence of dark circles under the eyes might be a sign of food sensitivities.

Unlike food allergies, evidence of food sensitivities may not show up in conventional testing. If a doctor orders a conventional skin-scratch test or blood test, it's quite possible nothing significant will show up, even though your immune system may be having an adverse reaction to a whole range of foods. Likely, you'll feel mystified because it's obvious that when you eat that certain food, an adverse reaction occurs—even though the lab test doesn't support what seems obvious.

The fact is, food sensitivities—also known as food intolerances—often do not show up on conventional allergy tests. Some people don't exhibit reactions to certain food items until two or three days have passed.

Because the tests are so unreliable in these situations, if you don't have life-threatening reactions to foods, I wouldn't even bother with a conventional food-allergy test. There's a good chance you'll make far more progress by using the information provided in this section. In addition, many holistic doctors and natural health practitioners are skilled in dealing with food sensitivities or intolerances.

## SENSITIVITY SITUATIONS

Why do some people have these sensitivities in the first place?

There are several explanations. Usually—that is, in 80 to 90 percent of the cases—food sensitivities are "acquired." Only a small percentage appear to be genetic. If a patient is having a reaction to apples or bread, often this is a new development, something that he or she did not experience as a child.

One reason for the development of food sensitivities is that people eat the same 15 or 20 foods all the time. With so little variety in the diet, for some reason the immune system develops a sensitivity to the frequently eaten foods.

Think about your own diet. Chances are you have "standard" breakfast, lunch, and dinner meals that you eat almost every day. Even snacks are the same. Once your body begins to become sensitive to these foods—whatever the reason— that sensitivity actually increases the more you eat these foods.

Another contributing factor is that people's digestive systems tend to get weaker as they get older. The typical digestive system is subject to a wide range of weakening forces, including the Standard American Diet (SAD!), stress, medications like antibiotics—and, with some people, alcohol and smoking.

Yet another cause with some people could be a condition that many health practitioners have identified as "leaky gut syndrome." A lot of people who have leaky gut syndrome are unaware they have it or what it is—but essentially, it's a condition that leads to maldigestion and poor absorption of food in the digestive tract. Food proteins do not get broken down efficiently enough, and larger-than-normal protein molecules get absorbed across the small intestine. The immune system "sees" these larger-than-normal proteins as foreign invaders and attacks them. In this sequence of counterattack, inflammatory chemicals are released in the body, resulting in many different types of physical and mental symptoms—all adding up to food-sensitivity reactions.

## APPROACHES TO CONSIDER

If you suspect you have food sensitivities but haven't tracked down what's causing your problems, there are some logical steps you can take to identify the foods you're reacting to.

One way to find the culprits is with the elimination/reintroduction diet. Begin by eliminating the most common causes of food sensitivity. These include cow's milk, wheat, sugar, chocolate, soy, citrus fruits, and peanuts. You should eliminate all of these from your diet for one to two weeks.

At the end of the period of total sanctions, begin to introduce one food at a time every two to three days and see if you notice a reaction. Do this until you have gone through all the foods.

True, two weeks may seem like a long time if you're on such a restricted diet. However, the elimination diet is quite accurate.

As an alternative approach, I more often recommend a modified version of the elimination diet that's less stressful. I've found that the foods people crave the most are also the foods to which they're most sensitive. So you might shortcut the deprivation process if you just eliminate the foods you crave the most. If you stop having symptoms such as runny nose, headaches, or bloating while you're off those foods, then you can assume those are the ones most likely involved in causing your sensitivities.

## MORE HELP

Another technique is to see a practitioner who practices Applied Kinesiology. The practitioner touches a food to some part of your body while testing muscle strength in that area. (Typically, the area tested is the arm or shoulder.) If the muscle tests weak, it can indicate sensitivity to that food.

A more elaborate version of this method that many practitioners use is the NAET (Numbudripad Allergy Elimination Technique). This system involves the use of Applied Kinesiology to identify food and environmental sensitivities. Once that's done, the practitioner then uses chiropractic and acupressure or acupuncture to desensitize the body to the offending food.

Another popular technique that I work with is the use of electrodermal testing, also referred to as electroacupuncture testing. Developed by a German medical doctor decades ago, it involves the testing of the electrical resistance of the skin to whatever food you want tested. A current runs through the testing machine and through a probe, which touches the patient's skin. It doesn't cause any pain, but the machine picks up subtle bioelectric changes that are caused by the food.

Though electroacupuncture testing may sound like something out of a science fiction book, I've found that it works well, and at least one controlled study lends support to this type of testing. In the study, the test proved accurate and reproducible when compared against conventional tests.

Another testing resource are the laboratories that provide special blood tests for people who have food sensitivities or allergies. These blood tests measure immediate and delayed reaction to foods by measuring antibody response (IgE and IgG4).

# AVOIDANCE MECHANISMS

No matter what technique you choose to help identify your food sensitivities, there are some common ways to desensitize yourself from these foods. Here are the steps to consider:

1. Avoid the food you are being desensitized to for one to two weeks to give your immune system a break.

2. Increase the variety of foods you're eating. In fact, try to double the number of different kinds of foods you are eating regularly. This will not only help to prevent sensitivities, but will increase the spectrum of nutrients you get.

3. Take supplements that will help improve your digestive power. The better you break down foods, the less you're likely to react to them. Microbial-enzyme supplements can be taken with meals to aid your digestion. The typical adult dose is two capsules with meals. Also, a probiotic supplement (contains acidophilus and other good bacteria, as well as FOS, a type of sugar that feeds good bacteria) will help to replenish the good bacteria in your digestive tract, which aids in digestion and works to repair a "leaky gut." Herbs such as gentian root, dandelion root, and ginger also stimulate digestive function. Look for herbal digestive formulas that contain these herbs and take them with meals.

4. Take betaine HCl to increase stomach acid. I generally reserve its use for seniors (who have very low stomach acid) or those who do not respond to other digestive supplements.

5. Use constitutional hydrotherapy to strengthen the digestive system (see HYDROTHERAPY, page 260).

Beyond these treatments there are ways to specifically get desensitized to foods you react to. Homeopathic remedies can be used. For example, if you are sensitive to apples, you can take a homeopathic apple remedy that, over time, can desensitize your immune system. Look for homeopathic desensitization drops that have the name of the food on the label. Most of these remedies can be found in a health food store or obtained from a homeopathic practitioner.

If you want to explore the NAET technique of desensitizing yourself to foods, you can see a practitioner who specializes in this technique or check the Web site *www.NAET.com*. Many people have had success on the NAET program.

General strengthening of your overall health, what practitioners call "constitution," can reduce your susceptibility to food sensitivities. Homeopathy and traditional Chinese medicine are ideal ways to help strengthen the constitution. Consult with a practitioner for individualized treatment.

---

# FOOD-SENSITIVITY THERAPY
## RECOMMENDATIONS FROM THE NATURAL PHYSICIAN FOR . . .

### ∾ ADD/ADHD

Many children with behavior and attention problems show some improvement when food sensitivities are treated. For instance, it's well known that sugar aggravates Attention Deficit Disorder (ADD) and Attention Deficit Hyperactivity Disorder (ADHD) symptoms in some children.

### ∾ Allergies

I have seen many patients who thought their allergy symptoms were due to something in the environment, but their symptoms cleared up after food sensitivities were treated. Though of course other factors can contribute to allergies, you may find that environmental allergies diminish or disappear entirely when a food sensitivity is treated.

### ∾ Arthritis

Food sensitivities can cause flare ups of many types of arthritis, especially rheumatoid arthritis.

### ∾ Asthma

With cases of asthma continually on the rise, especially among children, it makes sense to look at every possible cause. Food sensitivities are often associated with this condition, especially reactions induced by milk and wheat products. Artificial sweeteners and preservatives are suspect as well.

### ∾ Autism

Reactions to wheat and milk products have been reported to cause some cases of autism. Many aspects of a child's behavior may improve when these foods are removed from the diet. Some practitioners have noted great improvements in learning, behavior, and emotional responses. Since there are no conventional treatments for autism, it's always worthwhile to try dietary changes that might have a positive impact.

### ∾ Autoimmune Conditions

Since food sensitivities affect the immune system, treating those sensitivities is just one way of taking some burden off an already-imbalanced system. Conditions such as multiple sclerosis and lupus can be helped to some degree with food-sensitivity therapy.

*(continued)*

---

### ✇ Bloating

Have you ever wondered why you sometimes feel bloated within seconds of eating certain foods? This is a food sensitivity reaction—and when you treat it, you'll probably have a lot fewer problems with bloating.

### ✇ Bronchitis

Chronic cases of bronchitis can be due to food sensitivities, especially in children. Children who have milk sensitivity are especially likely to get frequent cases of bronchitis.

### ✇ Candida

I have many patients come to my office convinced that they have yeast (candida) overgrowth in their bodies. Symptoms can include—among other things — mood swings, depression, digestive upset, weakened immune system, and skin eruptions. In many cases, their symptoms were actually due to food sensitivities and disappeared when they were given food-sensitivity therapy.

### ✇ Constipation

If you're eating lots of fiber but still suffer from constipation, it's quite possible your food sensitivities are causing the bowels to slow down. Wheat can often be one of the offending foods.

### ✇ Depression

Depression can sometimes be caused or worsened by a chemical imbalance due in part to food sensitivity. If chemical imbalance is a salient factor, it will improve if you have food-sensitivity therapy. Pay special attention to this therapy if you notice that your depression gets worse after meals (though this can also be a sign of hypoglycemia).

### ✇ Diarrhea

If you have chronic diarrhea, it could be associated with regular consumption of foods that are causing negative reactions. Children, for instance, are often sensitive to fruit juices and react by getting diarrhea. (The symptoms might go away if you dilute the fruit juice with water or try various types of juices.)

### ✇ Ear Infections

Want to increase your child's chances by at least 50 percent of never getting another ear infection? Want to break that vicious cycle of antibiotic therapy? Then identify and treat the child's food sensitivities.

Foods such as cow's milk can cause fluid buildup in the middle ear. This provides a perfect breeding ground for viruses and bacteria. Wheat, sugar, soy, and citrus fruits are also commonly involved.

### ✇ Eczema

Food sensitivities might eliminate the underlying cause of this condition (though you should also consider fatty-acid imbalances as a possible cause). Eczema is not a cortisone-cream deficiency: You're not treating the cause if you just stop the irritation and itching with an over-the-counter ointment.

### ✇ Fatigue

There can be many causes of fatigue. A comprehensive protocol should also address diet and the role of food sensitivities.

### ✇ Gallbladder Problems

Dr. Jonathan Wright, a respected holistic medical doctor, states that in his experience most cases of gallstones do not need surgery. He reports that the patients in his care often recover from gallstones if their food sensitivities are

*(continued)*

addressed. By removing certain foods from your diet, you may be able to prevent inflammation of the bile duct.

## ◌ Headache

Many people get headaches immediately after eating certain foods. My wife has that problem with tomatoes. Chronic migraine headaches can be caused by food sensitivities.

## ◌ Heartburn

Instead of popping an antacid all day long to prevent or treat heartburn, it's a good idea to look at the role of diet. Food sensitivities might be a cause. Unless you have an underlying stomach infection, foods and stress are likely causing your symptoms—which may immediately improve when you identify the culprits.

## ◌ Hemorrhoids

One of my colleagues in Portland, Oregon, Dr. Steve Gardener, has a practice devoted almost exclusively to the natural treatment of hemorrhoids. To avoid flare-ups, he says, just follow the procedures to identify your food sensitivities, then avoid the foods that are causing problems. Most common on his list are citrus fruits, tomatoes, wheat, and sugar. This agrees with my own observation of the common-problem foods.

## ◌ Hypoglycemia

Reactions to food sensitivities can cause blood-sugar changes. If you suffer from hypoglycemia, investigate the role foods can be playing.

## ◌ Immune Deficiency

Food sensitivities waste immune power. If you are prone to getting sick easily or have an illness (such as HIV or tuberculosis) that leaves you open to secondary infections, then food-sensitivity therapy is highly recommended.

## ◌ Inflammatory Bowel Disease

Crohn's disease and ulcerative colitis can be greatly helped with food-sensitivity therapy. As you cut out the offending foods, you'll probably note a sharp decrease in the variety of digestive symptoms you're experiencing. I have seen some patients become symptom-free as a result of a change in diet.

## ◌ Irritable Bowel Syndrome

This is really another name for stress, poor digestion, and food sensitivities. Dramatic improvements are generally seen when the reactive foods are identified and treated.

## ◌ Psoriasis

Many people with this condition experience improvement with food-sensitivity therapy. Although I have seen mixed results, it's worth trying.

## ◌ Schizophrenia

Dr. Abraham Hoffer, a leading authority on the natural treatment of schizophrenia, has found that food sensitivities can be a major contributor to this disease. Wheat and milk are high on the list of common food offenders.

## ◌ Sinusitis

I have found chronic sinusitis often involves wheat and/or cow's milk allergy.

## ◌ Skin Rash

Any unexplainable skin rash can be a result of food sensitivities.

## ◌ Vaginitis

Chronic cases of vaginitis can be related in part to food sensitivities. Milk and sugar are commonly involved.

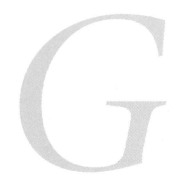

# Garlic

It isn't hard for me to believe that garlic *(Allium sativum)* is one of the best-selling supplements in North America and Europe. I would estimate that half of all my patients over the age of 50 are taking garlic supplements, whether or not I've recommended it for them. But it's actually appropriate that so many people are taking garlic supplements or eating more garlic for their health, as it's one of the most well-researched herbs in the world.

Even my grandmother is a garlic-taking advocate. As a child, she got into the habit of eating raw garlic every day, and she continues the habit to this day. She says that whenever she feels a cold or sore throat coming on, she just eats more garlic and she doesn't get sick.

To date, more than 200 human studies and at least 800 animal studies have contributed to our understanding of the effects of garlic. Many of these studies have pointed to the conclusion that garlic is a powerful aid in the fight against heart disease and cancer—so, it's natural that so many people are motivated to use this clinically proven wonder herb.

Garlic has many extraordinary attributes both as a food and supplement. Garlic's main medicinal uses are for cardiovascular protection, as it improves cholesterol levels, lowers blood pressure, inhibits blood clots, and improves circulation. In fact, it is one of the premier herbs for protection against cardiovascular disease and infectious diseases as well as cancer.

## GOOD BURN

A member of the lily family, garlic is in the same genus *(Allium)* as onion. The Latin translation of *Allium* means "hot" or "burning," and the word "garlic" translates to "spear plant." This refers to the leaves of the garlic plant that have a spearlike shape.

Garlic is a staple in the diets of many different cultures. It has long been recognized for its valuable medicinal properties. We know from Sanskrit records that are 5,000 years old that Middle Eastern people have long cultivated garlic and used it as a medicinal remedy. It was widely traded throughout the Middle East, and the Ancient Greek and Roman physicians relied on garlic to treat a host of conditions including low energy, parasites, respiratory ailments, and poor digestion. It also became an important part of traditional Chinese medicine.

In 1858, Louis Pasteur confirmed garlic's antibacterial properties. In both World Wars, soldiers relied on this herb's powerful antiseptic properties to help prevent gangrene. In fact, it was so widely used among Russian soldiers in World War II that it earned the nickname "Russian penicillin."

## GOOD CONSTITUENTS

Garlic has had many different constituents identified. Raw garlic cloves contain a high amount of a sulfur-containing compound called alliin, as well as the enzyme alliinase. When raw garlic is chewed or crushed, the alliin comes into contact with the alliinase enzyme, which forms the compound allicin. When alliinase is heated, however, it becomes inactive—so cooked garlic is not nearly so therapeutic as the raw form (although it still has some medicinal effect). Garlic also contains amino acids, vitamins, and minerals such as selenium and germanium.

Allicin is broken down in the body into other compounds, including one called diallyl disulfide. Allicin, diallyl disulfide, and other "metabolites" (the products of meteabolism) are responsible for garlic's strong smell and pungent taste as well as many of the medicinal benefits. But these series of metabolic conversions only occur when you eat raw garlic. Chopped, dried, and cooked garlic lose a lot of the valuable allicin.

If you eat raw garlic, of course, the fragrance lingers for a long time. For that reason alone, many people prefer to take garlic supplements in a form such as ground garlic powder contained in a capsule. If that's your choice, however, try to find supplements that are as close to raw garlic as possible.

Many of the supplements have enteric coating, which is a special coating that allows the tablets to go through stomach acid without being broken down. This is important because allicin is deactivated by stomach acid. The garlic powder needs to travel intact to the small intestine where the conversion to allicin occurs.

## DOSAGE

Raw garlic provides the highest medicinal properties. Not many people chew raw garlic, but if you do, the recommendation is one-half to one whole clove daily.

More commonly, garlic is used in cooking, but as I've mentioned, some of the benefits are lost when garlic is heated.

To take the more conventional route, you can find garlic supplements in supermarkets and pharmacies as well as health food stores, and they do have the distinct advantage of being odor-free. Capsules and tablets contain the ground powder, while soft gels are made up of garlic oil. Each form contains different active constituents of garlic and have various medicinal effects depending on the product.

For therapeutic purposes I recommend my patients use an odor-free, enteric-coated garlic powder supplement that is standardized to a dose between 4,000 to 5,000 micrograms of allicin (usually 600 to 900 milligrams per tablet). This is equal to the amount of one clove (4 grams) of fresh garlic. Your healthcare practitioner may recommend higher dosages depending on your body weight and condition.

## WHAT ARE THE SIDE EFFECTS?

Garlic has no known toxicity. However, some people experience digestive upset from eating garlic or taking garlic supplements. (Unfortunately, I happen to be one of them—but I'm the exception rather than the rule.)

Garlic does have natural blood-thinning effects, so you should discuss its use with your doctor if you are on blood-thinning medications such as aspirin, coumadin, and others. Also, if you are planning to have surgery, discuss your garlic use with your surgeon beforehand. He or she may advise you to cut down on the dose.

Breast-feeding mothers should be cautious about eating a lot of garlic or taking a lot of garlic supplements. Garlic can contribute to colic because it passes from the breast milk into the baby's intestinal system.

# GARLIC
## RECOMMENDATIONS FROM THE NATURAL PHYSICIAN FOR . . .

### ❧ Antimicrobial Effects

Garlic exerts a wide spectrum of antimicrobial activity against viruses, bacteria, fungi, and worms. I find that garlic usually works best to build immunity and prevent infections, rather than treating acute conditions—with the exception of respiratory tract infections like sore throat, bronchitis, and pneumonia. (A number of patients have told me that when they get an upper respiratory tract infection, they just load up on garlic and soon feel better.) Garlic is excellent on a long-term basis for those with an overgrowth of yeast in their systems and for women who have vaginal yeast infections.

People who have immune suppressive conditions such as HIV/AIDS and tuberculosis, are at serious risk of developing secondary infections from many different organisms. Garlic is one natural option to help with protection from these infectious agents.

### ❧ Aorta Elasticity Problems

Long-term use of garlic helps to protect the elasticity of the aorta. The aorta is a huge blood vessel that carries oxygenated blood out of the heart, branching out into other arteries to feed blood to the rest of the body. Stiffening of the aorta is associated with aging as well as with high blood pressure and cholesterol imbalances.

Elasticity is particularly important to help prevent an aortic aneurysm, a life-threatening event. (If the blood vessel wall weakens, losing its integrity and flexibility, there's a chance the aorta may burst.) Researchers who conducted a 1997 study of garlic's properties came to the conclusion that "garlic intake had a protective effect on the elastic properties of the aorta related to aging in humans."

### ❧ Blood Clotting

Garlic has a direct effect on the blood's clotting activities. It is known to prevent the clumping of platelets, which are cells that cause blood clotting to occur. Excessive clumping (medically termed as aggregation) is linked to cardiovascular disease because it contributes to poor circulation.

Garlic also lowers fibrinogen, a protein that is involved in blood clotting, which is also highly associated with cardiovascular disease.

### ❧ Cancer

Population studies have shown that garlic reduces the risk of cancer of the colon, esophagus, and stomach. One study looked at 41,000 American women and found that one or more servings a week of garlic was associated with a 35 percent decrease in the risk of colon cancer. It is thought that garlic's sulfur compounds are key in preventing these types of cancers by helping to control carcinogens (cancer-causing substances).

### ❧ High Blood Pressure

High blood pressure is recognized as one of the leading causes of heart disease, and garlic has been shown to have mild blood-pressure–lowering effects. Clinically, I would not rely on garlic alone to lower blood pressure. It should be used in conjunction with corrective changes in diet and lifestyle, and specific blood-pressure–lowering supplements such as hawthorn berry, ginkgo, magnesium, and calcium.

*(continued)*

### ❧ High Cholesterol

The most popular use of garlic is to protect against cardiovascular disease. Many studies have shown that garlic lowers total cholesterol, and scientists believe it does this by interfering with the manufacture of cholesterol in the liver.

Over 250 scientific studies have been published, most suggesting that garlic protects the cardiovascular system by lowering cholesterol and triglycerides, and inhibiting blood clots. In an overview of 16 prominent garlic studies, including a total of 952 people, researchers concluded that garlic lowered total cholesterol levels by 12 percent after one to three months of treatment. Eleven of the studies used dried garlic powder at a daily dosage ranging from 600 to 900 milligrams.

Garlic had a similar positive effect in the trials that looked at triglyceride levels, lowering health-threatening levels of triglycerides by as much as 13 percent, without having an adverse effect on the level of HDLs (the "good" cholesterol).

Other studies have shown that garlic can lower the LDLs ("bad" cholesterol) while also increasing HDLs. Garlic has also been shown in studies to reduce the oxidation of cholesterol, which is now recognized as a way to help control the development of heart disease.

I usually advise patients to take garlic for at least a few months. It takes at least that long, I've found, before garlic has a significant impact on cholesterol levels.

### ❧ Systemic Toxicity

Garlic is one of the best foods and supplements to use to promote detoxification. The high sulfur content helps the liver to detoxify various substances so that they can be metabolized and excreted from the body.

# Gelsemium

Tori, a 29-year-old mother who had just come down with flu, described the muscle ache as being "like someone had beaten me."

She had other symptoms as well. "I have the chills and a little diarrhea. It was hard getting out of bed to get to your office."

But she was strongly motivated to come see me. Her daughter's birthday was just two days away.

Tori's appearance wasn't promising. Her eyes looked heavy and droopy. Even in the warm examination room, she kept on her jacket to ward off the recurrent bouts of chills.

But I was glad she'd come. I didn't know whether homeopathic gelsemium would help her recover in the requisite 48 hours. But I did know, if she took it, she'd be feeling a lot better by the day of the party.

I made my recommendation and, as I requested, Tori called me the next afternoon to report how she was feeling. She said that her chills had subsided, muscles were much less achy, and her energy had improved. I was happy to find out later that she had recovered well enough to host her daughter's birthday party.

Gelsemium is the homeopathic preparation of yellow jasmine. Most homeopathic practitioners know it as a major flu remedy. It is also a top remedy for fatigue and headaches. It's also the remedy commonly recommended by naturopathic and homeopathic physicians for neurological conditions such as multiple sclerosis and tremors. Gelsemium is also the most common remedy for stage fright.

As with every homeopathic remedy, there are specific symptoms that suggest someone will readily benefit from gelsemium. People requiring gelsemium tend to exhibit four symptoms, referred to as the 4 D's: dizziness, drowsiness, droopiness, and "dumbness." The last refers to the fact that the person feels too tired to concentrate. These symptoms help you pick this remedy whether a person has the flu or a more complicated illness such as chronic fatigue syndrome.

## DOSAGE

For acute illness such as the flu, I recommend two pellets of 30C potency to be given two to four times daily. Lower potencies can also be used and may be effective with some people.

You usually don't have to take the remedy for more than two or three days. Practitioners often give one dose of a higher potency such as 200C, which is enough to help the body recover from acute illness.

For chronic health conditions such as chronic fatigue syndrome, I recommend a lower potency, such as 6C, taken one to two times daily. The pellets of this concentration can also be taken on an "as needed" basis, whenever they provide relief or improve your condition.

## WHAT ARE THE SIDE EFFECTS?

As with most homeopathic remedies, side effects are not a concern. When I recommend gelsemium for acute illnesses, I find that it either helps or there is no effect at all. I do recommend, however, that anyone with a chronic condition such as multiple sclerosis or chronic fatigue syndrome consult with a homeopathic practitioner in addition to your regular medical doctor.

Gelsemium is safe to use with children without the worry of side effects.

# GELSEMIUM
## RECOMMENDATIONS FROM THE NATURAL PHYSICIAN FOR . . .

### ❧ Anxiety

You can take gelsemium if you have anxiety caused by anticipation of a future event, such as an exam or speaking (a *very* common concern!). This is the main homeopathic remedy for stage fright, especially when the fear is so intense that it causes diarrhea. If you find you actually tremble from anxiety about an upcoming event, then this is the best remedy. It's also helpful to take if you have anxiety about an upcoming plane flight.

### ❧ Diarrhea

Gelsemium is indicated for acute illness, such as the flu, where diarrhea occurs. It is a specific remedy for diarrhea caused by anxiety.

### ❧ Fatigue

Patients who have endured chronic fatigue for months or years may recover completely if they take this remedy. The person who needs gelsemium feels apathetic, weak (especially the legs), and wants to sleep all day. If you're so tired it's hard to keep your head up, I recommend this remedy. It is also used to help recover from jet lag.

### ❧ Flu

Gelsemium is the most common remedy for the flu. If you do not know which homeopathic remedy to use, try gelsemium first. You'll probably get good results if you're feeling as if your muscles are bruised, you have a low-grade fever

with no thirst, and you have chills that run up and down your back.

### ❧ Headaches

This is an excellent remedy for the kinds of headaches that begin in the back of the head or neck and then radiate to your forehead. A unique symptom that suggests this remedy will help is if your headache improves after urinating. I also recommend taking it if your tongue and head feel heavy.

### ❧ Mononucleosis

Gelsemium is a main remedy for mononucleosis and can help you cope with all the fatigue that goes with it. This remedy works well against viral infections like mono. It is also indicated in cases where a person has had mono at one time, but never felt well since then.

### ❧ Multiple Sclerosis

Gelsemium is one of the main homeopathic medicines for multiple sclerosis. It improves the symptoms in some cases. Some people respond very well to the remedy and, in rare cases, become symptom free. It can be helpful for the neurological changes such as blurred or double vision and loss of balance.

### ❧ Vertigo

Gelsemium is helpful for vertigo, a condition in which you feel like the room is spinning around you.

# Gentian Root

"It just doesn't make sense, Dr. Mark," said Darrel, a 40-year-old business executive. "For the past two years, I've been eating an excellent diet. I rarely have junk food. I avoid fast-food restaurants and stay away from red meat and sugar. My wife prepares almost all my meals. But I still have this problem with bloating."

Darrel described how, after a meal, he always had to undo his belt and unbuckle his pants. Along with bloating and gas, Darrel sometimes got abdominal cramps that were extremely painful.

"I've seen two different gastroenterologists, and they can't find anything wrong," Darrel told me.

"How is your stress level—low, medium, or high?" I asked.

"It's low." He must have thought I looked skeptical, because he quickly added, "It really is. I had a lot of stress three to four years ago from my business, but things are great now."

Following our appointment that day, I had the lab do a comprehensive stool analysis for Darrel. We met later so we could go over the results of this and other tests.

I told him that the stool analysis showed he was not breaking down protein very effectively and he had some yeast overgrowth in his intestine. Briefly, I explained that the "overgrowth" simply meant his body—or the undigested food in his intestine—was producing an overabundance of yeast that could potentially cause health problems.

"Why didn't those other doctors find this out?" Darrel asked.

"Well, the average stool test is pretty basic. The report leaves out quite a bit, unless the doctor asks for specific tests. In your case, the test was done by a lab we often use that specializes in stool analysis. So the test was very comprehensive."

"How did I get these problems?"

"Based on your history and this test, I think the stress you experienced three to four years ago took its toll on your digestive system. You said you never had digestive problems until a few years ago, suggesting to me that the problems began earlier, during that stressful period."

I went on to explain that when your body is under stress, you have less blood flow to the digestive organs and more to the brain and muscles. There's also less nerve stimulation, which affects the organs of the digestive tract. When digestive organs don't work at peak efficiency, you don't break food down so well.

"In your case, you're not breaking down protein very well. As a result it causes the digestive symptoms you are experiencing," I concluded.

"Why am I still having problems, even though I'm not stressed anymore?" asked Darrel.

"Even though your stress level is no longer a problem, your digestive tract has not recovered. We need to get your nervous system and digestive organs back into gear again. Then we can do that with natural medicines."

"Good. What should I take?" asked Darrel.

"I get really good results with herbal medicines, particularly one called gentian root. It stimulates the digestive organs to work more effectively. It's great for stimulating the stomach to produce more hydrochloric acid, which is mainly what breaks down protein. After a couple of months of taking gentian root, your digestive organs will be retrained to work more efficiently."

"That sounds great," said Darrel. "Now, what should I do about the yeast?"

"Don't worry about that. The yeast is feeding off the byproducts of poor digestion. Once we get your digestive system working better, the yeast will die off because it will have nothing to eat."

As Darrel went on a regimen of gentian root over the next two months, he noticed that his digestive symptoms were constantly improving. He no longer had to loosen his pants after he ate. A follow-up stool analysis, four months later, showed normal levels of yeast in his stool.

## GETTING BETTER WITH BITTERS

The Bible makes several references to the health benefits of bitter herbs such as gentian root (*Gentian lutea* and related species). The plant grows wild in Europe and throughout Asia. In many cultures in these areas, people recognize the health benefits of gentian and other bitter herbs. They are used to help digest large or fatty meals, and to increase the digestive powers of the elderly or those with chronic disease. Gentian is considered to have cooling and drying qualities, which is significant to practitioners of Chinese medicine who help their patients "balance out" one body system by introducing food and herbs that have opposing qualities. (So someone with a warm constitution would benefit from the cooling effect of gentian root.)

Historically, bitters have always been taken in the form of liquid, so that one would taste the bitterness on the tongue. Gentian happens to be one of the most bitter substances known. According to Dr. Rudolf Weiss, "The bitter taste (of gentian) persists even in a dilution of 1:20,000. It is the most important of all European bitters. . . ."

It is believed that when bitter receptors on your tongue are stimulated, a reflex occurs that stimulates the vagus nerve. This nerve is known to stimulate the digestive organs to produce the enzymes necessary for digestion.

Studies have shown that gentian can also stimulate stomach function even if you don't actually put it on your tongue and taste it. This is an important issue for those who prefer to avoid the bitter taste and take gentian root in capsule form. I have used it in capsule form with good results.

One study involving 205 people found that gentian root capsules gave quick and dramatic relief of constipation, flatulence, appetite loss, vomiting, heartburn, abdominal pain, and nausea. Gentian is particularly good for improving stomach function.

## DOSAGE

The recommended dosage is 10 to 20 drops in a small amount of water (2 ounces) or 300 to 600 milligrams of the capsule form taken 5 to 15 minutes before meals. With this "lead time," the digestive juices can begin to kick in before you start eating.

I have found that gentian can still be helpful to stimulate the digestive system when taken with or shortly after meals. It can also be taken in tincture formulas that mask the bitter taste.

Gentian works well in combination with other bitter herbs such as wormwood. It also works well with scutellaria, which relaxes the nervous system and stimulates stomach function.

## WHAT ARE THE SIDE EFFECTS?

Gentian should be used with caution by those who have active ulcers, which can be aggravated by the herb.

Pregnant women and nursing mothers should also avoid it, since the effects on an unborn infant are not known.

# GENTIAN ROOT
## RECOMMENDATIONS FROM THE NATURAL PHYSICIAN FOR . . .

### ᘯ Anemia

Vitamins and minerals that are essential to your health can't be absorbed very well if your stomach acid is low. By boosting the action of your stomach acid, gentian root can help ensure that you don't suffer from some deficiencies—particularly from vitamin $B_{12}$ and folic acid—which could conceivably cause problems like fatigue, poor memory, and poor circulation.

Also, the iron that comes from food is not absorbed very efficiently when your stomach acid is low. Gentian root improves the levels of acid in the stomach.

### ᘯ Candida

Many people take drugs or supplements to kill intestinal *candida*, which is an overgrowth of yeast. While there may be initial improvement if you take this approach, many people experience relapses.

I learned many years ago that most cases of intestinal yeast overgrowth are in large part due to poor stomach and digestive function. By using gentian, and thus improving digestion and absorption, you stop the development of metabolic toxins that feed the yeast. Once their food supply is cut off, they die.

### ᘯ Constipation

Aside from not having enough dietary fiber, water, and exercise, some people suffer from constipation because the digestive organs and colon are not receiving enough nerve and hormonal stimulation, and peristalsis does not occur. Gentian root has a tonic effect on the entire digestive tract.

Also, the stimulation of bile flow from the gallbladder improves stool movement through the intestines and colon.

### ᘯ Food Allergies and Food Sensitivities

Many cases of food sensitivities are the result of poor digestion, especially due to inadequate protein breakdown. I have found that gentian is a valuable, long-term treatment for food sensitivities.

### ᘯ Headaches

Gentian is often prescribed for people who get frontal headaches, especially when the headaches are related to eating.

### ᘯ Indigestion and Irritable Bowel Syndrome

Since gentian targets all the major organs of digestion, it can be used as a tonic for many digestive complaints. Europeans often use gentian or other bitters to prevent indigestion after eating large or rich meals. It's especially helpful to have gentian along when you're having a big holiday meal.

### ᘯ Low Appetite

Interestingly, gentian has been used as an adjunctive treatment for anorexia because it stimulates appetite. It is also good to use for people with chronic illnesses who have reduced appetite because of the disease or medicine they're taking.

I have prescribed gentian root to children who had flu or pneumonia, which are infections that often cause them to lose their appetite. Their appetite soon comes back with gentian—which is important for nutritional reasons.

# Ginger Root

"I just got back from Mexico and I think I got poisoned!" said Ned, a patient of mine, over the phone.

"What do you mean?"

"For the past two days I have had watery diarrhea and now I have sore throat. I am feeling chills in my back as well. It must have been something I ate—or something in the water."

"Ah, the old Montezuma's revenge!"

Momentarily felled by the problem, Ned was staying with his sister-in-law in Los Angeles. The diarrhea was so bad that he didn't think he could make it into my La Jolla office, and asked me if I could recommend something that would be readily available.

"Have your sister-in-law pick up some fresh ginger root from the local grocery store," I suggested. "Cut a half inch and steep it in one cup of water for ten minutes." I recommended that he drink one cup of the ginger tea every couple of hours. "That should help the diarrhea and sore throat."

The next day I had another call from Ned. "Ninety percent better," he reported. "Hard to believe I was getting ready to go to the emergency room yesterday!"

From what Ned was telling me, it wouldn't be necessary to see him. But I did make a recommendation for his next trip to Mexico: "Take along some acidophilus and garlic supplements," I said, noting that it would prevent infection of the digestive tract. I didn't have to tell him to also keep some fresh ginger root on hand for just such an emergency.

## NOT JUST FOR COOKIES

For centuries, ginger *(Zingiber officinale)* has been widely valued as a medicinal herb. It is one of the most widely prescribed herbs by practitioners of Ayurvedic and Chinese traditional medicines. The botanical name for ginger is "zingiber," which, in Sanskrit, means "shaped like a horn." Technically speaking, the root is actually a rhizome, a stem that runs underneath the surface of the ground.

It's most commonly used to treat digestive disorders and arthritis in all the healing traditions. It is known as a warming herb, especially suited to people with "cold constitutions," and it's said to enhance circulation. Chinese herbalists use fresh ginger to "warm the lung and stomach."

Ginger is prescribed in Chinese medicine for the common cold, flu, coughs, vomiting, nausea and general digestive upset, and bleeding. It also reduces the toxicity of other herbs, so it's essentially an antidote to plants that might have side effects. Also, as Ned's case demonstrates, ginger can help protect an intestinal tract that has been ravaged by tainted or toxic food.

To practitioners of traditional Chinese medicine, every form of ginger root has certain distinct properties. Fresh ginger has a warming effect on the exterior of the body, while the dried ginger is apt to be recommended for warming the middle of the body.

One of the more intriguing Chinese medicine cures is quick-fried ginger, which is made by frying ginger until the surface is slightly blackened. Practitioners say this is the type that's effective for stopping bleeding and treating conditions that affect the lower abdomen.

Today, ginger is used by herbalists and physicians to treat colds, arthritis, digestive conditions, respiratory tract infections, headaches, motion sickness, and cardiovascular disease.

As with many herbs, ginger has many different active constituents. Dried ginger root contains between 1 and 4 percent volatile oils, which account for the strong taste and aroma. (The volatile oils include bisabolene, zingiberene, and zingiberol.) Two of the pungent principles—gingerol and shogaol—are believed to be responsible for a lot of the medicinal effects.

Ginger also contains proteolytic enzymes that help to digest proteins and reduce inflammation. Many commercial products are standardized to the constituent gingerol.

## DIGESTIVE POWER

Ginger has the unique ability to improve many organs that are involved with digestion. Known as an "aromatic bitter," it tonifies the intestinal muscles and stimulates the digestive organs. It also stimulates secretion of bile from the liver and gallbladder, which helps digest fats. Ginger is also a well-known carminative, meaning that it can reduce gas and bloating.

## ANTIINFLAMMATORY

Ginger acts as a natural antiinflammatory by inhibiting the release of prostaglandins and other chemicals in the body that promote inflammation and pain. Unlike nonsteroidal medications such as aspirin, it does not have the potential to damage the stomach, liver, and kidneys. For centuries, people used ginger as an antiinflammatory without knowing how or why it worked. Modern tests have now proven the herb's antiinflammatory powers.

## CIRCULATION AND CARDIOVASCULAR HEALTH

Ginger promotes cardiovascular health by making platelets (cells responsible for blood clots) less likely to clump together. This preventive action allows the blood to keep flowing smoothly and helps prevent hardening of the arteries.

Studies have shown that this protective effect is achieved by inhibiting the formation of thromboxanes, substances that promote blood clotting. Other substances in ginger promote the synthesis of prostacyclin, a component that helps prevent platelets from "aggregating" or clumping together.

Animal studies have also shown that ginger improves the pumping ability of the heart.

## DOSAGE

Fresh ginger root can be made into tea. It's also sold in capsules, tablets, and tinctures. I have found all these forms to work with patients and myself.

The tea is relaxing and works well for digestive upset, as do the capsule and tincture forms. For the treatment of inflammatory conditions, I recommend a standardized capsule to get high levels of the active constituents that reduce inflammation.

The typical capsule dosage is 500 milligrams two to four times daily. If you're taking the tincture, I recommend 20 to 30 drops two to three times daily.

## WHAT ARE THE SIDE EFFECTS?

Side effects are rare with ginger, though some people (my wife among them!) report heartburn after taking it. In the short term, pregnant women can take ginger for nausea and vomiting related to morning sickness. One to two grams appear to be safe and effective.

Ginger stimulates bile production, so some herbal experts recommend that you should avoid this herb if you have gallstones.

Although I have seen no human studies on drug interactions and ginger, it theoretically may cause a problem with blood-thinning medications such as coumadin. So check with your physician before using high doses of ginger if you are on a blood-thinning medication.

One last piece of advice you may not find in many books is that ginger root by itself may aggravate those who are very warm-blooded. If you are the type of person who gets warm and sweats easily, then long-term use of ginger is not recommended just because it can cause discomfort by making you even warmer.

## GINGER ROOT
### Recommendations from the Natural Physician for . . .

#### ❧ Arthritis

Many herbal medicine experts mention that ginger is effective in treating arthritis, but in day-to-day treatment of patients, I have not found this to be true. Ginger by itself does not usually provide substantial relief. That said, however, it can be helpful to some people as part of a comprehensive herbal formula, such as practitioners of Chinese herbal formulas have created for patients with a "cold constitution."

#### ❧ Bloating and Flatulence

Ginger is the remedy par excellence for relieving bloating and flatulence, which is the common result of what I call SAD (Standard American Diet). It reminds me of one lady who came up to me after a talk, looked around to make sure no one else was listening, and asked if there was anything I could recommend for her 36-year-old son who was having trouble with a lot of gas. It turns out this son was newly married, and his mother was worried that his flatulence would cause marital problems.

I recommended she give her son a bottle of ginger capsules to use with meals. Hopefully it rescued the young groom from some embarrassment—or possibly saved the marriage!

#### ❧ Cardiovascular Disease

Since ginger is a natural blood thinner, it promotes good circulation and therefore improves cardiovascular health. Animal studies show that it helps with the pumping action of the heart. To me, it is most beneficial as a synergestic herb—one that makes other herbs more effective rather than working by itself.

#### ❧ Diarrhea

There's a specific type of diarrhea, called "cold diarrhea" in Chinese medicine, that ginger seems to help significantly. This is the kind that gives you a case of the chills as well as loose stools. (What's called "hot diarrhea," as you might expect, is the kind where loose stools are accompanied by a feeling of feverishness.)

*(continued)*

### ❧ High Cholesterol

In animal studies, ginger has been found to lower cholesterol levels in rats. Unfortunately, it doesn't show exactly the same effect in humans. But if you're taking ginger for other conditions, there is a possibility that it could also help lower your cholesterol.

### ❧ Morning Sickness

Ginger has actually been studied as a relief for severe morning sickness. In 19 of the 27 women who took ginger for nausea and vomiting, both symptoms became less frequent within four days of treatment. The dosage of ginger-root capsules was 250 milligrams taken 4 times daily.

Since publication of the earliest studies, which were done in 1990, many conventional doctors have started to recommend ginger root for morning sickness. (My wife's obstetrician, for instance, recommends it to her patients.) However, I don't advise that women take more than one gram daily during pregnancy, and there's no reason to continue taking it after the morning sickness passes.

### ❧ Motion Sickness

Ginger has received a lot of attention for its ability to prevent and treat motion sickness. A study in 1982 revealed that ginger was superior to the drug Dramamine™ for reducing motion sickness. Not every study, since then, has supported this finding, but some excellent research done in 1994—involving 1,741 people—confirmed that ginger was indeed very effective in treating motion sickness.

The 1994 study was done with a group of people who were taking a whale-watching trip. Before boarding the boat, people were asked to take various kinds of motion-sickness remedies, ginger among them. (None of the passengers knew which remedy they were being given.) The study showed that 250 milligrams of ginger was just as powerful as the pharmaceutical medications, but without side effects such as drowsiness.

### ❧ Nausea and Vomiting

Bad food, flu, chemotherapy, and surgical treatments are just a few of the possible causes of nausea and vomiting. No matter what the cause, however, ginger has been shown to be an effective remedy.

In two studies, ginger helped reduce nausea and vomiting in patients who had just undergone surgery where they received anesthesia. (Anesthesia makes some people very nauseated.) If you are scheduled to have surgery, talk with your surgeon about taking one gram of ginger before and after surgery.

# Ginkgo Biloba

Not long ago, a 45-year-old female patient came to me for the treatment of painful feet. Shawna had seen many doctors—and none had been able to explain the problem or give her an effective treatment.

As with all patients, I talked to her at length—not just about the pain in her feet but also about her lifestyle, her everyday habits, moods, family illnesses, and many other questions that, to some other listener, might have seemed totally unrelated to the pain in her feet. I did not for a moment doubt that the pain was "real." Nor did I doubt that her doctors had done the best they could to diagnose her problem. But something had been missed along the way—obviously, since the unresolved condition continued to aggravate her and cause intense discomfort.

I was struck, however, by one remark she made almost in passing—that her feet often "felt cold." Later on, when I examined her feet, that was the first thing I noticed. She wore practical shoes and thick socks, and she had been sitting in a warm room, yet when I felt her feet they were almost literally like icicles.

But something else was wrong as well, as I discovered when I took the pulse in her feet. Normally, of course, the doctor checks the pulse in your wrist or the side of your neck, where it's strongest. That's usually sufficient, since an M.D. usually checks for pulse rate. But what I was trying to measure was the *strength* of Shawna's pulse—and when I touched the part of her ankle where the arterial blood flows close to the surface, the area where the pulse should be strongest, I felt almost nothing.

Clearly, her feet were chilly because she had a circulation problem. The flow of warming blood to these extremities was so slight that it wasn't even doing its job of warming her feet from heel to toe. Quite likely, the lack of circulation could also account for the pain.

But what could I "prescribe" that would improve her circulation? Many pharmaceuticals are available, from the powerful blood-thinning agents that are injected into heart-attack victims to common, everyday, over-the-counter aspirin, with its milder blood-thinning properties.

What I recommended Shawna, however, was a simple extract that comes from the leaf of a very ancient tree—ginkgo biloba.

She took 180 milligrams each day, in doses of 60 milligrams three times daily. We kept careful track of her progress during the next few weeks. The circulation to her feet steadily improved. The pain, as well as the chilliness, began to subside.

Shawna's feet were pain free at the end of two months. She continues taking ginkgo to this day—and has never had a recurrence of the chronic foot pain that originally brought her to my door.

What Shawna didn't realize at the time is that ginkgo biloba is one of the most all-round beneficial herbs that anyone could possibly take for his or her health. The power to cure cold feet is only one small fraction of its many powerful attributes.

## A POWER PLANT

While ginkgo may well be the most widely publicized herb to come along in the past 50 years, the history of its healing powers certainly predates its current popularity. In fact, the Chinese have known about it and have used it for over 3,500 years.

Ginkgo ranks among the top five herbs that I prescribe to patients on a daily basis. Millions of people around the world use ginkgo every day. In countries such as Germany and France, where doctors are accustomed to writing herbal prescriptions, ginkgo is among the most commonly prescribed medicines. European doctors use it to treat a wide range of conditions—from memory impairment, dizziness, and ringing in the ears (tinnitus) to headaches and depression. There are even more uses—as Shawna discovered—such as a blood mover for improved circulation.

If ginkgo trees could speak for themselves, some would give first-person accounts of Aztecs, Vikings, and the Battle of Hastings, since the grandparents of the species have lived as long as 1,000 years. Some reach a height of 120 feet, with a girth of 48 inches. Apart from longevity, ginkgoes boast venerable ancestors.

Fossil records show that the ginkgo is the world's oldest living species of tree. It's very hardy, able to thrive in extreme heat and cold, and to withstand the sinus-hammering pollution of downtown Los Angeles or New York. It's also almost pest-proof: There doesn't seem to be an insect that can do serious damage to this hardy tree.

The leaves, the source of ginkgo medicinals, are fan-shaped and bilobed, resembling the maidenhair fern. The resemblance is so close, it's sometimes called the "maidenhair tree."

## TURNING OVER AN OLD LEAF

Researchers in the 1950s, having heard of the medicinal powers of ginkgo leaves, began mashing and distilling the components in search of the so-called active ingredients—that is, the chemical compounds that seemed to have potential healing power. What are believed to be the key medicinal ingredients have now been identified. I know it would be rash to say these are *all* the active, healing constituents—certainly more will be discovered—but at least we're starting to understand how some of the ginkgo-leaf ingredients make important contributions to improved health.

While the active constituents are important, however, I remind people that it's best to use the whole herb rather than focus on one ingredient or component.

Studies have shown that the whole herb plus standardized active constituents are more effective than just using the isolated active constituents.

The two groups of active components include flavone glycosides and terpene lactones. Quality ginkgo products are "standardized" to 24% flavone glycosides and 6% terpene lactones—which is a virtual guarantee that the products contain at least these proportions of those particular ingredients. Such products have the same proportion of these ingredients as the extract that's used in clinical studies.

## POTENT CELL PROTECTOR

Flavone glycosides are types of bioflavonoids, the plant-based compounds that are found in oranges and other fruits and vegetables. With bioflavonoids, ginkgo has been blessed with the potent powers of an antioxidant. That means if you take ginkgo, you're less likely to suffer the cellular damage caused by free radicals—unstable molecules that are a result of metabolic activities in the body and environmental pollution.

Many researchers believe that ginkgo produces more antioxidant activity than many of the better-known vitamin antioxidants such as C, E, and beta carotene. Several studies have demonstrated that ginkgo exerts antioxidant activity in the brain, eyes, and cardiovascular system. This could easily explain why ginkgo seems to be effective in the prevention and treatment of diseases that affect those parts of the body—including Alzheimer's disease, strokes, cataracts, macular degeneration, and diabetic retinopathy.

Ginkgo bioflavonoids also protect blood vessels by strengthening and reducing inflammation of their elastic walls. So that's an additional benefit of this herb—significant in helping to relieve varicose veins and reverse the effects of cardiovascular disease.

## KEEPING UP CIRCULATION

In addition to the bioflavonoids, ginkgo has another component, unique to this plant. A family of terpene lactones—specifically called ginkgolides and bilobalides—give ginkgo an extraordinary ability to increase circulation to the brain and extremities. The substances cause the blood vessel walls to relax and dilate, which permits increased blood flow. They also have what's called a "tonifying effect" on the venous system, allowing for the more efficient return of blood to the heart.

Ginkgo also has a natural blood-thinning effect. It helps to prevent blood platelets from sticking together—and platelets are the cells that form blood clots.

The way ginkgo improves circulation is particularly impressive. In one study where researchers measured the blood flow through capillaries in healthy adults, they found a 57 percent increase in blood flow among those who were regularly taking ginkgo. This finding is particularly important to seniors. As we age, we're more likely to have blockages in the blood flow that reaches the brain and other parts of the bodies. These problems are directly attributable to plaque buildup in the arteries. Ginkgo acts as sort of a bypass mechanism, helping the blood make its way through partially clogged arteries.

## NERVE RENEWAL

The ginkgolides also help protect nerve cells from being damaged. This is important for people who are recovering from a stroke. In addition, some ongoing research will probably show whether ginkgo has the benefits that it's reputed to possess for people who are recovering from brain trauma. What's certain is that nerve cells need the kind of protection that ginkgo provides—particularly people (such as those with diabetes) who have problems with neuropathy (nerve disorder).

## DOSAGE

As a standard dosage, I recommend a ginkgo extract standardized to 24% flavone glycosides and 6% terpene lactones. Dosages used in studies range from 120 milligrams to 360 milligrams daily. Most of my patients take 60 milligrams two to four times daily, for a daily total of 120 to 240 milligrams. The vast majority report beneficial results.

For severe cases, like early-stage Alzheimer's disease, I recommend that people take 240 to 360 milligrams daily.

If you start to take ginkgo for a particular condition or for general health, I suggest you continue taking it for at least eight weeks to assess its therapeutic effect. Most of my patients who take it to improve their memory or help their circulation (like Shawna, the woman who came to me with foot pain) notice the beginnings of improvements within about a month.

Ginkgo supplements are available in capsule, tablet, and tincture form.

# WHAT ARE THE SIDE EFFECTS?

Doctors, researchers, and practitioners have noted very few adverse effects among people who take ginkgo. A small number—less than 1 percent of those who take it—have reported mild digestive upset.

Other rare side effects mentioned in the literature include headaches and dizziness. I've had very few patients who complained of these problems, and in those few cases, the side effects disappeared when I lowered the dosage.

One warning, however. If you're taking a blood-thinning medication such as coumadin or aspirin, be sure to notify your doctor. These medications, like ginkgo, have a blood-thinning effect—and the cumulative doses might be more than you need. Your doctor can monitor how well your blood is clotting through regular blood work, by taking blood samples and testing them in the lab.

---

## GINKGO BILOBA
### RECOMMENDATIONS FROM THE NATURAL PHYSICIAN FOR . . .

**∾ Attention Deficit Disorder (ADD)**

Although I have not seen any studies on ginkgo and Attention Deficit Disorder, I have had parents tell me that it helps their children with concentration and memory with schoolwork. These are specifically children with memory and concentration problems—*not* hyperactivity.

**∾ Alzheimer's Disease**

Ginkgo has shown to be of benefit in cases of senility and Alzheimer's disease. In fact, it has been approved for the treatment of Alzheimer's disease by the German government. While it's not a cure—none exists—ginkgo has been shown effective in delaying the mental deterioration that often occurs rapidly in the early stage of the disease.

A study done in 1994, involving 40 patients who had early-stage Alzheimer's disease, demonstrated that 240 milligrams of gingko biloba extract taken daily for 3 months produced measurable improvements in memory, attention, and mood.

Most of the patients I see do not have Alzheimer's, but they experience a general decline in short-term memory and concentration. Ginkgo is at the top of the list for safe and effective supplements I recommend. Plus, it is not overly expensive—about $12 to $16 per month at the dosage I recommend—so you won't break the bank if you take it regularly.

**∾ Circulatory Diseases**

Ginkgo is one of the best medicines in the world for improving circulation to the hands and feet. For this reason it's an effective treatment for intermittent claudication.

People who have intermittent claudication—which is really a circulatory problem—experience pain and severe cramping in the lower legs,

*(continued)*

particularly while walking. This condition is particularly prevalent among the elderly. Many clinical studies have shown ginkgo can help alleviate the condition in 3 to 6 months if you take daily dosages of 120 to 160 milligrams.

Ginkgo has also been shown to improve the condition of people who have Raynaud's disease, a condition where the hands or feet instantly turn blue if you just reach for something in the freezer or step outside on a cold day. (For some reason, women are much more likely than men to suffer from this condition.) Again, the problem is circulatory. I have frequently recommended ginkgo—and achieved positive results—when patients were bothered by cold hands and feet.

Finally, people with diabetes are particularly prone to have poor circulation in their extremities. Supplementing with ginkgo is certainly beneficial.

### ❧ Depression

Ginkgo is an effective natural antidepressant when the depression is related to poor blood flow to the brain. When blood flow improves, more oxygen and nutrients naturally reach the brain cells as well as extremities.

Ginkgo also improves the activity of neurotransmitters, the brain's chemical messengers. A study of elderly patients who took doses of 240 milligrams of ginkgo extract daily showed that many experienced significant improvements in mood after only 4 weeks. The improvements were even more dramatic after 8 weeks of taking the same concentration of extract.

### ❧ High Blood Pressure

Ginkgo is one of the main herbs I recommend to patients who have hypertension or high blood pressure. It helps to relax the artery walls, thus reducing pressure within the blood vessels. A typical dosage would be 120 to 180 milligrams daily.

### ❧ Impotence

Impotence occurs in the vast majority of cases because there's poor circulation to erectile tissue. Instead of recommending Viagra® to patients with impotence problems, I usually start with a prescription of ginkgo biloba (and sometimes some ginseng as well). Ginkgo works very well, is much less expensive, and doesn't have any side effects—unlike Viagra®.

Because ginkgo improves penile blood flow, it provides the physiological basis for an erection. In one study, 50 percent of patients treated for impotence using 60 milligrams of ginkgo per day regained potency.

I generally recommend 180 to 240 milligrams of ginkgo in the treatment of impotence. If ginkgo doesn't help, I'll have the patient tested for the hormones DHEA and testosterone. If these hormones are deficient, I'll recommend they be used in therapeutic dosages.

### ❧ Memory Loss

Even if you don't remember things so well as you used to, the awareness of memory loss is not a signal of oncoming Alzheimer's disease or senility. Memory loss is quite common—and understandable, given the fact that we do tend to lose some memory capacity as we age and that we are quite susceptible to distractions.

"Cerebral vascular insufficiency" is a phrase that's often used to describe poor blood flow to the brain. Often, the problem gets worse as people get older because people gradually experience atherosclerosis—hardening of the arteries—which sharply decreases the efficiency of blood flow. Simply put, when the brain doesn't get enough oxygenated, nourishing blood, we're more likely to have memory loss. (Depression, as noted, can also be related to restricted blood flow.) Given its power to improve blood flow, ginkgo biloba is the

*(continued)*

treatment of choice. Once the brain cells get the oxygen and blood sugar needed to help them function properly, memory improves. Clinical studies have confirmed that significant change can occur as rapidly as 8 to 12 weeks.

### Premenstrual Syndrome (PMS)

For women who experience cramping, pain, and breast tenderness around the time of their periods, ginkgo may also provide some benefits. I have been surprised to learn that these typical symptoms of PMS might respond to gingko. Studies have shown that ginkgo can be helpful in alleviating breast tenderness and fluid retention.

### Radiation Effects

After the Chernobyl nuclear accident in 1986, Russian scientists tried a wide variety of treatments to help workers and residents who had been exposed to radiation. Researchers discovered that ginkgo helped combat the effects of radiation. It was found to be a potent agent in fighting free-radical damage to the cells, providing the same antioxidant benefits that help protect normal body cells from the effects of rapid aging.

### Ringing in the Ears (Tinnitus)

Studies have been done to test the effectiveness of ginkgo in relieving the condition known as tinnitus, which is simply ringing in the ears. Results have been mixed. I feel it is worth trying if there's the possibility that tinnitus is the result of poor circulation. Sometimes the condition is related to the fact that insufficient blood is reaching the inner ear. In other cases, however, tinnitus occurs when people are exposed to excessive noise—and in those cases, ginkgo doesn't seem to help very much.

Ginkgo can be helpful if you've had acute hearing loss as a result of pressure changes or sound trauma. Even if you don't know the factors that have contributed to loss of hearing, taking this herb might produce some positive effects.

### Stroke

Ginkgo is valuable both in the immediate treatment of stroke and in helping stroke victims during the months or years of recovery. One of the keys to the prevention of stroke is keeping the blood thin. Again, the objective is to improve circulation so sufficient blood gets to the brain. New research is also showing that therapeutic doses of antioxidants may be an important treatment for strokes. As I mentioned, ginkgo provides antioxidant activity as well.

Many doctors who are oriented toward holistic medicine—treatment of the whole patient rather than a single "problem"—often recommend ginkgo to people who are particularly susceptible to a stroke. Among those who need to take special care are anyone with a personal or family history of high blood pressure, atherosclerosis, diabetes—particularly if you're a smoker or if you've had a previous stroke. But remember: Many doctors prescribe pharmaceutical blood-thinning medications after a stroke, so if you're taking one of these, you need to talk to your doctor and have some blood work done before you start taking ginkgo, too.

### Vision

Ginkgo is also useful in the prevention and treatment of macular degeneration and diabetic retinopathy. If left untreated, both conditions can result in blindness. Macular degeneration, often associated with age, is the result of nerve degeneration in the particularly sensitive light-receptor cells of the eye. Diabetic retinopathy is a serious eye disease that can lead to blindness.

Ginkgo has been shown to be helpful in both conditions. I also recommend ginkgo as part of a natural treatment for cataracts.

**218**

# Ginseng

"I have been taking ginseng for about two months. Shouldn't my energy be better by now?"

An electrician who was used to working long hours on an irregular schedule, Will had been taking regular doses from a bottle of ginseng that his wife picked up at the pharmacy. Both of them had read that ginseng was a good energy booster, and Will was expecting to see some improvement.

"It depends on a few things," I replied. "We have to figure out what was causing your low energy. But I'll also need to know what kind of ginseng you're using, and the quality of the ginseng product."

Will had the bottle with him. I glanced at the label, then set it aside while I got a more thorough history. I also ordered some blood work.

Later, I returned to the subject of ginseng.

"I'll bet you've been feeling more irritable and restless since you've been taking the ginseng from that bottle," I speculated.

"That's true!" Will looked startled. "How did you know?"

"You have been taking Chinese ginseng, also called *Panax* ginseng. This can be quite a warming and stimulating herb. You told me that you get warm and sweat very easily. Based on your constitution, Chinese ginseng is not very compatible. It is too warming and stimulating for you and I would have expected that it would aggravate your symptoms."

Like many people who buy off-the-shelf ginseng, Will's wife had no idea there were different types of ginseng, and of course she didn't have a clue what would be best for her husband.

I briefly described the characteristics of each of the most common kinds—Chinese, Siberian, and American.

"You would do much better on Siberian or American ginseng instead of Chinese," I told him. "Because you are so physically active and warm, I am going to recommend the American ginseng."

Two weeks later, Will reported that the switch to American ginseng had the desired effect. He had noticed a distinct improvement in his energy level.

I recommended that he stay on a regular dose as long as it produced the desired effects—improving his energy levels and decreasing the effects of stress at work—and he continued to do so.

# HUMMING WITH GINSENG

Fatigue and stress are universal health problems, and ginseng has a well-earned reputation for addressing both. But the situation with my patient Will is quite typical of what happens when people don't know which kind of ginseng to select.

All varieties are what we call "adaptogens," herbs that essentially help the body to adapt to changes in environment and resist the effects of stress. This term was first used by two Russian scientists to describe the effects of Chinese ginseng and later to its relative, Siberian ginseng. Here's how these adaptogens can help your body cope with the effects of stress and also help with energy production—each in its own, unique way.

## ∾ *Chinese Ginseng (Panax ginseng)*

The Chinese translation for ginseng is "root of man," and the root of this plant is what's used to make the herbal medicines that are so widely used throughout China and Southeast Asia. The "grandparent of ginsengs," and possibly the most well-known herb in the world, is *Panax* ginseng. This comes in two types: "white" and "red." White ginseng is the dried root, and is more cooling and less stimulating than the more potent form of red ginseng, which is steamed and cured (dried over a fire or in the sun). These types of *Panax* have had numerous common names including Asian ginseng, Korean ginseng, Red ginseng, and Ren-Shen.

The word *Panax* is Latin for "panacea"—appropriately enough, as this type of ginseng is highly revered by the Chinese for its health-enhancing effects. The *Panax* variety used to grow wild in China, Japan, Korea, and the eastern portion of Russia; now it's widely cultivated for commercial use in Asia, the United States, and Canada.

Chinese herbalists will tell you that the root of the wild plant is more potent than the cultivated kind. But wild ginseng is now so rare that you'd have to travel to China or Korea on a wild-root-chase to find it—and you'd probably end up paying thousands of dollars if you tried to buy the real thing. In my experience, the commercially grown varieties work fine, as long as the herbal preparations are taken appropriately.

*Panax* ginseng has been used for over 5,000 years in traditional Chinese medicine. Historically the elderly seized upon it as a rejuvenating tonic. Among its "tonic" effects, *Panax* improves sexual function, increases energy and vitality, helps speed the recovery from illness, and even slows the aging process.

In the not-so-distant past, traditional Chinese herbalists wouldn't even prescribe ginseng for younger people. They recommended "saving" this potent medicine for the elderly. Today, however, *Panax* ginseng is prescribed by Chinese herbalists for anyone who suffers from shock or collapse, heart palpitations, insomnia, or forgetfulness. It's also used to strengthen the lungs —particularly for people with asthma, for improving digestive function, and for combating diabetes. (While it can help Type 1 or Type 2 diabetes, I mainly recommend it for Type 2.)

The exact mechanism of how Chinese ginseng works is not completely understood. Animal and human studies have shown that it supports and strengthens the function of the adrenal glands. These are sometimes called stress glands because they produce stress hormones that enable the body to respond to stress, danger, or threats.

*Panax* ginseng has a balancing effect on the stress hormones, and it improves the cells' ability to "burn" oxygen as fuel, thus improving energy production and enhancing physical performance. In addition, it helps muscles utilize glycogen, which is the "stored" form of blood sugar or glucose.

A group of compounds known as ginsenosides are thought to be responsible for many of the therapeutic effects of Chinese ginseng. The ginsenosides Rg1 and Rb1 have been most intensively studied. Rg1 has been shown to stimulate brain and central nervous system activity, allowing increased energy and

## Good Roots for Athletes

All three types of ginsengs can be used to enhance athletic performance, but Chinese and Siberian ginsengs have produced the best results in research tests.

Chinese ginseng has been shown to increase endurance and quicken recovery time after workouts. A placebo-controlled, double-blind, 20-week trial with male athletes supplementing 200 milligrams of a standardized Chinese ginseng extract found that it increased performance significantly.

In a study of Siberian ginseng, 12 male athletes were given either the herb or a placebo. Athletes who took Siberian ginseng showed a 23.3 percent increase in total exercise duration and stamina as compared with only 7.5 percent among those who were taking a placebo. Athletes who take Siberian ginseng generally notice improved performance and quicker recovery from workouts and competition.

improved intellectual performance. Rb1 has been shown to relax brain activity and lower blood pressure. So, these two constituents represent both sides of the "adaptogenic" properties of Asian ginseng.

Other ginsenosides, as well as polyacetylenes and polysaccharides, activate the immune system and also prompt anticancer activity. Undoubtedly, other active constituents of ginseng are still to be discovered.

Today, Chinese ginseng is commonly recommended for fatigue, immune enhancement, improved mental alertness, cardiovascular disease, and diabetes. It also serves as a sexual tonic, an athletic-performance enhancer, and a "soother" that helps fight stress. Holistic doctors also recommend it to lower high cholesterol, provide support for the immune system if someone is undergoing chemotherapy and radiation, and for the control of anxiety and depression.

Although there have been at least 400 published studies on Chinese ginseng, the vast majority of experimental work was done on rats. However, researchers are beginning to undertake more human studies.

## ∿ Siberian Ginseng (Eleutherococcus senticosus)

When it was reported that a Russian Olympic athlete had taken supplements of Siberian ginseng to improve his endurance and speed his recovery from training, many athletes from other countries took notice. This type of ginseng—or eleuthero, as it's sometimes called—is hardly a novelty. It has long been used by the Siberian people to enhance their quality of life and to reduce their susceptibility to infections.

Though this isn't the same species as Chinese ginseng, it's popular in many of the same countries where *Panax* is used, including northern Korea and Japan. It's been used for over 2,000 years in China as a tonic for energy and vitality, as well as to prevent respiratory tract infections, cold, and flu.

The Russian medical doctor I. I. Brekhman, the researcher who coined the word "adaptogen," completed many studies of the medicinal effects of Siberian ginseng—paralleling his investigations of *Panax*—in the 1940s and 1950s. He was interested in eleuthero because he could see that its properties were similar to those of *Panax*, though the Siberian variety is more economical to grow commercially. Intensive research continued on Siberian ginseng for the next 30 years.

Eleuthero appears to be the perfect adaptogen. In addition to being a favorite with many athletes, it has also been used by Russian cosmonauts to improve energy and help adapt to their new environment—and by many other Russian workers who appreciate its energizing powers. Interestingly, after the Chernobyl accident, many Russians within range of the fallout area were given Siberian ginseng to counteract the effects of radiation.

While there have been over 1,000 studies on *Eleutherococcus,* most are in Russian. As with *Panax* ginseng, Siberian ginseng seems to support adrenal gland function and oxygen utilization by the cells. Though Brekhman and other researchers have identified similar healing properties in both the Chinese and Siberian forms, the known active constituents of Siberian ginseng are completely different from those found in Chinese ginseng. The active constituents of Siberian ginseng that have received the most attention are a group of saponins known as eleutherosides.

While there are many different eleutherosides, the forms known as B and E have received the most attention. Siberian ginseng also contains polysaccharides, which are believed to help support immune function.

One of the nice things about Siberian ginseng is that it has a neutral temperature—that is, taking it doesn't necessarily make you warmer or chillier. It seems to be well tolerated by many people, and it can be taken for extended periods of time.

## ✑ *American Ginseng (Panax quinquefolius)*

In contrast to Siberian ginseng, which has a neutral temperature, and Chinese ginseng, which is warming and more stimulating, the species known as American ginseng is a cooling herb.

*Panax quinquefolius*—the genus and species name of American ginseng— translates as "five-leafed *Panax*." Indigenous to North America, it grows wild in forests of northern and central United States, as well as parts of Canada. It is also commercially grown in the United States, China, and France. Historically, Native Americans such as the Iroquois and Cherokee used American ginseng for a wide variety of medicinal purposes. They used it to treat fevers, improve digestion, heal wounds, and ease menstrual problems. It was also used to relieve shortness of breath.

American ginseng was imported by China in the 1700s and became a highly esteemed herb in the vast formulary of Chinese botanical medicines. Today, most American ginseng still travels from the United States to China, though a small amount is raised in Southeast Asia. Despite the lively export business, it wasn't until lately that the healing benefits of American ginseng were recognized on its home continent.

Chinese doctors value the herb because it's more cooling than Chinese ginseng and can be applied to more health conditions. During hot summer weather, Chinese physicians prescribe it regularly as a cooling tonic.

Despite the differences between American and Chinese ginseng, there are some striking similarities as well. Their appearance is similar, American ginseng being a smaller-looking version of the Chinese root. Also, both these ginsengs need to mature for four years before the roots are ready to be harvested. (Chinese ginseng is best between the fourth and sixth years.)

Both the American and Chinese versions contain similar, active constituents—namely, ginsenosides, which support adrenal gland function. However, the ratio and types of ginsenosides are different. American ginseng contains much more of the Rb1 group, which are less stimulating than the Rg1 group found in Chinese ginseng. The Rb1 ginsenosides in American ginseng are believed to give off nerve-relaxing, antiinflammatory, antifatigue, fever-reducing, blood-pressure–lowering, pain-relieving, and digestive-tonic properties.

When I recommend either herb to patients, it's often for similar health problems. Both can decrease the effects of stress, and both types of herb help to support the immune system. But because it contains more Rb1 ginsenosides, American ginseng is considered to be the superior herb for treating digestive problems, especially ulcers. It is much better suited for the person who gets warm easily, is "uptight," but not suffering from burnout. Chinese ginseng, by contrast, is preferred for people who are chilly, totally exhausted and depleted, and feeling burned out.

Siberian ginseng is somewhere in the middle, just as its temperature is in the middle range between Chinese and American. Siberian ginseng is for people who are still fairly healthy and need extra support to help combat the effects of stress, athletes being a prime example.

## DOSAGE

### ∾ *Chinese Ginseng*

I recommend using a product that is standardized between 4% to 7% ginsenosides. The dose is 100 milligrams two to three times daily.

Be sure to check the label of any product you purchase. On the standardized extract label it will say *Panax* ginseng C. A. Meyer. This refers to a specific type of Chinese ginseng and the one used in most studies. It was named by C. A. Meyer in 1843 to differentiate it from other ginsengs native to China and North America.

If you can't find the standardized version, I recommend consulting with a reputable Chinese herbalist to make sure you get a quality product and take the proper dosage. *Panax* ginseng, like the other ginsengs, is typically taken for 3 weeks straight. Some herbalists recommend taking a break every 4 to 8 weeks before resuming its use.

### ∾ *Siberian Ginseng*

In most studies where Siberian ginseng has been proven effective, people take 8 to 10 milliliters of an alcohol extract two to three times daily.

I have also seen good results with a standardized capsule extract containing 0.4% eleutherosides at a dosage of 300 milligrams taken two to three times daily. For long-term use, I typically have people take Siberian ginseng for 4 weeks before taking a week off. You can repeat this cycle as often as necessary, as long as you continue to get benefits from the ginseng.

### ∾ *American Ginseng*

There is currently no ideal standardization recommended by researchers or herbalists. In my experience, the most effective dosage is 1,000 to 2,000 milligrams daily of the capsule or 30 to 60 drops (1 to 2 milliliters) of the tincture taken two to three times daily.

## WHAT ARE THE SIDE EFFECTS?

### ∾ *Chinese Ginseng*

If you overdose on Chinese ginseng, you may detect symptoms of anxiety and insomnia, as I've witnessed with a few patients. Also, be cautious with this herbal remedy if you have high blood pressure.

Women should not take Chinese ginseng during pregnancy unless they're under the guidance of a practitioner of Asian medicine. (Sometimes, it's helpful to a woman in pregnancy, but its use needs to be monitored by a practitioner.).

I recommend staying away from any other stimulants, including caffeine, when you're taking Chinese ginseng.

Women who have heavy menstrual flow or fibrocystic breast syndrome should avoid this herb unless they have the guidance of a practitioner of Asian medicine.

It is best to not take *Panax* ginseng before bedtime.

## ❧ Siberian Ginseng

People rarely have side effects from Siberian ginseng, though I've had patients who have trouble sleeping when they take it just before bedtime.

The German Commission E says people with high blood pressure should not use this herb. (I don't agree, since I've seen studies showing that Siberian ginseng can reduce high blood pressure.)

In general, I would caution against taking Siberian ginseng before bedtime, and I recommend that it should be avoided during pregnancy.

## ❧ American Ginseng

Side effects to American ginseng are uncommon. Similar to the other ginsengs, some people who are sensitive may notice too much stimulation and require a lower dosage—so I recommend that people avoid taking it before bedtime.

At least one study has demonstrated that American ginseng may lower blood-sugar levels, and the authors of that study concluded that people should take it with meals. This would make even more sense for people with diabetes—but if you have diabetes, be sure your doctor knows you're taking it.

Like the other ginsengs, the American variety should not be taken during pregnancy unless you're under the care of a doctor or practitioner who knows how and when to recommend it.

---

# GINSENG
## RECOMMENDATIONS FROM THE NATURAL PHYSICIAN FOR . . .

### ❧ Aging

Nothing can stop aging, of course, nor is it a "health problem" like arthritis or diabetes. Nevertheless, there are certain herbs with adaptogenic qualities that can be reasonably classified as "anti-aging herbs"—and two types of ginsengs are among the best. Studies show that the Siberian and *Panax* ginseng have a balancing effect on stress hormones. Prolonged, high levels of hormone such as cortisol have been shown to accelerate aging as do the relative

deficiency of hormones such as DHEA. Balancing of these hormones with ginseng is a safe way to slow down the aging process.

In addition, all three types of ginseng have been shown to have good antioxidant activity, which is also thought to slow the aging of cells. (The ginsenosides in Chinese and American ginseng are particularly effective.)

The ginsengs have proven themselves to restore vitality. Of course, vitality is a subjective feeling that is hard to quantify with lab tests,

*(continued)*

but in controlled clinical trials, people taking ginseng (without their knowledge) reported feeling more vital and full of energy than people who were taking a placebo. There are also ways to measure energy in terms of physical response. In one trial with 49 elderly people, the results demonstrated that 1,500 milligrams of *Panax* (red) ginseng improved coordination and reaction time as well as increased alertness and more energy.

### ✎ Asthma

American ginseng is a good tonifying herb for the lungs and benefits some people with asthma and allergies. It is best used under the guidance of a natural healthcare practitioner.

### ✎ Cancer

Ginseng may have protective effects against cancer. One Korean study found that those taking *Panax* ginseng had approximately half the risk of cancer as those in the control group who did not take it. They found that the preventive effects seemed to apply to all types of cancer, not just one kind.

In a study of one type of ginsenoside, researchers showed that this component of ginseng had a suppressive effect on the growth of prostate cancer cells.

Another study compared the effects of American ginseng and estrogen on breast cancer cells. Estrogen was shown to increase the proliferation phase of cancer cell formation while American ginseng decreased the cell proliferation phase and had no adverse effect on breast cancer cells.

Russian and German cancer clinics commonly use Siberian ginseng to reduce the side effects of chemotherapy and radiation and to improve immune function. One Russian clinic studied the effects of Siberian ginseng on 80 women undergoing chemotherapy and radiation treat-

ment for breast cancer. Half of the women received Siberian ginseng and the others received no additional treatment. Women who took the Siberian ginseng had a significant reduction in side effects.

Natural healthcare practitioners often report benefit in people receiving chemotherapy treatment and Siberian ginseng. Apparently, the ginseng helps to normalize the ratio of white blood cells in the body.

Much more research needs to be done in this area, but ginseng should at least be considered for the complementary treatment of cancer, and certainly to help protect anyone who's receiving chemotherapy and radiation treatments.

### ✎ Diabetes

A study done by the University of Toronto in early 2000 found that American ginseng reduced blood-sugar levels in people with Type 2 diabetes. It was also found that ginseng significantly reduced blood-sugar levels when taken 40 minutes before patients with diabetes were injected with a glucose solution— but not when the ginseng was taken at the same time as the injection. If you have diabetes, and your doctor is in agreement, I recommend taking ginseng 40 minutes before your meals.

Chinese ginseng is also used in formulas to treat diabetes.

### ✎ Fatigue

Historically, as I've mentioned, Chinese ginseng was used to help improve fatigue and restore vitality to those who were chronically tired, especially the elderly. Different studies have shown that the various ginsengs can improve fatigue, presumably through their benign action on the adrenal glands. When your adrenal glands function more efficiently, your body uses

*(continued)*

oxygen and stores energy more effectively. The result is increased energy.

I've found that the ginsengs can be helpful to restore energy levels, though that doesn't mean it's fast-acting. In people who have chronic fatigue, it can take weeks before improvement begins to show. But by strengthening adrenal gland function with ginseng, people with chronic fatigue are less likely to suffer relapses.

### ❧ Heart Failure

In one Chinese study, doctors looked at the effects of Chinese ginseng on heart function. Selecting 45 patients who had suffered heart failure, doctors gave one group the heart drug digoxin, a second group was given Chinese ginseng, and the third received Chinese ginseng plus digoxin. (None of the groups, of course, knew which treatments they were actually getting.)

The most significant improvements occurred in groups two and three. The combination of Chinese ginseng and digoxin had the best results of all. The authors of the study stated that this drug–herb combination was safe and effective.

### ❧ Immune System Problems

German research has shown that Siberian ginseng increases immune function, particularly the activity of lymphocytes, the bodies that combat infection. Chinese ginseng has also been shown to improve immune function.

### ❧ Memory Problems

A few human studies show that Siberian and Chinese ginsengs improve mental function, including both memory and concentration. It is now accepted that high, prolonged levels of the stress-hormone cortisol destroy brain cells and can cause memory problems, and it's possible that additional stress even contributes to the development of Alzheimer's disease.

It's quite possible that ginseng, with its hormone-balancing, stress-reducing effect, also improves mental function. Perhaps memory and concentration improvements might be the result of better circulation and increased brain oxygenation, which is another benefit of ginseng.

### ❧ Menopause Symptoms

When a woman enters menopause, her adrenal glands help to produce the hormones that no longer come from the ovaries. Siberian ginseng can be helpful in relieving menopause symptoms such as fatigue and depression, and American ginseng is even better because it has cooling properties.

I have seen some commercial menopause formulas that contain Chinese ginseng. In my view, this is not a good choice if a woman is experiencing problems with menopausal hot flashes, since the Chinese form is likely to make the hot flashes more severe rather than milder.

### ❧ Reduced Libido

I have not seen any good human studies of lowered sexual desire, but my patients report that they've gotten some benefits, especially from Chinese and Siberian ginsengs. The Chinese species can be helpful for both men and women. The Siberian, in my view, mainly helps men.

Herbs such as the ginsengs and tribulus (puncture vine) are a good first line of treatment for people with low libido, and I'd certainly recommend any of these before resorting to hormone replacement.

In younger males, Chinese ginseng can sometimes be too stimulating and the sex drive actually increases to the point of excess. The Chinese who are familiar with traditional treatments have great respect for the ability of Chinese ginseng to improve libido and sexual performance, especially among aging men.

*(continued)*

### ❧ Stress

The ginsengs are, without question, the best possible herbs to combat the effects of stress. Of course, exercise and proper nutrition are also essential—and prayer is a proven stress-reliever. But along with these measures, ginsengs allow you to be more proactive in reducing the effects of stress on the body.

### ❧ Toxins

Siberian and Chinese ginsengs have been reported to help the body deal with toxins. Both have also been shown to protect against the side effects of radiation exposure.

# Glandulars

Thousands of years ago, people would eat the organ of an animal with the hope that the healthy organ would treat the corresponding diseased organ in the human body. For example, if you had liver disease, why not eat a cow's liver to help recover? The practice was so common that the traditional Chinese doctors introduced "glandulars" into their herbal medicine formulas. In fact, glandulars have been part of their formulas for over 4,000 years.

Today, glandulars are still used as nutritional treatments for the prevention and treatment of disease. The term "glandulars" refers to supplements that are available to "tonify" and support the function of the major organs of the body.

Julieta, a 31-year-old teacher, came to my clinic to consult with me for help with her thyroid. She had been experiencing symptoms of fatigue, PMS, weight gain, and chilliness for the previous two years. Her doctor ran many lab tests, including a "thyroid panel"—that is, a complete examination for thyroid problems—but all the tests proved negative. Believing that there was nothing physically wrong with Julieta, her doctor simply told her to get more rest. He surmised that the stress of teaching was likely the cause of her symptoms.

After my initial exam of Julieta, I asked her to take her body temperature each morning for five days in a row. The temperatures she reported were on the low side of normal, averaging about 97.4 degrees Fahrenheit rather than 98.0 to 98.6 degrees. I recommended that we put Julieta on a nutritional protocol that included two kinds of glandulars: thyroid and adrenal extracts. The idea behind this treatment was to nourish and stimulate her glands so that they would work more effectively.

Julieta had what holistic doctors call "subclinical" symptoms of thyroid and adrenal insufficiency. That is to say, her hormones are not so low that they showed up as abnormal on standard lab tests, but on the other hand they weren't high enough to be at optimal level.

The adrenal glands and thyroid gland work in tandem to help control the body's metabolism—that is, the way it burns energy. Those glands also help the body adapt to stress.

Julieta felt her energy begin to improve within a few weeks after she started the glandular therapy. I recommended that she stay on the glandulars for at least three months. After two months of use her temperature had increased to an average of 97.8 degrees. The nighttime chills were less of a problem, and she felt that her PMS symptoms were beginning to improve.

## THE BEST OF THE BEASTS

The glandular preparations sold in the health food market have usually been purified to adjust the concentration of cells from the animal's organ or to ensure that there's no contamination. The most reliable and safest source of glandulars, from most reports, are New Zealand sheep. These sheep reportedly have the lowest amount of contamination from hormones, antibiotics, pesticides, and other undesirable chemicals.

Of course, there are other sources as well, and some companies use bovine (cow) as the source for their glandular products. Using such products raises the specter of contamination with the virus that causes Mad Cow Disease, a deadly infection of the brain, and few people think that taking a glandular is worth that kind of risk. Nonetheless, there has not yet been a case of infection resulting from glandular products sold in North America. (Britain has been the most-publicized location of Mad Cow Disease.)

I have not seen any solid scientific evidence to explain how glandulars work. It is thought that the amino acids and polypeptides (chains of amino acids) are absorbed through the small intestine and exert either a stimulating effect on the organ being treated or have a minor, hormone-altering effect. It has also been postulated that the amino acids are incorporated into the gland cells' DNA and then act to help regenerate the cells. In addition, very small amounts of hormones may still be left intact in the glandular extracts.

Also, some practitioners have suggested that glandulars act like a crude form of homeopathy—that is, "like cures like." That's a possibility, but, at this point, we can only say that the scientific mechanisms of glandulars are still unknown. What we do know is that many doctors and health practitioners have seen successful outcomes when they treated patients with glandulars.

## DOSAGE

Glandular products, like most supplements, have various different potencies. However, the general adult dosage is 1 to 2 capsules or tablets taken two to three times daily. Both tablets and capsules have the same effect. But the greater your body weight, the higher the dosage you'll need.

It is best to take glandulars between meals, although they're almost as effective when you take them with food. Some people begin to see positive results after a few weeks, but for others, glandular therapy may take several months or more.

## WHAT ARE THE SIDE EFFECTS?

A small percentage of people get digestive upset from glandulars. If that happens, try taking the supplements with meals instead of between meals.

People who take adrenal glandular extracts tend to have the most problems with other side effects, such as headaches, heart palpitations, anxiety, and insomnia. Generally, the side effects will diminish or stop entirely if you reduce the dosage. For people sensitive to supplements and medicines, it is always best to start at a low dosage—one capsule or tablet daily—and build up to a higher dosage over time.

Of course, glandulars are not compatible with vegetarianism since all are made from animals. But there is an alternative to animal-derived glandulars in homeopathic preparations of the glandulars known as isopathy or organopathy. These homeopathic preparations are effective with some people, and they're compatible with a vegetarian diet.

There are a variety of different organ-specific glandulars available. Following are some of the common ones, with their recommended uses.

# GLANDULARS
## RECOMMENDATIONS FROM THE NATURAL PHYSICIAN FOR . . .

### ~ Adrenal Glands

Adrenal glands, located on the top of each kidney, are the organs that help us survive stress. They secrete a variety of hormones including epinephrine (adrenaline), cortisol, DHEA, and others.

Adrenal glandulars are used for people who are "burned out," either from too much physical activity or from emotional stress. Excess secretion of one kind of hormone—such as cortisol—may create an imbalance. That gives an opportunity for other illnesses to set in.

People with chronic fatigue syndrome may benefit from adrenal extracts. These extracts are also recommended for chronic inflammatory illnesses such as rheumatoid arthritis, lupus, and ulcerative colitis. By supporting stress-hormone production, the adrenals keep inflammation to a minimum.

However, I don't advise anyone to use adrenals as substitutes for prescription medications such as prednisone (cortisone). Rather, they're an excellent supplement if you're coming off prednisone and other steroids, helping to ensure that the adrenals do not become "lazy."

You may also need adrenal support if you have allergies or asthma. Women can benefit from adrenal glandulars during menopause, when the ovaries quit producing hormones and the adrenals have to "take up the slack."

Other nutrients that act synergistically with adrenal glandulars include pantothenic acid, vitamin C, zinc, licorice root, and the ginsengs. All of these related therapies help to support adrenal function.

### ~ Liver

Liver glandular is used to support the detoxification properties of the liver. I have recommended them in cases of hepatitis and cirrhosis. They can also help with the liver detoxification process.

### ~ Ovary

Since the ovaries are responsible for the production of hormones as well as ovulation, good ovary function is critical to hormone balance. I have seen women who have hormone imbalances respond very favorably when they were given ovarian glandulars for PMS, menopause, and ovarian cysts.

### ~ Pancreas

The pancreas is responsible for producing and secreting enzymes that break down food in the small intestine. A different section of the pancreas produces hormones such as insulin and glucagons that control blood-sugar levels. I have mainly seen pancreatic glandular used for people with chronic pancreatitis (inflammation of the pancreas) with modest results.

### ~ Pituitary Gland

The pituitary gland, located in the brain, releases many different hormones that help regulate other hormones in the body. For example, the pituitary hormone LH signals the ovaries to ovulate every month. It also secretes a hormone called TSH (thyroid stimulating hormone), which signals the thyroid gland to release thyroid hormone.

I have mainly used pituitary glandular to increase the activity and metabolism of the thyroid gland. There are many hypothyroid products available that contain pituitary and thyroid glandulars together, which makes a lot of sense.

*(continued)*

### ❧ Spleen

A fist-sized organ located underneath the left ribs, the spleen is a filter for blood cells. It's also an important part of the immune system because it produces white blood cells and destroys bacteria and other microbes.

When I've recommended spleen glandular, it's usually for people who need immune-system support, especially if they have had their spleen removed. According to naturopathic physician Michael Murray, the spleen produces two immune-enhancing compounds known as tuftsin and splenopentin. Since these compounds are important to the vital functioning of the immune system, Murray says, "Spleen extracts should probably be viewed as a necessary medicine for people who have undergone a splenectomy."

### ❧ Testicles

The testicles produce the hormone testosterone, which is responsible for a man's sex characteristics. Testicular glandular—often labeled as orchic glandular—is typically used for conditions such as low libido, impotence, and poor sperm production (infertility). (The Chinese used to use tiger testicle and tiger penis in herbal formulas to increase sexual performance in elderly men—but sale of these formulas is now, thankfully, outlawed to protect the tiger population. Bovine glandular, from bull testicles, is generally used instead.)

### ❧ Thymus Gland

The most well-studied glandular is the thymus, which is located just behind the breastbone. The thymus gland in the human body is responsible for the production of T-lymphocytes, especially in children. Anyone who needs extra immune support may benefit from thymus.

Because it appears to have a balancing effect on the immune system, thymus extract is particularly recommended for people who have cancer, HIV, rheumatoid arthritis, and allergies. Some chiropractors and naturopathic doctors say they've seen very good results when they gave thymus extracts to children who were getting reoccurring ear and throat infections.

### ❧ Thyroid Gland

It is amazing the number of patients who have been diagnosed with low thyroid. There are many more who have subclinical hypothyroidism—that is, a slight deficiency of thyroid that is too small to detect, yet has an impact on health.

The lack of exercise, stress, emotional traumas, hormone imbalance (among estrogen, progesterone, pituitary hormones, and adrenal hormones), and environmental toxins have a lot to do with the pandemic of low thyroid.

Thyroid glandular can work well for mild cases of hypothyroidism. Many women who have been newly diagnosed with low thyroid by their doctors assume they will need to begin a medication such as Synthroid, the most commonly prescribed pharmaceutical for hypothyroidism. But thyroid glandular is another option.

For more severe cases I recommend Armour Thyroid—a thyroid prescription medication that's rarely prescribed by nonholistic doctors. Armour Thyroid, contains thyroid glandular as well as thyroid hormones. I find it works better than Synthroid in most cases because it has a glandular effect, which Synthroid does not have. Also, it contains a wider spectrum of thyroid hormones than Synthroid.

Because thyroid glandular contains very little thyroid hormone, you might have to take it quite a while before you begin to see benefits. I have had patients who feel better in a week with thyroid glandular supplementation, but more often, it needs to be taken for months to get the full benefit.

# Glucosamine Sulfate

Can glucosamine sulfate combat osteoarthritis?

Over 40 million Americans would urgently like to know the answer to that question. That's the number of people—most over the age of 45—who have osteoarthritis, the most common of nearly 100 different forms of this widespread problem.

Fortunately, the answer is yes. Osteoarthritis is the form that glucosamine is tremendously effective in treating.

More than 7 million people visit their doctors every year to seek relief from the swollen and stiffening joints that are caused by arthritis. A degenerative disease, osteoarthritis is characterized by the breakdown of joint cartilage—the spongy, cushioning tissue that protects the ends of the bones. Bones rub against each other when cartilage breaks down. The pain can be intense. Movement is usually restricted. Other common symptoms include tissue swelling and crepitus (creaking of joints), and feeling very stiff in the morning.

This type of arthritis mainly occurs in weight-bearing joints, such as the hips, knees, and spine. But people get it in their finger joints as well—which makes sense, since the fingers are in such constant use.

The exact cause of osteoarthritis is unknown, but researchers have seen an association with many other common health problems. This type of arthritis is associated, for instance, with obesity—which makes sense, since the joints have to carry excess weight. It's also associated with aging (joints are simply "wearing out") and with joint damage (the result of sports injuries, for instance). There also seems to be a genetic factor, because you're more likely to have osteoarthritis if a close relative has had it.

From my own observations, I'd say there are other associated factors as well. Biomechanics can be part of the problem, because it seems as if people are more likely to develop arthritis if they have flat feet or if the spine is out of alignment. Other factors that seem to contribute are poor digestion, high concentration of toxic substances, food sensitivities, hormonal imbalances, and nutritional deficiencies (if you're not getting enough vitamins, minerals, or essential fatty acids, for instance).

## FROM PAIN TO RELIEF

Several well-designed studies have proven that glucosamine sulfate is just as effective as standard drug therapy for relieving the symptoms of osteoarthritis—and, in some cases, the supplement is even *more* effective than conventional medicines.

In a number of double-blind studies, researchers have demonstrated that glucosamine sulfate can be beneficial for people with osteoarthritis. Many of these studies compared glucosamine sulfate head-to-head with standard NSAIDs (nonsteroidal antiinflammatory drugs), the pharmaceuticals that are often prescribed to reduce pain by reducing inflammation. Glucosamine was shown to produce better long-term results than these conventional medicines.

For example, in one 4-week study, scientists compared glucosamine sulfate (1,500 milligrams daily) to ibuprofen (1,200 milligrams daily). All the people in the study had osteoarthritis affecting their knees. The ibuprofen group experienced pain relief faster—but by the end of the second week, the people who were taking glucosamine were getting just as much pain relief as those in the ibuprofen group.

There were drawbacks to taking ibuprofen, however. Those in the ibuprofen group experienced significantly more side effects—35 percent, as opposed to just 6 percent in the glucosamine group.

Other trials support the benefits of glucosamine. In a study that involved 252 doctors and 1,506 patients, each patient was given 1,500 milligrams of glucosamine sulfate every day for about 7 weeks. When asked to judge the improvement in their patients, the doctors reported "good" results for about 59 percent of the patients and "sufficient" improvement in an additional 36 percent of them. Both doctors and patients rated glucosamine sulfate as being significantly more effective than previous treatments, which included NSAIDs, vitamins, and cartilage extracts.

Glucosamine is not a pain reliever, per se, so in general it doesn't work so swiftly as conventional drugs. But in the long run, I've found it relieves pain just as effectively as NSAIDs.

## BETTER BUILDING MATERIAL

This supplement has another asset as well. Glucosamine helps rebuild cartilage or, at least, prevent further loss of cartilage. In this respect, it's quite different from the commonly used drugs, which tend to combat pain and can actually increase cartilage degeneration.

The body naturally manufactures its own glucosamine, but apparently our ability to produce the substance begins to wane as we age. (One theory holds that nutritional deficiencies may be a contributing factor.) When the body does not produce so much glucosamine as it once did, supplementation is in order.

Glucosamine supplements are made from chitin, which comes from shellfish. It has an absorption rate of 90 to 98 percent, so most of the supplements' ingredients are effectively incorporated into the joint cartilage.

There are additional benefits when you take these supplements in the form of glucosamine sulfate. Glucosamine sulfate stimulates the repair and growth of proteoglycans, an important component of cartilage. Also, the sulfur portion of this complex is thought to stabilize joint tissue and cartilage. In this respect it's like SAMe—the one other supplement I recommend to help the body build more cartilage.

## DOSAGE

The typical adult dosage is 1,500 milligrams daily. But the optimum dosage depends to an extent on body size and weight. For people who are overweight, I usually recommend 2,000 milligrams daily to achieve full benefits.

Of the different types of glucosamine available, I prefer glucosamine sulfate for two reasons. First, most studies have been done with this supplement, so we know how well it's absorbed and how well it works. Second, as I've mentioned, the sulfur content helps ligaments and tendons as well as cartilage.

## WHAT ARE THE SIDE EFFECTS?

Glucosamine sulfate is extremely safe. On rare occasions, some people get mild, digestive upset accompanied by diarrhea. Even these symptoms tend to go away if you take glucosamine with meals.

Some people who are allergic to sulfite and sulfates wonder whether it's safe for them to take glucosamine sulfate. My answer is always "yes." Glucosamine sulfate contains the mineral sulfur, which is a normal constituent of the body, while sulfites and sulfates are preservatives.

Similarly, I've been asked about adverse affects by people who take sulfa drugs. But with these medications, too, the source of the drugs is different from the mineral sulfur found in glucosamine sulfate. Even though the name suggests sulfur, this is a completely different chemical from glucosamine sulfate.

People who are allergic to shellfish sometimes worry that the chitin in glucosamine supplements comes from shellfish. But the usual allergic reaction is caused by the protein found in shrimp and crabmeat, not from a reaction to the shell material. There have been no reports of severe reactions to glucosamine sulfate. (If you are concerned, however, you can test a small amount on the tip of your tongue while in the presence of your doctor before taking a regular dose.)

# GLUCOSAMINE SULFATE
## Recommendations from the Natural Physician for . . .

### ⌇ Osteoarthritis

In my view, given the risk of osteoarthritis that faces most of us, this is one of those supplements that nearly everyone over age 45 should be taking. Glucosamine sulfate is a superior long-term treatment for osteoarthritis, far outweighing the power of conventional medications such as aspirin, the NSAIDs such as Tylenol®, and commonly prescribed steroids. All of these pharmaceuticals only mask the pain while cartilage degeneration continues. (In fact, there's evidence that NSAIDs and aspirin actually destroy cartilage by suppressing the cells and enzymes that should help to build it!)

As for the side effects of medications, it is a well-known fact that long-term use of a steroid like prednisone can damage the body's tissue, bone, immune system, and joints. Also, people who are committed to long-term use of NSAIDs and aspirin run the risk of kidney and liver damage. Aspirin is also one of the leading causes of hospitalization for bleeding stomach ulcers.

Given all the benefits of glucosamine, and the deleterious side effects of so many medications, it's a possible solution for anyone with chronic arthritis problems. It can be used by people who have diabetes or blood-sugar imbalances such as hypoglycemia. It's also safe for people who have high blood pressure. (However, I recommend sodium-free glucosamine sulfate products for anyone concerned about sodium intake.)

If you begin with a 1,500-milligram dosage of glucosamine sulfate, you may be able to cut back after a while. It really varies, depending on the individual. Some of my patients are able to cut back to 500 milligrams daily after a few months of taking 1,500 milligrams, while others regress after cutting back their dosage and have to resume the higher level. Studies show that benefits wear off after a few months if you completely discontinue glucosamine supplementation.

If you're already taking antiinflammatory medications, it's safe to take glucosamine sulfate as well. In fact, I have many patients who do this all the time. Just be sure to let your doctor know you will be using this supplement. Chances are your doctor will be able to decrease your medications after 8 weeks of use.

Ever since publication of *The Arthritis Cure*, people have asked about the benefits of taking glucosamine sulfate and chondroitin sulfate together. In my experience, I've found that most people do well by just supplementing with glucosamine sulfate—and there have been fewer

*(continued)*

studies on the chondroitin sulfate. Occasionally, however, when I have a patient who doesn't respond so well as I would like to glucosamine sulfate, I'll also recommend a combination with chondroitin sulfate—and sometimes the two, taken together, produce a better effect.

There's certainly no harm in trying the combination (though cost may be a consideration). The daily dosage recommended for chondroitin sulfate is 1,200 milligrams.

Other supplements may be beneficial as well. For some patients I recommend MSM and SAMe in additional to glucosamine sulfate. You may also want to consider taking antioxidants such as vitamins C and E, selenium, and lipoic acid, or natural herbal antiinflammatories such as bromelain, boswellia, and cat's claw. To help relieve pain—and possibly improve the condition of cartilage—you can apply ointments that contain MSM or capsaicin.

# Goldenseal

"I don't want to take antibiotics, but all this mucous congestion in my nose and throat is driving me crazy. If I weren't in another state right now, I'd be headed for your office to see you."

Jonathan, a patient of mine, was calling me from his cell phone between sales calls. Was there anything he could pick up at a nearby health food store that would help him get through the next few days?

"Pick up some goldenseal," I advised. "Take 20 drops mixed in a quarter cup of water, three to four times a day for the next few days. But if you don't feel better after a few days, you'll have to see a local doctor to make sure the infection is not getting worse," I added.

Three days later, Jonathan called to leave a message with my receptionist. He was doing 80 percent better. His message?

"Thanks!"

## GOING FOR THE GOLDENSEAL

We have the Native Americans to thank for a lot of our current knowledge of goldenseal (*Hydrastis canadensis*). The Cherokee, Iroquois, Crow, Seminole, Blackfoot, and other tribes used goldenseal for many different medicinal effects, including respiratory tract infections, eye infections (eyewash), skin cancer, skin disorders (acne, wounds, ulcers), pelvic bleeding, and liver disease. This knowledge was passed on to pioneers, who used the popular herbal medicine for many different ailments. Eventually, a Jesuit priest collected the advice in a single volume that was published around 1650.

Among eclectic physicians and homeopaths in the 1800s, goldenseal was often recommended as a digestive stimulant and tonic for the mucous membranes. It is one of the few North American herbs that can positively affect these two systems of the body simultaneously. When I recommend goldenseal, it's usually for one or both of these benefits.

Goldenseal is a bitter-tasting herb. In herbal medicine, bitters are known to stimulate digestive secretions, which is helpful if you have a weak digestive system. In many European countries it's common to take some "bitters" before meals as a time-honored method of improving digestion and elimination. (Dandelion and gentian root are also favored as bitters.)

When the "bitter receptors" on the tongue are stimulated, there's a reflexive reaction from the nervous system that stimulates the digestive organs such as the stomach, liver, gallbladder, and pancreas. So if you take goldenseal before your meals, over time it will help build up the power of the digestive system. A small dose of 5 to 10 drops is all that is needed to stimulate digestion.

## MORE MUCUS

As a tonic for the mucous membranes, goldenseal provides benefits to many different areas of the body—the sinuses, respiratory tract, digestive tract, urinary tract, and vagina. Herbalists have stated that goldenseal has an "alterative action" on the mucous membranes. That means it literally alters the action of the membranes, stimulating the secretion of more mucus when there is not enough.

As a fluid that helps keep things flowing, mucus is an important part of the immune-system response to allergies and infection. It transports immunoglobulin A (IgA), which binds to foreign invaders and helps block infection. By stimulating secretions that produce extra IgA, goldenseal helps carry away viruses or bacteria that could cause infections.

That stimulating effect only lasts for a day or so, however. After that, goldenseal has a drying effect. This makes it effective for combating sinusitis, sore throats, bronchitis, pneumonia, colitis, vaginitis, and urinary tract infections.

Goldenseal is often referred to as a natural antibiotic, but this description is somewhat misleading. It hasn't been proven to directly kill bacteria. It does, however, contain very small amounts of a group of constituents known as alkaloids, including berberine, hydrastine, and canadine. These are considered the active substances, and often, they're the constituents that are tested.

## THE BERBERINE FACTOR

There has been a lot of research on berberine, but usually in the form of berberine sulfate, which is much more concentrated than the amount present in goldenseal. Berberine sulfate has been shown in test-tube studies to have antimicrobial power, so it can help wipe out many bacteria, fungi, and parasites. But no one's sure whether the berberine in goldenseal has the same antimicrobial power as the more concentrated form that's found in berberine sulfate. In fact, berberine is poorly absorbed when it comes from goldenseal.

My thought is that goldenseal may have a direct "killing" effect on microbes if it's applied directly to certain tissues. If you use it as an eyewash, for instance, it actually helps block infection—and it may have a similar effect on the mucous membranes if you take it in tincture form for a sore throat. But whatever its power as a microbe-killer, goldenseal definitely stimulates IgA secretion, so it optimizes the immune response against pathogens.

In traditional Chinese medicine—where the energy of each herb is considered—goldenseal is regarded as a cooling herb. Bacterial infections tend to cause "heat," in the view of Chinese practitioners, and that heat is best treated with the application of cooling herbs.

Without question, goldenseal is one of the more popular medicinal herbs, but this has had an unfortunate ecological impact. Due to the tremendous demand for herbal supplements by the public, goldenseal has become endangered in a number of different states. As a result, some suppliers are cultivating goldenseal in an attempt to meet retail demand.

There are some good alternatives if goldenseal is unavailable. First on my list is Oregon grape root, which contains berberine along with a number of alkaloids not found in goldenseal. Like goldenseal, Oregon grape root also works to improve digestion and fight infections, and I actually prefer it for the treatment of acne. I find it works quite well, especially when combined with burdock root and hormone-balancing herbs such as vitex. Other goldenseal substitutes include coptis, also known as gold thread, and barberry.

## DOSAGE

There is no agreed-upon standardization for goldenseal, so the concentrations of alkaloids like berberine will vary.

Most people take goldenseal in the form of a tincture or capsule, though you can also drink goldenseal tea. The typical adult dosage for acute infections is 15 to 30 drops of the tincture, or one 500-milligram capsule taken three to four times daily. As a digestive stimulant, I recommend you put 5 to 10 drops of the tincture in a glass of water and drink it before meals.

To make an eyewash, dilute 10 drops of tincture in a half ounce of saline solution and place 2 drops in each eye three to four times daily.

Many people use a combination of goldenseal and echinacea to combat infections.

Goldenseal is generally used for a limited time, so my usual recommendation is to continue using it until the condition improves. For acute infections this may be a week or so, and for digestive tonification, up to a few months.

## WHAT ARE THE SIDE EFFECTS?

If you take too much goldenseal, it can dry out mucous membranes or cause irritation along the digestive tract. Also, some people get heartburn and digestive upset unless they take it with meals.

It is best to not use goldenseal in the beginning stages of a cold. If you take too much at the onset of a cold, it can suppress mucus formation, and you need as much mucus as possible for a healthy immune response.

Don't take goldenseal during pregnancy. Alkaloid-containing herbs or drugs may cause harm to the baby or cause miscarriage.

Some authors state that long-term use of goldenseal can destroy good bacteria in the body, but this claim has not been supported by any studies. Research findings have shown that the active ingredient berberine—when tested apart from goldenseal—doesn't destroy beneficial bacteria.

# GOLDENSEAL
## RECOMMENDATIONS FROM THE NATURAL PHYSICIAN FOR . . .

### ✌ Acne

The hair follicles secrete an oily substance called sebum. When sebum gets blocked up and infected with bacteria, the result is acne. Goldenseal is sometimes found in acne formulas. Perhaps it fights bacteria, though that's unknown. In any case it helps stimulate a sluggish liver and improve digestion, which are underlying causes of some cases of acne. So goldenseal may be worth a try, though, as mentioned, I've found that Oregon grape root generally works better.

### ✌ Common Cold

It is best to not use goldenseal in the first stages of a cold so that mucus can flow freely. However, it can help to clear up the end stages of a cold where there is excess mucus. If you have just started to have cold symptoms, wait a day or two before you take goldenseal to fight it.

Similarly, if you have a case of the flu, I don't advise taking goldenseal right away. Wait a couple of days—after that, it can help speed your recovery.

### ✌ Diarrhea

Goldenseal does help with many cases of bacteria. In studies, berberine sulfate (one of the active substances in goldenseal) has been shown to kill different bacteria such as *E. coli*.

### ✌ Digestive Disorders

Goldenseal stimulates the digestive organs so that food can be broken down and assimilated more effectively. It can be used for irritable bowel syndrome, Crohn's disease, and ulcerative colitis. Because goldenseal helps stimulate a sluggish liver and gallbladder, it assists your body in breaking down fats more effectively.

### ✌ Eye Infections

Goldenseal works well for eye infections. Be sure to dilute it with a sterile saline solution before applying it topically to the eyes.

### ✌ Parasites

Many herbalists and natural doctors use goldenseal in a blend of herbs—including wormwood, garlic, and coptis—to eradicate parasitic infections.

### ✌ Respiratory Tract Infections

The most popular use for goldenseal here in North America is for respiratory tract infections, including sore throats, bronchitis, and pneumonia. It works best when there is excess mucus—but for a serious infection like pneumonia, you will need the advice of a doctor. I have treated strep throat using goldenseal and other herbs effectively, but I do not recommend you do this by yourself.

### ✌ Urinary Tract Infections

Goldenseal has a history of use for urinary tract infections. I like to use it in formulas with herbs such as echinacea, uva ursi, horsetail, and marshmallow.

# Green Tea

"Darla, it's pretty simple. You need to cut down on the amount of coffee you're drinking."

Darla, the 55-five-year-old owner of a jewelry store, had just told me she was drinking about nine cups a day. Clearly, all that caffeine was contributing to her insomnia and anxiety. Though she valued coffee for its stimulating effect, it was also contributing to her fatigue—because the "caffeine high" was invariably followed by plummeting energy levels. Another, unrecognized side effect was going on in her skeleton. By drinking a lot of the caffeinated beverage, she was excreting more calcium than normal whenever she urinated. All that coffee was speeding the hidden process of bone loss or osteoporosis.

Like many coffee drinkers, Darla questioned how she could possibly give it up, or even reduce her consumption. "Caffeine is what keeps me going during the day," she told me. "I *can't* give it up!"

"Well, there's a way you can still get in some caffeine without causing damage to your body. It's called green tea," I replied.

Darla had heard about green tea. She had a few friends who drank it occasionally. "But I've never tried it," she confessed.

Briefly, I described its assets. Green tea has many antioxidants that help provide protection against heart disease and cancer—and it also helps the liver with detoxification. With about half the amount of caffeine as coffee, green tea provides a reasonable energy boost, without the sharp "ups" and "downs" so often experienced by coffee drinkers.

I suggested that, over time, Darla could reduce her coffee intake to a couple of cups in the morning. "The rest of the day," I suggested, "have green tea instead."

"If you think it's important, I'll give it a try," replied Darla.

Over the next few months Darla was able to cut down her coffee consumption to the recommended two cups per morning, shifting to green tea the rest of the day. (A number of her friends and coworkers also adopted this change.) Darla noticed almost at once that her insomnia and anxiety improved.

## TEA FOR YOU

Green tea *(Camella sinensis)* comes from the same leaves of *Camella sinensis* that are used to make oolong and black tea—but, compared with those, green tea undergoes the least amount of processing.

To make green tea the fresh-picked leaves of *Camella sinensis* are lightly steamed or sometimes lightly pan-cooked. This process inactivates enzymes that would otherwise degrade the tea and reduce the antioxidant activity. The green tea leaves are then rolled and dried.

By comparison, oolong tea is allowed to partially oxidize, which gives it a stronger taste but interferes with its antioxidant activity. Black tea is allowed to oxidize even more, by exposing the rolled-up leaves to air until they're oxidized to black. This gives black tea the strongest flavor of all three, but the long drying time reduces the antioxidants because of the oxidation that occurs.

## THE GREENING OF AMERICA

Millions of people drink green tea every day—but until recently, most green-tea consumption seemed to be confined to the Far East. Among the Chinese, for instance, green tea is actually held in high esteem. Almost 90 percent of the Chinese population has at least one cup of green tea every day.

While Chinese records mention the use of tea as a medicinal beverage around 300 B.C., it has also been popular in Japan and India. Made popular by emperors in these countries, it eventually became the drink of choice at almost all social and spiritual gatherings. In the early 1600s, Dutch traders brought green tea to Europe, and from there the beverage made its way (via the Dutch and English) to America.

In the U.S., it's probably most popular in its cold form—that is, iced green tea. But you can now find green-tea extract supplements in many supermarkets, health food stores, and pharmacies.

## POWERING UP WITH POLYPHENOLS

The group of antioxidants that have helped give so much fame to green tea is known, collectively, as polyphenols. Polyphenols prevent free radicals (unstable molecules) from damaging body tissues and genetic material inside the cells. These phytonutrients are even more powerful than the vitamins most commonly taken as antioxidants—vitamins C and E.

Diseases such as cancer, heart disease, and many other chronic conditions are linked to the damage caused by free radicals, so any antioxidants that help prevent this damage will also help guard against these diseases. In fact, every aspect of aging is associated, in part, with various kinds of free-radical activity.

When the green tea polyphenols go to work in your body, they offer some powerful protection against the ravages of free radicals. Polyphenols contain flavonoids such as catechin, epicatechin, epicatechin gallate, epigallocatechin gallate (EGCG), and quercitin. Of all these, EGCG appears to have the strongest antioxidant and anticancer activity. The polyphenols have been shown to have a protective effect on vitamin E, helping to maintain vitamin E levels in the body rather than allowing it to become depleted.

Green tea also contains vitamins C, D, K, and $B_{12}$. It has ample supplies of minerals, too—including calcium, magnesium, chromium, manganese, iron, copper, zinc, molybdenum, selenium, and potassium.

Green tea enhances the liver's ability to detoxify and also protects liver cells from damage. It helps the liver process carcinogens.

# DOSAGE

### ❧ Tea Form

To prevent disease and maintain wellness I recommend two to three cups of green tea daily. This approximates the average green-tea consumption of three-cups-a-day that people drink in many Asian countries. (Many of the population studies of green tea have been done in Asia, so this consumption is considered the minimum standard for producing benefits.) Each cup of green tea contains 50 to 100 milligrams of polyphenols.

Many companies now offer organic green tea, which ensures that it has not been contaminated by pesticides or other chemicals. Decaffeinated green tea is also available, in case you happen to be sensitive to caffeine.

### ❧ Supplement Form

Green-tea extract is available in capsules or in whole-food formulas. If you're getting a supplement, check the label for standardization. Look for formulas standardized between 80 to 90% polyphenols and 35 to 55% epigallocatechin gallate. The typical capsule dosage is one 500-milligram capsule taken one to three times daily.

The supplemental form of green tea usually has the caffeine removed.

## WHAT ARE THE SIDE EFFECTS?

Regular, caffeinated green tea can cause the usual effects associated with caffeine, such as irritability, insomnia, nervousness, and tachycardia (fast heart rate). The longer the tea is steeped, the higher the amount of caffeine. Of course, if you're concerned about caffeine or don't like the side effects, you can always choose decaffeinated green tea instead.

---

## GREEN TEA
### RECOMMENDATIONS FROM THE NATURAL PHYSICIAN FOR . . .

---

### ꙮ Cancer

Green tea provides protection against some of the organic processes that increase your risk of cancer. The strong antioxidant activity of polyphenols helps to protect the DNA against damage, thus providing some protection for the critical genetic material in every human cell. The polyphenols also block the formation or reduce the cancer-causing activity of nitrosamines—that is, nitrites and nitrates. These are the agents in processed meats such as hot dogs, bacon, and ham that are associated with an increased risk of stomach cancer. Researchers have found that if you want the most protective effect of this kind, you should drink green tea before any meal that might contain nitrites and nitrates. (You'll get some benefits from drinking the tea afterward, as well, but it's more effective if you drink it before your meal.)

Lastly, green tea polyphenols prevent certain enzymes (specifically, cytochrome P450) in the liver from activating carcinogens during the detoxification process.

Most of the excitement about the cancer-prevention properties of green tea has come about because of population studies. In general, it's been found that in populations of people who consume green tea on a regular basis, people have a much lower incidence of cancer than in populations where people drink other kinds of tea or none at all. In Japan, for example, researchers have noted significantly lower cancer rates. In large part, they feel, that's attributable to the high consumption of green tea.

One study looked at 472 women in various stages of breast cancer (labeled I, II, or III, depending on how far the cancer had progressed). Increased green-tea consumption was associated with a decreased risk of lymph node metastasis in premenopausal women with stages I and II cancer. The researchers also found that if women with these stages of breast cancer consumed 5 cups a day of green tea on a long-term basis, they were more likely to be in remission 6 months later when the follow-up study was done.

Green tea appears to target some specific cancers. Researchers say that it may help protect against breast, prostate, esophagus, stomach, colon, lung, skin, liver, bladder, and ovarian cancers. It also seems to help guard against leukemia and oral leukoplakia.

Summing up their recommendations, a group of Japanese researchers concluded that green tea is potentially beneficial to anyone who takes it to help prevent cancer. "We suggest

*(continued)*

246

drinking green tea may be one of the most practical methods of cancer prevention available at the present," the Japanese team concluded.

### ∾ Cardiovascular Disease

It seems the French drink red wine to prevent heart disease while the Japanese drink green tea to prevent heart disease. Meanwhile, North Americans don't seem to drink anything that prevents heart disease.

Cholesterol is one of the factors involved with heart disease. Animal studies have shown that green tea polyphenols, especially EECG, prevents cholesterol from being absorbed from food into the body. By resisting absorption, you also reduce the risk of heart disease and other kinds of circulatory diseases that are so closely associated with high cholesterol.

A study of 1,371 Japanese men showed that a high consumption of green tea (more than 10 cups daily) was associated with lower total cholesterol levels. This quantity of green tea actually raised the level of HDL, which is "good cholesterol," while sharply lowering the concentration of lower LDL or "bad cholesterol."

Green tea was also shown to reduce the oxidation of LDL cholesterol, which is implicated in the initial development of atherosclerosis.

Also, green tea has natural blood-thinning properties. Doctors in China use high-potency green tea extracts for this purpose. (Blood thinners help lower high blood pressure and reduce the risk of stroke.)

### ∾ Detoxification

While helping to support the liver—your body's chief detoxifier—green tea also prevents the formation of cancer-causing substances. I recommend using green-tea extract as part of a detoxification program, or simply drink the tea on a regular basis so that toxins do not build up in your body.

Wisely, many whole-food supplements—often dubbed "green drinks"—contain green-tea extract in their formulations.

### ∾ Digestive Health

According to *The Green Tea Book*, "Green tea promotes a healthy digestive tract by altering the intestinal environment to make it favorable to the growth of the friendly bacteria and less favorable to the growth of undesirable bacteria."

One Japanese study demonstrated that a special green-tea extract improved the levels of the good bacteria *Lactobacilli* and *Bifidobacteria* in nursing home patients. It also lowered the levels of certain kinds of potentially harmful bacteria.

### ∾ Tooth Decay

Green tea contains small amounts of fluoride that can help prevent tooth decay. Animal and human studies have shown that the polyphenols found in green tea prevent the growth of bacteria that cause cavities and plaque. In one study with human subjects, researchers discovered that green tea polyphenols decreased plaque deposits even when the volunteers just took the green tea, without bothering to brush or floss their teeth.

### ∾ Weight Loss

Most people know that caffeine is a stimulant, but not everyone realizes that this stimulant can help promote weight loss. I am not an advocate of using caffeine products as a "quick fix." The supplements themselves are not a shortcut to weight loss. But some preliminary research has shown that green tea can help stabilize blood sugar. Indirectly, then, green tea might help promote weight loss by preventing insulin spikes from occurring. As long as insulin doesn't shoot up, you're less likely to store excess fat. But so far, we still aren't sure that green tea can really prevent these spikes. More research needs to be done.

# Guggul

• • • • • • • • • • • • • • • • • • • • • • • • • • • • • • • • • • • • • • • • • • • • • • • • • • • • • • • • • • •

Mention the condition "high cholesterol," and most natural healthcare practitioners will think of the herb guggul *(Commiphora mukul),* often referred to as guggulipid.

Cholesterol imbalance is one of the major risk factors for heart disease which, in turn, is the leading cause of death in the U.S. With this in mind, the promise of guggul is obvious. It offers a safe and effective alternative to cholesterol-lowering drugs.

In several well-designed human studies, guggul has been shown to lower the "bad markers" of cardiovascular disease, such as total cholesterol, LDL, and VLDL cholesterol. Simultaneously it increases the level of the "good marker" HDL cholesterol.

Guggul has a storybook history. In the 1960s, an Indian researcher read about the medicinal effects of guggul in the ancient Ayurvedic medical text called *Sushrutasamhita.* This classic text described the effectiveness of guggul for the treatment of obesity and disorders of fats. Inspired by the text, researchers began to conduct studies to determine the effects of guggul on animals that had heart disease. The early animal studies showed that guggul resin significantly reduced high cholesterol and offered protection against atherosclerosis.

During the next four decades, in numerous trials with people who had high cholesterol, guggul extract proved to be a potent herbal therapy, helping to reduce not only high cholesterol but also triglycerides. Studies show it to be as effective— or even more effective—than many cholesterol-lowering drugs. It's much safer, too. It is approved by medical authorities in India as a lipid-lowering drug.

## A TREE GROWS IN BANGLADESH

Guggul is a small, thorny tree native to India and Bangladesh. The resin is extracted from underneath the bark where yellow fluid oozes out. Guggul resin contains a mixture of lipid steroids termed guggulipid, which exerts the cholesterol-lowering and antiinflammatory effects.

Within guggulipid are guggulsterones. Guggulipid also contains other compounds that exert a synergistic effect.

In traditional Ayurvedic medicine, guggul is indicated as a potential cure for arthritis, diabetes, gout, and skin disorders. It's also recommended to improve immune function, appetite, and digestion. Since it's been reputed to help prevent dental problems, it's also used as a mouthwash.

Guggul reduces cholesterol by "prompting" the liver to metabolize or "burn up" excess cholesterol. It also inhibits the cholesterol that's produced by the liver.

Animal studies show that guggulsterones stimulate the thyroid gland, so it may also be helpful for people who have low thyroid. It's an interesting connection between this thyroid effect and the metabolism of cholesterol. It's known that low thyroid function leads to reduced cholesterol metabolism by the liver—so thyroid stimulation would theoretically reduce cholesterol levels. There's ample evidence for this, since thyroid hormone medications reduce high cholesterol when given to people who have low thyroid function.

Guggul extracts also prevent platelet aggregation—the clumping of platelets that can lead to blood clotting—so it may prevent strokes.

In general, I favor this type of treatment over pharmaceutical, cholesterol-lowering drugs. I've found that the pharmaceuticals carry the risk of liver toxicity, so even though they may help reduce the risk of heart disease, they can aggravate other health problems.

## DOSAGE

For cholesterol and triglyceride reduction, I recommend 500 milligrams of a 5% guggulsterone standardized extract three times daily. This is equivalent to 25 milligrams of guggulsterones three times daily.

An equivalent dosage that some products contain is 1,000 milligrams of a 2.5% guggulsterone standardized extract taken three times daily. Researchers recommend the extract be taken for at least 4 weeks before reevaluating blood cholesterol and lipid levels. I find it may need to be taken for 2 to 2½ months before reasonable improvements are seen with lab testing.

I typically recommend that guggul be taken in combination with other cholesterol-balancing supplements such as niacin (*Inositol hexaniacinate*) and garlic. In Canada a supplement known as Policosanol is very effective as well.

## WHAT ARE THE SIDE EFFECTS?

Guggulipid has been shown to be nontoxic, but a small percentage of people experience minor digestive upset when they take it. It should not be used during pregnancy or by women who have heavy uterine bleeding. You probably shouldn't use it in combination with cholesterol-lowering pharmaceutical medications either, though the interaction with such drugs hasn't been studied in detail.

Those on thyroid medication should be especially monitored while taking guggulipid (and should be monitored even if *not* on guggulipid).

---

## GUGGULIPID
## RECOMMENDATIONS FROM THE NATURAL PHYSICIAN FOR . . .

### ◆ Atherosclerosis

Animal studies have shown that guggul extract both prevents and reduces existing atherosclerosis. More studies are needed before we know for sure that the herb holds the same benefits for humans.

### ◆ Cholesterol and Triglycerides

As mentioned, guggulipid extract has been shown to decrease LDL, VLDL, total cholesterol, and triglyceride levels while increasing the protective HDL cholesterol. One 12-week study demonstrated that 1,500 milligrams of guggulipid had average reductions in serum cholesterol of nearly 22 percent, while triglycerides were reduced about 25 percent in people who took it regularly.

Another scientific study involving 233 people with elevated cholesterol or triglyceride levels (or both) showed that guggulipid worked better than the cholesterol-lowering drug clofibrate. People taking guggulipid had the added benefit of seeing some improvements in HDL, the "good cholesterol"—an effect that wasn't in evidence with the pharmaceutical. As for the length of time the benefits lasted, it was about the same—approximately 20 weeks—for those who took the herb and those who took the drug.

As researchers have identified some very specific types of high cholesterol, they have conducted studies to see which types are best treated with guggulipid. One study showed that guggulipid works best for people who have high-cholesterol readings of the type IIb (increased LDL, VLDL, and triglycerides) and type IV (increased VLDL and triglycerides).

---

# Gymnema Sylvestre

. . . . . . . . . . . . . . . . . . . . . . . . . . . . . . . . . . . . . . . . . . . . . . . . . .

"My doctor told me I need to lose twenty five pounds. He told me to quit eating at McDonald's and get more exercise. And if I don't improve my blood-sugar levels over the next two months, my doctor says I'll have to go on drugs for diabetes."

Stephen, a new patient, was obviously chagrined at the program his doctor had outlined for him. To me, it sounded like pretty sound advice—though of course I didn't like the idea of diabetes drugs any better than Stephen did.

"That's good, basic advice," I assured him. "But I'd like you to get on a more thorough program. You're thirty-five years old. That's pretty young to be having Type two diabetes. If you do what I suggest, I think we can get your blood-sugar levels back in the normal range. Type two diabetes can be completely reversed with proper nutrition and exercise. Throw in effective herbs and nutritional supplements, and your progress will be even better."

Stephen's lifestyle is fairly typical. Like a very large segment of the U.S. population, he's ready to admit that he probably watches too much T.V., and eats too many sweets and white bread. Most of his exercise is turning the steering wheel of his sports car.

Not surprisingly—given this general lifestyle pattern—the statistics on Type 2 diabetes have become alarming. In recent years, the largest increase among those who have "adult-onset diabetes" occurs in people ages 30 to 39.

To help Stephen, I gave him a more detailed diet plan than he'd gotten from his doctor. If he followed my recommendations, he would be eating a lot of complex carbohydrates, getting more of his protein from quality sources, and consuming more essential fatty acids. I also asked him to restrict simple carbohydrates such as breads, pastas, and sugar products.

Recognizing that he needed some kind of regular exercise program, Stephen started walking 20 minutes a day. He also followed my supplement recommendations, including daily doses of the herb gymnema sylvestre. This herb helped Stephen to control his appetite for sweets. It was just one of the tactics we used to help bring his blood-sugar levels under control.

## TAMING THE SWEET TOOTH

Also known as gurmar, or "sugar destroyer," gymnema sylvestre has been embraced by many physicians who practice Ayurvedic medicine. Somehow, it has the ability to block the taste of sweetness, so it helps to stave off the "craving for sweets" that leads to overeating of simple-carbohydrate foods.

Gymnema grows in the forests of India and has been used by local healers and Ayurvedic physicians for the treatment of blood-sugar imbalances for more than 2,000 years.

Gymnemic acids are thought to be the important active constituents in gymnema. But this herb contains other important components as well, including resins, saponins, stigmasterol, quercitol, and the amino-acid derivatives betaine, choline, and trimethylamine.

**251**

A number of mechanisms seem to be activated when gymnema goes about its business of balancing blood sugar. Two animal studies found gymnema extracts doubled the number of insulin-secreting beta cells in the pancreas and returned blood sugars to almost normal. Gymnema also increases the activity of enzymes responsible for glucose uptake and utilization.

## WATCHING WHAT HAPPENS

Since the 1930s, scientists have been trying to figure how gymnema can provide botanical therapy for Types 1 and 2 diabetes.

In a controlled study, a standardized gymnema extract was given to 27 people with Type 1 diabetes, all receiving a dose of 400 milligrams daily for periods ranging from 6 months to 2 1/2 years. Thirty-seven of the other people in the study continued to take the usual insulin therapy without the addition of gymnema. Among those who took the herbal extract, researchers found that insulin requirements fell off dramatically. In addition, there was a statistically significant decrease in the blood-sugar marker that tests long-term blood sugar. Those in the control group showed no significant decreases in blood sugar or insulin requirement.

In another study, 22 people with Type 2 diabetes were given 400 milligrams of gymnema extract every day for 18 to 20 months while they also continued to get their usual medication for hypoglycemia. Average blood-sugar levels improved significantly in this group, along with another sugar-related blood factor (glycosylated hemoglobin). Results also showed that there was an increase in pancreatic release of insulin among the people who got gymnema. People in the study were able to reduce their medication, and five were able to discontinue their drugs entirely.

As these studies show, gymnema has the ability to make quite an impact on blood-sugar metabolism. It is even more effective when combined with exercise and proper diet.

Several animal studies have also confirmed the blood-sugar lowering effect of gymnema sylvestre.

## DOSAGE

A therapeutic dose of an extract is standardized to contain 24 to 25% gymnemic acids. I usually recommend 400 to 600 milligrams daily of the capsule form. I typically have patients take divided doses throughout the day before or with meals.

Gymnema also works well in combination with other blood-sugar balancing herbs such as bitter melon and fenugreek.

## WHAT ARE THE SIDE EFFECTS?

No side effects have been reported, but researchers have not established whether this herb is absolutely safe for pregnant women.

Be cautious using this herb if you're taking pharmaceutical medications (oral hypoglycemics or insulin) for diabetes. The combination of gymnema and these medications can lower blood-sugar levels to potentially risky levels. If you're already taking diabetes medications, it's extremely important to work with a physician before supplementing with gymnema because the physician needs to closely monitor blood-sugar levels. In many instances, your doctor will need to lower the dosage of the pharmaceutical medication you are on.

## GYMNEMA SYLVESTRE
### RECOMMENDATIONS FROM THE NATURAL PHYSICIAN FOR . . .

**◌ *Diabetes***
Gymnema can be effective for people who have either Type 1 or Type 2 diabetes, although I mainly recommend it for Type 2.

**◌ *Insulin Resistance***
When there's a high level of blood sugar, the body produces more insulin, which is the hormone that helps shuttle blood sugar into the cells of the body. But as too much insulin is produced, the body's cells become resistant to it—hence, the term "insulin resistance." When that happens, blood sugar remains high.

Many people who have insulin resistance gain weight, no matter what their diet. Gymnema may help. It improves the cells' uptake of blood sugar and helps the body utilize it.

**◌ *Syndrome X***
The term "Syndrome X" describes a whole cluster of health problems that increase the risk of diabetes and heart disease. (Many older Americans, as you might expect, show many of the symptoms of Syndrome X.) Insulin resistance is the underlying factor in this condition. As a result, people who have Syndrome X often show signs of glucose intolerance, obesity, high blood pressure, and elevated levels of cholesterol and triglycerides.

Since gymnema helps improve blood-sugar uptake and utilization, it is the herb I recommend for Syndrome X.

# H

# Hawthorn

· · · · · · · · · · · · · · · · · · · · · · · · · · · · · · · · · · · · · · · · · · · · · · · · · ·

Hawthorn is truly a superstar when it comes to the heart and cardiovascular system. Millions of people can benefit from the medicinal effects of this herb, including anyone who suffers from high blood pressure, coronary artery disease, angina, or heart arrhythmia.

Since cardiovascular disease is the number-one killer in this country, hawthorn is a crucial treatment when it comes to herbal prevention and natural treatment of this pandemic disease. Chances are high that nearly all of us will suffer from one or more of these heart-related conditions by the age of 60—so you might also think of hawthorn as the anti-aging herb for the heart.

## ONE FOR THE HEART

I love to prescribe hawthorn to patients. Most people begin feeling much better, almost from the first instant they take it. The herb improves oxygenation, and thus has an immediate, beneficial impact on energy levels. In addition, it improves blood flow through the coronary arteries (the vessels that supply blood to the heart), increases strength of heart contractions, prevents plaque buildup in the arteries, relaxes blood vessels so that blood flows more efficiently, and helps prevent pressure buildup inside the arteries. No wonder so many European doctors and North American "natural doctors" prescribe hawthorn on a daily basis. As far as I am concerned, every cardiologist should be recommending this lifesaving heart tonic to patients.

Many parts of the plant—leaves, flowers, and berries—are used medicinally, although most extracts are mainly from the berry. Researchers have found that the active ingredients in this herb seem to be a group of flavonoids that provide unique benefits to the cardiovascular system. A leading characteristic of these powerful flavonoids is their incredible ability to improve blood flow to the heart.

Hawthorn is the premier cardiotonic in European herbal medicine, meaning that it's often prescribed simply to support normal heart functions.

## DOSAGE

Practitioners commonly use standardized extracts of 2.2% flavonoids or 18.75% procyanidins. In many of the studies where patients showed the greatest improvement, researchers were administering between 160 and 900 milligrams daily of the capsule extract.

With serious heart conditions like congestive heart failure, it's important for anyone taking hawthorn to get the benefit of its therapeutic effects as quickly as possible. For those taking it in tincture form, I have seen good results with doses of 30 to 60 drops three times daily.

The tea form is also available, but I prefer to use capsule or tincture with my patients. (I have no experience with hawthorn tea.)

## WHAT ARE THE SIDE EFFECTS?

While there are no adverse side effects, hawthorn does provide one bonus—it enhances the heart drug digitalis, making it more potent. The herb may also increase the effectiveness of beta blocker drugs that are used to treat high blood pressure.

If you're being treated for a heart-related condition by a conventional doctor, be sure to let your physician know if you're also taking hawthorn, because it has a mild blood-thinning and diuretic effect. With close monitoring by your doctor, you may be able to use a lower dosage of the pharmaceutical medications—which is an advantage, because so many of them have side effects.

# HAWTHORN
## RECOMMENDATIONS FROM THE NATURAL PHYSICIAN FOR . . .

### ∿ Angina

Angina pain, according to patients, is like having your heart squeezed until it hurts. The pain can be brought on by stress, but it might also be caused by a shortage of oxygen reaching heart tissue. That's one thing that happens when you have arteriosclerosis, more commonly known as hardening of the arteries.

I have seen hawthorn help numerous patients with angina. For the most severe conditions, I recommend taking hawthorn in combination with the herb cactus (*Cereus grandiflorus*).

In a 3-week study that confirmed the benefits of hawthorn for people with angina, researchers demonstrated that daily doses of 180 milligrams had a significant effect on blood flow to the heart. Though 78 percent of these people had "abnormal" endurance readings before the study, those who took hawthorn quickly showed a 25 percent improvement in their exercise tolerance—whereas those in a control group (who received no hawthorn) showed no improvement at all. The conclusion I drew from this study is that a simple supplementation program of hawthorn can make an incredible difference in oxygenation to the heart and help treat the underlying cause of angina.

### ∿ Arrhythmia

Almost anyone who has a mild case of heart arrhythmia can be helped with hawthorn. Better yet, in my view, is a combination that includes not only hawthorn but also the supplement coenzyme Q10, L-carnitine, and the mineral magnesium.

### ∿ Congestive Heart Failure

Researchers have focused on congestive heart failure in most of the studies on hawthorn. Symptoms of this condition include shortness of breath, poor exercise tolerance, fatigue, elevated heart rate, and swelling of the ankles (edema). This is the result of a loss of efficiency in the body's one and only blood-pumping organ, the heart.

But the problem doesn't originate in the heart itself. Rather, it's caused by arteriosclerosis, the condition where plaque buildup in the arteries prevents adequate blood flow into the heart, or from long-term high blood pressure.

For congestive heart failure, hawthorn comes highly recommended by the German Commission E that evaluates the effectiveness of a wide range of herbs. This official government agency based its recommendations on a number of supportive studies. One high-quality study, for example, showed that 8 weeks of hawthorn extract supplementation improved heart function and symptoms in people who had a moderate degree of congestive heart failure. In another study, researchers learned that hawthorn extract is just as effective as the drug catopril, a pharmaceutical medication that's custom-designed for people with high blood pressure who are prone to congestive heart failure. Among those who had a moderate degree of congestive heart failure,

*(continued)*

256

hawthorn reduced heart rate and improved exercise tolerance.

The latter study, which was done with 900-milligram daily doses of hawthorn extract, demonstrated that the potency of hawthorn is roughly equal to that of heart medications. But unlike the pharmaceuticals, hawthorn doesn't create unwanted side effects.

### ✺ Heart Attack Recovery

I routinely prescribe hawthorn to people who have a history of a heart attack. Of course, having been in and out of the hospital, and under the care of conventional doctors, these are people who are already taking their share of medications such as the blood-thinner coumadin or common aspirin. Frequently these medications are prescribed by cardiologists to help prevent a second attack.

A good case can be made for hawthorn supplementation as an adjunct to drug therapies. But hawthorn is more than a good assistant. It does something the pharmaceuticals can't accomplish—increases circulation to the coronary arteries. Since these small arteries feed the heart muscle, they're critical to the health of this organ. It's when your heart tissue isn't getting sufficient blood flow that a heart attack is most likely to occur.

Hawthorn by itself only has some of the healing properties that are needed for complete recovery. So in addition to this herbal supplement, I typically recommend others as well to heart attack survivors—including natural vitamin E, coenzyme Q10, magnesium, L-carnitine, and a host of antioxidants.

As long as your physician knows you're taking natural supplements that may have a mild blood-thinning effect, you can probably continue taking pharmaceuticals as well as the supplements. I have not had any drug–herb interaction problems among patients who took both.

### ✺ High Blood Pressure

Hawthorn alone is a good treatment for high blood pressure, but I see even better results when it's combined with ginkgo, viscum, dandelion leaf, and valerian.

Hawthorn has a mild diuretic effect, which reduces the amount of water in the blood, thus reducing blood volume and blood pressure. Hawthorn also relaxes blood vessel walls, which also helps lower blood pressure.

### ✺ Preventing Heart Disease

Most people will develop heart disease in their lifetime. The statistics are irrefutable.

Improving lifestyle factors can make some difference—and I certainly recommend exercise, stress reduction, adhering to a quality diet, and not smoking or drinking. But, in addition, if you're over the age of 50, I'd advise you to take hawthorn supplements on a long-term basis. Not only does it improve heart circulation, but hawthorn also contains potent flavonoids that protect the heart and cardiovascular system from oxidative damage.

# Horse Chestnut

Most patients who have varicose veins have read all about the possible remedies, and they've tried a number of pills and powders. So the question I'm most frequently asked is this: "If you had to pick one supplement for varicose veins, which one would it be?"

The list of possibilities is fairly extensive. I've had good results with ginkgo, grape seed, bilberry, hawthorn, witch hazel, pycnogenol, and vitamin C. But at the top of my list is horse chestnut.

As the baby-boom generation continues to age, conditions like varicose veins will receive more attention from the medical and natural health communities. This condition occurs when the minuscule valves in veins begin to weaken. Instead of supporting the flow of blood that's making a return trip to the heart, the tiny valves allow a backwash that results in pooling. This leads to the engorgement of veins, especially in the legs where gravity is exerting a strong, downward pull.

Varicose veins are not harmful, but people occasionally have a problem with a related symptom called thrombophlebitis, where veins become painfully swollen and inflamed. With this condition—commonly called phlebitis—there's a risk of blood clot formation, a potentially serious situation.

Fortunately, the seeds of horse chestnut *(Aesculus hippocastinum)* produce a tonic effect on veins—and, indeed, on the entire circulatory system. In addition, horse chestnut has natural antiinflammatory properties, so it's also helpful for the treatment of swelling and edema, bruises, arthritis, and backaches.

While the seeds are the seat of the horse chestnut's power, I don't recommend eating them. Before they're ready for human consumption, the seeds must be specially processed to remove harmful, naturally occurring components.

## THE ROOTS OF CHESTNUT LORE

As with many of today's popular herbs, horse chestnut has a rich history in Europe. As a matter of fact, the main active constituent that has been identified, called aescin, is a registered drug in Germany. German doctors recommend it for edema and muscular injuries, and it's also given by injection for head trauma. Not surprisingly, the German Commission E—a government body that holds responsibility for herb-testing—has approved horse chestnut for the condition called "venous insufficiency," which simply means lack of blood flow through the veins. Commission E also endorses the herb for nighttime leg cramps, swelling, and itching of the legs.

Horse chestnut is native to Asia but can also be found throughout the United States and Europe. The seeds come from the fruit that is picked each September.

Horse chestnut has an interesting mechanism of action. The active constituent aescin helps strengthen the vein walls and valves, as well as capillaries. Aescin also decreases the permeability of the tiniest blood channels, the capillaries, by preventing key enzymes from breaking the walls of capillaries. Research has shown that these enzymes are at much higher levels in people with varicose veins—presumably causing a faster breakdown of capillary walls—so aescin helps put the brakes on this process.

Horse chestnut also improves circulation and reduces edema by promoting fluid drainage from the tissues into the capillaries. This is important, since excess fluid in the tissues accumulates around and in the veins—and when the veins become distended, they're a less efficient circulation mechanism.

Finally, horse chestnut contains small amounts of a blood-thinning agent called coumadin. When blood becomes thinner, it flows more easily and swiftly, which helps explain why this herb helps to improve circulation and relieve congestion.

## DOSAGE

I recommend patients use a standardized capsule of horse chestnut at the same dosage used in clinical studies, which was 600 milligram daily. This is equivalent to 100 milligrams daily of the active constituent, aescin. Topical gels containing horse chestnut are also available.

## WHAT ARE THE SIDE EFFECTS?

Side effects are rare. A small percentage of people get digestive upset, and some patients have reported skin itching and headaches. Since horse chestnut has a natural blood-thinning effect, be sure to check with your physician if you're on blood-thinning medications or have any kind of bleeding disorder. If you have concerns about such conditions, you can always use the horse chestnut gel, applied directly to the surface of the skin (rather than taken internally).

## HORSE CHESTNUT
### RECOMMENDATIONS FROM THE NATURAL PHYSICIAN FOR . . .

### ❧ Back Pain

European doctors use horse chestnut for the relief of back pain. Though I don't have any experience using it for this condition, I have treated people with the homeopathic form called aesculus. (Aesculus is specific for pain that radiates to the low back and hips.)

### ❧ Hemorrhoids

Hemorrhoids are really a collection of varicose veins that are distended and protruding. Horse chestnut is a popular herb that's often recommended by naturopathic doctors and herbalists to shrink hemorrhoids and alleviate pain and itching.

### ❧ Varicose Veins

Most of the research with regard to horse chestnut has been focused on varicose veins. One study of 240 people found that horse chestnut was just as effective as the treatments most often used in conventional medicine—combining compression therapy (heavy, elastic, custom-fitted stockings) with daily doses of a diuretic (a medication that reduces body fluids by increasing the need to urinate).

In my own practice, I have seen good results in people with mild to severe cases of varicose veins. It's especially recommended in severe cases, because varicosity can lead to thrombophlebitis. I also recommend horse chestnut for people who have had vein surgery, so that the varicosities do not return.

# Hydrotherapy

"My chest hurts, especially when I breathe in. I also have a lot of mucus coming up, which makes me cough even more. I don't want to see my family doctor. I know she will give me antibiotics."

Sherry was speaking from experience. The year before, she'd had several courses of antibiotics for various infections—and each time, she'd suffered the side effects of yeast infections and bloating. This time, she wanted to make sure she tried the alternatives if she could.

"You can help me, right?" asked Sherry.

"Let's see what is going on with you and then I will let you know what I can do," I replied.

I listened to her lungs, then ordered X-rays and blood work. The results confirmed my suspicion that Sherry had bacterial pneumonia. She was 39 years old, and I would have considered her a healthy individual, except that she got bronchitis or pneumonia a couple times every winter. But if she continued to get antibiotics for these problems, I felt there was a real risk that she would eventually get a bacterial infection that couldn't be fought off with conventional antibiotic medications. She, too, knew about this risk, which was why she'd asked me to treat her with natural medicine.

But the need for treatment was urgent and immediate. Bacterial pneumonia is a serious condition, and we had to bring it under control right away.

To Sherry's question of "What next," I proposed an aggressive treatment protocol. Perhaps the most important part of the plan would be constitutional hydrotherapy.

## HOT AND COLD

Naturopathic doctors have used constitutional hydrotherapy for over 100 years. Essentially, it means alternating heat and cold by applying water-soaked towels over the chest and back.

I was quite sure that constitutional hydrotherapy would increase Sherry's white blood cell count, which would enhance her body's natural ability to fight off the bacterial infection. At the same time, the treatment with hot and cold would be likely to reduce congestion and inflammation of the lungs by improving circulation. I also prescribed an herbal formula and homeopathic remedy to accompany the hydrotherapy treatments.

Sherry's husband helped her with the hydrotherapy treatment at home.

Sherry returned to the clinic for follow-up visits at 3-day intervals. Sherry noted that after a hydrotherapy treatment, she was able to cough up mucus that seemed to be deep in her lungs. When she had therapy in the evening, she noted that it also enabled her to sleep better that night.

Sherry was showing evident improvement at each visit. Nine days into the therapy, she had returned to work and felt that she was close to being her old self.

# WATER TREATMENTS—WITH GUIDANCE

I would never recommend that anyone try to treat bacterial pneumonia without the help of a physician, and I know many medical doctors who might think I was crazy to recommend hydrotherapy for Sherry. Then again, many doctors who readily prescribe antibiotics are not completely informed about the powerful natural healing therapies that can be very effective in fighting many kinds of disease.

Hydrotherapy simply refers to the use of water for healing. The actual treatments can take many forms. Steam inhalation and a wet sauna are forms of hydrotherapy. So are baths or hot tubs, and hot and cold applications with towels, compresses, or gel packs. Some practitioners use colonic hydrotherapy, which means "flushing out" the colon with sterile water to remove toxic or harmful substances.

Hydrotherapy is very common in European countries. Even in the U.S., however, many health spas have extensive hydrotherapy programs. There are many medical doctors as well as naturopathic physicians who advocate various forms of hydrotherapy treatments for certain conditions.

The healing powers of water have been recognized for thousands of years. Hydrotherapy treatments were certainly well known to Ancient Egyptians and Babylonians. The Greeks and Romans emphasized the importance of baths and the healing power of natural springs.

# WATER EXPLORER

If any single individual were to be described as the founder of this therapy, it would have to be Vincent Priessnitz, who lived from 1799 to 1852. Born a peasant in a small European mountain village in what was the former Czechoslovakia, Priessnitz observed how an injured animal instinctively headed for a nearby creek when it had an injury. The cold, flowing water healed its injuries.

Priessnitz experimented with different forms of hydrotherapy on injuries he sustained when he was working on the family farm. When he was 17 years old, Priessnitz was run over by a wagon carrying a heavy load of wood. A local surgeon evaluated his internal injuries and pronounced them untreatable. He seemed convinced that Priessnitz would never recover.

Undeterred by his surgeon's evaluation, Priessnitz went home and set his broken ribs by pressing his abdomen against the arm of a chair, then covered the injured ribs with cloths that were moistened with cold water. Ten days later, he had resumed his place on the farm with his previous rounds of chores.

Duly impressed with the effectiveness of his own self-treatment, Priessnitz became a strong advocate of hydrotherapy, using the treatments with the sick and injured who came from far and near for treatments. His fame spread until medical authorities became jealous of the popularity and success of his practice. But their efforts to get him to halt his practice were futile, even when they resorted to legal means. In the view of the court, Priessnitz was just making use of a natural substance, water, and was not using medicine.

In one instance, when a patient was called as a trial witness, the judge asked specifically who had helped the patient. The patient replied, "They have all helped me. The doctors, the apothecaries, and Priessnitz. The former helped me to get rid of my money, and Priessnitz, to get rid of my illness."

Eventually, Priessnitz's critics were muted by his record of success with such patients. In the end, the Austrian Emperor gave Priessnitz a gold medal for civic merit, the highest mark of distinct in Austria.


## TAPPING INTO HYDROTHERAPY

As I have noted, there are many different types of hydrotherapy. The one I recommend most frequently, known as constitutional hydrotherapy, was taught to me by Dr. Jared Zeff of Portland, Oregon. Dr Zeff, in turn, had inherited his knowledge and ability from older generations of naturopathic doctors.

Constitutional hydrotherapy benefits the whole body. Among the many benign effects of this type of therapy, it helps to produce the following results:

1. Optimizes circulation
2. Detoxifies and purifies the blood
3. Enhances digestive function and elimination
4. Tonifies and balances the nervous system
5. Stimulates and enhances the immune system.

Constitutional hydrotherapy is best done with an assistant, who is needed to lay the wet towels on various parts of the body and replace the towels as they cool. The usual sequence of events is as follows:

1. Lie in bed on your back.

2. The assistant covers your bared chest and abdomen with two thicknesses of towels that have been placed in hot water and wrung out. (If it's a child who's being treated, rather than yourself, you need to make sure the water is tolerably warm. Before you give a full-scale treatment, be sure to place a small section of the towel on the child to make sure the cloth isn't too hot.)

3. The assistant should cover the wet, hot towels with a dry towel.

4. Blankets go on top of the dry towel. Once you're bundled up, the towels and blanket should stay on at least 5 minutes.

5. After 5 minutes, remove the hot towels and replace them with a single thickness of a thin towel that has been run under cold water and then wrung out. (There should still be some moisture left in the towel.)

6. Place the cold towel on the bared chest and abdomen. Cover with a dry towel and blankets. Leave the towel on for 10 minutes, which is about how long it takes to reach body temperature. (If it takes longer than that to warm up, leave it on longer and don't make the towel so cold or wet next time.)

7. Your assistant may have to take off the cold towel (depending on what part of your body it covers). After it's off, turn over and lie on your stomach.

8. Repeat the same procedure on your back while lying on your stomach—following 5 minutes of hot towel treatment with 10 minutes under a thin, cold towel.

The contrast between hot and cold is the effective part of this therapy. Heat dilates the blood vessels, while cold initially constricts and then dilates them. The alternating dilation and contraction creates a pumping action that improves circulation through the superficial and deep blood vessels.

## DOSAGE

I recommend one or two treatments daily if you have an acute condition. For a chronic condition, once a day is sufficient. After each treatment, drink at least 8 ounces of purified water and rest for at least 15 minutes.

If you're giving treatments to an infant, be sure to follow the guidelines of a natural or holistic doctor.

Do not eat large meals before a hydrotherapy treatment.

# WHAT ARE THE SIDE EFFECTS?

Hydrotherapy is not recommended if you have an asthma condition. Also, it should only be done with the guidance of a naturopathic or holistic doctor if you're pregnant or have diabetes.

## CONSTITUTIONAL HYDROTHERAPY
### RECOMMENDATIONS FROM THE NATURAL PHYSICIAN FOR . . .

### ❧ Arthritis

Constitutional hydrotherapy is effective for all types of arthritis. It improves circulation and reduces inflammation of the joints. It also addresses the underlying cause of many cases of arthritis such as toxicity and poor digestion. Local applications of hot and cold, or alternating hot and cold, help to soothe and relieve pain.

### ❧ Bronchitis and Pneumonia

Hydrotherapy is one of the best therapies for respiratory tract conditions. If you apply alternating hot and cold directly over the bronchial area, you may be able to see very rapid results.

### ❧ Cancer

The stronger your immune system, the greater your ability to resist cancer. Hydrotherapy helps your immune system in a number of ways: aids detoxification, improves digestion, and stimulates immune-cell activity. This therapy also helps with lymphatic drainage that is so important for a healthy immune system.

I advise patients who have cancer to use constitutional hydrotherapy as part of a comprehensive program coordinated by the doctor who's overseeing the treatment. It does not interfere with any conventional treatments such as chemotherapy or radiation.

### ❧ Detoxification

You cannot be healthy in today's world without efficient detoxification. Constitutional hydrotherapy stimulates circulation through the liver and kidneys to eliminate toxins. It also brings blood flow to the skin to help with the toxin-elimination process. In addition, it improves digestion and, therefore, elimination.

If you're already on a detoxification program, I advise adding constitutional hydrotherapy as part of the therapy. As a matter of fact, some naturopathic doctors get amazing results by detoxifying people with hydrotherapy combined with dietary changes.

### ❧ Fever and Infections

Constitutional hydrotherapy stimulates the white blood cells, increasing their number and their activity. This makes it an excellent therapy for fevers and infections. As a matter of fact, the fever may increase slightly, and temporarily, with hydrotherapy treatments, a sign the immune system is "kicking in." Soon after, the fever drops below where it started, a sign that the infection is calming down.

*(continued)*

### ∾ Digestive Conditions

When hydrotherapy is applied to the abdominal area, there's a great increase in circulation to the digestive organs, including stomach, intestines, colon, liver, gallbladder, and pancreas. The improved circulation helps to heal inflamed or damaged tissues, promotes better function of the digestive organs, and improves elimination through the colon. I commonly recommend it for the following digestive conditions:

- *Constipation.* Hydrotherapy helps normalize the messages that travel from the nerve centers to the colon and digestive organs. It helps to stimulate and balance peristalsis— the wavelike contractions that move stool through the colon.

- *Crohn's Disease, Ulcers, and Ulcerative Colitis.* Tissues are inflamed and damaged with these diseases. I have seen a lot of people with these problems have long-term improvements from constitutional hydrotherapy. If the condition is serious, it may take months of treatments to heal the damaged tissues, but consistent treatments are almost invariably effective.

- *Irritable Bowel Syndrome.* Often, this condition is the result of stress combined with poor digestion. Hydrotherapy helps to tonify the system, which usually produces good improvements. This therapy is also good for treatment of acute symptoms associated with irritable bowel syndrome, such as abdominal pain, gas, and bloating.

### ∾ Headaches

Chronic headaches can be greatly improved or relieved with constitutional hydrotherapy. People suffering from toxicity, maldigestion, and poor liver function are most helped with this therapy. A more effective treatment for acute headaches is foot hydrotherapy.

While there are different versions of foot hydrotherapy, I've found the following sequence to be effective:

At the onset of a headache, place your feet in a bucket or tub of hot water. (The water should be as hot as possible, but still tolerable to the touch.) Then place a cold cloth on your forehead or an ice pack on the back of your neck.

With this combination of hot and cold, your body diverts blood flow to the feet and away from the head, thus reducing head congestion. The treatment can also be helpful for sinusitis.

### ∾ Skin Conditions

The skin is the largest organ of elimination. Therefore, internal toxicity often shows up on the skin. Such is often the case with chronic skin rashes and eczema. I have seen constitutional hydrotherapy help to clear up longstanding cases of skin rashes.

# I

# Ignatia

......................................................................

"Dr. Mark, I am so stressed out! With all the things going on at my job and with my kids, I'm embarrassed to say that my husband and I are having problems again. I just don't know if I can handle it anymore."

These were the words of Jacqueline, a patient whose family I had consulted with over the years. In the past, I had helped her children with various health problems. Now Jacqueline felt the time was right to get her own health in order.

During Jacqueline's visit, she described herself as a very caring person whose feelings are hurt very easily. She takes her work and home life very seriously—perhaps too seriously, as she admitted. As a result, she suffered from tight shoulder and neck muscles, which could trigger excruciating tension headaches.

"I get very moody," she observed, when I asked her to talk about her emotions. She went on to say that she would occasionally lose her temper with her kids or husband over trivial matters that had never bothered her in the past. Jacqueline often felt like crying, sometimes for no apparent reason, and she spoke of "walking around with a lump in my throat." Even in our first interview, I noticed that from time to time, she would sigh heavily as if she was trying to bear up under a great load of stress.

Jacqueline's situation is hardly unique. Many women feel themselves in similar situations, with similar reactions. My prescription, in these cases, is the homeopathic remedy ignatia.

In fact, many women and men in our society would benefit from taking ignatia (*Ignatia amarus*), along with using a number of stress-reduction techniques. Frequently prescribed by homeopathic physicians for the effects of stress, it's especially effective when people are suffering grief of any kind. This could be grief from

## A Jaw-Saving Remedy

One of the most dramatic cases of homeopathic healing I have ever seen involved a 30-year-old patient of mine, Laura, who had a severe case of TMJ. As a matter of fact, it was so severe her doctor was recommending jaw surgery. In an attempt to forego surgery, Laura was getting regular chiropractic, massage, and acupuncture treatments. All gave her temporary relief, but no permanent escape. A few hours after each treatment, her jaw muscles would tighten up again and the unbearable pain would set in.

After taking her case, I found out that she and her husband were very stressed about having children. Laura had an emotionally traumatic history of miscarriages. Many people who have TMJ can trace the onset to some physical trauma like a car accident. But in Laura's case, the TMJ problem began about the same time as her first miscarriage.

Coincidence? Perhaps, but even so, I felt ignatia was worth trying.

Five minutes after Laura took her first dose of ignatia 30C, she noticed improvement of her TMJ discomfort. She called me immediately, very excited about the improvement. Of course, I simply recommended that she continue taking it as needed.

Over the next week, Laura found that she had to take ignatia a few times a day to prevent the muscle tightness and TMJ from flaring up. But about two weeks later, after receiving a number of encouraging reports from her, I got a panicked call.

"The remedy is not working any more. My TMJ is killing me!"

"All right," I replied. "I want you to take the 200C potency of ignatia and call me back in 30 minutes."

After about a half hour of suspense, Laura called to say the higher potency was effective. Triumphantly, she announced that the TMJ pain went away in about 5 minutes after taking the stronger dose.

Miraculously, Laura has only had to repeat the high-potency ignatia a couple of times in the ensuing 5 years. I spoke to her much less frequently, but at last report, she was no longer suffering from TMJ syndrome.

the death of a loved one, grief from a turbulent relationship or divorce, or grief from some kind of misgivings.

The connection between stress and grief is obvious. Anyone who's grieving has all sorts of stored emotions that may cause her to "tighten up." These emotions can be expressed in many different ways—crying, mood swings, or tightening muscles. All these factors contribute to what homeopathic physicians call an ignatia state.

But there may be other factors as well. I often find the person requiring ignatia to be a perfectionist. Living in an imperfect world leads to easily hurt feelings and a lot of disappointments. The feelings of disappointment and grief are suppressed, which leads to a very interesting ignatia symptom—the sensation of a lump in the throat.

As strange as it may sound, many patients requiring ignatia have said almost exactly the same thing—that they felt a "lump in the throat." Now, whenever I hear of this characteristic symptom, the remedy ignatia immediately comes to mind.

But there's another unique symptom that suggests the need for this remedy—sighing. I realize that no conventional doctor would ask a patient, "Are you sighing a lot?"—but we all recognize, and know intuitively, that sighing is a very real expression of an emotion. As I have learned in Chinese medicine, symptoms of suppressed grief often show up in the lungs, with sighing being an outlet for this contained grief.

By the way, Jacqueline responded very nicely to ignatia. After only two days she felt "calmer" and in the following two months, her muscle tightness greatly decreased and that "lump in the throat" feeling went away. She felt that she was now in more control of her feelings and that the ignatia definitely was helping.

## DOSAGE

The typical dosage for ignatia is to take a 30C potency twice daily for a week or longer, or until the user has experienced substantial relief of symptoms. When symptoms have been acute, most people notice a difference in one or two doses. Homeopathic practitioners often give a single dose of 200C or higher in the belief that it will have a deeper effect. I have noticed that some patients respond better to a higher potency of ignatia.

## WHAT ARE THE SIDE EFFECTS?

Ignatia has no side effects at all with some people. If it's not helpful, however, you can simply stop using it. If you have questions about whether or not you should use ignatia in the first place, you'll want to consult a homeopathic practitioner.

---

# IGNATIA
## RECOMMENDATIONS FROM THE NATURAL PHYSICIAN FOR . . .

### ◌ Depression

Ignatia works quite nicely to relieve depression when it comes on after a grief or disappointment. A common example is a person who is suffering in a relationship where things are not going well, and depression sets in from the suppression of grief. Ignatia helps to release the suppressed grief and relieve some of the symptoms of depression.

### ◌ Grief

Ignatia remedy comes in handy when grief occurs suddenly, in unforeseen circumstances. If a loved one has died suddenly, people may ask me what kind of natural therapy can help ease the shock and pain of the moment. Ignatia is the first remedy to try. Obviously, it will not take away all the emotions that naturally accompany a tragedy. But for those who are very sensitive, who have a hard time coping, it helps reduce that "heart pain." With ignatia, you can avoid the use of tranquilizing and antidepressant medications.

Many practitioners of homeopathy, as well as psychologists and counselors, have observed that patients who are undergoing counseling for deep-seated emotional traumas recover more

*(continued)*

quickly when they are also given the indicated homeopathic "grief" remedy like ignatia. I have seen this with patients who have made little improvement with various counselors over the years. When given ignatia, they make dramatic changes in their outlook on life.

Ignatia works to help remove emotional blockages. For example, I remember one 44-year-old patient, Minnie, who had a bad case of multiple sclerosis (a serious condition where the immune system attacks the body's nervous tissue). Minnie related to me that her condition had started right after her divorce four years previously. Although she had tried various natural and conventional therapies, her condition was getting worse.

Based on the fact that her illness began after the trauma of her divorce, I prescribed ignatia. Two weeks after taking ignatia, Minnie came to see me, as she was feeling very emotional. She found herself crying a lot and losing her temper more than usual. My comment to her was "Great!"

"What do you mean, great?" she shot back. "I feel like an emotional basket case, I haven't felt like this in years!"

"This is probably similar to how you felt during your divorce," I suggested. After a moment's hesitation, she agreed.

"That's an excellent sign," I went on. "You need to heal emotionally before you can heal physically."

The intensity of Minnie's symptoms began to diminish over the next week. She felt a commensurate increase in her energy level, another sign the remedy was working.

Over the next two months, her muscle weakness and visual problems ceased to be a problem, and during the next three years, Minnie lived without symptoms of multiple sclerosis. Apart from taking repeated doses of ignatia during times of severe stress, she takes no other medicines.

### ❧ Headache

As most of us have learned by experience, stress contributes to the most common type of headache, known as a tension headache—an experience of pain that patients sometimes describe as a "vice tightening around their head." Tension headaches are related to tight neck and shoulder muscles.

Since ignatia helps to reduce the effects of stress, and also reduces muscle tightness, it's a remedy worthy of consideration any time you have a tension headache. It is particularly indicated when the headaches occur on the left side of the head.

### ❧ Muscle Spasm

If you're prone to muscle tightness as the result of stress, the tightness usually occurs in the neck and shoulders. Ignatia, as well as massage, works nicely to prevent the tightness and muscle spasms in this area.

In addition, ignatia can save a lot of trips to the chiropractor. My wife, who is also a naturopathic physician, treated one woman who had chronic, severe fibromyalgia, a painful condition of the muscles and joints. After my wife administered one high-potency dose of ignatia, the woman discovered that her symptoms were alleviated—permanently!

### ❧ PMS

Premenstrual syndrome can be greatly helped by ignatia. It is indicated when symptoms of crying, mood swings, and jealousy come out during the premenstrual days.

### ❧ TMJ Syndrome

This is not something you will find in too many books, but I have found ignatia to help a number of patients who have temporomandibular joint disorder (TMJ), a painful condition of the jaw joint.

# Ipecacuanha

"I might need to go home soon. I woke up this morning feeling nauseated, and it hasn't gone away. Do you have a homeopathic that can help me?" asked Val, the office manager at our clinic.

"Sure, but are you pregnant?" I asked half-jokingly.

"No I'm not. It feels like I may be coming down with the flu," replied Val.

"Here you go. Take two pellets and let's see how you do over the next fifteen minutes," I said.

As I walked by the front desk five minutes later, Val stopped me.

"It's amazing," she said. "The nausea is all gone. Can it work that fast?"

"Yes, homeopathics can be pretty incredible," I said.

"They really can be. What was the one you gave me?" inquired Val.

"It's called ipecac."

"Isn't ipecac used to make people throw up?"

"Regular ipecac is used for that; but homeopathic ipecac has the opposite effect. It relieves nausea and vomiting."

The next day, Val reported that she had felt fine for the rest of the evening.

## ROOTS FROM THE NEW WORLD

Ipecacuanha is the homeopathic preparation from the leaves of the ipecacuanha shrub from Brazil. The leaves of this shrub have a bitter, nauseating taste. Thus, it has been used in Brazil since 1648 as an emetic (to make people throw up to expel ingested poisons). The standard medicine is found in medicine kits and in pharmacies. The homeopathic has the opposite effect, and helps to relieve nausea and vomiting.

Homeopathic ipecacuanha, referred to by homeopaths as ipecac, is the main remedy for nausea and vomiting, no matter what the cause. This could be the result of the flu, as in Val's case, or intestinal problems that result from spoiled food, bronchitis, or a condition where there is marked nausea and/or vomiting such as from a migraine headache.

Ipecac is also commonly recommended for women who have nausea associated with pregnancy. In addition, I've recommended it as a remedy for hemorrhaging—such as uterine hemorrhage—as well as for bronchitis and asthma.

**271**

As with any homeopathic remedy, physicians look for certain key symptoms. In the case of homeopathic ipecac, the telltale symptom is constant nausea that is unrelieved by vomiting. But there may be another symptom as well—the tongue looks clean despite constant vomiting.

This is definitely a remedy that belongs in every first-aid kit.

## DOSAGE

Dissolve two pellets of the 30C potency (or whatever potency you have on hand) in your mouth every 15 minutes for the relief of symptoms. Two to three doses should be sufficient for acute cases.

*Note:* The dosage is the same for all age groups.

## WHAT ARE THE SIDE EFFECTS?

There is no concern about toxicity or side effects with homeopathic ipecacuanha. As with any homeopathic remedy, take it as needed for relief of symptoms.

---

## IPECAC
### RECOMMENDATIONS FROM THE NATURAL PHYSICIAN FOR . . .

**∾ Asthma and Bronchitis**

Ipecac is useful for a rattling cough that is accompanied by gagging and vomiting resulting from increased mucus. These symptoms might indicate a case of bronchitis or asthma. Symptoms are worse at night, when eating, and when in a warm room. The person feels better in the open air, after coughing up mucus, and being in a cool room.

Homeopathic ipecac is a common remedy for childhood asthma.

**∾ Hangover**

Ipecac can help reduce the nausea and vomiting that occur the "morning after" indulging in too much alcohol.

**∾ Hemorrhage**

Ipecac is a good remedy for uterine hemorrhage or heavy menstrual flow, accompanied by nausea and vomiting.

**∾ Migraine Headache**

The severe nausea and vomiting caused by migraines can be alleviated with ipecac. The headaches tend to be on the left side. It's most likely to be effective if you have a migraine headache that makes you want to remain still and if you feel better with fresh air.

(continued)

**🙰 Morning Sickness**

Ipecac is one of the main remedies to help relieve the classic nausea and vomiting that some women get during pregnancy. The nice thing about homeopathic ipecac is that there is no risk of side effects that would harm the baby.

# Ipriflavone

"Here is what I am taking."

Mary, a 55-year-old restaurant owner who had come to see me about her osteoporosis, lifted a supplement-filled plastic bag to my desk. As I watched in wonderment, she methodically arranged twenty-one bottles of supplements single file along the edge.

"Is that *all?*" I asked, when she had added the last bottle to the row.

Mary looked chagrined at the note of awe in my voice. "I've been looking forward to this day. I really have no idea what I should or should not be taking. The trouble is, I read a whole lot of health magazines, and I have a friend who works in a health food store. Adding up all the advice I get from one place or the other, well—" she paused, waving her hand. "Here's where I am."

Reading the formulations on each bottle, I made some notes, then asked, "Suppose you could reduce the number of supplements from twenty-one to five? Would you do it?"

"Wouldn't that be nice!" She hesitated. "But I want to make sure I'm not missing anything. I saw what my mother went through when she had a hip fracture in her seventies. She was never the same after that. I know a lot of women who worry about osteoporosis, but it seems to be a particular problem in our family. I don't want to end up with a hip fracture like my mother did."

In principle, Mary was absolutely right to be concerned about her osteoporosis. A recent bone-density study showed that she was below average for her age, and she had the beginnings of osteoporosis (decreased bone density).

But her supplement program was out of control. As I told Mary, I would help her simplify that program, but at the same time, I wanted to add one important supplement to it. "It's called ipriflavone," I said.

"It sounds like something all women such as myself should be taking," Mary observed.

"Probably," I replied, "and it can help men's bones too."

## A MASTER BUILDER

Ipriflavone increases the activity of the cells that form fresh bone. At the same time, it decreases the activity of bone cells that aid in the destruction of the bone. This supplement also raises the levels of a hormone that helps to increase the amount of new bone that's constantly being created by a healthy body.

So ipriflavone really has two effects. It helps *maintain* bone density, and, when it's combined with calcium and other substances in your body, it does even more—it helps to *increase* bone density.

Ipriflavone is still being scrutinized, and not all studies support its effectiveness. For instance, as this book was going to press, a negative study about ipriflavone appeared in the *Journal of the American Medical Associations (JAMA)* indicating that ipriflavone combined with calcium was no better than a placebo in slowing bone loss. However, as with most drug or supplement studies, it is common to have a certain percentage of studies that are not favorable. In general, clinical studies over the past 15 years on ipriflavone have been positive. Over 150 studies of its safety and effectiveness, in both animal and human studies, lend support to its use.

In fact, the use of ipriflavone is likely to become more prevalent. One out of every three women in North America develops osteoporosis, and researchers expect that the percentage of Americans with osteoporosis is going to continue to climb steadily as baby boomers move into their elder years.

An estimated 7 to 10 billion dollars each year are spent treating the complications that arise from this disease—such as the hip fracture that Mary's mother endured. Broken bones are debilitating when they happen to older people. Statistics show that after a hip fracture occurs, approximately 15 percent of patients die within one year. (Often, the problem is some complicating factor, such as a blood clot that's related to prolonged immobility.)

Ipriflavone is an isolated copy of an important chemical found in soy, called isoflavone daidzein. First discovered in 1930, ipriflavone has been widely studied in humans, though it really didn't become widely used until the mid 1990s.

## BARRING BREAKDOWNS

Bone continually remodels itself. Bone cells are constantly being eroded by cells called osteoclasts, while new bone is being formed with the help of other cells called osteoblasts. The key to good bone health? Just replace as many or more bone cells than are lost.

But, of course, that replacement and rebuilding process requires assistance. That's where ipriflavone comes in.

Ipriflavone has been found to have its own receptor site on immature osteoblasts—the bone-building cells. It directly stimulates the activity of these cells, which in turn promote bone-cell formation. And ipriflavone does not have an estrogenic effect. That's an advantage, because estrogen produces a number of side effects and has been shown to increase the risk of breast cancer as well as other kinds of cancer.

In one study, 15 postmenopausal women were given ipriflavone or a placebo. Various hormones, including estrogen, were measured after a single oral dose of 600 or 1,000 milligrams, and after 7, 14, and 21 days of treatment with 600- or 1,000-milligram doses. By the end of the study, there was no elevation of estrogen among any of the women. Clearly, the ipriflavone did not have the effect of increasing estrogen levels.

Studies do show that ipriflavone acts synergistically with estrogen to normalize calcitonin secretion. In other words, it helps open the pathway for more active bone growth.

## DOSAGE

I recommend ipriflavone be supplemented at 600 milligrams daily. This is the same dosage used in the osteoporosis studies.

It's important to note, however, that calcium was given to many of the people who participated in the studies, so the bone-strengthening benefits were really the result of dual supplementation.

Take ipriflavone with meals to enhance absorption. For maximum effectiveness, I always recommend taking it with other vitamins and minerals known to play a role in bone metabolism. Calcium, magnesium, and vitamin D are the most important. But there are other important supplements as well, including zinc, silicon, manganese, vitamin C, vitamin B$_6$, boron, vitamin K, vitamin B$_{12}$, and folic acid. All these can be found in bone-building formulas offered by many companies, so you don't have to purchase them separately.

## WHAT ARE THE SIDE EFFECTS?

In general, ipriflavone appears to be very safe. In a study that was launched in 1997, researchers showed the long-term safety of ipriflavone for periods ranging from 6 to 96 months, when the supplement was taken by 2,769 people.

The most common side effect is digestive upset, but this symptom is likely to go away if you take ipriflavone with food. Other symptoms observed, to a lesser extent, included skin rashes, headache, depression, drowsiness, and rapid heartbeat (tachycardia). A small percentage of people, when tested, showed minor abnormalities in liver, kidney, and blood, but the abnormalities were quite minor and they rapidly disappeared.

I advise caution with ipriflavone, however, if you're taking the drug theophylline for asthma. In one case, someone who was already taking theophylline had excessive levels of this substance in her blood when she started taking ipriflavone along with her regular asthma medication. Animal studies have found that ipriflavone may inhibit certain liver enzymes that break down theophylline, leading to higher-than-normal blood levels.

For anyone who's had kidney failure, I advise close monitoring before supplementing with ipriflavone, although it appears to be safe in those with mild kidney disease. Researchers recommend lower doses (200 to 400 milligrams daily) in patients with more advanced renal failure. Further study is required to determine absolute safe dosages for those with kidney disease.

Lymphocyte levels should also be watched by a doctor. In one study of 132 women who were taking ipriflavone, 29 of the women in the group developed a reduction in lymphocytes, a type of white blood cell that is an integral component of the immune system. According to some researchers, the reduction in lymphocytes in this study is not clinically significant. However, to be safe your doctor can measure your lymphocyte levels with a simple blood test every 6 months to make sure your levels are within normal ranges. Optimally, blood work would be done at the onset of starting ipriflavone and every six months thereafter.

# IPRIFLAVONE
## Recommendations from the Natural Physician for . . .

### ❧ Hyperparathyroidism

In this condition, high levels of parathyroid hormone cause calcium to be withdrawn from the bone and cause elevated levels of blood calcium. As a result, bone health suffers from calcium loss. One study showed that 1,200 milligrams of ipriflavone daily resulted in significant reduction of bone turnover. Researchers interpreted this to mean that there was increased bone formation among those who took ipriflavone.

### ❧ Kidney Failure

Ipriflavone is not a supplement for the treatment of renal failure. It may, however, be of value if someone is losing bone minerals because of kidney failure (known as renal osteodystrophy). One study of 23 people on kidney dialysis with decreased bone mineralization due to renal failure were given ipriflavone (400 to 600 milligrams daily) and observed for a period of one to nine months. Researchers found evidence that there was significantly less breakdown of bone and significant increases in bone formation. No adverse side effects were reported. But I would want to see more research before recommending ipriflavone for anyone with a kidney condition.

### ❧ Osteoporosis

There have been over 60 human studies in the past 10 years, many of which are double-blind and placebo-controlled—meeting the standards for scientific validity.

The most significant study I've run across involved 100 postmenopausal women between the ages of 53 and 65, whom researchers tracked for a full year. Each woman received 200 milligrams of ipriflavone three times a day after meals. They were also given 1,000 milligrams of calcium daily. Ninety women completed the study, and the results indicate that bone-mineral density was increased by 2 percent after 6 months and 5.8 percent after 12 months!

During that time, pain symptoms also decreased and mobility improved. Only three women dropped out of the study because of problems with digestive upset. This study is even more remarkable when its outcome is compared with what happens with other kinds of drug therapies. Most pharmaceutical drugs only slow down the loss of bone, and usually, when calcium is added as a supplement, the rate of bone loss increases, but the calcium supplement doesn't help increase bone density. Researchers came to the conclusion that ipriflavone was the decisive factor in improving bone density.

Researchers have explored in a number of studies the possibility of combining ipriflavone with estrogen for the treatment of osteoporosis. Some of these studies have, indeed, shown that bone density improves more significantly when people get a combined dose of ipriflavone and estrogen. With the combination treatment, it's feasible to take lower doses of estrogen—which is a benefit, since that may reduce the risk of estrogen-related cancers.

For example, in one controlled, 1-year study, 83 postmenopausal women were divided into three groups. The first group received neither estrogen nor supplements; the second received estrogen; and the third got ipriflavone along with estrogen. At the end of the 12 months, those who got the combination treatment showed a significant increase in bone-mineral density. Though bone density decreased or increased only slightly in the

(continued)

other groups, it was up 5.6 percent among those who had a combination of estrogen and ipriflavone. These results have been supported by other human studies as well.

Ipriflavone can also help women who have had their ovaries removed (ovariectomy). Typically, the removal of the ovaries results in rapid bone loss because there's a sharp decrease in hormone production. A study of 32 women who had recently had ovariectomies showed that ipriflavone appeared to protect them from sudden bone loss. In the study, the women received 500 milligrams of calcium and 600 milligrams of ipriflavone daily for 12 months.

### ∾ Otosclerosis

There are sometimes small but significant changes in the structure of one of the bones involved with hearing—a very tiny structure called the stapes. This condition leads to gradual hearing loss, the condition known as otosclerosis. It's sometimes accompanied by another type of hearing problem, tinnitus, which is essentially "ringing in the ears."

Otosclerosis can be treated surgically, and a hearing aid can help compensate for some hearing loss. To find out whether ipriflavone could help this condition in some way, researchers tried a small study of patients who had tinnitus due to otosclerosis.

All the patients also had stapedectomies—that is, removal of the inner ear bone. People in the ipriflavone study received 200 milligrams of the supplement four times daily. Supplementation began three months before the operation, then continued at the same dosage for three months afterward. During the preoperative phase, tinnitus was stopped in four of nine patients. (Only one out of seven in the placebo group experienced relief of tinnitus.) Postoperatively, all patients in the ipriflavone group, but only 50 percent of the patients in the placebo group, experienced relief of tinnitus.

Though researchers can't explain why the ipriflavone was beneficial in this study, it will almost certainly lead to further exploration.

### ∾ Paget's Disease

This is a disorder of the skeleton where bone turnover is increased to an abnormal rate. As a result, bones develop in abnormal ways, people have more fractures, and some of those with Paget's disease have severe bone pain. Almost 3 percent of people over the age of 40 have this disease, though the cause is unknown.

When doctors studied 16 patients who had this disease, they found that ipriflavone supplementation reduced the evidence of bone breakdown—which means the "turnover" was slowed. Bone pain was also reduced. Dosages used in the study were 600 to 1,200 milligrams daily.

# Iron

Iron has paradoxical qualities. It can be a healing therapy, but it can also be toxic, causing illness. A simple health-giving goal is to get the most out of iron and avoid the potential risks.

We need iron to live. It enables our red blood cells to carry oxygen to the cells. It also is involved in different enzyme reactions, one of which is to produce energy. However necessary, though, it can create problems if you get too much iron in supplements or if you suffer from a genetic condition like hemochromatosis—which means, simply, that your body absorbs abnormally high amounts of iron. An excess of iron definitely causes side effects, and researchers think it's also connected with certain diseases. There's some evidence that there is a correlation between excessive iron levels and increased risk of heart disease and cancer.

There are two sources of dietary iron, referred to as heme and nonheme. Heme iron is found in animal products and is the form that our bodies absorb most efficiently. Nonheme iron is found in plant foods and is not absorbed so well.

Your body stores iron in the liver, spleen, and bone marrow.

## SOME IRONIES

Though it's easy to get iron in the diet or in supplements, iron deficiency is the most prevalent type of nutrient deficiency in the United States—and it has consequences. Iron-deficiency anemia, as the name implies, is a direct result. If you have this kind of anemia (there are other kinds as well), your red blood cells lose some of their capacity to carry oxygen. From that microscopic change in transport capabilities, you can end up with a whole range of serious problems, including fatigue, poor memory and concentration, learning problems, paleness, increased menstrual loss, and weakened immunity.

Symptoms of chronic, severe iron deficiency are even more pronounced. Some people get a condition called pica, a craving for substances, such as dirt, ice, or pencils, that have no nutritional value. Cracks in the corner of the mouth, or cheilosis, is another common problem. People with severe deficiency may also develop spoon-shaped fingernails and toenails.

There are serious consequences of iron deficiency in children. Studies show that approximately 9 percent of all children in the U.S. between the ages of 12 months and 36 months have iron-deficiency anemia. The prevalence is higher among children living at or below poverty level, and it's also higher among black or Mexican-American children.

When children are iron deficient, they may have delayed physical growth, slow mental development (as evidenced by lower IQ scores and poor short-term memory), and behavioral disturbances such as hyperactivity and problems with social interaction. Unfortunately, if the iron deficiency continues beyond age 5, these changes can be irreversible.

Growth spurts in children and teenagers can lead to an increased demand for iron and thus iron-deficiency anemia.

Severe iron deficiency also has consequences for adults. Among women, iron deficiency can lead to prolonged menstrual bleeding. For adults of either sex, if you frequently feel tired, or if you can't sustain activity for a prolonged length of time, these symptoms of fatigue may be due to iron deficiency.

## BLOOD BOTHERS

The question is, how do we become deficient in iron in the first place?

The most common cause for adults is blood loss. For women this is mainly due to heavy menstrual flow. A vicious cycle occurs when a menstruating woman is anemic, because the iron-deficiency anemia actually leads to even more bleeding. In some cases, the bleeding is continuous, not just cyclical. So a woman with this condition needs to raise her iron levels and get the anemia improved to correct the underlying cause of the heavy menstruation. But the underlying problem—and what leads, ultimately, to iron deficiency—could be a hormone imbalance.

Shelly is a good example of what women can go through with this condition. A 22-year-old college student with a 4-year history of heavy menstrual bleeding, Shelly had become severely anemic. I could see indications of that, even before I did an examination. Her face was pale and she had purple circles under her eyes. Suspecting iron deficiency, I checked the inside of her eyelids—which were as pale as her face—and felt her hands, which were chilly.

Shelly's medical doctor had put her on high doses of iron tablets. Though she was taking 150 milligrams a day, the therapy wasn't helping. In fact, these large doses of iron caused severe constipation. Her cyclical menstrual flow had been heavy, but with the addition of large doses of iron, it turned into continuous bleeding that was uninterrupted throughout the month. It was not heavy every day, but there was always some blood loss.

Her doctor had then recommended the next, usual step in conventional medicine: prescribing a birth-control pill to help regulate Shelly's menstrual cycle. These pills, however, gave her severe migraine headaches, and she stopped using them—whereupon her doctor told her that the only option left was a hysterectomy. At that point, Shelly knew she wanted to try other resources, and upon the advice of a friend, she came to see me.

The first lab test revealed immediately that the anemia was very severe. I switched her over to 50 milligrams a day of a more absorbable form of iron. I also asked her to take other nutrients to help build her blood—among them, vitamin C (which improves iron absorption), folic acid, and vitamin B$_{12}$. Finally, I gave her homeopathic ferrum phos 6x and the herb vitex for hormone balancing.

Things did not improve overnight, but over the next two months, Shelly could feel that progress was being made. She felt more energetic. I continued to do the lab work necessary to monitor her blood —and the results showed a steady increase of iron. After three months of treatment, the bleeding was under control. We were eventually able to get her off the iron and other supplements, and she made a full recovery.

## Minding Your Iron Mine

Good sources of iron include beef, organ meats, and eggs. Good plant sources include lima beans, tofu, legumes, kelp, green leafy vegetables, whole grains, Brewer's yeast, pumpkin, and nuts.

It's important to keep in mind that the iron you get from meat is much more easily absorbed than the kind that comes from plant foods. Approximately 30 percent of heme iron (from meat) is absorbed while only 2 to 10 percent of nonheme iron (from plant foods) makes its way into your cells. This does not mean that people living on a vegetarian diet are destined to become iron deficient. You can get all the iron you need without eating meat. On a vegetarian diet, however, it's important to get plenty of iron-contributing plant foods or to supplement your diet with a well-absorbed form of iron.

How much iron do you need on a daily basis? Following are the Recommended Dietary Allowances for iron. While some people may need more than these recommended daily amounts, they are usually adequate.

Birth to 6 months: 6 milligrams

6–12 months: 10 milligrams

1–10 years: 10 milligrams

Males 11–18 years: 12 milligrams

Males 19 and older: 10 milligrams

Females 11–50 years: 15 milligrams

Females 51 and older: 10 milligrams

Pregnant Females: 30 milligrams

Lactating Females: 15 milligrams

Whether or not you show physical, external signs of iron deficiency, your doctor should give you a regular blood test for iron. The test is quite simple, and children, in particular, should be screened regularly. It also makes sense for your doctor to run a ferritin test, which measures the amount of stored iron in the body.

## LINKS AND CAUSES

Iron deficiency is often a problem in pregnant women. The growing baby uses much of the mother's iron stores and so she is prone to iron-deficiency anemia, which can lead to complications if the condition isn't identified and treated. The rate of premature delivery is twice as high for a mother who has iron-deficiency anemia, and the birth weight of the newborn tends to be much lower. Infants who are born prematurely are also much more prone to iron deficiency than those who reach full term.

Among men who have iron deficiency, the most common cause is what's known as chronic occult bleeding—the medical term for internal bleeding. (Women may have chronic occult bleeding as well, though it's a less common cause of iron deficiency than menstrual bleeding.) Adults of either sex may have bleeding in the gastrointestinal tract, related to polyps or ulcers, or by hemmorrhoids. Internal bleeding may be associated with drugs that irritate the gastrointestinal lining, such as aspirin. There's also a risk that the bleeding can be caused by cancer.

Among infants and children who have iron deficiency, the main cause is obvious—lack of iron in the diet. But there's another, lesser-known cause: The consumption of cow's milk may cause gastrointestinal bleeding.

Some people simply don't absorb iron so efficiently as they need to. In some cases, particularly among the elderly, the problem is low production of stomach acid. Similar problems can arise if you take a lot of antacids, because the antacid neutralizes stomach acid.

## DOSAGE

Since dosages depend on the severity of iron deficiency, you should work with a nutrition-oriented doctor when supplementing iron so that it can be monitored correctly. A typical adult dosage is 25 milligrams of elemental iron taken twice daily, but you'll probably need higher dosages if you have severe anemia. I recommend taking the iron supplement with meals to avoid digestive upset.

Iron supplements can be absorbed on an empty stomach and some studies show that it has a higher absorption taken this way. Vitamin C enhances the absorption of iron so it is prudent to take a couple hundred milligrams with every dose of iron. I commonly recommend homeopathic ferrum phos 6x and the herbs yellow dock and nettles for blood building as well.

There are some supplements that can interfere with the absorption of iron, including calcium carbonate, magnesium, and zinc—so don't take them at the same time you're taking iron. Antibiotics can also interfere with absorption: If you have a prescription, take it as recommended, but wait at least a couple of hours before you take iron. Plant foods have phytates, which can also decrease absorption, so you'll get more benefit from the iron supplement if you don't take it immediately before or soon after a meal.

Some iron supplements are much more well-absorbed than others. I recommend that you avoid taking iron sulfate (ferrous sulfate), which is commonly prescribed by conventional physicians. It is not well absorbed, it irritates the digestive tract, and it also causes constipation.

Constipation is probably the worst for pregnant women. Pregnant women are often given a cheap, prenatal vitamin containing iron sulfate as a way to help prevent iron-deficiency anemia, and the supplement worsens constipation problems. (It can also contribute to other health problems during pregnancy such as headaches and hemorrhoids.) When giving iron to pregnant women, I recommend other forms that are more absorbable and that don't produce so many side effects.

Good forms of supplemental iron include iron citrate, iron glycinate, iron succinate, and iron fumarate. The form of the supplement should be clearly indicated on the label.

I do not recommend taking a multivitamin that contains iron. If you're not iron deficient, the extra iron may cause oxidative damage and liver toxicity. If you are iron deficient and need that extra iron supplement, then you don't want to be taking it along with other minerals that might impede its absorption. Depending on the brand of multivitamin, you can usually find one that's iron free.

## WHAT ARE THE SIDE EFFECTS?

Current research is showing that excessive levels of iron in the body promote oxidative damage. Researchers believe that high iron levels increase the risk of heart disease, cancer, and possibly other serious conditions. More definitive research is being done in this area.

You should avoid iron supplementation if you have hemochromatosis, a genetic condition where there is increased iron absorption from the diet.

Iron poisoning can be very serious for children. If you're taking iron supplements, be sure to keep them in a secure cabinet where children can't reach them. An overdose of iron can lead to digestive tract damage, nausea, vomiting, liver failure, and possibly death. Iron is the most common cause of accidental poisoning in children.

# IRON
## RECOMMENDATIONS FROM THE NATURAL PHYSICIAN FOR . . .

### ❧ Fatigue

Many people believe they should take iron supplements if they have fatigue, but that's only true in some cases. While fatigue can be a major symptom of iron deficiency, lack of the mineral is only one possible cause. If your fatigue has another cause, but you start taking iron anyway, the supplement can actually make your fatigue worse.

### ❧ Iron-Deficiency Anemia

Obviously, it makes sense to take iron supplements if you know for sure you have this condition. Be patient, though, because it may take months for more severe iron deficiencies to be brought back to the normal ranges. If you're seeing a conventional medical doctor for this condition, be sure to ask about the more absorbable forms of iron supplements—that is, iron citrate, glycinate, succinate, or fumarate.

### ❧ Low Thyroid

Iron deficiency may impair the body's ability to manufacture thyroid hormone. Have your doctor check your iron status if you have low thyroid. If you do need iron, make sure you don't take it along with your thyroid medicine. Iron can interfere with thyroid-hormone absorption—but that will be less of a problem if you take the iron supplement at a different time of the day.

### ❧ Pregnancy

I generally recommend iron be taken during pregnancy to prevent iron-deficiency anemia. The usual dosage is 25 to 30 milligrams of elemental iron daily—that is, the usual adult dosage—which is perfectly adequate for pregnant women as long as they don't have anemia. Prenatal vitamins contain iron. Again, look for formulas that do not contain ferrous sulfate, which is constipating.

### ❧ Restless Leg Syndrome

Iron deficiency in the elderly may cause restless leg symptom. Supplementation can help improve this condition. Note, however, that other minerals may also be lacking—particularly zinc, calcium, and magnesium—so you may need additional supplementation to help the condition.

# Juicing

It doesn't take a rocket scientist, as they say, to figure out that anyone can make delicious, refreshing, and nutritious drinks by squeezing fresh fruit and vegetables until their juice pours out. But beyond the good taste, there are proven rewards for health and vitality.

Today, more people than ever are benefiting from the healing power of juices. Even I got pumped up after seeing the "juice man" himself, Jay Kordich, on late-night infomercials praising the miracles of juicing. He looks like he has more energy and enthusiasm than my three-year-old son!

What is so great about juicing? Well, it's a way to get vitamins, minerals, enzymes, and phytonutrients all in one drink that happens to be "highly absorbable." What that means is, when you get your nutrients in this form, they're readily incorporated through your digestion into your bloodstream, and from there to the cells of your organs and tissues.

Studies show that most people consume woefully small amounts of fruits and vegetables in their daily diets. Yet, nutritional experts and researchers keep turning up evidence that our bodies can get a lot of protection from these same plant foods, if we just eat enough of them. The beauty of juicing is that it gives us a different way to get these life-enhancing nutrients in a very concentrated and tasty form, without carrying around bushel baskets of fruits and vegetables each day.

# TURNING ON THE JUICE

The typical juicer extracts the juice and expels the pulp or fiber. This makes juice easy to digest and assimilate. You can completely control taste by varying the ingredients you put in. But there's a downside to using this type of juicer. When you extract the fiber, you're leaving something out that's essential for digestion and for assimilation of the nutrients.

Fiber slows down the rate at which your body absorbs sugar, taking it from the digestive tract and pouring it into the bloodstream. If you don't have the fiber that helps control that assimilation, you could end up with a blood-sugar imbalance. For this reason, I recommend that you drink juice with meals: The fiber and bulk in your food helps with the blood-sugar regulation.

But I also advocate using a juicer that doesn't remove fiber, such as the one that's branded Vita-Mix®. I mention this machine in particular because it uses the whole plant—pulp as well as juice—blending the fruit or vegetable into a juice that has fiber as well as liquid. Of course, some people just don't like juice that's full of "chunky stuff," but if you're experimenting, be sure to try it for a while. Having the pulp and juice all blended together really makes an appetizing drink—almost a meal in itself.

Of course, you can also buy packaged juices. These juices are great if no sweeteners have been added (the label will tell you), but even the "purest" of packaged juices aren't so healthful and nutritious as fresh juices. That's because pasteurization destroys enzymes, and oxidation destroys some of the nutrients. (Oxidation is essentially a speeding up of the ripening process, and it accelerates as soon as organic material—like fresh food—is crushed and exposed to air.)

People who have heard about juicing sometimes ask me whether they can get the same benefits from "whole-food supplements," that is, freeze-dried and packaged supplements that are created from the original juices. You'll find these supplements in the form of "green drinks" in many health food stores. The reference to "green" in the label usually indicates that these supplements contain plant material with high nutritive content such as wheatgrass, barley grass, chlorella, and spirulina. But the label shouldn't be taken too literally, as many formulas contain other plants, such as carrots, beets, and various herbs, that are not green.

The advantage of these formulas is that they are ready to be used and require little effort to prepare. They include a blend of vegetables, fruits, and herbs that would be hard to cram into a single fresh drink—so you get the benefit of a wide variety of food extracts. The drawback, of course, is that the green drinks aren't made up of fresh foods, so you do lose some of the nutritive value of fresh juices. But they are helpful, easy, and convenient—and you can get green drinks in powder or capsule form.

One of the major reasons I recommend juicing for patients is that it helps them to detoxify. The phytonutrients, vitamins, minerals, and enzymes in juices work at the cellular level to promote detoxification, and they also help detoxify the liver. I estimate that the vast majority of the population could benefit from concentrated foods that promote detoxification.

## DETOXING JUICING RECIPES

There are many different juicing recipes that help to promote detoxification. Following are two that I recommend:

### ❧ *Fresh juicing*

2 medium-sized carrots

1/2 apple

stick of burdock root or 1 small beet

In this formula the carrots provide a blend of carotenoids and the apple contains vitamin C and other nutrients. The burdock root, or beet, work to promote bile flow and liver detoxification.

Start with one glass daily with a meal; you can drink more than cup daily if you desire.

Another way I commonly use this mixture is to make the Natural Physician Shake. Mix in a blender:

1 to 2 cups rice milk (calcium-enriched)

1 banana

1/2 to 1 cup blueberries

probiotic (acidophilus) containing 2 to 4 billion organisms

1 tablespoon flaxseed oil or essential fatty-acid blend
such as flaxseed and evening primrose oil

2 digestive enzymes such as papain and bromelain

1 scoop soy or whey protein powder

This is a particularly good shake for people on the go. Rather than skipping breakfast in the morning, if you can take a few minutes to put this blend together, you'll have more energy throughout the day. It also helps normalize your appetite, so you're less likely to get hunger pangs or food cravings during the day. This blend is also good to take before or after workouts.

### ∿ Green Drink

Many different formulas labeled as "green drinks" can be purchased at health food stores and some pharmacies. I use a formula (all organic) that mainly consists of the "super green foods" such as wheatgrass, barley grass, alfalfa, spirulina, chlorella, and kelp. It also contains carrot juice, dandelion root, milk thistle, Siberian ginseng, pineapple extract, milk thistle, and natural sweeteners such as mango and stevia. I like to mix this powder in a glass of 3/4 apple juice and 1/4 water.

The combination of supergreen foods and detoxifying herbs such as milk thistle and dandelion root has helped many patients as part of a detoxification program.

## WHAT ARE THE SIDE EFFECTS?

Since juices can contain a lot of sugars, even if no sweeteners have been added, they can be hard on blood-sugar levels. As I've mentioned, that's why I recommend taking them with meals that slow sugar absorption or using a Vita-Mix® to ensure that the fiber is included in the drink.

Green drinks that contain spirulina and chlorella are good for people with blood-sugar problems as they contain a high amount of protein. Some people need to build up the amount of juice they are drinking gradually, as it may cause detoxing reactions such as skin eruptions, headaches, or digestive upset.

Make sure to use organic fruits and vegetables whenever possible, and wash the foods thoroughly before juicing. Remove seeds and pits before juicing—particularly apple seeds, which contain the poisonous substance cyanide. Do not juice carrot tops, which contain toxic substances.

# K

# Kava

· · · · · · · · · · · · · · · · · · · · · · · · · · · · · · · · · · · · · · · · · · · · · · · · · · · ·

Minnie, a 44-year-old business executive, was facing a stressful time at work, but she had already dismissed the idea of using sedatives to control her anxiety and insomnia. She had taken a prescription sedative several years before that had made her feel "all doped out."

"I'm not going to take that again," she told me. "It's hard to get things done when you're taking medicine that makes you feel like a zombie."

Nonetheless, Minnie still felt she needed some help to cope with stress, and a friend had recommended the herb kava. Before taking it, she wanted to know whether, in my view, it would be helpful for her.

"I'd like to give it a try if you think it would help me," she said. "But before I do, I want to make sure it's safe."

In all honesty, I could tell her that I had seen many people benefit from the use of kava. The benefits depended not only on the individual, but also on the dosage used and the quality of the extract.

As I took a more thorough history on Minnie, I realized she had other problems besides insomnia associated with her anxiety. She frequently got headaches and suffered from neck and shoulder tension that were obviously brought on by stressful conditions at work.

I agreed kava (or kava kava) would be very worthwhile for her to try. She was not currently taking any pharmaceutical drugs for her anxiety, so it was feasible for her to start kava right away. (With many drugs used to treat anxiety, phobia, or depression, it's essential to decrease dosages slowly, with advice and monitoring from the prescribing doctor.)

"Kava will be a good alternative to a pharmaceutical for the next couple of months to help you with all the stress and anxiety," I observed. "You'll probably find that it helps for those bouts of insomnia that you sometimes experience from work-related stress. It may also help with the neck tightness and headaches you get. I have successfully recommended it for those same problems with other patients."

I also let her know that kava's safety record was almost perfect.

"It is just as effective as common antianxiety medications, but without causing problems like poor concentration and drowsiness." But I also encouraged her to accept a broader program of treatment. "Keep in mind though that kava is not a replacement for stress-reducing techniques like exercise and prayer." If I was going to recommend kava for Minnie, I also wanted her to pursue the other kinds of self-treatment as well.

## A GIFT FROM THE ISLANDS

Kava *(Piper methysticum)* has a unique history. The natives of the South Pacific islands (Fiji, Tonga, Samoa, Vanuatu, New Guinea, and Hawaii) have used kava for thousands of years. Inhabitants of these islands mainly used it as a ceremonial drink and to increase sociability.

Though kava is relaxing, it doesn't create side effects, apart from the mild euphoria that some people experience. Tea-drinking tribesmen report trance-like states and greater clarity of thought. The Greek translation of kava is "intoxicating." The root was and still is ground up by natives and soaked in coconut milk or water.

Interestingly, Captain Cook and his crew discovered kava during his voyage to the South Pacific in 1768, but it wasn't until the early 1860s that kava was available on the European market. In the United States, Kava gained popularity after World War II for its calming properties. I noticed the popularity of kava began to soar in the American health food market in 1996 and 1997, probably because of all the media play it was getting. It seemed to become an overnight success as a natural stress, anxiety, and depression reliever.

Kava has a number of different constituents that are thought to have effects on various parts of the brain and nervous system. Animal studies have shown that kava influences GABA (gamma-amino-butyric acid) receptors. GABA is a neuro-transmitter, which promotes relaxation, and whole kava extracts appear to have a strong interaction with them. Although there are active constituents called kavalactones in kava, the whole herb has a greater effect than the constituents, so it seems reasonable to assume that this complex herb has more than one set of active constituents.

Kava has been shown to affect the part of the brain that influences emotions, known as the amygdala. It also prevents the hormone norepinephrine from initi-ating a stress response. The herb relaxes the muscles and reduces pain. It's been shown in laboratory studies to have some properties that are similar to those of antiepileptic drugs.

## DOSAGE

For stress and anxiety, I recommend the standardized capsule form with a base of the whole herb. This form has worked well with my patients, and it's been used in many studies.

The dosage is 70 milligrams of kavalactones two to three times daily. Remember that many products are labeled in total milligram amount and then a standardized extract percentage is given. For example, a 250-milligram capsule containing 30% kavalactones contains 75 milligrams kavalactones.

For insomnia, I recommend 2 capsules (usually 500 milligrams) one-half hour before bedtime. The dosage for muscle relaxation is 70 milligrams of kavalac-tones three times daily. If the tincture form is used, I recommend 20 to 30 drops in water three times daily.

*(Interesting note:* One typical bowl of kava drink—as consumed by the Polynias—contains approximately 250 milligrams of kavalactones. It's customary to consume many bowlfuls at one sitting.)

Kava is best used for short-term use (up to three months). I have not seen any reports that show it is harmful if used longer than three months. However, long-term studies have not been done.

## WHAT ARE THE SIDE EFFECTS?

The kava supplements purchased in North America are quite safe, with no side effects. When studies were done with the original kava drink, researchers found that some people occasionally suffered from an upset stomach, but none of my patients have had these side effects from the normal doses I've recommended.

It is assumed that some ingredient is present in the drink form that is not found in the capsule or tincture form. Some members of Captain Cook's expedition reported that they got a scaly skin rash and eye irritation from drinking kava, especially in large amounts, but the effects went away when they stopped drinking. This side effect has not been reported with the supplement form. Perhaps the extraction process removes the ingredient that causes the side effects.

Although no problems with pregnancy have been reported, I recommend that you avoid kava if you're pregnant or nursing, since we don't have any good studies about the effects on the fetus. Also, I advise that you don't combine kava with alcohol, mood-altering pharmaceutical medications such as antidepressants, or antianxiety medicines. In fact, if you're on any medications at all, consult with a doctor first before using kava.

If you are a first-time user of kava, I would advise you to try it in a situation where you don't have to drive. Though kava probably won't impair your driving ability, it never hurts to be on the safe side. I advise against using kava when you have to operate heavy machinery.

---

# KAVA
## RECOMMENDATIONS FROM THE NATURAL PHYSICIAN FOR . . .

### ❧ Anxiety

Many patients have reported that they felt reduced anxiety while using kava. The anxiety-relieving effects are borne out by studies.

One placebo-controlled study looked at 101 people with anxiety who were given an extract of kava three times daily (approximately 70 milligrams of kavalactones per dose). Psychological tests were given before, during, and after the study. Researchers found that kava was superior to the placebo for short- and long-term effectiveness, and most people improved within two months.

Kava was well-tolerated and side effects were very rare among the people in the study. As a matter of fact, more people on the placebo dropped out than those on kava. There were no physical side effects or adverse reactions among those who took kava.

In other studies, kava was shown to reduce stress as well as anxiety, and it proved to be just as effective as an anxiety-reducer as the antianxiety drug oxazepam. Also, in the comparison of the drug with the herb, researchers found that people who received kava had a greater reduction in fear and psychosomatic

*(continued)*

nausea and vomiting than those who were taking the drug.

Not surprisingly—given these studies—more and more doctors and psychiatrists are incorporating kava into their practice.

### Depression

Herbalists and naturopathic physicians often include kava in formulas for the treatment of depression. I have not found it to be so effective as St. John's wort. It is, however, an excellent complement to St. John's wort and other herbs and nutrients that are typically used for depression.

### Headaches

I have found kava to be the most effective for tension-type headaches. Kava can prevent or alleviate tension headaches by helping to relax the muscles in the neck.

### Insomnia

Kava is one of the better herbs to use for insomnia. It does not cause that "hangover feeling" that some people get the following morning when they've used pharmaceutical sleep aids the night before. It is a good option for someone who experiences grogginess or a hangover effect from the herb valerian.

Kava is best used on a short-term basis for insomnia, as it does not really address the underlying cause. Many natural-health insomnia formulas include kava as a principal ingredient.

### Muscle Tension and Spasms

In a clinic where I used to practice, a chiropractor and I both recommended kava to patients to help them reduce muscle spasms and tightness. We found that patients reported very good results, especially when their ailments were the result of stress or accidents.

### Pain

Many people report that kava helps to reduce pain, but I have found that its effects are usually minimal. However, it can help to relieve pain indirectly by reducing the spasms that cause some kinds of muscle pain.

### Panic Attacks

Several patients have told me that kava helps to ward off panic attacks if taken near the onset of the attack. For some patients with this disorder, I recommend the herb as a preventative. I recommend their taking kava regularly throughout the day (two times daily) to prevent an attack. This helps prevent acute attacks, but it's most effective when combined with counseling and homeopathic treatment.

# L

# Lachesis

· · · · · · · · · · · · · · · · · · · · · · · · · · · · · · · · · · · · · · · · · · · · · · · · · · · ·

Dr. Constantine Hering, a botanist and homeopath, was researching plants in Europe in 1828. He heard the legend about a gigantic, venomous snake known as the bushmaster *(Lachesis muta)* that lived in the bushes in tropical Latin America. According to natives, the bushmaster snake's venom was so deadly that a single drop could kill a person. In addition, the snake had a reputation. According to people who lived in the region, the bushmaster was not only very aggressive, it was also extremely protective of its territory.

When Hering traveled to Latin America, he offered to pay some of the local natives if they would help him catch the deadly bushmaster. His offer was universally declined. In fact, the natives thought Hering was crazy. Why would anyone want to capture this dangerous snake?

Among homeopathic researchers, however, there was logic in Hering's pursuit. If a bushmaster's venom could cause the symptoms of a deadly disease, perhaps the same substance—diluted to almost-invisible amounts—could be made into a homeopathic remedy that would cure human diseases when the victims had similar symptoms.

Hering steadily increased his offers of payment until the natives finally relented. A hunt for the bushmaster ensued, and one was finally captured. As Hering was extracting some of the venom, however, a few drops landed on his exposed skin. According to onlookers, he keeled over, unconscious, and was out cold for nearly 20 minutes. When he recovered, he had no memory of what had happened to him.

Returning to his home country, the United States, Dr. Hering continued to do research with lachesis venom, fully persuaded that it would be effective as a homeopathic remedy. Today, thanks to Dr. Hering's unrelenting efforts, lachesis is not only an accepted homeopathic remedy but one of the most important remedies in the homeopathic pharmacy for treatment of hormonal imbalances such as PMS and menopause, as well as circulation disorders.

## PERSONALITY TYPES

Like other homeopathic remedies, lachesis has proven to be most effective with people of a particular personality type—specifically, those who are most intense and suspicious. Their aggressiveness is the result of pent-up anger, and they seem ready to lash out at somebody else at a moment's notice—not unlike the bushmaster.

Sometimes, they're very possessive, keeping close tabs on the people in their lives and yearning for material possessions. If you try to come into their territory, look out, for they will attack (another characteristic of the jungle snake). If they don't get you in the heat of the moment, they will, for they long for revenge.

Jealousy and envy also characterize people needing lachesis. They may lash out physically, but more often, they're talkers, and they use verbal abuse to get out their frustrations. If you're in a large group of people and one of them is particularly loquacious, you know that's probably the lachesis personality. When you try to get a word in edgewise, the lachesis individual is likely to cut you off because he or she wants to be heard and knows what is right. Even when you say you have to leave, it's quite possible the lachesis type won't even get the hint. This type of person may keep talking right in your face even as you're placing your hand on the door to leave.

There are other characterstics as well of someone who requires this remedy. This type of person will never wear a turtleneck, for instance, because he or she can't stand to have anything around his or her neck—just as the person can't bear to have anyone touching him or her. Again, I think of the snake itself, which always tries to protect its own neck.

One last interesting note about the lachesis personality type is that the person has a fear of snakes!

## IN THE BLOOD

Lachesis, like all the snake remedies, has a pronounced affect on the circulatory system. The venom from the bushmaster snake acts to prevent blood from clotting, which is what normally stops blood flow. Without blood clotting, a person can't stop bleeding. But the mild homeopathic dose will not cause such a dire reaction, so it's sometimes prescribed for circulation problems. For example, massive purple blood clots that cause excruciating pain during a woman's menstrual cycle can be relieved with this venom remedy.

It also contains neurotoxins that cause a person to freeze up if he or she is bitten by the snake. Used in the mild dose of a homeopathic remedy, lachesis can have the beneficial effect of causing constriction of some blood vessels. It's valuable for hemorrhage conditions, such as an abnormally heavy menstrual flow or even something like a retinal (eye) hemorrhage. A woman in menopause, who is experiencing severe hot flashes, can get much-needed relief. Lachesis is also one of the best remedies for the heart, improving conditions such as heart palpitations.

A person who needs lachesis is someone who tends to have left-sided symptoms. I remember Jessie, a 58-year-old patient of mine, who came to see me for the natural treatment of her arthritis and headaches. She had arthritis. I wouldn't usually treat arthritis with lachesis, except in her case, the physical symptoms were on the left side. For example, it was only her left knee and left wrist where her arthritis occurred. In addition, she had headaches, and these primarily afflicted her in the left temple.

There was another clue—body temperature. Those requiring lachesis tend to have a higher body temperature than most people. Even though it was winter, Jessie wore light clothing that seemed to keep her quite comfortable.

For all these reasons, I prescribed lachesis for Jessie's conditions. Over the next three months, the lachesis totally eliminated Jessie's headaches, and her arthritis improved tremendously.

## DOSAGE

For the treatment of long-term conditions I prefer to use low dosages of lachesis, such as potencies of 6C that can be taken two to three times daily for a few weeks—and, thereafter, on an as-needed basis. A much higher potency, 30C, is commonly available at health food stores and pharmacies, but if you're taking 30C, try it one or two times daily for just a week or two to see if your symptoms improve. I recommend taking it regularly for one week, then on an as-needed basis after that.

You can take 200C potency for certain acute conditions, but don't take more than one dose.

# WHAT ARE THE SIDE EFFECTS?

As with other homeopathic remedies, side effects are not a real concern. If the potency or frequency are too high, you might get a temporary aggravation of symptoms. But symptoms will return to normal if you just stop the remedy.

---

# LACHESIS
## RECOMMENDATIONS FROM THE NATURAL PHYSICIAN FOR . . .

If you suffer from any of the conditions listed below, lachesis is worth trying. I find it invaluable for women's health problems such as PMS, menopause, menstrual cycle abnormalities, ovarian cysts, and left-sided headaches. I also find it works better than hormones for some menopausal symptoms.

### ❧ Alcoholism

Anyone with a history of alcoholism certainly needs counseling, but some people are helped by homeopathic remedies as well. The "lachesis personality type"—that is, someone who might be helped by lachesis treatments—is the person who tends to become violent when drinking. This includes verbal as well as physical violence. The person who swears and makes wild accusations while under the influence of alcohol is usually a lachesis type.

### ❧ Asthma

Lachesis is especially effective in people who have the type of asthma that's worst when they first wake up from sleep or when they're in a warm room—but the asthma improves when someone is cold. If you have asthma that wakes you with a suffocating feeling, lachesis might help. It's "very indicated," according to homeopathic physicians, when the asthma starts after feelings of jealousy.

### ❧ Ear Infections

Lachesis is a main remedy for left ear infections in children. The child has severe ear pain and feels hot. The left ear is all red and feels better with cold applications. If your child has a left-sided earache, then lachesis is worth trying and usually works quite well.

### ❧ Endometriosis

Lachesis can be quite helpful and sometimes curative when a woman's endometriosis symptoms match the remedy. Lachesis helps to balance the hormones, which are almost always a root problem in this condition.

### ❧ Hemorrhage

Lachesis is one of the main remedies to use for hemorrhage or when you have a susceptibility to hemorrhage. I typically use it when a woman says she's been having heavy menstrual cycles and blood clots that have a purplish color.

### ❧ Hypertension

As mentioned, lachesis can be used to help the circulatory system. Many practitioners have found that it helps reduce high blood pressure.

### ❧ Hyperthyroid

Lachesis is indicated for hyperthyroid, especially in the early stages. I recommend it if the person has flushes of heat and heart palpitations.

*(continued)*

**297**

Sometimes these symptoms are accompanied by left-sided thyroid gland pain.

### Manic-Depression

Many cases of manic-depression have been reported to be helped with lachesis. For this condition, however, you will need the supervision of an experienced doctor.

### Menopause

Lachesis is one of the five most common remedies used in menopause. I recommend it if you have hot flashes, heavy uterine bleeding, and increased feelings of suspiciousness and jealousy. Menopausal women who benefit from lachesis often have one uncharacteristic symptom: Unlike many women in menopause, the sex drive usually stays very high for those requiring lachesis.

### Migraine

This remedy is the main homeopathic for left-sided migraine headaches. Recently, a woman came to me for the natural treatment of migraine headaches. When she told me these headaches usually began on the left side, I immediately recommended lachesis, which is an excellent nondrug treatment, especially for prevention of these types of headaches. It balances the hormones and normalizes circulation. The pastor told me she was pregnant when she started to develop these headaches, but lachesis is so safe that a woman can use it during pregnancy.

### Ovarian Cyst

Lachesis is the main remedy for left-sided ovarian cysts. Gynecologists are baffled when their patients, who have had ovarian cyst problems for years, take a homeopathic remedy like lachesis and the ultrasound shows they have disappeared! But seeing is believing! I have seen many chronic, painful cases cured with this remedy.

### PMS

Symptoms of irritability, jealousy, and depression are relieved with lachesis. One peculiar symptom that differentiates it from other remedies is that menstrual cramps disappear once the flow begins.

### Shingles

Painful, burning blisters that pop up on the left side of the body respond to lachesis.

### Varicose Veins

Lachesis is one of the best remedies for varicose veins that have a purplish discoloration and look like they could burst at any moment.

# L-carnitine

L-carnitine is a substance that's involved in the transportation of a particular kind of fatty acids into the mitochondria (energy factory) of cells. It's often called "carnitine"—which is the same thing.

Think of it as part of the transport system that shovels coals into the fire for burning. The "burning of fats" by the mitochondria is important, as this process fuels the energy that reaches your heart cells and your muscle cells.

Because carnitine is such an integral part of this fueling process, it's particularly valuable as a preventative and therapeutic supplement. If you have a problem related to energy production, carnitine can come to the rescue. Because it helps get energy to the heart muscles, it also assists with several cardiovascular conditions.

Other conditions that seem to benefit from supplementation of L-carnitine include anorexia, chronic fatigue, hypoglycemia, male infertility, and muscular myopathies. Also, L-carnitine is showing promise for premature infants, dialysis patients, and HIV-positive individuals.

You have three sources of carnitine. First, the body manufactures carnitine from the amino acid lysine. But there are other important substances involved in this process as well. These include methionine, SAMe, magnesium, vitamin C, vitamin $B_6$, niacin, and iron.

You can also get carnitine in your diet. Meat is the major dietary source. Carnitine comes from animal protein—with red meat being the richest source.

Plant foods, unfortunately, contain little or no carnitine, which is a cause for concern if you're a strict vegetarian. But fortunately, there's a third possible source of carnitine that can be used by vegetarians and others. The supplement form of L-carnitine is available and commonly recommended by nutrition-oriented doctors.

## DEFICIENCY NOTICE

L-carnitine deficiencies do occur, though some cases are more severe than others. There are a number of possible causes, such as:

- *Genetic defect.* Due to some genetic defect that prevents the body from synthesizing carnitine, some people simply don't get enough.

- *Deficiency of certain amino acids.* If lysine and methionine are missing—or if either one is lacking—you'll have a problem getting adequate carnitine.

- *Deficiency of "cofactors."* I have already mentioned the other substances required for synthesis of carnitine, including SAMe, magnesium, vitamin C, vitamin $B_6$, niacin, and iron. These are called cofactors, and if any of them are missing, you may have problems assimilating carnitine.

- *Strict vegetarianism.* Since there's no carnitine in plant foods, supplementation is required.

- *Formula-feeding babies.* Most infant formulas do not contain carnitine, which is naturally present in breast milk.

- *Liver or kidney disease.* When the liver or kidneys aren't functioning properly, your body can't produce adequate carnitine. People with kidney disease receiving dialysis are almost certain to need supplementation.

- *Severe infections,* such as chronic bronchitis.

- *Increased metabolic stress,* such as the kind caused by heavy physical exertions or chronic disease.

- *Intestinal malabsorption.* If you've had a portion of the small intestine removed (a resection), you'll need carnitine supplementation.

- *Side effects from medications.* Some people will have an increased need for carnitine when they're taking certain kinds of medications.

## Get Up and Go for Athletes?

Studies on the benefit of carnitine and the improvement of athletic performance have been mixed. It appears carnitine is most indicated for those involved in endurance sports such as long-distance running. Also, those athletes with a preexisting carnitine deficiency benefited most from supplementation.

Theoretically, it makes sense to have an adequate body supply of carnitine to burn fatty acids efficiently for muscle energy. I find many athletes who undergo intensive training respond favorably to a comprehensive nutritional supplement support program—and I include L-carnitine in my recommendations for such a program.

There are a number of leading signs of carnitine deficiency. I always suspect it when patients report muscle fatigue and cramps. If their lab tests show a deficiency of carnitine in the tissue and red blood cells, I know supplementation will be necessary.

If there's a severe chronic carnitine deficiency—that is, over a long period of time—one may see symptoms of low blood sugar, fatigue, and nervous system disorders. Also, tests will show that the transport of fatty acids is impaired—a condition called impaired lipid (triglyceride) metabolism—resulting in an increase in triglycerides. That's because carnitine is required to shuttle fatty acids into the cells.

When the condition is chronic, fatty acids are likely to accumulate in the muscles and liver.

The heart muscle is affected. This buildup of fats in the muscles causes progressive muscle weakness. So a chronic deficiency of carnitine can lead to serious conditions related to the heart, such as cardiomyopathy and congestive heart failure. It can also contribute to liver enlargement (hepatomegaly) and brain swelling (encephalopathy).

Children appear to be very susceptible to carnitine deficiency. I'm particularly concerned about infants who only get infant formula. Most of these formulas do not contain L-carnitine. In susceptible children, this may hinder their growth and development.

## DOSAGE

I typically recommend an adult dosage of 1,000 milligrams taken two to three times daily. You can take higher dosages, up to 2,000 milligrams per dose—but it appears that this is the maximum that can be absorbed and utilized at one time. For this reason, I recommend divided doses—taken several times during the day if necessary—rather than large single doses.

If you have heart disease, consider a formula that contains L-carnitine in combination with CoQ10. This is a powerful supplement combination for treatment of a number of related conditions including cardiomyopathy, angina, or congestive heart failure. I recommend the L-carnitine form—which is the designation of most of the carnitine supplements. The D,L carnitine form is also available, but I don't recommend it, as it is not biologically active and can cause side effects.

(**Note:** I have only seen the L-carnitine form in health food stores and pharmacies.)

## WHAT ARE THE SIDE EFFECTS?

Carnitine is a very safe supplement. Occasionally, people get digestive upset, but if you reduce the dosage or take carnitine with your meals, you can usually resolve the problem.

Don't supplement with carnitine if you're taking the respiratory stimulant drug pentylenetetrazol.

# L-CARNITINE
## RECOMMENDATIONS FROM THE NATURAL PHYSICIAN FOR . . .

### ❧ Alzheimer's Disease and Memory Problems

A different form of carnitine known as acetyl-L-carnitine (ALC) has been shown in studies to be valuable in the treatment of Alzheimer's disease, senile depression, and memory loss associated with aging. ALC occurs naturally in the body. Biochemically speaking, it is L-carnitine bound to acetic acid. You can purchase ALC supplements in many places where carnitine is sold, and it's specific for the memory and for the health of the brain.

ALC benefits brain function in many ways. It improves energy metabolism in the brain cells and also improves the transmission of nerve impulses. It is one of the few substances that improves communication between the two hemispheres of the brain, and it also acts as a potent antioxidant for brain cells, helping to slow the aging process.

One of the unique features of ALC is that it is structurally similar to a substance called acetycholine, a vital neurotransmitter that's needed for many different brain functions including memory. Interestingly, many Alzheimer's drugs are designed to increase acetycholine in the brain.

One double-blind, placebo-controlled study of people diagnosed with Alzheimer's disease were given 2,000 milligrams twice daily of ALC or a placebo. Those receiving ALC scored better on all the assessment tests and had a slower rate of deteoriation than those taking the placebo.

Another double-blind study demonstrated that ALC was effective for the elderly with age-associated memory impairment. It has also been shown in studies to be effective for senile depression.

**Note:** The dose for someone suspected of having Alzheimer's disease is 500 milligrams three to four times daily between meals. For prevention, 250 milligrams is generally considered a good daily dosage. This amount will also help optimize brain function.

### ❧ Angina

Several studies have shown that L-carnitine is effective in the treatment and prevention of angina. In a well-controlled scientific study of men and women taking L-carnitine, researchers found that 22 percent of angina patients given L-carnitine became angina-free during the study. That was more than twice the percentage of those in the placebo group—that is, the ones who were not taking L-carnitine. Those taking carnitine also experienced increased exercise tolerance. When doctors did follow-up electrocardiogram tests, they found that the patients taking L-carnitine showed evidence that there was less restriction of blood flow in their arteries.

Another study looked at what happened when scientists gave L-carnitine supplementation of 2,000 milligrams daily to 100 randomly selected patients with stable angina over a 6-month period. The carnitine was given in addition to the therapy already started. Researchers found improvements in a number of important indicators of heart health. Those receiving L-carnitine were found to be more likely to have their cardiac medications reduced.

I find that carnitine, in addition to CoQ10, vitamin E, magnesium, hawthorn berry, and cactus (Cereus grandiflorus) are excellent for the prevention of angina.

*(continued)*

### Anorexia

In patients with anorexia nervosa, the combination of carnitine and vitamin $B_{12}$ accelerates the gain of body weight and helps normalize gastrointestinal function. Anorexia is best treated by a specialist, but nutritional support has proven helpful to many. With L-carnitine, people have a resource that helps them fight fatigue and improve mental performance.

The combination of $B_{12}$ with carnitine has been proven helpful for infantile anorexia. It appears nutritional support with supplements such as carnitine, $B_{12}$, as well as zinc are important to include as nutritional support to hasten the recovery process. But again, you'll need the help of a specialist before giving treatment to an infant.

### Arrhythmias

Double-blind studies have shown that carnitine supplementation helped patients to receive lower dosages of their antiarrhythmic drugs, indicating that carnitine has a beneficial effect.

### Cardiomyopathy

Children with this form of heart disease and who had carnitine deficiency responded favorably to carnitine supplementation. Along with CoQ10, it should be used with anyone who has cardiomyopathy to improve heart performance.

### Chronic Fatigue Syndrome

One of the challenges with chronic fatigue syndrome is that it can have many different causes. Among the possible causes are viral infection, digestive disturbances, nutritional deficiencies, adrenal burnout, and hormone imbalances.

I find nutritional supplements such as carnitine act as complementary treatments to more primary treatments such as detoxification and homeopathic treatment. This observation is supported by one study that showed clinical improvement in 12 of 18 people with chronic fatigue syndrome.

### Congestive Heart Failure

Nutrition-oriented doctors such as myself routinely recommend carnitine to patients with congestive heart failure. This is a condition where the heart is failing to pump out efficiently.

In one study, 21 people with congestive heart failure were given 1,000 milligrams of carnitine twice daily for 45 days along with conventional drugs. The participants showed improvements in levels of triglyceride and cholesterol, heart rate, edema, and breathing. Supplementation also allowed for lower daily doses of digitalis.

### Diabetes

L-carnitine supplementation makes sense for people with diabetes who are predisposed to cardiovascular and neurological disease.

### Down's Syndrome

Although Down's syndrome is a genetic condition, one 90-day study found that ALC supplementation was beneficial in improving visual memory and attention in children who had the syndrome.

### Deficiencies from Drug Interactions

Anticonvulsant drugs such as phenobarbital, valproic acid, phenytoin, and carbamazepine significantly lower carnitine levels. So does the drug pivampicillin. If you're on any of these medications, you should talk with your doctor about supplementing with carnitine to prevent deficiencies.

L-carnitine may prevent heart complications in people with cancer who receive interleukin-2 immunotherapy and the chemotherapy drug

*(continued)*

**303**

adriamyacin. And it appears to also have a protective effect on the cell mitochondria for people with HIV using the drug zidovudine (AZT).

### Heart Attack Recovery

L-carnitine has been helpful for people recovering from a heart attack. One study of 160 people who recently suffered a heart attack showed significant improvements in blood pressure, heart rate, angina attacks, and other markers of heart function. The dosage used in the study was 4,000 milligrams of L-carnitine, taken in divided doses throughout the day. Studies have also shown that victims of heart attacks are more likely to survive if they take carnitine supplements during the next 24 hours.

With such positive results, supplements like carnitine really should be routinely prescribed for heart attack victims. It only makes sense as carnitine helps the heart produce energy so that it can function more effectively.

### HIV

A few studies have shown that carnitine supplementation can be helpful in improving the immune status (CD4 and CD8 counts) in people with HIV.

### Kidney Disease

People undergoing dialysis for kidney disease are often deficient in carnitine. Supplementation helps to reduce triglyceride levels while increasing the good HDL cholesterol.

### Liver Disease

Carnitine helps metabolize fatty acids in the liver. In people with liver cirrhosis it has been shown to reduce triglycerides, increase the good HDL cholesterol, and decrease elevated liver enzymes. It works to reverse fatty liver disease caused by alcohol.

### Male Infertility

Carnitine is required to help improve the motility and number of sperm. Supplementation of L-carnitine can improve sperm quality in some patients with idiopathic asthenospermia (defective sperm motility of unknown cause).

Researchers provided 100 patients with 3,000 milligrams daily of L-carnitine for four months and found improvements in all assessed parameters of sperm motility, as well as an increase in the total sperm count. Other nutrients that I recommend to increase sperm count and motility include vitamin C, arginine, CoQ10, vitamin $B_{12}$, vitamin E, and zinc.

### Premature Infants

Carnitine appears to be important to supplement to the mother if it is suspected or known that a premature delivery is inevitable. Carnitine is involved with the activation of surfactant, a substance that promotes proper function and maturation of the infants' lungs.

One study showed that women have healthier babies who are less likely to have respiratory distress syndrome if the expectant mothers are given carnitine along with the drug betamethasone during the prenatal period. The trial showed how the combination of supplement and pharmaceutical can reduce both the incidence of respiratory distress syndrome and the mortality of premature newborns. In the trial, some mothers were just given the prescription drug, while others got carnitine as well. For the mothers who took both, the incidence of respiratory distress syndrome among the infants was about half of that for the drug-only group. For mothers who took carnitine, the mortality rate of infants was 1.8 percent, while it was 7.3 percent for mothers who took the betamethasone alone.

# Ledum

Years back, my mother got a needle biopsy for a breast lump her doctor discovered. My mother anticipated some pain from the procedure and when she asked my sister whether there was any way to avoid the after-effects, my sister approached me with the question. "Mark, is there anything we can give Mom to help with the pain from her biopsy?"

"Yes. Give her a couple doses of ledum right after the procedure," I said.

After the biopsy—which proved to be negative—my sister gave Mom the ledum *(Ledum palustre)*, a homeopathic remedy specific for puncture wounds. My mother said that in the following days she could not feel any pain where the needle was inserted.

In my view, surgery clinics and medical offices would serve their patients well if they would just make ledum available to patients. Every time a person gets an injection or gets blood drawn, a dose of ledum can help reduce the pain and speed tissue healing.

Ledum is the homeopathic preparation of an herbal preparation from wild rosemary, a small shrub. It is commonly recommended by homeopathic practitioners as an acute remedy for bites, stings, and wounds. It is also a good arthritis remedy.

## DOSAGE

A few doses of the 30C potency or a single dose of 200C is helpful for acute situations that require ledum. Chronic cases like arthritis are generally treated with a 6C or 30C potency a couple times daily.

## WHAT ARE THE SIDE EFFECTS?

None of my patients have suffered from any side effects from taking ledum.

# LEDUM

## RECOMMENDATIONS FROM THE NATURAL PHYSICIAN FOR . . .

### ꙮ Arthritis

Linda was a 53-year-old patient of mine who was consulting with me for natural treatment of multiple health problems. One of her most immediate concerns was the arthritis she suffered in her left foot. Chiropractic and acupuncture had helped slightly, but the pain was really concerning her.

Upon further examination, I found that the foot looked bruised, and Linda told me that it also felt hot at times. We discovered that ice water made the foot feel better, at least temporarily, whereas warm applications worsened the pain and inflammation. All these key symptoms suggested that ledum would be the best remedy.

Within one week of beginning the treatments, Linda felt what she described as "70 percent improvement!" Over the next few months, Linda reported that the pain in her left foot was almost gone.

Ledum is one of the remedies to consider when arthritis occurs in the feet and ankles. It is also one of the better remedies to use to treat flare-ups of gout.

### ꙮ Bruises

Ledum is useful for bruises to the soft tissues, similar to arnica. I find it helpful for patients who get bruised from blood draws in the clinic. It helps reduce the pain and swelling the same day, often within a matter of minutes.

### ꙮ Mosquito Bites

I have recommended ledum on several occasions for people who react strongly to mosquito bites. Some people have very sensitive skin, and they get large, boil-like, itchy, painful lesions from normal mosquito bites. For them, I recommend mixing a couple pellets of ledum (any potency such as 6C or 30C) with water in a spray bottle. In a mosquito-infested area, it's best to spray the solution on the skin every hour. The itching will be more bearable, and the bites will not flare up so badly.

Ledum can also be used for relief from bee stings, especially the kind that are relieved by cold applications.

### ꙮ Puncture Wounds

Before the creation of the tetanus vaccine, practitioners used to give ledum to prevent wound infections. In addition to cleaning a wound, you can help prevent infection by taking a dose of ledum for faster tissue healing.

But whether or not there's a risk of infection, ledum can be a pain-reliever for puncture wounds. I remember taking it myself when I received a vitamin $B_{12}$ injection that was administered by a colleague of mine, Dr. Steve Nenninger. This was in his early days of practicing medicine—and both of us were just beginning to develop our skills as physicians. I felt a tremendous amount of pain after the injection. Fortunately, one dose of ledum quickly relieved this intense, sharp pain.

### ꙮ Sprains

Ledum is often given after a sprain, such as an ankle sprain. I typically use it if arnica does not reduce the swelling and discomfort in the ankle.

# Licorice Root

By the time Ray, a 44-year-old salesman, came to see me for the treatment of his peptic ulcers, he had already spent two frustrating years trying to relieve his stomach pain with many different types of medications and natural remedies. Again and again he tried new pills, capsules, and formulas, each of which seemed to work for a while before gradually losing its effectiveness, leaving him to relapse into agony.

In the long list of remedies he'd taken, however, I discovered that one—the most effective of all—was conspicuously absent. This gave me the clue I needed to help him attack his problem. Besides having Ray reduce his coffee intake and increase his exercise as part of a stress-reduction program, I prescribed licorice root (DGL form). He was to chew two capsules at least 15 minutes before each meal every day.

The result? On the very next visit he reported his ulcer was healed! I knew better, of course. Even though he felt much, much better, it takes longer than two weeks to declare a complete victory over an ulcer, so I recommended that he continue using DGL for another four weeks.

Now, after six months, Ray still shows no sign of relapse.

## THE ALL-PURPOSE REMEDY

In my experience, licorice root is the most versatile of all the herbs. Native to both Asia and the Mediterranean, it has been used by practitioners of Ayurvedic and Chinese medicine for over 5,000 years.

In fact, close to 50 percent of all Chinese herbal formulas contain licorice root. The ancient Chinese texts say it can suppress coughs and moisten the lungs, relieve spasms, and soothe the digestive tract. It is also called a "harmonizing" herb. This means that it helps other herbs to work more effectively to reduce their toxicity when used in a formula.

Licorice also helps detoxify the liver, supports the adrenal glands (your body's major guardians against stress), balances the hormones, and has powerful antiinflammatory effects.

**307**

## IMMUNITY BOOSTER

Licorice contains two substances, glycyrrhizin and glycyrrhetinic acid, that have been shown in animal studies to increase the body's supply of one of nature's most powerful antiviral agents: interferon. Interferon helps to keep viruses from reproducing and stimulates the activity of other beneficial immune cells, as well. That's probably why licorice root is found in so many Western, Chinese, Japanese, and Ayurvedic formulas for treating infectious disease.

Licorice root is highly regarded among European physicians as one of the top herbal medicines for combating viral hepatitis. They use the intravenous form for the treatment of both Hepatitis B and C.

## DELICIOUS DETOXIFIER

The Chinese have found through many centuries of using licorice that it reduces the toxicity of other herbs, so they add it to many of their remedies. For example, traditional Chinese herbal formulas containing Ma Huang, (containing the chemical ephedrine, which helps open respiratory passageways but can also cause stimulant effects, such as fast heart beat, sweating, and anxiety), almost always contain licorice root, which helps to prevent these unwanted side effects.

**Note:** The Chinese species of licorice root is *Glycyrrhiza uralensis*. I find it works very similar in action to the kind used in North America—*Glycyrrhiza glabra*.

## DOSAGE

For most conditions, I recommend taking licorice in tincture, capsule, or tablet form. As a tincture, take 10 to 30 drops two to three times daily. As a capsule, take 1,000 to 3,000 milligrams daily.

DGL comes in tablet form. Chew one or two tablets (380 milligrams per tablet) 20 minutes before meals or take between meals.

## WHAT ARE THE SIDE EFFECTS?

High dosages of licorice root (3,000 milligrams daily of the powdered extract or more than 100 milligrams of the constituent glycyrrhizin) taken over many days can have effects similar to those associated with the hormone aldosterone. These include sodium and water retention, and potassium loss, which can lead to high blood pressure. We saw this problem occur when practitioners began recommending very high dosages of licorice root for adrenal burnout and chronic fatigue (which it can help).

Overall, I feel the risk of developing high blood pressure from using licorice is greatly exaggerated. Historically, herbalists have used this root in formulas for thousands of years. The trick is to use it in small amounts.

I do hear the occasional story of someone who feels that taking small amounts of licorice root has caused an increase in his or her blood pressure. This is perfectly possible for people who are very sensitive to licorice root or are low in potassium. As a matter of fact, anyone concerned about high blood pressure should

### Treat or Trick?

The Greek translation of licorice is "sweet root" or "sweet wood," and it's aptly named. The sweetness of licorice root is 50 to 100 times that of sugar! But oddly, the one place you won't find any licorice root is in American licorice candy, which actually contains anise oil and simple sugars such as glucose and fructose, and artificial dyes, sweeteners, and preservatives that can wreak havoc with the brain. The known active constituents of real licorice include glycyrrhizin, glycyrrhizinic acid, glycyrrhetinic acid, flavonoids, sterols, amino acids, coumarins, and volatile oils.

Unfortunately, most of the licorice root imported to the United States is used as an additive in tobacco products, since it is sweet and soothing. (I doubt tobacco manufacturers included it to reduce the toxicity of the over 100 toxic chemicals found in cigarettes.) The Europeans and Chinese, on the other hand, do give licorice root to their children as a healthy substitute for sugar candy.

increase his or her intake of potassium-rich foods (bananas, orange juice, vegetables, etc.) and decrease the intake of sodium-containing foods (table salt, canned foods, and restaurant foods). Using table-salt substitutes, which usually contain potassium, can help reduce sodium intake. Multivitamins also contain potassium.

Unless instructed to do so by a natural healthcare practitioner, people who have kidney failure and hypokalemia (low potassium blood levels) should avoid using licorice root. Likewise, pregnant women and people with high blood pressure should use it with caution and under medical supervision. Whole licorice extract should not be combined with digitalis and diuretic medications. Taking only the DGL extract (for ulcers) eliminates most of the potential risk for high blood pressure.

# LICORICE ROOT

## Recommendations from the Natural Physician for...

### ❧ Coughs

Licorice is an excellent herb to use for coughs, both wet and dry. Licorice has a moistening and soothing effect for dry coughs. It also has a direct cough suppressant effect and is a common ingredient in throat lozenges.

### ❧ Detoxification

Licorice is one of the herbs to consider when undergoing a detoxification program. As I mentioned, it helps support the liver and should be considered along with herbs like milk thistle and dandelion root. It also works to heal a damaged digestive tract, which is key to long-term detoxification success.

### ❧ Eczema and Psoriasis

Creams containing glycyrrhetinic acid are used to treat inflammatory skin conditions such as eczema and psoriasis. Its effect is similar to that of topical cortisone, and some studies have found it more effective. However, I do not recommend topical treatments (whether natural or pharmaceutical) as the main therapy for skin conditions, as they can simply mask a symptom without treating its underlying cause (e.g., food sensitivities, poor digestion, nutritional deficiencies, etc.). Topical treatments are fine, so long as you also address the internal imbalances that are creating the symptom.

### ❧ Fatigue

People who experience high levels of stress for long periods of time can suddenly find that their adrenal glands can no longer produce balanced levels of stress hormones, such as DHEA, pregnenolone, and cortisol. As a result, fatigue, poor memory, blood-sugar problems, decreased resistance to illness, and hormonal imbalance can occur.

Some doctors immediately recommend using hormone replacement, and in some cases this is necessary. However, it is worth trying a gentler approach, using supplements such as licorice root, especially to balance out cortisol levels. A typical adult dosage would be 1,000 to 2,000 milligrams of licorice root extract taken daily for two months or longer.

Other supplements that work synergistically to treat this condition include adrenal glandular, ginseng, pantothenic acid, vitamin C, beta carotene, and zinc. In more serious cases, hormones such as DHEA, pregnenolone, and even cortisol may need to be used.

### ❧ Hormone Imbalance

Licorice is one of the better hormone-balancing herbs. It appears to have a balancing effect between estrogen and progesterone, and reduces excess testosterone levels. It is commonly included in formulas for PMS and menopause.

### ❧ Infections

As mentioned earlier, licorice root is very good for the immune system. The soothing and anti-inflammatory effect of licorice makes it especially good for respiratory tract infections.

### ❧ Inflammation

Licorice has potent antiinflammatory properties. Glycyrrhizin is an important constituent that improves the effects of cortisol in the body (powerful antiinflammatory and antiallergy effects), without the side effects seen with pharmaceutical antiinflammatory agents such as prednisone. It also inhibits the formation of prostaglandins, which are substances in the body that cause inflammation.

*(continued)*

**310**

### ∾ Inflammatory Bowel Disease

Licorice root is often included in formulas designed to heal conditions such as Crohn's disease and ulcerative colitis.

### ∾ Mouth Sores

Mouth sores, also called aphthous ulcers, can be helped by licorice root. One study of 20 people found that a DGL mouthwash improved the symptoms of 15 of the participants by 50 to 75 percent within 1 day, and complete healing of the sores within 3 days.

### ∾ Ulcers

One of the most popular uses of licorice extract is for ulcers of the digestive tract. The recommended form is DGL. It has an interesting mechanism of action: It stimulates cell growth of the stomach and intestinal linings, increases the natural mucous lining of the stomach, increases blood flow to the damaged tissues, and decreases muscle spasms.

In a single-blind study of 100 people with peptic ulcers, participants took either DGL (760 milligrams three times daily) or the medication Tagamet® (cimetidine). Both groups showed equally significant healing of ulcers after 6 and 12 weeks, demonstrating that DGL is as effective as pharmaceutical medications for this condition. Another study of 874 people also demonstrated that DGL was as effective as antacids and the antiulcer drug cimetidine in persons with duodenal ulcers.

More important, DGL actually works to heal ulcerated tissues instead of simply suppressing stomach acid in the way antacids and drug medications do. Remember, with insufficient stomach acid, you cannot digest proteins, minerals, and other nutrients very efficiently. Stomach acid also acts as a natural barrier that keeps bacteria, parasites, and other microbes from penetrating the digestive tract.

# Lomatium

Scientists are in a race to find drugs that can eradicate bacteria, which are becoming more and more resistant to antibiotics. They are also frantically looking to develop drugs that fight off viruses as well, especially in light of HIV, ebola, herpes, hepatitis, and the ever-changing strains of the flu.

Scientists are looking increasingly to the plant kingdom and reviewing the historical use of plants as medicines to fight off invading microbes. One of these plants is lomatium.

Lomatium (*Lomatium dissectum*) is an herb that has been known about for almost a century, but has been used by only a small percentage of natural healthcare practitioners. Recently, it has become more popular as a commercial immune-system enhancer to fight off pathogens such as viruses, bacteria, and fungi.

For almost a decade, I have been using lomatium for my patients, and quite often with extraordinary results. It ranks with some of the other well-known immune-system herbal therapies such as echinacea and astragalus.

Lomatium grows in British Columbia, Alberta, southern California, New Mexico, Colorado, eastern Oregon, eastern Washington, Idaho, and the Columbia Plateau. It is also referred to as desert parsley.

# A HEALING INDIAN ROOT

Once again, we have the Native Americans to thank for our present use of lomatium. Historically, it was one of the most important medicinal plants used by several tribes of the western United States.

Lomatium was used to treat infections of the respiratory and urinary tracts, as well as of the eyes. The species used by the Indians and the one still popular today is *Lomatium dissectum*. The Native Americans would also eat the shoots and roots. For medicinal use, a decoction was made by boiling the root in water. This decoction was also used topically for sores, rashes, and cuts. A poultice of lomatium was used for swellings, joint pain, and sprains.

One of the interesting historical notes about lomatium is that it was used by Native Americans during the Spanish flu epidemic of 1917–1918. This is the epidemic that killed over 22 million people worldwide, and over 500,000 people in the United States. A doctor noticed that Native American Indians in the Nevada desert were recovering from the Spanish flu. He found they were boiling and ingesting lomatium root. He learned how to use the herb from the Indians and began using it, as did other doctors who saw similar healing effects from using lomatium. However, the interest in lomatium dramatically decreased after the epidemic ended.

Several earlier in vitro studies have shown lomatium to have direct killing effects on many different types of bacteria and fungus, including *Candida albicans*. It is also believed that phytochemicals found in lomatium have the ability to inhibit viruses from replicating. Studies have shown these phytochemicals to be effective against DNA and RNA viruses—two major categories of viruses.

Practitioners of natural medicine find lomatium root effective against several types of viruses including Epstein-Barr, herpes, flu, common cold, cytomegalovirus, and *condyloma acuminata* (genital warts).

## DOSAGE

Lomatium is available in tincture form. I recommend taking 30 drops (0.5 milliliters) every two to three hours for acute infections. For chronic viral infections, I recommend 0.5 milliliters or 500 milligrams twice daily. I use lomatium in formulas that contain herbs such as echinacea, astragalus, reishi, and licorice. It also combines well with herbal cough formulas for a more aggressive treatment.

## WHAT ARE THE SIDE EFFECTS?

The only side effect to be aware of is that a very small percentage of users will develop a measleslike rash. The rash is not serious, and will disappear after a few days if you stop taking lomatium.

## LOMATIUM
### RECOMMENDATIONS FROM THE NATURAL PHYSICIAN FOR . . .

### ❧ Common Cold and Flu

One of the most common uses of lomatium is for colds and flu. I have found it to have one of the strongest antiviral effects of all the herbs I have used. When taken at the onset of a cold or when you feel the first flu symptoms coming on, you'll find that it can greatly decrease the severity of symptoms. Also, you're likely to get over these viral infections more quickly: I have seen patients with severe cases of the flu show great improvement within 24 hours of taking lomatium.

### ❧ Epstein-Barr

This virus is noted for causing mononucleosis as well as some cases of chronic fatigue syndrome. Practitioners find that lomatium is one of the best herbs to use to eradicate this virus. (It is

certainly a better protocol than the traditional one, which is generally bed rest.)

### ❧ Herpes and Genital Warts

Lomatium is popular for the natural treatment of herpes—both the kind that occur on the mouth (Type 1) and genitals (Type 2). It's also effective as a treatment for genital warts. Again, this herb appears to have a direct effect of blocking viral replication as well as assisting the immune system's antiviral weaponry. It is taken internally in both cases.

People with herpes find that if they take lomatium at the first symptoms of an outbreak, it helps to suppress the outbreak or reduce its severity. Those with genital warts should use lomatium only with the supervision of a physician.

*(continued)*

∾ **Respiratory Tract Infections**

Lomatium was used in the past for bronchitis, pneumonia, and even tuberculosis. Today, naturopathic physicians frequently use it in a blend of herbs for respiratory tract ailments.

∾ **Urinary Tract Infections**

Lomatium can be used by itself or in combination with herbs that are specific for urinary tract infections, such as uva ursi and goldenseal.

# Lycopodium

George, a 44-year-old lawyer, came to see me for treatment of chronic digestive problems and fatigue.

"No matter what I eat, I produce tremendous amounts of gas," he said. He went on to describe how difficult it was for him at work, where he had trouble restraining himself when he was meeting with clients. "At my desk," he added, "I have to loosen my belt and pants because of the abdominal pressure from the bloating."

Fatigue was also a problem, though he didn't know whether or not it was related to digestion. "It is getting more and more difficult for me to get up in the morning. Then, I get tired at 8 P.M., so it's difficult to stay awake. My wife is upset over my lack of sociability. I also find that I'm very irritable with my secretary and short tempered with my family."

I recommended lycopodium.

It worked wonders for George. Over the next couple of months, his flatulence and bloating were greatly improved; he felt more energy upon awakening, and although he still had a short temper, his wife commented that he seemed more patient.

## AN EARTHY SOLUTION

Lycopodium, the homeopathic dilution of club moss, is one of the best homeopathic remedies for digestive problems. It is prescribed specifically for bloating and distension of the abdomen that is relieved by passing gas and burping.

People requiring lycopodium usually have very large appetites, and eating makes the bloating and gas worse. They find that warm drinks have a soothing effect on the digestive system, while cold drinks do not. It is also one of the more common remedies for heartburn.

People who respond well to lycopodium tend to have a strong craving for sweets. Another peculiar problem is that many of their symptoms worsen between 4 and 8 P.M., as was the case with George and his fatigue. Patients often say their digestion is fine until evening, and then it acts up.

There's another symptom, too, that could indicate a need for lycopodium. Physical problems tend to occur on the right side of the body. For example, one patient of mine had chronic headaches that always occurred in the right temple area. Lycopodium cleared up this chronic problem for her.

The mental profile of someone requiring lycopodium is unique and fits a lot of people in our "power hungry" society. These people want to be in control. Often, they are people who act bossy, arrogant, irritable, and domineering. (The typical schoolyard bully would benefit from lycopodium.)

## DOSAGE

The typical dosage is 30C potency twice daily for the relief of acute symptoms such as gas or bloating, or right-sided headaches. Long-term treatment is best done with a lower potency, such as 6C, taken two to three times daily.

## WHAT ARE THE SIDE EFFECTS?

Side effects are not a concern with lycopodium. If you are not sure whether you should use it, consult a homeopathic practitioner.

## LYCOPODIUM
### RECOMMENDATIONS FROM THE NATURAL PHYSICIAN FOR . . .

**∾ Arthritis**

Typically, lycopodium is helpful for arthritis that is alleviated with warm applications and that affects joints on the right side of the body.

**∾ Colitis**

Lycopodium has an amazing ability to heal the digestive tract. It has helped many people who have digestive problems such as colitis, Crohn's disease, and irritable bowel syndrome (IBS).

*(continued)*

### ❧ Headaches

Whenever a patient complains of a right-sided headache, I immediately think of lycopodium as a possible remedy. The headache may be worse between 4 and 8 P.M.

### ❧ Hepatitis

Lycopodium also has an affinity for the liver. It is one of the main remedies to use for liver problems such as hepatitis.

### ❧ Impotence

Lycopodium is the main homeopathic remedy for impotence and premature ejaculation. It is well indicated when the sexual problems of the man are psychological in origin, due to low confidence. I have seen this remedy help several of my male patients.

### ❧ Ovarian Pain

Right-sided ovarian pain is an indication for lycopodium. Women with ovarian cysts respond well to this remedy. It not only takes the pain away, but also helps in preventing the cysts from developing again.

### ❧ Respiratory Tract Infections

Right-sided respiratory tract infections often require lycopodium. This includes asthma, bronchitis, pneumonia, and sinusitis. I treated a 1-year-old child who was having trouble breathing at night. On listening to his lungs through a stethoscope, I discovered that he had congestion in the right lobe only. I recommended lycopodium—and the treatment was successful.

# Lysine

I was summoned to the phone.

"Dr. Mark, it's Rick calling. I'm on vacation in Hawaii and my mouth started breaking out with cold sores yesterday. I hope there's something you can recommend to clear them up. It feels awful and looks like the start of a bad outbreak. I haven't had a case like this in years."

"Go to a pharmacy or health food store," I said, "and pick up the supplement lysine. Take 1,000 milligrams three times daily between meals. Get started right away, and it should help clear things up pretty quickly."

Then I recalled how much Rick liked to party. I was forced to add, "By the way—try to keep away from alcohol for the next few days."

"I'll get the lysine right away. Thanks, Dr. Mark."

(I noticed he didn't acknowledge my request to watch his alcohol intake—but I think he'd heard me nonetheless.)

The next time I saw Rick, he told me that the lysine had helped to keep the cold sore outbreak at bay. A few large cold sores did pop out, but they healed up quickly in four days. He also mentioned that this particular outbreak was significantly less intense than what he had experienced in the past.

## LOOKING AT LYSINE

Lysine—also called L-lysine—is an essential amino acid. This means you must consume it in your diet as your body cannot synthesize it or make enough of it to function properly. Actually, the bacteria in the gut produce amino acids, including lysine in very small amounts. This amino acid is highly concentrated in muscle tissue.

Foods high in lysine include chicken and wild game, cottage cheese, and wheat germ. Most fruits and vegetables, except for avocados, contain little lysine.

Lysine is involved in many different metabolic activities in the body. It is required for growth, particularly in children. It is thought to be important for bone health, and some consider it a supplement for the treatment and prevention of osteoporosis.

Lysine helps to fight lead toxicity. It is required for the body's synthesis of carnitine, an amino-acidlike substance that's particularly essential for good heart function.

The primary use of supplemental lysine is to prevent or treat herpes outbreaks. A lysine deficiency can impair the immune system. It is one of the amino acids that are depleted from the body when it is under stress. People who have Parkinson's disease, hypothyroidism, kidney disease, asthma, and depression have been found to have low levels of lysine.

## DOSAGE

A typical dosage is 1,500 to 3,000 milligrams for the acute treatment of herpes outbreaks (both Type 1 and Type 2). Lower dosages are used by some practitioners for the prevention of outbreaks, usually 500 to 1,000 milligrams daily.

A number of nutrients help your body absorb and use lysine. Among the nutrients involved in this process of lysine metabolism are niacin, vitamin $B_6$, riboflavin, vitamin C, glutamic acid, and iron. Interestingly, B vitamins and vitamin C are commonly recommended for the treatment of herpes as well.

# WHAT ARE THE SIDE EFFECTS?

L-lysine is well tolerated. Studies have shown that people can take up to 8,000 milligrams without any problems. However, taking high doses of lysine for long periods of time may deplete the levels of the amino acid arginine.

Lysine should not be taken at the same time you're taking antibiotics.

---

## L-LYSINE
### RECOMMENDATIONS FROM THE NATURAL PHYSICIAN FOR . . .

#### ∾ Herpes

L-lysine is a common treatment for people suffering from herpes outbreaks. Research on the herpes virus showed that in a culture dish, the amino acid arginine stimulated growth of the virus while the addition of lysine inhibited growth.

A study was conducted on 45 patients who experienced frequent herpes outbreaks. They received 312 to 500 milligrams of L-lysine for 2 months to 3 years. The dosage was increased to 800 to 1,000 milligrams for acute outbreaks, and foods high in the amino acid arginine—such as chocolate, various kinds of seeds, and nuts—were restricted. This therapy reduced the frequency of outbreaks and greatly accelerated the recovery from acute outbreaks.

Another study found that 1,200 milligrams of L-lysine significantly reduced the recurrence of herpes simplex outbreaks. L-lysine is effective for both oral and genital herpes. I recommend that persons with herpes reduce their intake of foods containing arginine during acute outbreaks. These include chocolate, nuts, seeds, peanuts, and grains (wheat).

#### ∾ Osteoporosis

Animal studies have shown that lysine deficiency increases calcium excretion. While lysine deficiency is rare, it is theorized that a low-grade deficiency may lead to bone loss. Lysine is used by the body to form collagen, an integral component of bone. More research is needed to see if lysine supplementation would be helpful for increasing bone density.

# M

# Magnesium

·····················································································

Fifty-six-year-old Gina said she often had muscle cramps and spasms during the day, but they were worse at night.

"My doctor can't find anything wrong," she continued. "My blood work didn't show any thing out of balance. I was told to take some calcium, but it hasn't been helping."

"Does your calcium supplement also contain magnesium?" I asked.

"No, my doctor didn't mention anything about magnesium," she replied.

"That's likely to be the problem," I said. "Calcium and magnesium both help to relax the muscles. Some people with muscle spasms respond better to higher levels of magnesium, while some respond better to calcium. In any event, both should be taken, as both are commonly deficient. Also, you need magnesium for your bones as well."

An extra 500 milligrams of magnesium did the trick for Gina. Within three days, her muscle cramps and spasms subsided, and she found that she slept better as well.

## THE MIGHTY MINERAL

Magnesium is the second most abundant mineral in the cells after potassium. Sixty percent of the body's magnesium is found in the bones, while the muscles contain approximately 27 percent; and the rest is found in the tissues and blood. The body maintains a narrow range of magnesium blood levels, and will draw it from the bones if blood levels are low.

Magnesium is required as a cofactor for hundreds of enzymatic reactions. This includes energy production, lipid and protein synthesis, nerve impulses, muscle contraction and relaxation, and bone formation by helping to regulate calcium metabolism.

It is also necessary for the cardiovascular system. It is required for heart function and relaxes blood vessel walls, so blood pressure is reduced.

## MISSING MAGNESIUM

Most children and adults do not get adequate amounts of magnesium in their diets. They tend to eat processed foods, and processing destroys the magnesium content. Only a small percentage of the population eats whole grains, legumes, nuts, and green leafy vegetables on a regular basis.

A magnesium deficiency can cause many different symptoms. These include muscle cramps, spasms, and weakness; fatigue; irritability and personality changes; confusion; loss of appetite; poor coordination; and cravings for sweets.

Conditions or diseases associated with a magnesium deficiency include high blood pressure, kidney stones, insomnia, premenstrual syndrome, hair loss, swollen gums, and reduced heart function.

Aside from poor diet, factors that could cause magnesium deficiency include digestive disorders (such as malabsorption or chronic diarrhea), kidney disease, use of diuretics, diabetes, and alcoholism.

Medications known to deplete magnesium include digoxin, corticosteroids, birth-control pills, theophylline, and warfarin.

Standard blood tests do not pick up a magnesium deficiency until it is very severe, usually after a serious condition has developed. Therefore, symptoms and diet analysis help to determine if there is a magnesium deficiency.

## DOSAGE

Even though the Recommended Daily Allowance (RDA) is somewhat lower, the optimum dosage I recommend for most adults is 500 milligrams of magnesium daily. You can meet this goal by taking a multivitamin and/or a calcium/magnesium complex or bone health formula.

I recommend that children take 250 to 500 milligrams daily. These supplements should be taken with meals.

When someone needs a very high dosage of magnesium (such as a person with fibromyalgia), then magnesium may be taken by itself. Magnesium glycinate is a good form to use for a high dosage (750 milligrams or higher) as it is less likely to cause diarrhea. Otherwise, magnesium citrate or other chelates are well absorbed.

Vitamin B$_6$ and magnesium work synergistically in many different enzymatic reactions.

## WHAT ARE THE SIDE EFFECTS?

The most common side effect is loose stools or diarrhea. This tends to happen when the dosage is above 500 milligrams. I find some people need to start at a lower dosage (such as 250 milligrams) and slowly increase the amount over a few weeks until they reach their desired therapeutic dosage. Magnesium chloride, sulfate, carbonate, and oxide are more likely than magnesium glycinate and magnesium citrate to cause this problem.

People with kidney and heart disease should not use a magnesium supplement unless instructed to do so by a physician. It should not be taken at the same time as the drugs fosamax, cimetidine, ranitidine, and tetracycline; these substances should be taken a few hours apart.

## MAGNESIUM
### RECOMMENDATIONS FROM THE NATURAL PHYSICIAN FOR . . .

#### ✑ Angina
This is a heart condition where a person feels a heaviness or squeezing sensation in the chest, often accompanied by a feeling of suffocation. In this condition there is a lack of blood flow and oxygen to the heart tissues, or spasm of the coronary arteries. Magnesium is important as it helps relax and dilate the arteries that feed the heart. Nutritional doctors also use magnesium intravenously for this condition. I find the oral supplement works best when taken in conjunction with CoQ10, L-carnitine, hawthorn berry, L-arginine, vitamin E, and other targeted support for the heart.

#### ✑ Arrhythmias
Magnesium is often recommended for those with heart arrhythmias. It can reverse the condition in some people. I also recommend CoQ10 and calcium as well. If you are taking medication for heart arrhythmia, you must check with your doctor before using a magnesium supplement.

*(continued)*

### Asthma

Magnesium promotes the relaxation of the bronchial muscles. Using a magnesium supplement helps to reduce the incidence of asthma attacks.

Doctors have found that an oral supplement does not help in an acute asthma attack. However, if a doctor gives it intravenously, magnesium may be effective in relieving an acute asthma attack.

### Cardiomyopathy and Congestive Heart Failure

When someone has cardiomyopathy, the heart is weakened by a viral infection or some other cause. Cardiomyopathy can lead to congestive heart failure—a condition in which the heart fails to pump blood adequately. Magnesium helps to support energy production and improve the pumping action of the heart.

One study showed that persons with congestive heart failure who had normal levels of magnesium had longer survival rates than those with lower magnesium levels.

### Diabetes

Magnesium, along with vitamin $B_6$, is important for the proper functioning of insulin so that glucose can get into the cells properly. It also helps to prevent complications of diabetes such as heart disease and retinopathy. (It has also been shown that children with insulin-dependent diabetes have lower levels of magnesium than other children.)

### Fatigue

Magnesium is involved in the production of energy; it helps to prevent and treat fatigue. Studies have shown magnesium to benefit those with chronic fatigue syndrome.

### Fibromyalgia

I routinely recommend magnesium along with calcium to help patients with this disorder affecting the muscles and joints. It helps to reduce muscle soreness and tightness, as well as relieve other symptoms such as fatigue and insomnia. The dosage I recommend for fibromyalgia is up to 1,000 milligrams taken in divided doses throughout the day.

### Glaucoma

This is an eye condition in which there is increased pressure within the eyeball. If left untreated, blindness can result. One study showed that a dose of 141.5 milligrams taken twice daily for one month improved the visual fields of people with glaucoma.

### High Blood Pressure

Studies have shown magnesium to be helpful in the treatment of hypertension. I always recommend it along with the mineral calcium and CoQ10. It seems to help for long-term treatment of hypertension.

### Kidney Stones

Most kidney stones are composed of calcium oxalate. Magnesium makes calcium more soluble in the urine, and thus inhibits the formation of calcium-oxalate crystals. One study examined 55 people with reoccurring kidney stones, who were given 500 milligrams of magnesium daily for up to 4 years. The study showed that 85 percent of these people remained stone-free compared with 41 percent of a group of people who did not receive magnesium supplements.

Taking vitamin $B_6$ in conjunction with magnesium works even better as it aids in oxalate metabolism. I recommend 500 milligrams of

*(continued)*

magnesium citrate and 50 milligrams daily of B$_6$ for the prevention of kidney stones.

### ∾ Migraine Headaches

Magnesium is helpful for the prevention of migraine headaches for some people. Those who suffer from chronic migraine headaches should supplement 500 milligrams of magnesium daily.

### ∾ Mitral Valve Prolapse

Magnesium has been shown to be helpful for this condition. It should be taken with L-carnitine and CoQ10 by anyone who has mitral valve prolapse.

### ∾ Osteoporosis

Many researchers feel that magnesium is as important for the prevention and treatment of osteoporosis as is calcium. Remember, magnesium is of critical importance for the proper utilization of calcium by the bones. Magnesium should be part of a comprehensive supplementation protocol. A dosage of 500 to 1,000 milligrams daily is recommended.

### ∾ Pregnancy

Studies have shown magnesium to be helpful in preventing preeclampsia, a condition characterized by increased blood pressure, fluid retention, and protein in the urine. Preeclampsia can cause fetal growth retardation and premature delivery. Magnesium is often given intravenously for treatment when this condition is acute. I recommend that all pregnant women take a magnesium and calcium supplement.

### ∾ Premenstrual Syndrome

Magnesium levels have been shown to be lower in women with PMS than in those without this condition. One double-blind study found that 200 milligrams per day of magnesium supplementation alleviated PMS symptoms such as breast tenderness, abdominal bloating, weight gain, and swelling of the extremities. Another study found that magnesium was effective in relieving premenstrual mood changes.

Magnesium is one of the cofactors required for estrogen metabolism. An imbalance between estrogen and progesterone is one of the main theories as to why PMS occurs.

# Melatonin

"I just can't get to sleep," said Glen, a 59-year-old retired pilot.

"What therapies have you tried for your sleep problems?" I asked.

"My doctor prescribed many different drugs. Most didn't help, or if they did, it was temporary. With a couple of them, I couldn't handle the side effects—like feeling hung over in the morning."

Glen went on to name some natural remedies that his chiropractor had suggested, including kava and valerian.

"I also tried acupuncture," Glen continued. "That worked well for my back, but did nothing for my sleep."

"Well, you certainly have tried a lot of remedies. What about melatonin?"

Though Glen had heard of it, he hadn't tried it.

I explained how it works.

"Melatonin is a hormone produced by a gland in your brain that is released when it's dark, in the night, and it promotes sleep."

"How well does it work?" asked Glen.

"It's like everything else—it works for some people, and not for others. But overall, I have found it to be reasonably effective. Since it is a hormone, I use it when other natural therapies aren't helping. However, I would say it's a heck of a lot safer and usually more effective than sleeping pills."

"I'm ready to try it," said Glen.

It was a few days before Glen called, but when he did, he reported that he no longer had a problem sleeping. Melatonin had done the trick.

## FOR THE REST OF IT

Melatonin is a hormone produced by a pea-sized structure called the pineal gland, located in the center of the brain. Interestingly, it was once thought that the pineal gland had no function. Today, we know that the melatonin released by this gland helps to set the rhythms of waking and sleeping. Taken as a supplement, melatonin has been used as a potent antioxidant as well. For some people, it reduces jet lag.

Some preliminary research suggests that melatonin can strengthen the immune system, play a role in the prevention and treatment of cancer, and help people recover from heart disease. It is also recommended by some holistic doctors for people who have HIV and chronic infections. In addition, it is thought by some researchers to have "anti-aging" properties.

## THE DARK SIDE

Melatonin synthesis is stimulated by exposure to darkness, while it's suppressed by exposure to light. When light enters the eye, it activates a series of signals that are transmitted to the pineal gland, which cuts back on production of melatonin. In darkness, however, the eye sends a contrary signal, activating melatonin production.

Melatonin is actually produced from the amino acid tryptophan. Tryptophan is converted to a chemical called 5-hydroxytryptophan (5-HTP), then to the neurotransmitter serotonin, and finally into melatonin.

There are several substances that can decrease your body's production of melatonin. These include alcohol, aspirin, caffeine, and ibuprofen. The presence of nicotine also depresses melatonin production, so you have a problem if you smoke regularly. A number of prescription medications also reduce melatonin production, including beta blockers, calcium channel blockers, and tranquilizers.

Stress-reduction techniques such as prayer and meditation increase your body's level of melatonin.

Melatonin is found in foods such as oats, sweet corn, rice, ginger, tomatoes, bananas, and barley.

Some research has indicated that melatonin levels decrease as we age, but not all the studies are in agreement. I don't think all elderly people should take melatonin, but I do know it's helpful to some. It can greatly improve sleep quality.

Not surprisingly, shift workers have been particularly interested in melatonin. Working the night shift is hard on the biological rhythms of the body, because it's difficult to get proper sleep during the day when the sun is out. Melatonin has been particularly helpful for people who work the "graveyard shift." By regularly taking melatonin just before the "sleep time" in the morning, their biological rhythms and sleep patterns usually improve. Usually, it takes about a week for complete adjustment to take place.

## DOSAGE

As with any hormone, it is best to use the lowest possible dosage to get the desired effect. This is especially true when using it for insomnia.

I find that a dose of 0.1 to 0.3 milligrams may be all that is needed to promote sleep for those with insomnia or for people using it to regulate sleep cycles as a result of time-zone changes (jet lag) or shift work. Some users will require higher dosages up to 3 milligrams, or occasionally 5 milligrams.

Dosages of 20 to 50 milligrams and higher are prescribed for immune-system enhancement and for the treatment of cancer. These high dosages should only be taken with a physician's guidance.

Melatonin is available in capsule, tablet, and liquid forms, as well as in time-release and sublingual forms.

Vitamins $B_3$ and $B_6$, and the minerals calcium and magnesium are important for melatonin synthesis. Many of my patients report that taking calcium or magnesium (or both) in the evening improves their sleep.

## WHAT ARE THE SIDE EFFECTS?

Melatonin appears to be a safe hormone with relatively little toxicity, but unfortunately, there have not been good, long-term human studies.

Because it hasn't been adequately tested, I don't advise pregnant women or nursing mothers to take melatonin. If you're a woman who's trying to conceive, you'll want to avoid melatonin because high dosages have been shown to suppress ovulation.

It should not be used with children—again, because the long-term effects are not known.

People taking steroid medications such as dexamethasone and cortisone should avoid using melatonin unless a doctor prescribes it. Also, people with autoimmune diseases or cancer should use it only under the guidance of a doctor.

## MELATONIN
### RECOMMENDATIONS FROM THE NATURAL PHYSICIAN FOR . . .

### ❧ Aging

Researchers feel that melatonin may help prolong youth through several mechanisms such as reducing free-radical damage of cells, improving immune-system function, normalizing circadian and biological rhythms, improving sleep and repair, and through the stimulation of growth-hormone production.

More research needs to be done before we can say for sure that melatonin has an "anti-aging effect," but it seems to be promising.

### ❧ Cancer

Melatonin is recommended by some cancer specialists, though they usually advise taking it in conjunction with chemotherapy or radiation. It's thought to be helpful for treatment of various cancers, especially breast, prostate, lung, and skin. It also appears to have an antiproliferative effect on certain kinds of hormone-dependent cancers, helping to prevent the spread of those cancers to other organs or parts of the body. The antiproliferative effect seems to apply to estrogen-dependent breast cancer and androgen-dependent prostate cancer.

Also, melatonin has been shown to increase the efficacy of chemotherapy and reduce the toxicity of the treatments.

*(continued)*

### ∾ Insomnia

Many studies have shown that melatonin is effective for those with insomnia, both in young adults and the elderly. It has also been shown to improve the sleep quality of people with chronic schizophrenia. I advocate the use of melatonin to help wean people off addictive benzodiazepine drugs that are used for insomnia.

Melatonin has been shown to help normalize the sleeping patterns of blind people. Since the pineal gland is light sensitive, blind people are often "out of sync" with the usual patterns of wakefulness during daylight hours and sleepiness at night. By pacing the way they take melatonin, they can adjust so they don't suffer from daytime sleepiness.

Low doses of melatonin are often the most effective. It should always be taken at night.

### ∾ Jet Lag

If you need to choose between melatonin and pharmaceutical sleeping pills for fighting jet lag, I'd recommend the melatonin. Sleeping pills may help one fall asleep but they do not help reset the body's "clock." Also, sleeping pills can be addictive and cause drowsiness.

To combat jet lag, take melatonin one hour before your normal bedtime, in the time zone where you'll be landing.

### ∾ Radiation Exposure

Melatonin may become a common therapy for the prevention and treatment of radiation exposure. One study found that it protected human white blood cells 500 times more effectively than the potent antioxidant (DMSO) that was used for comparison.

# Mental Imagery

"Part of our treatment for your anxiety will be to imagine yourself in a beautiful, pleasant environment with a calm setting. Think of a place you have been before, where the atmosphere was very calming to you. A couple times a day, or when you feel your anxiety coming on, I want you to sit and envision yourself in this place. Take some deep, slow breaths and really see yourself in this place with in your mind."

Thirty year old Allison had long been seeking an alternative treatment for her anxiety disorder. Though she had experienced the limitations of pharmaceutical medications, I wasn't sure whether she was quite ready to accept the practice I was suggesting—mental imagery—as the answer to her problems.

But whatever her unspoken skepticism, it vanished when she began using the technique I described. She soon found that this technique helped to keep her anxiety at bay. During times of stress, she could feel the anxiety coming back. That's when she would go off by herself to a quiet place and use mental imagery to relax and calm herself.

## MENTAL FIX

Mental imagery is simply envisioning what you want something to be. In the health field, the practice of using mental imagery for healing has become well accepted. Much evidence has turned up in the field of oncology—the study of cancer—showing that cancer patients tend to live longer, and certainly have a better quality of life, if they are associated with programs where mental imagery is regularly practiced.

Some leading cancer clinics such as Cancer Treatment Centers of America, a national chain, have mental imagery programs available to patients. The term most often used to describe these programs is "mind–body medicine," or, in more scientific terms, "psychoneuroimmunology." "Psycho" refers to thought, emotions, and mood; "neuro" refers to the nervous system; and "immunology" refers to the immune system. So the translation of psychoneuroimmunology means the effect of the mind on the nervous system and immune system.

Your thoughts and feelings affect the chemistry of your nervous system and ultimately all the cells in your body, including the immune system. Studies have proven what many have always believed for ages. Yes, the thoughts in our minds and the images that we *bring* to mind do have direct effects on the cells of our bodies.

In one study that included 10 men and 10 women, researchers explored the effects of visualization, or mental imagery, on immune-system response in people who had depressed white blood cell count. When white blood cells are "depressed," it means the body is more susceptible to the invasion of some disease. The patients in this study had a variety of health problems ranging from cancer and AIDS to viral infections.

When the patients in the study used mental imagery, their white blood cell count (the measurement of improved health) showed significant increases over a 90-day period.

## A HEALTHY PRACTICE

Mental imagery isn't just for the sick. If it can have such a positive effect on health, that's ample reason to recommend it to those who are healthy. Using mental imagery can be a powerful way to maintain health and prevent illness.

How do you go about this? Well, picture in your mind what you want to look like and how you want to feel. The first time you try this imagery, it may seem like a mere exercise and you may well wonder how it will ultimately shape your future health and vitality. But with repetition, it does.

I saw a good example of this positive effect when I recommended mental imagery to a friend of mine, Jason, who had suffered many years ago from reoccurring bronchitis and pneumonia. After a long bout of pneumonia had left him feeling depleted and unwell, he started to find out whether he could use mental imagery to "turn the corner." During quiet periods of reflection, he told himself he would never get pneumonia again. He envisioned his lungs and respiratory system becoming impervious to infection.

Treating this almost as an experiment, Jason did nothing else to materially improve his health. He didn't start taking new supplements, nor did he change his diet and lifestyle. Nonetheless, he discovered that just the change in his mental outlook made a very significant difference. From that day to the last time I saw him—very recently—he has not had any reoccurrence of pneumonia or bronchitis.

## DOING IT YOUR WAY

Whatever illness you may have, you can picture "in your mind's eye" your body recovering.

When you practice mental imagery, try to get as detailed as you can. For example, if you have osteoarthritis of the knees, see your cells creating new cartilage in the knee joints. Also, envision yourself with less pain and with greater mobility.

If you have high blood pressure, envision yourself in a calm and serene environment. Then see your blood vessels relaxing and the pressure decreasing within the blood-vessel walls.

When you're using mental imagery, it's also good to use your other senses to make the positive images as real as possible. For example, if you picture yourself relaxing on a beach in Hawaii, then also smell the salt spray of the ocean, feel the warmth of the sun on your skin, and hear the waves on the shore.

Many different mental-imagery techniques are advocated by different specialists. If you want help learning the process, you can find psychologists, hypnotherapists, counselors, pastors, and doctors who specialize in mental-imagery practices. But it's also something you can train yourself to do. Of course, whether you see a specialist or teach yourself, the day-to-day exercise of mental imagery is up to you. But the evidence is steadily mounting that this is one of the most effective healing techniques we know about.

# Milk Thistle

Most people in the U.S. have an overabundance of toxins in their bodies, and their livers are overburdened.

Take a hard look at the toxins in our environment, and the reasons for these health problems are hardly a mystery. According to the U.S. Environmental Protection Agency, an estimated 2.2 billion pounds of environmental toxins were released into the environment between the years 1987 and 1994—and that's just counting industrial waste. If you also add over-the-counter and prescription medications that we consume, along with the additives in many food products, our bodies are dealing with a staggering number of chemicals that we're not equipped to handle.

Hence, the need for milk thistle *(Silybum marianum)*. At one time or another, nearly everyone can benefit from this potent herb that has the power to protect and revitalize the liver, our major organ of detoxification.

## SIZING UP THISTLE

Milk thistle has been used for its medicinal properties for over 2,000 years. Over the span of those two millennia, herbalists have come to admire the beneficial effect it can have on the liver and gallbladder. In Germany, where doctors routinely prescribe herbal treatments, it's one of the favored treatments for liver problems. That may be news to many people in the United States, but even here, it's getting increasing attention among health practitioners and the general public.

The "milk" in the name refers to the white sap that leave markings on the leaf—but it also has the prickly, spiny appearance of a typical thistle. It grows wild in parts of Europe, Russia, Asia, and North Africa. English colonists brought it to North America.

It's the milk thistle seeds that have medicinal properties. The seeds contain a group of flavonoids that are collectively known as silymarin. Within this group are silibin, silidianin, and silychristin.

## A COMPLEX SUBJECT

All the flavonoids in the silymarin complex have the combined power of antioxidants that can prevent free-radical damage from the toxic substances that enter the liver. Silymarin has been found to be ten times more potent of an antioxidant than vitamin E, the single vitamin most renowned for its antioxidant power. It's silymarin that has the unique ability to slow down the rate at which the liver absorbs toxic substances.

Additionally, milk thistle is one of the few substances that can increase the glutathione content of the liver. This is important as glutathione, one of the body's most important antioxidants, is critical for efficient detoxification. Milk thistle also increases the levels of another potent antioxidant known as superoxide dismutase (SOD).

Milk thistle stimulates the regeneration of liver cells. This makes it valuable for conditions such as hepatitis, fatty liver, and cirrhosis of the liver. Treatment with milk thistle is essential for anyone who has been poisoned by eating the death-cap mushroom (Amanita phalloides). In 49 reported cases where people with deathcap poisoning received an injectable form of milk thistle (silibin), physicians reported full recovery—even when treatment came as late as 36 hours after the poisoning occurred.

Milk thistle extract also has been shown to stimulate kidney-cell regeneration.

Milk thistle is also one of the better herbs for stimulating the flow of bile, which is essential to good digestion. For this reason, it's helpful for improving the digestion of fats and also helpful in improving bowel elimination.

## DOSAGE

I recommend one take a 200- to 250-milligram capsule of a standardized extract (80 to 85% silymarin) three times daily. This is equivalent to 480 to 600 milligrams of silymarin daily.

If you suffer from digestive problems, then take it 15 minutes before or with a meal. A special form of milk thistle bound to phosphatidylcholine, known as Phytosome®, has been shown to increase absorption. The dosage for the tincture form is 20 to 30 drops three times daily.

## WHAT ARE THE SIDE EFFECTS?

The only major concern with milk thistle is that a very high dosage can cause loose stools due to increased bile flow. If you have a sensitive digestive system, start with one capsule and gradually increase the dosage. If you experience loose stools or diarrhea, then cut back on the dosage.

## MILK THISTLE
### RECOMMENDATIONS FROM THE NATURAL PHYSICIAN FOR . . .

**❧ Alcohol and Drug Addiction Recovery**

When recovering from addiction, the liver is working overtime to cleanse the tissues and regenerate its own tissues—and milk thistle helps with both these processes. I also find that it helps to improve mood and energy levels, which are essential in the recovery process.

**❧ Allergies**

If you have chronic allergies, especially multiple-chemical sensitivity, you may respond well to milk thistle. It enables the liver to process environmental allergens more effectively.

**❧ Circulation**

Herbalists and naturopathic doctors historically used milk thistle for the treatment of hemorrhoids and varicose veins. Blood is continually flowing through the liver, and if you have a "sluggish liver" that doesn't process blood very efficiently, it tends to back up in the rectum and

in the veins of the legs. In theory, at least, improved liver function and metabolism also improve the rate at which venous blood returns to the heart, so there's a reduction of hemorrhoid and varicose vein problems.

I have not used milk thistle by itself for these conditions, but I do, at times, incorporate it into a comprehensive protocol.

**❧ Cirrhosis**

Cirrhosis refers to severe liver damage. Liver tissue can be scarred by the effects of alcoholism, drugs, or liver infections such as hepatitis. When blood tests demonstrate elevated liver enzymes, it's an indication that liver scarring or cirrhosis has probably occurred.

In a well-controlled study of 105 people with cirrhosis, researchers compared those who took 420 milligrams of silymarin with those who (unknowingly, of course) were taking a placebo. After an average of 41 months, it was found those in the placebo group had almost twice the mor-

*(continued)*

tality rate as those in the silymarin group. While the researchers acknowledged that milk thistle does not cure cirrhosis, this study provided compelling evidence that silymarin can improve the survival rate of people with this disease.

### Constipation

The stimulation of bile secretion by milk thistle improves elimination. For people who eat enough fiber, get enough fluids, yet still have sluggish bowel movements, I recommend milk thistle supplementation to help increase bile flow.

### Depression

One of the traditional ways to help alleviate depression is by improving liver function—which makes sense, when you consider the liver influences the biochemistry of the body as it metabolizes hormones and neurotransmitters. In traditional Chinese and naturopathic medicine, physicians and acupuncturists regularly incorporate milk thistle with other therapies that are designed to improve liver function.

### Detoxification

Everyone can benefit from detoxification. A month or two of milk thistle supplementation "does a liver good"—and, of course, the results are even better when supplementation is combined with a good program of diet and exercise. There are benefits for the immune system, as well, since it is not so burdened with toxins.

In fact, I'd be wary of any detoxification formula that does *not* contain milk thistle. It does such a superior job that most high-quality detoxification supplements will include it as one of the main ingredients in a formula.

### Gallstones

Since milk thistle improves bile flow, it decreases the saturation of cholesterol in bile. (High cholesterol saturation in bile is what leads to gallstone formation.) That said, I'd advise caution for those diagnosed with moderate to large gallstones. Use milk thistle or other bile-stimulating herbs under the guidance of a healthcare professional.

### Hepatitis (Viral)

Silymarin has been shown to be effective in the treatment of acute and chronic viral hepatitis. In a study of chronic viral hepatitis, silymarin not only lowered elevated liver enzymes, but liver cell damage was also reversed as demonstrated by a liver biopsy.

I have had numerous patients with hepatitis C who responded favorably to milk thistle supplementation. I've found it helps to normalize or lower elevated liver enzymes. Just as important, the patient looks better and feels more energetic.

With such encouraging results, I think milk thistle treatment will become much more widespread. It is estimated that 3.9 million Americans and up to 3 percent of the world's population are infected with hepatitis C, and conventional medical treatments with alpha interferon are often unsuccessful.

In addition to milk thistle, there are other safe and effective supplements that I consider better options for long-term treatment of hepatitis C. Among the others I recommend are licorice root, reishi, and selenium.

### Hormone Imbalance

Although not thought of as a hormone-balancing herb, milk thistle can give indirect benefits by improving liver function and metabolism of hormones. This makes it helpful for conditions such as PMS or even prostate enlargement.

### Indigestion

One of the many functions of bile is to digest fats. When patients tell me they get indigestion only after eating fried or fatty foods, I know

*(continued)*

their bile production is deficient. I recommend taking milk thistle several times daily, with meals, for a few months.

### ☙ Liver Protection

I recommend milk thistle supplementation to those who require long-term use of prescription medications. Such medications can damage the liver, and milk thistle seems to provide some protection from this side effect.

In a double-blind, placebo-controlled study of 60 people, researchers found that silymarin protected against the long-term use of drugs used for mental illness. The benefits came with doses of 800 milligrams per day of silymarin. There was evidence that these doses reduced the blood levels of MDA (malon-dialdehyde), which is the "marker" that shows the liver has been damaged by long-term use of psychotropic drugs.

I also recommend milk thistle to anyone who's exposed to toxins in the workplace. A classic example would be a welder, who is exposed to smoke and other contaminants.

People who can't quit smoking may be able to limit the liver damage by supplementing with milk thistle.

I commonly recommend milk thistle extract for those undergoing chemotherapy or radiation treatments for cancer. Metabolic waste products are produced by these treatments, and the liver must metabolize the waste before it can be safely eliminated.

### ☙ Skin conditions

Chronic cases of skin rashes, acne, eczema, and even some cases of psoriasis greatly improve when people take milk thistle. While improving the liver's detoxification ability, milk thistle helps remove toxins from the bloodstream, which can, in turn, help prevent skin eruptions. This is why it is sometimes referred to as a "blood cleanser."

# MSM

I remember one of my professors in medical school saying that if you can't relieve a patient's pain quickly, the patient will not be coming back to your office.

It's true.

No one wants to experience pain—and when you're afflicted with it, all you want is relief. Yet chronic, ongoing pain is a major problem for many people. It's been estimated that one-third of all Americans have to deal with it, often as the result of disease.

I can't claim that the supplement called MSM will help everyone. But I do know we're fortunate to have it around. It's one of those breakthrough supplements that, for many people, works very effectively to reduce pain and inflammation.

MSM is the abbreviation for methylsulfonylmethane. It was originally discovered when research was being done on DMSO—dimethylsulfoxide, a related compound that was known to alleviate pain. One problem with DMSO is that it has a very strong and disagreeable odor.

MSM doesn't have the odor problem and it seems to be just as effective as DMSO—or even more so. Most of the research on MSM has been done by Dr. Stanley Jacob of Oregon Health Sciences University in Portland and Dr. R. Lawrence of UCLA in California. Both have treated many thousands of people who are afflicted with painful conditions with DMSO and MSM.

In their book, *The Miracle of MSM*, they report that MSM can deliver numerous benefits, including:

- Pain relief
- Reduced inflammation
- Increased blood flow
- Control of overactive nerve impulses
- Reduced muscle spasms
- Softening of scar tissue

## Media Treatment of MSM

On one edition of *Larry King Live*, the talk show host was interviewing a panel of experts about natural treatments of arthritis. One of those experts was Dr. R. Lawrence, who advocated the use of MSM.

When a caller asked if MSM could be used for a child who had rheumatoid arthritis, Dr. Lawrence replied that it would be fine to try the supplement with the child, but certainly less than an adult dose.

A medical expert from CNN, who was also on the panel, said he could not agree with this recommendation. According to the CNN expert, the use of MSM was not supported by enough studies. Then the CNN medical expert went on to say that the standard steroid treatment would be the best option for this child.

Unfortunately, the discussion moved on before it was thoroughly explored. But I found myself cringing at the thought that if the parents took this advice, their child would be deprived of a nontoxic supplement that millions of people have used—a supplement, further, that was recommended by medical doctors like Lawrence and Jacob, and which had no proven side effects. In exchange, the child would probably be given many doses of steroids, whose side effects are established to be profound and long-lasting.

In addition, MSM has an antiparasitic effect—that is, it helps to resist the invasion of unfriendly parasites. It also has a normalizing effect on the immune system, which means it's useful in treating autoimmune diseases like rheumatoid arthritis and lupus.

MSM is a component of many foods, including green vegetables, and it's a natural part of living organisms, including plants and animals. As the name implies, MSM is a source of the mineral sulfur.

The body uses sulfur for many different functions. It is an integral component of amino acids, the building blocks of protein. Amino acids are essential in numerous biological functions, from building enzymes, hormones, and immune cells to building tissues like the skin and hair.

Sulfur is particularly important for the three sulfur-containing amino acids methionine, cysteine, and cystine. It's also an important mineral for detoxification. Food sources of sulfur include meat, eggs, poultry, fish, and milk. Plant foods that contain sulfur include garlic, onions, broccoli, cauliflower, cabbage, legumes, and sunflower seeds.

## PAIN CONTROL WITHOUT SIDE EFFECTS

MSM is not the only supplement that has powerful, direct, antiinflammatory and pain-relieving effects. Others that I recommend are bromelain, tumeric, boswellia, and white willow. But I would have to say that none of these are so quick in their pain-relief action as MSM.

While some medications are just as fast-acting as MSM, most pain and antiinflammatory medications cause serious side effects. For example, aspirin is one of the leading causes of ulcers, and can damage the kidneys and liver. It also accelerates cartilage destruction.

Other NSAIDs (nonsteroidal antiinflammatories) are known for their side effects. Research has shown that corticosteroids such as prednisone have been associated with emotional disturbances, osteoporosis, liver and kidney toxicity, weight gain, and suppression of the immune system. Long-term use of such pharmaceuticals can sometimes be worse than the disease itself.

MSM provides relief of pain and inflammation without causing damage to the body. This has enabled many people to work with their doctors to reduce or totally eliminate the use of pain medications.

## A CASE OF ARTHRITIS

Joe was one of the many patients whom I have treated for arthritis—and his story is a good example of what MSM can do.

When I first saw Joe, he could not walk without limping. There was no mystery about the cause of his pain. For years, he'd endured osteoarthritis that was progressively getting worse, and in recent days, the arthritis in his left knee had flared up. The pain was almost unbearable.

Though only 55, Joe wondered how much longer he would be mobile—and he envisioned having a knee transplant in the not-too-distant future. He had been on a regimen of painkillers prescribed by his doctor, but he stopped taking them when he discovered they caused ulcers and other digestive problems.

When I told Joe that many of the medications he had used in the past may actually accelerate the degeneration of cartilage in his joints, he replied, "Oh great. Why didn't my doctor tell me that?"

Though not particularly overweight, Joe was a large man, weighing 210 pounds, and he needed a higher-than-usual dose. I started him on 4,000 milligrams of MSM, taken daily in tablet form, and also recommended topical applications of MSM as a cream. Within two days Joe noticed a dramatic reduction in his knee pain.

For the next two months, Joe continued with the high dosage of MSM, then—at my recommendation—reduced to a maintenance dosage of 2,000 milligrams daily. The pain, he reported, was "80 percent improved," and he said there was noticeable improvement in his mobility.

I later added glucosamine sulfate to his protocol to help rebuild his knee cartilage. Some researchers believe that MSM helps to rebuild cartilage, which is possible because it has chemical properties that help to incorporate fluid in the joint tissue. But I wanted to ensure that Joe was also taking a supplement that would help reverse the deterioration of knee cartilage.

## DOSAGE

For preventative purposes, I recommend 1,000 to 2,000 milligrams daily. When using it for therapeutic purposes (e.g., pain relief) the dosage varies depending on body weight, sex, and individual need. Usually, somewhere between 3,000 to 8,000 milligrams is effective. I typically have patients start at 3,000 milligrams and gradually increase the dosage until they begin experiencing relief. Most find they begin to feel a lot better when the range is somewhere between 3,000 and 5,000 milligrams. MSM is available in capsule, tablet, crystal, lotion, cream, or gel. If you're taking the crystal form, be sure to add it to water for dilution, as the crystal is very bitter tasting. Or you can take it with juice to make it more palatable.

It is best to take MSM with meals to avoid the chances of stomach upset. I tell people to avoid taking MSM before bedtime because the supplement can keep you awake. Liginsul® MSM is the brand of MSM used in clinical studies.

## WHAT ARE THE SIDE EFFECTS?

Most people experience no side effects from MSM, though there have been some reports of digestive upset on high doses. A few people are sensitive to MSM, and have stomach upset, cramping, or diarrhea—so I recommend people start at a lower dosage and then gradually increase the dose every few days. This helps the body adjust to the MSM and reduces the chance of side effects.

If you do have an adverse reaction, you'll probably find that the symptoms go away if you reduce the dosage or—if necessary—stop taking MSM.

I am commonly asked if people allergic to sulfites or sulfa antibiotics can use MSM. The answer is yes. Sulfites and sulfa antibiotics don't have the same chemical make-up of MSM, which contains the mineral sulfur.

For children, I start with a very small dose of MSM. The gel or cream is particularly good to use with children for joint or muscle injuries.

The authors of *The Miracle of MSM* state that the supplement is safe to take during pregnancy, but I concur with their recommendation that a pregnant woman should consult with a physician first before using it.

Although it has not been studied, the authors also caution against using MSM in conjunction with blood-thinning medications such as heparin. If you are on a blood-thinning medication, consult with your doctor before using MSM.

## MSM
### RECOMMENDATIONS FROM THE NATURAL PHYSICIAN FOR . . .

#### ∾ Allergies and Asthma

Some patients have reported that MSM calms down pollen allergies. I certainly see many patients in the San Diego area with these problems, reacting to year-round influxes of different kinds of pollen. I haven't found that MSM is a cure for these allergies, but it effectively reduces the symptoms.

With its natural, antiallergy powers, MSM is also useful for asthma, which is often triggered by pollen allergies. People with chronic sinusitis may be helped because this, too, is a condition often associated with allergies.

*(continued)*

Dr. Jacob also reports that MSM has helped reduce food-allergy symptoms in the people he has treated.

### Arthritis

While MSM is particularly effective for treatment of osteoarthritis, it can also be used to take care of rheumatoid and other types of arthritis.

I find that most people with osteoarthritis who take MSM supplements notice a decrease in their pain within two to three weeks. Some report improvements within a day or two, especially when the cream or gel is applied to affected joints.

Small clinical studies have been done on MSM. In one of these, reported in the *International Journal of Anti-Aging Medicine*, 16 patients ranging in age from 55 to 78 were randomly assigned to two groups. All of the patients had degenerative joint disease and had chronic severe pain. When researchers compared the outcome of people taking 2,250 milligrams daily of MSM with those who were getting a placebo, it was found that those taking MSM reported over 80 percent improvement after six weeks. By comparison, those taking the placebo had less than 20 percent improvement.

### Autoimmune Diseases

MSM can offer a lot of pain relief to people with autoimmune conditions such as rheumatoid arthritis, lupus, scleroderma, and interstitial cystitis. While the supplement is not a cure, it does help many people manage the inflammation caused by these diseases and allows them to lead more normal lifestyles.

The supplement works even better when you take the precaution of combining it with nutritional changes and some natural therapies like homeopathy or acupuncture. With MSM supplementation, many people have lowered antiinflammatory or steroid medications. This of course needs to be done under the supervision of a doctor.

One of the outspoken fans of MSM is actor James Coburn, who had rheumatoid arthritis for many years. He claims MSM made a dramatic improvement in his arthritic pain and, the last I heard, continues taking it every day.

### Fibromyalgia

We still don't know what causes the painful muscle condition known as fibromyalgia, but my own clinical experience has shown that natural therapies work quite well for most people. Ongoing treatment with natural therapies is a far better long-term approach than trying to deal with the problem by administering megadoses of drugs. MSM is one of the supplements I recommend to help reduce the muscle pain.

### Hair and Nail Health

People report that MSM improves the strength and sheen of their hair, and also helps to preserve harder, shinier nails. In one study, 21 patients were assessed by a certified cosmetologist under the direction of a medical doctor, then given supplements, and finally, assessed again at the conclusion of the study. Both the patients and investigators were unaware of whether the "supplements" they received were actually MSM or placebo pills with no active ingredients. Dosages were 3,000 milligrams daily of Liginisul® MSM.

Those given supplemented MSM, evaluated by the cosmetologist, had shown significant improvement in hair health while those on placebo showed few or no changes. Participants as well as the investigators could see clear improvements in those who used MSM.

*(continued)*

A similar study, done with dosages of Liginisul® MSM, showed similar improvements in nail health. The 11 patients in the study, the examining cosmetologist, and the investigators were unaware of which patients had received MSM and which got placebos. When the study was done, and nails were measured for length, thickness, luster, and general appearance, those receiving MSM had shown significant improvement. The overall improvement rate was near 80 percent.

### ❧ Headaches

MSM helps to reduce muscle spasm and tension, so it is helpful to prevent tension headaches.

### ❧ Heartburn

MSM helps to relieve heartburn in some people, though researchers haven't yet discovered why it helps. MSM is certainly a better option than antacid medications that might provide temporary relief but also reduce the important stomach acid needed to digest food.

### ❧ Muscle and Sports Injuries

MSM is one of the best sport-injury supplements to use. It is the arnica of nutritional supplements. Apply it as a cream to sprains, strains, or other athletic injuries. It helps to reduce muscular soreness after workouts and competitions.

# Multivitamins

Years go, patients would customarily ask me if a multivitamin was really necessary as part of their preventative health program. Today, after all the current studies that have been released regarding nutritional deficiencies, many people understand that they are at risk for such deficiencies. Regular use of multivitamin supplements is much more common.

For optimal health, people need to consume certain amounts of vitamins and minerals on a regular basis. The Recommended Dietary Allowances (RDAs) have been used as a guideline since 1941. The goal of the RDAs is to reduce the incidence of diseases that occur as a result of severe nutritional deficiencies.

A classic example is scurvy. Once the scourge of sailors and arctic explorers who had to go long periods without any sources of vitamin C (such as fresh fruits and vegetables), scurvy has virtually been eliminated because vitamin C is so easy to get under normal condition. If you get at least the RDA of vitamin C, it's a virtual guarantee that you'll never have a problem with a vitamin-C–deficiency problem such as scurvy.

The criticism of the RDA by nutrition-oriented doctors like me is that it often does not promote optimal health or take into account the nutritional requirements of each individual. While the guidelines may be adequate for most people, some require higher daily amounts of certain vitamins and minerals than the amounts designated as "acceptable" in the RDA guidelines.

For example, people who have homocysteinuria (a genetic condition where the amino acid methionine is converted to the potentially toxic compound homocysteine), have a much greater risk of heart disease and stroke. These people need higher amounts of vitamins $B_6$ and $B_{12}$ and folic acid to prevent the buildup of this toxic metabolite. Following the RDA guidelines will not work for most people with this condition.

## OTHER FACTORS

Environment is a factor as well. People regularly exposed to environmental toxins require antioxidants such as vitamin C at higher levels than specified by the RDA guidelines. Athletes, or those with physically demanding jobs, are others who often require higher amounts of many vitamins and minerals.

It is also becoming better understood how certain pharmaceutical medications deplete vitamins and minerals. For example, the birth-control pill and various types of antibiotics deplete vitamins $B_6$ and $B_{12}$ and folic acid. Cholesterol-lowering drugs such as lovastatin deplete CoQ10.

More people are becoming aware of the new Dietary Reference Intakes (DRI) that have been released by the Food and Nutrition Board of the National Academy of Science. Again, these values offer information on protecting society as a whole against nutritional deficiencies, but still come up short for many people.

## AND ONE TO GROW ON

All pregnant women should take prenatal vitamins; most obstetricians now recommend them. They not only keep the pregnant woman healthier and prevent conditions such as anemia, but they could have lasting benefits for the baby as well. It is very important that women of childbearing age take a multivitamin before becoming pregnant as folic acid and $B_{12}$ help prevent birth defects.

Most children should be on a full-spectrum multivitamin. A wide variety of vitamins and minerals are required for growth and development. It makes sense to prevent a nutrition-related disease than to treat one. In one study, 60 children ages 12 to 13 were examined for the effect of a multivitamin on intelligence. Each child was given either a multivitamin or placebo for eight months. Only the group receiving a multivitamin showed improvement in nonverbal intelligence.

## GOOD HEALTH INSURANCE

I like the analogy of comparing a multivitamin to an insurance policy. Seeing that vitamins and minerals are required for life, and that when used properly they do not pose toxic side effects, it makes sense to take one.

One of the problems with multivitamins is that people don't always feel a difference when taking them. In other words, some multivitamin users do not feel a tremendous surge in energy, or improvement in mood or concentration.

Remember that most chronic diseases take years to develop. Long-term nutritional deficiencies are often at the root of these chronic maladies.

The immune system requires many vitamins and minerals to function optimally. This is especially true in the elderly. One study examined the effect of a multivitamin on the immune function in the elderly. Those who received the multivitamin supplement had significantly fewer infections compared with those who received placebo.

Another study found that a multivitamin and trace element supplement resulted in stronger immune cell markers, as compared with those who took placebo, whose showed a reduction in immune-cell parameters.

Many of my patients who have no major illnesses often notice improvements such as healthier hair and nails, better skin health, and fewer cravings for sweets and other junk foods. However, I do not find, nor do I expect, that multivitamins by themselves make a major noticeable impact on existing disease. For example, it is rare to see a patient with arthritis who starts taking a multivitamin and notices that his arthritic pain dramatically improves.

## DOSAGE

The term "multivitamin" refers to a supplement that contains the essential vitamins and minerals. Look for a formula that contains a wide blend of vitamins and minerals. Ask your natural healthcare provider or pharmacist to recommend a high-quality product. There are a wide range of products on the market, varying in quality and potency. Following is an example of an adult full-spectrum multivitamin and mineral formula:

## ∾ *Vitamins*

Vitamin A: 1,000 to 5,000 IU

Beta carotene: 2,500 to 25,000 IU (mixed carotenoid complex is even better)

Vitamin D: 200 to 400 IU

Vitamin E (d-alpha tocopherol): 400 IU

Vitamin K: 650 to 200 micrograms (not allowed in Canadian formulations)

Vitamin C: 100 to 1,000 milligrams

Vitamin $B_1$ (thiamin): 10 to 100 milligrams

Vitamin $B_2$ (riboflavin): 10 to 50 milligrams

Vitamin $B_3$ (niacin): 10 to 100 milligrams

Niacinamide: 10 to 50 milligrams

Vitamin $B_5$ (pantothenic acid): 25 to 100 milligrams

Vitamin $B_6$ (pyridoxine): 25 to 100 milligrams

Folic acid: 400 to 800 micrograms

Vitamin $B_{12}$: 400 to 800 micrograms

Choline: 10 to 100 milligrams

Inositol: 10 to 100 milligrams

## ∾ *Minerals*

Calcium: 250 to 1,000 milligrams

Magnesium: 250 to 500 milligrams

Chromium: 200 to 400 micrograms

Copper: 1 to 2 milligrams

Manganese: 5 to 15 milligrams

Molybdenum: 10 to 25 micrograms

Selenium: 200 micrograms

Boron: 1 to 3 milligrams (not allowed in Canadian formulations)

Silica: 1 to 20 milligrams

Vanadium: 50 to 100 micrograms

Zinc: 15 to 30 milligrams

I prefer capsules and powders to tablets for improved absorption, although some tablets are absorbed well (depending on the brand). Most high-potency multivitamins require 2 to 6 capsules or 2 to 4 tablets daily. Beyond obtaining a high-quality multivitamin, the most important consideration is consistency in taking it.

## WHAT ARE THE SIDE EFFECTS?

Some people may experience digestive upset. This can be avoided by taking the supplement with meals and by using a high-quality product. Also, users can occasionally be sensitive to an ingredient in the multivitamin. This is more of a risk with cheap brands that use fillers, colorings, or other added chemicals. Choose a hypoallergenic multivitamin formula.

I recommend that you avoid a multivitamin that contains iron, unless your doctor has determined that you have iron-deficiency anemia. Iron supplements are suspect in causing oxidative damage when used by those who do not have an iron deficiency.

Pregnant women should not take vitamin A in dosages above 2,500 to 5,000 IU.

Occasionally, I have a patient who cannot tolerate multivitamins. For these patients I either recommend starting with a multivitamin that comes in lower dosages (for example, a formula where four capsules equals the daily dosage, and have the patient start with one capsule daily and slowly increase their dosage), or using whole food supplements.

Some people's livers cannot handle higher dosages of vitamins and minerals, and they may require a detoxification program first before using a multivitamin.

# N

# Nettle

· · · · · · · · · · · · · · · · · · · · · · · · · · · · · · · · · · · · · · · · · · · · · · · · · · · · · · · · ·

"Is there something you can recommend for my mother?" Todd asked. "She has terrible hayfever symptoms this spring."

Though Todd was a long-term patient of mine, I had never met his mother. Nevertheless, he couldn't go wrong with a remedy that used to be part of every home herb garden.

"Stinging nettles," I suggested.

Todd looked at me as if I'd just offered to poison his mother.

"Don't worry," I assured him. "When you take these nettles in the supplement form, they don't really sting. You can pick them up from the health food store. Have her start with two capsules taken three times daily."

A few weeks later, when I saw Todd again, I asked how his mother was doing with her hayfever.

"She noticed an improvement in three days," Todd said. In fact, his mother had asked him to pick up another bottle of nettles, to make sure she didn't miss a single dose. "She doesn't want to run the risk of her allergies coming back," he told me.

"Great. At some point she can probably cut down the dose and still get the same benefit," I replied.

## UNSTUNG HERO

Though stinging nettle (*Urtica dioica*) is a threatening-looking plant, the roots and leaves have the components of a remarkably effective herbal medicine.

Curiously, each part of the plant has different medicinal uses. The leaf is used for allergies. A rich source of minerals, it also serves as a mild diuretic, and it's often recommended for arthritis. The root has become popular for the treatment of prostate enlargement.

The Latin name of *Urtica* means "to sting." The plant does, indeed, have small fibers or spines that sting the skin, and it can be seriously irritating. But as I explained to Todd, the herbal supplement has no such properties at all.

There are many different species of nettles, but most herbalists use *Urtica dioica*. (You should find the species name on the label of any supplement package you buy.) Though it's native to Europe, similar species grow in North America. When I was attending National College of Naturopathic Medicine in Portland, Oregon, students regularly plucked leaves from some of the nettles growing around the campus courtyard.

Nettle has been used as a medicinal food for many centuries. It's often taken in Europe for arthritis, kidney disease, anemia, and skin ailments. Native American women, when pregnant, boiled nettles to make a nutritive tonic that ensured the baby's health and was also reputed to ease labor. The tradition of giving nettle tonic during pregnancy continues to this day: Naturopathic obstetricians often recommend it to pregnant women to prevent anemia and fatigue.

Herbalists and naturopathic physicians often recommend nettle leaves as an essential part of any detoxification program. In fact, it was so often given to patients in springtime that it became known, literally, as a "spring tonic." Part of this "tonic" effect may be the natural diuretic action, which removes toxins through the kidneys.

## GOOD GREENS

Herbalists recommend the young greens rather than mature plants. Naturopathic physician Sharol Tilgner has specified that nettle should never be harvested after the flowers appear as it may cause urinary tract irritation.

Young nettles can be prepared like a vegetable. When steamed or simmered in water, nettle looks like spinach, and the taste is similar. If you like the taste, you can use them in soups or salads.

Nettle has many active or beneficial constituents including lignans, sterols (including beta sitosterol), polysaccharides, histamine, acetylcholine, potassium, calcium, magnesium, carotenoids, iron, vitamin C, and silicic acid. The plant is also a good source of chlorophyll.

Most of the vitamins and minerals are located in the leaves, which also harbor the compounds that help prevent allergies. Lignans and sterols are found in the root. These are the compounds that seem to be so important in relieving the symptoms of an enlarged prostate.

## DOSAGE

### ∾ *Nettle Leaf*

I recommend two capsules of 600 milligrams taken two or three times daily. The freeze-dried capsules are best.

Nettle-leaf tincture is also available. Take 30 drops or 0.5 milliliters two or three times daily.

Alternatively, you can take two or three cups of nettle leaf tea.

### ∾ *Nettle Root*

For capsules, try to get a total of 320 to 1,200 milligrams daily.

**Note:** Nettle root is often combined in formulas containing saw palmetto that are sold in capsule form.

The recommended dose of nettle root tincture is 0.5 milliliters (30 drops) two to three times daily.

If you're taking nettle root tea, drink two to three cups daily.

## WHAT ARE THE SIDE EFFECTS?

Nettle is very well tolerated. Occasionally, people may experience digestive upset, which may be resolved if the nettle is taken with a meal.

If you're on diuretic medications, however, you should avoid taking the leaf form of nettle. Excessively large dosages should be avoided during pregnancy. The maximum dosage recommended during pregnancy is 2 to 4 capsules daily or 20 drops of the tincture twice daily, taken with guidance from your doctor.

# NETTLE
## Recommendations from the Natural Physician for . . .

### ✎ Anemia

Nettle is one of the most widely used herbs for the treatment of anemia. It is often referred to as a "blood builder" as it contains iron and many other minerals.

It can be used safely by anyone who is susceptible to anemia, including women who have heavy menstrual flow. Pregnant women can safely take 600 to 1,200 milligrams daily of nettle leaf. It combines well with the herb yellow dock, which improves iron absorption.

### ✎ Arthritis

Nettle leaf has often been used as an external and internal treatment for rheumatoid arthritis and osteoarthritis. It has also been popular for relieving tendonitis and sciatic pain. In one clinical study, researchers found that the combination of nettle leaf and a pharmaceutical antiinflammatory (diclofenac) was as effective at relieving the pain of arthritis as a full dose of the drug. Though the drug diclofenac is considered ineffective at dosages below 75 milligrams per day, many participants in the study were getting good results with just 50 milligrams of diclofenac when the drug was combined with stewed nettles. This is a good indication that nettle has a significant effect on pain relief. Other studies have shown that nettle blocks the release of inflammatory chemicals.

I generally find that long-term use of nettle works well for chronic conditions such as arthritis. I also find it works best in formulas that contain other effective supplements for arthritis.

### ✎ Edema

Since the herb has a mild diuretic effect, it can be beneficial if you have water retention or swelling—such as edema from pregnancy or varicose veins. It should not, however, be combined with diuretic drugs.

### ✎ Gout

Nettle leaf is one of the herbs that has been used by European doctors to reduce uric acid buildup associated with gout. It can be given every two hours to relieve acute gout attacks and works well when taken on a long-term basis to prevent uric acid buildup. Combined with this treatment, I also recommend a plant-based diet—and no alcoholic drinks—for anyone who is prone to gout.

Historically, a related species of nettles, *Urtica urens*, was commonly used for the treatment of gout. In the early part of the twentieth century, Dr. Burnett of London was so successful treating gout with nettle that he drew patients from the farthest reaches of the United Kingdom, eventually earning the nickname "Dr. Urtica."

### ✎ Hair Problems

Nettle has been used historically for hair loss and to improve hair health. This has not been scientifically studied, but my guess is that the minerals, particularly silica, are responsible for this effect.

Hair loss can be a symptom of anemia, so those who are anemic and take nettle leaf may indirectly notice hair improvement.

### ✎ Hayfever

When someone asks what one herb I consider most effective for hayfever, my immediate response is nettles. I find about 50 percent of people who use freeze-dried nettles for hayfever notice a substantial improvement. Take 2 capsules three times daily until the symptoms are under control. *(continued)*

**348**

After a week or two you may be able to reduce the amount by half and continue taking it as a maintenance dosage. Again, side effects are not an issue—which makes nettle very attractive for people who suffer drowsiness and other side effects from prescription antihistamine medications.

In a randomized, double-blind study, scientists looked into the effects of freeze-dried nettles on people who had hayfever ("allergic rhinitis"). It was found that after one week of use, 58 percent of the participants were helped by this herbal extract.

## ❧ Pregnancy

There are few herbs I recommend women use during pregnancy. Nettle leaf is one of them. It helps to prevent and treat anemia. In fact, midwives and naturopathic obstetricians routinely recommend nettle during pregnancy as a nutritive herb. It also helps some women with the overwhelming fatigue that can accompany pregnancy. It can also help to alleviate muscle cramps. (In all likelihood, this benefit comes from the many minerals in nettle, including calcium, magnesium, and potassium.) It can also help relieve constipation associated with pregnancy.

As mentioned earlier, very high dosages are not recommended during pregnancy—so don't exceed 2 to 4 capsules daily (600 to 1,200 milligrams) or 20 drops of the tincture twice daily, and only with the consent of your doctor.

## ❧ Prostate Enlargement

Based on published clinical studies, nettle root has become very popular for the treatment of benign prostatic hyperplasia (BPH). Approximately 50 percent of men over the age of 50—and close to 90 percent of men in their 80's—have BPH. Common symptoms of prostate enlargement include an increasing need to urinate frequently, especially at night, and reduced force of the urinary stream.

Researchers found that men with BPH could reduce the symptoms of urinary frequency and nighttime urination in the span of 10 weeks if they took nettle. In one study, for instance, over three-quarters of the men who took nettle reported "good" or "very good" results.

Nettle root is often used in formulas that contain other effective herbs for the prostate such as saw palmetto and Pygeum africanum. I typically recommend that it be used this way to make the most of synergistic effects among these herbs.

There have been some positive studies that show the combination of saw palmetto and nettle root works well for the treatment of prostate enlargement. One randomized, double-blind study found the combination of nettle root and saw palmetto worked as effectively as the pharmaceutical drug finasteride, which is commonly used to reduce the symptoms of BPH. Participants either took the combination of 240 milligrams of nettle root with 320 milligrams of saw palmetto extract—or took 5 milligrams of finasteride daily for 48 weeks. (None of the men knew whether they were getting the herbs or the drug.) Researchers noted the herbal combination had fewer side effects than were experienced by men taking the pharmaceutical drug.

Another landmark study showed that the combination of saw palmetto and nettle root worked to shrink enlarged prostate tissue. This has been the first study to confirm that these two common herbs can have such an effect.

When men are using herbs like nettle root or saw palmetto, I always recommend that they continue on regular dosages for at least 6 to 8 weeks. It takes at least that long to see whether these herbs are having a positive effect.

# Nux Vomica

Nux vomica is a homeopathic remedy required by tens of thousands of people every day in the United States. This remarkable remedy is the diluted extract of poison-nut. While the nut is very toxic and causes a multitude of symptoms that range from vomiting, cramps, and nerve reactions, the homeopathic remedy is completely safe. It's an extremely diluted form of poison-nut extract—so diluted, that only the vibrational frequency of the plant remains. No material is left in it. In this form, the extract from the nut can treat numerous symptoms, especially those related to intestinal problems or insomnia.

Miles, a 41-year-old patient of mine, suffered both from chronic heartburn and from insomnia. Before coming to me he had been through the full gamut of conventional therapies—including heartburn medications and a whole range of sleep medicines. He had even been to a world-renowned sleep clinic where he was treated for insomnia, but with no improvement.

Miles fit the profile of what homeopathic physicians call a "nux vomica personality." Friendly and outgoing, he was also a hard-driving businessperson, who owned two successful businesses and liked to be very involved. He was also a beer drinker—another nux vomica trait. Emotionally, he tended to get irritable and impatient, and he could be easily angered.

For Miles, nux vomica provided an incredible response. When he started taking it, the incidents of heartburn greatly decreased in frequency and intensity. Insomnia ceased to become a problem. He told me he could finally get a sound night's sleep.

## A QUESTION OF DIGESTION

Nux vomica has a specific action on the digestive system. It is one of the best remedies for heartburn, ulcers, cramps, hiccups, food poisoning, and constipation. It also has a detoxifying effect on the liver.

There are also beneficial effects on the nervous system. Nux vomica has a relaxing and calming effect, so it helps reduce the effects of stress, including muscle spasms and cramps.

In addition, nux vomica is commonly used to cure hangovers. Many years ago, after a friend's wedding, I recall giving nux vomica to quite a few members of the wedding party. Fifteen minutes after taking the remedy, people were coming to me with the question, "What *was* that remedy?" In that very short time, they were already feeling better.

Translated from German, nux vomica simply means "no vomit."

## DOSAGE

For acute relief of symptoms, I recommend a 30C potency to be taken every 15 to 30 minutes. (If 30C is not available, you can use other potencies at the same interval.) For chronic health problems, I recommend a dose twice daily for two weeks and then as needed.

## WHAT ARE THE SIDE EFFECTS?

I have never seen side effects with this remedy.

---

# NUX VOMICA
## RECOMMENDATIONS FROM THE NATURAL PHYSICIAN FOR . . .

### ❧ Alcoholism

Nux vomica helps reduce the craving for alcohol and facilitate the recovery process. It also helps recovering addicts to detoxify more effectively.

### ❧ Allergies

This remedy is effective with hayfever and other inhalant allergies. If you sneeze frequently and have a runny nose when you wake in the morning, nux vomica is the remedy of choice.

### ❧ Back Pain

Many practitioners are not aware that nux vomica helps to relieve back pain. While it is particularly effective if taken just before you go to bed,

it can also help relieve back spasms and cramps during the day.

### ❧ Bladder Infection

Consider nux vomica for the relief of bladder symptoms when you have a constant urge to urinate. If you find that hot baths help relieve the pain, then nux vomica can probably provide further relief.

### ❧ Chemotherapy

Nux vomica helps people undergoing chemotherapy to experience fewer symptoms of nausea, vomiting, and constipation. It is the second most-common remedy that I prescribe

*(continued)*

to prevent or treat chemotherapy side effects. (The other remedy I prescribe is cadmium sulph.)

## Colic

Nux vomica is an excellent remedy for colic symptoms. If you have a baby who is typically constipated, irritable, and arches the back during bouts of colic, the infant is a good candidate for nux vomica. It is not uncommon for the infant to improve within seconds or minutes after receiving the remedy.

## Colitis

This remedy provides relief for people suffering from digestive conditions such as ulcerative colitis, Crohn's disease, and irritable bowel syndrome (IBS). It helps prevent and relieve symptoms of abdominal cramps that may be brought on from feelings of anger, poor food choices, or stress. When tight clothes around the waist make the symptoms worse—and warm applications and warm drinks help provide relief—nux vomica is an excellent remedy as well.

## Constipation

Nux vomica is the most common homeopathic remedy for constipation. Even if you're getting plenty of fiber and water in your diet, nux vomica can provide further relief. It's the remedy to use when constipation occurs while traveling.

## Flu

Nux vomica leads to faster recovery from the flu, particularly if you're feeling very chilled, nauseated, and achy.

## Hangover

For anyone who's had a few too many drinks, nux vomica can alleviate symptoms of nausea, vomiting, fatigue, headache, and cramps. (Of course, the surest prevention is to drink in moderation or not at all.)

## Insomnia

Nux vomica actually treats the biochemical imbalances that lead to insomnia. If you've had trouble sleeping because you've been thinking about work, nux vomica is particularly effective. Another "nux vomica symptom" is waking between 3 and 4 A.M.

## Ulcer

I have had fantastic results in treating ulcers with this remedy. Patti, a 42-year-old patient of mine in Canada, exemplified the kind of success that someone can have with this remedy. She actually had to visit the emergency room because of extreme pain from stomach ulcers—and when she called me afterwards, she was still in pain.

After she had described her symptoms, she tried one kind of homeopathic remedy, then I switched her to nux vomica, which brought her relief the same day. Over the next two weeks, the nux vomica completely healed her ulcer.

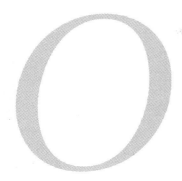

# Onion

Often, practitioners of natural medicine focus on looking for the "new." It's exciting to discover a potent healing supplement that is being researched or developed for the first time—or the newly discovered healing power of some food.

However, sometimes old news is the best news. There are certain foods that have been around for centuries. Their potent medicinal effects are no secret, their story deserves to be told again.

Such is the case with the lowly onion *(Allium sativum)*.

Most cultures around the world use onions as a seasoning that lends pungency to many dishes. It has also been a medicine for many centuries, particularly in Chinese and Ayurvedic medicines. But whether you consume onion for its flavor or value its medicinal properties, there's no question that you get hearty benefits from the allium every time you take a bite.

During the Civil War, General Ulysses S. Grant requested and received a shipment of onions to treat the soldiers who had dysentery.

Just a generation ago, it was common for people to make an onion poultice to help cure sore throats—a practice that proved its usefulness from the wild frontier to the urban landscapes of America.

Today, the scientists who have explored the components of the common onion have discovered that it does, indeed, possess medicinal properties that are very similar to those of garlic. It has antimicrobial qualities, reduces blood pressure and elevated cholesterol, and helps lower elevated blood-sugar levels.

Onions contain dozens of powerful medicinal ingredients, including:

- Sulfur compounds called thiosulfinates, which are thought to have strong antiinflammatory effects and help with detoxification
- Flavonoids
- Phenolic acids, sterols, pectin, and volatile oils
- Vitamin C

You don't need to restrict your appetite to one particular type of onion, either. Other members of the allium family are beneficial, too. Scallions—often called spring or green onions—contain even more vitamin C than white or yellow onions. The green kind are also high in folate, which is one of the essential nutrients. The small onions called shallots are very rich in vitamin A as well.

Onions have been shown to have strong antioxidant effects. They are a good source of the flavonoid quercitin, which is valued as a potent antioxidant. It is estimated that a medium-size onion contains as much as 50 milligrams of quercitin. It is possible to get therapeutic amounts of this antioxidant if you eat onions every day.

## DOSAGE

Choose firm, small-necked onions with brittle outer leaves. Avoid dark spotted or sprouting bulbs. To maintain good health, try to eat the equivalent of one-half to one cup of chopped onions every day.

Raw onions contain higher amounts of the disease-fighting chemicals, but cooked onions are also healthful.

## WHAT ARE THE SIDE EFFECTS?

Aside from getting burning, watering eyes when you chop them, some people experience digestive upset and heartburn from onions. If you have asthma, be wary of pickled onions, which may contain sulfites that can trigger asthma attacks.

Another side effect is "onion breath." Eating a sprig of parsley with your meal can help prevent bad breath that's associated with eating onions.

# ONION

## RECOMMENDATIONS FROM THE NATURAL PHYSICIAN FOR . . .

### ✺ Asthma

Onions have been traditionally used for the treatment of asthma. Animal studies have shown that phytochemicals within onions such as thiosulfinates and cepaenes inhibit inflammatory compounds associated with inducing asthma.

Nutrition-oriented doctors commonly prescribe high dosages of supplemental quercitin (1,500 to 3,000 milligrams) to help prevent asthma. As I've mentioned, onion is a natural source of quercitin. If you need a large dose, onions can't compete with a supplement (you'd have to eat too many), but for anyone with asthma, it's helpful to get as much quercitin as possible in your diet.

### ✺ Cancer

A French study of 345 women found that risk of breast cancer decreased as consumption of fiber, garlic, and onions increased.

A study examined the relationship between allium vegetable intake (including onion), and cancer of the esophagus and stomach in Yangzhong City, one of the highest-risk areas for these cancers in Jiangsu Province, China. The researchers suggested that allium vegetables, like raw vegetables, may have an important protecting effect not only against stomach cancer, but also against esophageal cancer.

Quercitin, which appears to be one of the key active substances in onions, has been shown to protect against colon cancer in studies involving animals.

### ✺ Cholesterol and High Blood Pressure

In clinical studies, researchers have found that onions decrease cholesterol and trigylceride levels. If you eat lots of onions, you can also help lower your blood pressure. In fact, if I see anyone with these conditions, I encourage the person to incorporate onions into his or her daily diet on a long-term basis. One medium onion a day—raw or cooked—can be helpful. You can't expect immediate improvements, of course, but over time, the ingredients in onions give you cumulative benefits.

### ✺ Diabetes

Studies have shown that onion reduces elevated blood-sugar levels. Along with garlic, onions are an excellent food for people with this condition to consume on a regular basis.

If you have diabetes, you should check with your doctor before introducing quantities of onion or making any changes in your diet.

### ✺ Immunity

Onion is helpful in protecting against bacterial, fungal, and worm infections. It is excellent to include in a soup or broth for sore throats and upper respiratory tract infections.

# P

# Passionflower

∙∙∙∙∙∙∙∙∙∙∙∙∙∙∙∙∙∙∙∙∙∙∙∙∙∙∙∙∙∙∙∙∙∙∙∙∙∙∙∙∙∙∙∙∙∙∙∙∙∙∙∙∙∙∙∙∙∙∙∙∙∙∙∙∙∙∙∙∙∙

"I have had insomnia for a few months now. At least a couple nights a week, I can't even fall asleep."

Tammy was a 40-year-old mother of three. All of her children were beyond the "crying baby" stage, but even so, she often found herself lying awake at night. For a while, she had tried the natural sleep aid valerian—but she didn't like it. "I felt groggy in the morning, like I was hung over," she said. So, she had come to me to ask for something that wouldn't have any side effects. "Is there anything else you'd recommend?" she asked.

"Let's start with passionflower," I suggested. "It is a gentle herb that has been used for centuries to help relieve insomnia."

Four weeks later Tammy reported that the passionflower had worked like a charm. She said, "Those nights I can't fall asleep I take the passionflower as you told me to, and within thirty minutes I am fast asleep. I also feel perfectly fine when I wake up in the morning."

## THE REST IS HISTORY

Passionflower (*Passiflora incarnata*) was used by Spanish explorers and missionaries who visited Peru in the early seventeenth century. They were intrigued by the plant's resemblance to a crown of thorns on top of a cross—suggesting volumes of religious meaning—and in 1605, one intrepid missionary sent samples of the symbolic flower to Pope Paul V. Along with a name that suggested "Christ's passion," the passionflower was also referred to as the Holy Trinity flower and passion-vine.

A climbing vine that can grow upwards of 28 feet, passionflower grows wild in the southern United States as well as South America. It's also found in the East Indies and in parts of Europe. Historically, Native Americans ate the leaves and fruit of the passionflower and used various parts of the plant to cure ailments. Today, all parts of the plant—root, leaf, stem, and fruit—are used medicinally, although it's mainly the flower parts that are included in capsules, teas, and tinctures.

Researchers believe that certain flavonoids are responsible for the nerve-relaxing properties of passionflower, although other constituents are likely involved as well.

## DOSAGE

I recommend 500 milligrams of the capsule form, or 20 to 30 drops (0.5 milliliter) of the tincture form, or one cup of the tea, taken two to three times daily.

## WHAT ARE THE SIDE EFFECTS?

I have not read any reports of side effects to passionflower, nor have my patients shown any sign of them. As with any herb, I do not recommend large dosages for pregnant women.

## PASSIONFLOWER
### RECOMMENDATIONS FROM THE NATURAL PHYSICIAN FOR . . .

### ✺ Anxiety and Stress

Passionflower is an excellent herb for anxiety and general stress. It helps to relax the nerves and muscles without any kind of sedating effect, so it's particularly effective if you want to take something during daytime hours to reduce the effects of stress and anxiety. Passionflower also helps to relax tight muscles.

### ✺ Heart Palpitations

This herb is commonly included in European formulas for treatment of heart palpitations, particularly when there's an underlying component of anxiety. It is often combined with hawthorn berry extract, which is used as a heart tonic.

*(continued)*

### ꙮ High Blood Pressure

I like to use passionflower or valerian in herbal hypertension formulas when stress and anxiety are at the core of a high blood-pressure problem.

### ꙮ Insomnia

Passionflower is particularly good for insomnia related to anxiety. People who experience side effects from sleep medications and even from valerian—as Tammy did—have no such problems when they take passionflower.

Passionflower does not cause the drowsiness associated with over-the-counter or prescription sleep medications.

If you are taking it primarily as a sleep aid, I recommend 30 drops of the tincture or 500 to 1,000 milligrams of the capsule form be taken a half hour before bedtime. It is commonly found in formulas that contain nerve-relaxing herbs such as kava, hops, chamomile, and valerian.

### ꙮ PMS and Menopause

Passionflower is sometimes used to help reduce the anxiety and irritability experienced by women who have premenstrual syndrome (PMS). We commonly recommend it for the relief of PMS symptoms in a formula that also contains hormone-balancing herbs such as vitex. It is also effective for relief of some menopause-related problems, such as relief from irritability, depression, and insomnia.

# Peppermint

"I have been following those diet changes you recommended as well as the digestive enzymes and have been feeling a lot better. But I still get some gas and cramps in my lower abdomen."

At the age of 29, Kristina had all the symptoms of irritable bowel syndrome (IBS), a painful digestive problem that often requires long-term treatment. The fact that she had already improved was significant—and for her remaining symptoms, I recommended peppermint (Mentha piperita).

"If it works as it should, you'll be pretty much symptom-free. The peppermint oil capsules help to relax the digestive tract and reduce spasms and gas."

Over the next month, Kristina experienced the same results as many patients with IBS who take peppermint. She found that this simple natural remedy made a tremendous difference in how she felt. It was just what she needed on days when she felt some "uneasiness" in her lower abdomen.

# MAKING A MINT

Mentha piperita has long been used to help digestive complaints such as digestive cramps and spasms, flatulence, colic, and gallstones. While it's one of the best herbs to use for irritable bowel syndrome, it also helps resolve problems with the upper respiratory tract. It can help relieve the symptoms of a cold and clear out sinusitis and bronchitis. Herbalists and holistic doctors have long used peppermint for the treatment of headaches, as well. When it's made into a cream, peppermint is an excellent topical ointment for relief of joint and muscle pain.

Other "mints"—and there are quite a number—share some of the healing powers of peppermint. They were used by ancient Greeks, Romans, and Egyptians as herbs for cooking and medicinal purposes. Peppermint has also been used for thousands of years by doctors who practiced traditional Chinese and Ayurvedic medicines. Introduced to western Europe in the 1800s, it remains popular among British and European herbalists to this day.

Peppermint is actually a hybrid of two other mints—spearmint *(Mentha spicata)* and watermint *(Mentha aquatica)*. It's the leaves that are used for medicinal purposes.

The key constituents of peppermint are essential oils that include menthol and menthone. Menthol is particularly important for its antispasmodic, gas-relieving, bile-stimulating, and pain-relieving qualities. Peppermint also contains flavonoids, tannins, tocopherols, carotenes, and other nutrients.

Peppermint is an aromatic herb that has a cooling effect on the body. According to traditional Chinese medicine, it has an affinity for the lungs and liver.

# DOSAGE

## ∾ *Tea*

I recommend an infusion of 1 to 2 teaspoons of the dried leaf per 8 ounces of water, one to three times daily.

## ∾ *Tincture*

I recommend 20 to 60 drops (approximately 0.5 to 1.0 milliliters) one to three times daily.

## ✒ Capsule

I recommend 1 to 2 enteric-coated capsules (0.2 milliliter per capsule) two to three times daily between meals. This is the form recommended for irritable bowel syndrome or digestive problems that occur in the lower half of the digestive tract (e.g., flatulence).

## WHAT ARE THE SIDE EFFECTS?

Peppermint may aggravate esophageal reflux (heartburn). It should also be avoided if you have cholecystitis (inflammation of the gallbladder) or severe liver disease. Peppermint essential oil—the kind that's sold for aromatherapy—should be used with caution in people with asthma. Inhaling the fragrance of the essential oil could cause a flare-up of asthma.

Note that peppermint essential oil, the kind used for aromatherapy, is for scent only. Like other essential oils, it should never be taken internally.

Use caution if you're applying peppermint oil externally as it may cause skin irritation. Don't use the oil topically around the eyes, especially with children.

I have found that too strong a concentration or too high amount of peppermint oil taken internally can cause digestive upset in children.

---

## PEPPERMINT
### RECOMMENDATIONS FROM THE NATURAL PHYSICIAN FOR . . .

### ✒ Cold and Cough

Peppermint has been used for thousands of years in traditional Chinese medicine for the treatment of the common cold when someone has symptoms of fever, slight chills, headache, cough, and eye redness. It is also commonly used as a topical or inhaled preparation (including menthol extract) to help ease breathing and open the respiratory passages.

Peppermint has been shown to possess antiviral qualities. In addition, it is a common ingredient in cough formulas.

### ✒ Gallstones

Menthol has been shown to be helpful in dissolving gallstones when combined with ursodeoxycholic acid. It's used in a proprietary formulation known as rowachol.

### ✒ Headaches

Peppermint is also used internally and as an oil externally to relieve headaches, particularly tension headaches.

*(continued)*

### ❧ Irritable Bowel Syndrome

Enteric-coated peppermint oil capsules have become very popular to reduce and sometimes eradicate the symptoms of irritable bowel syndrome (IBS). This common condition is characterized by constipation or diarrhea—or an alternation of these two symptoms—as well as flatulence and intestinal cramping.

Peppermint oil helps to relax the smooth muscle of the digestive tract. It has also been shown to have antimicrobial effects against yeast and other bacteria that are often involved with IBS.

Several studies have shown that peppermint oil is effective for IBS. One randomized, double-blind, placebo-controlled trial of 110 people with IBS found that peppermint oil improved symptoms of abdominal pain, distention, flatulence, and other symptoms. Peppermint oil was significantly more effective than placebo.

### ❧ Muscle and Bone Pain

Both peppermint oil and menthol have been shown to reduce pain when applied topically. For this reason they are commonly used in creams and gels for muscle pain and spasm.

# Phosphatidylserine

"Doctor, I am having terrible memory problems," said 57 year old Melanie. "I have trouble remembering my friends' phone numbers, and I'm always forgetting where I put things."

I noticed memory problems during her visit. She had difficulty with both short-term concentration and long-term recall. She had difficulty remembering names of people she knew well.

After completing a medical history, I prescribed phosphatidylserine—a dosage of 300 milligrams daily. (Melanie had already been taking ginkgo with limited results.)

She forgot her purse and car keys when she left my office. I dashed out to the parking lot to give them to her.

"This is always happening to me," she said with tears in her eyes.

Eight weeks later, Melanie reported excitedly that her memory was coming back. After five months, her memory had improved even more. No more forgotten keys!

## THE "NEW GINKGO"

Phosphatidylserine (also called PS) is being hailed as the "ginkgo for the millennium." Studies have shown that this phospholipid extract from soy is effective in improving mental alertness, and especially the memory, in people with age-related mental decline.

PS is an important phospholipid that is a building block for cell membranes. It is found in every human cell, but is a very specific brain nutrient, being most highly concentrated in brain cells.

It has the following functions: It normalizes brain chemistry, improves cell-to-cell communication, regulates nutrients that enter brain cells and waste products that exit brain cells, stimulates production and activity of neurotransmitters, and supports stress-hormone metabolism.

PS is found in foods such as rice, fish, soy, and green leafy vegetables. It is thought that the amount of PS people get from foods is not enough for many people as they age. It is estimated that the average person gets about 70 to 80 milligrams of PS daily from diet. Studies show that up to 300 milligrams is required for therapeutic effects. Using a PS supplement is a way to achieve required levels.

Dr. Paris Kidd, one of the world's leading experts on phosphatidylserine, has reviewed some 3,000 peer-reviewed research papers on PS. "It is the single best nutrient (really, the single best means of any kind) for safely conserving and restoring crucial higher functions of the brain," according to Dr. Kidd. "The remarkable benefits of PS and its safety in use are now established beyond doubt. What remains is to spread the message to the people who can benefit from PS."

## DOSAGE

I recommend starting with 300 milligrams daily for the first month. Optimally, 100 milligrams should be taken three times daily with meals. This initial dosage helps to saturate the brain cells with PS. After one month, most people can use a maintenance dosage of 100 to 200 milligrams. If one is suspected of having Alzheimer's disease or severe memory loss, then I would recommend not using less than 300 milligrams, and perhaps even a higher dosage such as 500 milligrams.

Make sure to buy phosphatidylserine and not phosphorylated serine. The latter is not the same and will not have the same effect. (Typically, this means looking for brands that have the Leci-PS logo.)

PS is available in formulas that contain other beneficial brain nutrients such as DHA, ginkgo, acetyl-L-carnitine, $B_{12}$, folic acid, and others.

It works even better when combined with the following holistic program for optimal brain health:

- Eat brain-fortifying foods (fish, nuts, seeds, fruits, vegetables, and whole grains).

- Take nutritional supplements, including acetyl-L-carnitine and ginkgo biloba.

- Practice stress-busting lifestyle habits (proper sleep, exercise, prayer, etc.).

## WHAT ARE THE SIDE EFFECTS?

There are no side effects to speak of, except digestive upset for a small number of people. However, I would recommend not taking PS before bedtime, as it keeps some people awake.

## PHOSPHATIDYLSERINE
### RECOMMENDATIONS FROM THE NATURAL PHYSICIAN FOR . . .

### ❧ Age-Associated Memory Impairment (AAMI)

Many people experience impaired memory as they age. Some researchers feel that AAMI is the beginning of a continuum of memory decline, with the worst case of deterioration ending in Alzheimer's disease. AAMI is the condition that brings many people to see me for their memory problems. Generally, I find people improve with PS. Many people try ginkgo first because it is less expensive than PS—and some patients are already taking ginkgo on their own before they see me. But I find PS especially helpful when patients do not respond to ginkgo.

In a 1991 study of phosphatidylserine among people aged 50 to 75, doctors found positive results when they used 100-milligram doses of PS, three times daily. Participants were given objective assessments at the beginning of the study and at 3-week intervals. Researchers found a 30 percent improvement in cognitive function that included memory, learning, recalling names, faces, and numbers. They also found that some people with the worst memory impairment were more likely to respond positively to PS.

In evaluating this supplement, Dr. Thomas Crook, a leading researcher on the effects of drugs and supplements on memory, concluded that PS is "by far the best of all drugs and nutritional supplements we have ever tested for retarding Age-Associated Memory Impairment."

### ❧ Alzheimer's disease

Alzheimer's disease is one of the most feared of all diseases. When someone has Alzheimer's, the progressive deterioration of the brain has an obvious impact on behavior. One loses the abili-

*(continued)*

363

ty to retrieve memory, learn, and reason. It is not well understood what causes this disease, although we do know that brain cells die.

Aside from ginkgo, PS is one of the few natural treatments that has been shown to delay the progression of the disease. Note that it delays the progression; it does not reverse or cure Alzheimer's. There is currently no treatment that does.

Several studies have shown that people who have Alzheimer's, especially in the earliest stages, experience an improvement in memory and cognitive function if they take PS.

### ✌ Attention Deficit Hyperactivity Disorder (ADHD)

PS is being recommended by holistic doctors as an alternative to pharmaceutical medications such as Ritalin®. In an article in *The Alternative Medicine Review*, Dr. Paris Kidd states, "In a physician in-office study of 21 consecutive ADHD cases aged 4–19, dietary supplementation with PS benefited greater than 90 percent of the cases. At intakes of 200–300 mg/day of PS for up to four months, attention and learning were most consistently improved. Oppositional conduct proved most resistant to PS."

### ✌ Brain Injury

Anecdotal reports from emergency room physicians confirm that PS helps quicken recovery from brain injuries. I had a patient who sustained a brain injury after falling off a tractor. PS helped improve his cognitive function after a month of use.

### ✌ Dementia

Alzheimer's disease is probably the best known of the brain-related diseases that fall under the category of dementia. All cases of dementia involve memory loss as well as loss of motor function, vocabulary, and judgment.

Dementia can result from various things—a stroke, Parkinson's disease, drugs, nutritional deficiencies such as $B_{12}$ or folic acid, or even brain trauma. Several studies have shown PS to be effective in alleviating various symptoms.

### ✌ Depression

PS has been shown to improve mood and alleviate depression. It has a balancing effect on the neurotransmitters of the brain, which are largely responsible for our moods.

### ✌ Stress and Fatigue

Cortisol, a hormone produced by the adrenal glands, plays a role in both stress and fatigue. When you have acute stress, cortisol is released in high amounts to help your body deal with it. With a rise in cortisol comes an increase in blood sugar and heart rate. Other physiological effects also occur. This type of response is required for normal functioning. However, prolonged elevation of stress leads to chronically elevated cortisol levels, which causes serious problems.

Prolonged elevation of cortisol kills brain cells, suppresses the immune system, and leads to a breakdown of the body. Stress, whether it be physical or mental, causes elevated cortisol levels. PS has been shown to have a balancing effect on the adrenal glands, the ones that control cortisol. It is one of the supplements to consider taking if you are under chronic stress or are recovering from chronic fatigue.

PS is also effective in helping athletes adapt to stress caused by exhaustive training.

# Phytonutrients

Phytonutrients, also known as phytochemicals, are naturally occurring substances that give plants their characteristic flavor, color, aroma, and resistance to disease.

We get our phytonutrients from plant foods such as vegetables, fruits, nuts, seeds, grains, and legumes. Thanks to a great deal of research that's been done over the last few decades, we know many of the health benefits of these substances—and there are more than we suspected. While hundreds have already been discovered, I suspect that thousands more will be identified in the future.

Some have been in the news. The phytonutrients known as isoflavones are found in soy, and seem to have a great number of health benefits. The carotenoids found in yellow-orange fruits and vegetables such as carrots and squash also have a great reputation, because they seem to help prevent cancer and heart disease.

Many phytonutrients have potent antioxidant activity, even exceeding the well-known antioxidant properties of such vitamins as E and C. In fact, the phytonutrients known as polyphenols, which are found in green and black teas, are some of the most potent antioxidants known.

## DETOX PROGRAM

Many phytonutrients promote detoxification in the body, which is critical to overall health and the prevention of disease. A great example is d-glucarate, which has been shown to help the liver metabolize pesticides, hormones, carcinogens, and other toxins. Certain phytonutrients also help damaged cells to repair themselves, which is important in treating conditions like arthritis.

When we don't consume adequate amounts of fruits, vegetables, and other plant foods, we're not only missing out on the benefits of fiber, vitamins, minerals, and enzymes—we're also losing the opportunity to eat some vital, powerful phytonutrients. So the first thing I recommend, if you want to get more disease-fighting phytonutrients, is to increase your consumption of plant foods.

The second best way to increase your levels of phytonutrients is to use whole-food supplements. In some cases it makes sense to take high dosages of supplemental phytonutrients for the treatment of certain diseases. For example, I highly recommend the phytonutrient lycopene for men with prostate cancer and help them shape their diets so they're getting as much as possible in their meals. Then I recommend lycopene supplements.

We already know a number of other phytonutrients that seem to be effective for treatment of specific health problems. Flavonoid-rich supplements such as grape seed extract or pycnogenol are excellent for varicose veins. Anthocyanosides as found in bilberry are excellent for eye conditions such as cataracts or poor night vision. Curcumin extracted from turmeric has potent antiinflammatory properties. Indole 3 carbinol is helpful for women with abnormal pap smears, indicating cervical dysplasia.

Studies are ongoing in regards to isolated phytonutrients and their benefit in the treatment of specific diseases.

## DOSAGE

The recommended dosage for the supplemental form really varies depending on the phytonutrient and what it is being used for. Consult the listing and description in this section.

## WHAT ARE THE SIDE EFFECTS?

Whether you're getting phytonutrients in food or taking specific supplements, side effects are rarely a problem. Some people have to be wary of grapefruit and grapefruit juice, however, because it affects the way the liver metabolizes certain drug medications. The fruit and concentrated juice have been shown to alter the blood levels of some heart medications and antidepressants, sometimes causing the drugs to have a greater than anticipated effect.

---

### PHYTONUTRIENTS
#### RECOMMENDATIONS FROM THE NATURAL PHYSICIAN FOR . . .

Some phytonutrients seem very effective in boosting general good health, while others are ones I'd recommend for specific conditions. The following list of recommendations is a summary of what we've learned about these nutrients so far.

❧ *Chlorophyll*
*Source:* green plants and other colored vegetables

*Properties:* antioxidant; contains vitamin K, which is needed for blood clotting and to build bone cells
*Conditions:* anemia; detoxification; burns and wounds, cancer prevention

*(continued)*

---

## ❧ Curcumin

Source: turmeric

Properties: antiinflammatory; antioxidant

Conditions: arthritis; inflammatory bowel disease; cancer

For more about the benefits of this nutrient, see TURMERIC, page 444.

## ❧ Ellagic Acid

Source: berries; grapes; apples; tea

Properties: detoxifies

Conditions: cancer prevention

## ❧ Flavoglycosides

Source: ginkgo; black tea

Properties: antioxidant; improves blood flow

Conditions: heart disease; kidney disease; varicose veins; depression; poor memory

## ❧ Fructooligosaccharides (FOS)

Source: Jerusalem artichoke; chicory root; garlic; bananas

Properties: detoxifies; increases beneficial bacteria

Conditions: digestive conditions such as irritable bowel syndrome, Crohn's disease, ulcerative colitis; yeast overgrowth; cancer; vaginitis

## ❧ Gallic Acid

Source: green tea; red wine

Properties: antioxidant; enhances immunity

Conditions: infections; heart disease

## ❧ Glucosinolates

Source: cruciferous vegetables (broccoli, cauliflower, kale, Brussels sprouts)

Properties: detoxifies; helps balance hormones

Conditions: cancer prevention; general detoxification

## ❧ Hypericin

Source: St. John's Wort

Properties: antiviral; may improve mood

Conditions: depression; anxiety; viral infection

For more about the properties of hypericin, see ST. JOHN'S WORT, page 430.)

## ❧ Indoles

Source: cruciferous vegetables (broccoli, cauliflower, kale, Brussels sprouts)

Properties: detoxifies; helps balance hormones

Conditions: cancer prevention (especially, prevention of hormone-dependent cancers such as breast and prostate)

## ❧ Isoflavones

Source: soy; red clover

Properties: helps balance hormones; lowers cholesterol; antioxidants; cancer prevention

Conditions: menopause; PMS; cancer prevention; high cholesterol

## ❧ Isothiocyanates

Source: broccoli; cabbage; cauliflower; horseradish

Properties: detoxifies

Conditions: cancer prevention

## ❧ Lignans

Source: flaxseed; walnuts

Properties: immune enhancement; helps balance hormones

Conditions: cancer and cardiovascular disease prevention

For more about lignans, see FLAXSEED, page 181.

## ❧ Limonoids

Source: citrus fruits and peels

Properties: detoxifies

Conditions: cancer and cardiovascular disease prevention

*(continued)*

ᔕ *Lycopene*

*Source:* tomatoes; red grapefruit

*Properties:* antioxidant

*Conditions:* cancer prevention and treatment (particularly prostate)

See also Carotenoid, page 89.

ᔕ *Organosulfur compounds*

*Source:* garlic; onions; chives

*Properties:* antioxidant; immune enhancing; detoxifies

*Conditions:* cancer and cardiovascular disease prevention; immune enhancement; general detoxifies

ᔕ *Phenolic Acids*

*Source:* broccoli; berries; tomatoes; cabbage; whole grains

*Properties:* antioxidant

*Condition:* cancer prevention

ᔕ *Silymarin*

*Source:* milk thistle

*Properties:* antioxidant; liver cell regeneration

*Conditions:* hepatitis; elevated liver enzymes; fat malabsorption

See also Milk Thistle, page 330.

ᔕ *Sulforaphane*

*Source:* cruciferous vegetables such as (broccoli, cauliflower, kale, and Brussels sprouts)

*Properties:* detoxifies; helps balance hormones

*Conditions:* cancer prevention

# Potassium

Fred, a friend of mine, had just finished his daily jog when he arrived at my house. Actually, he had been experiencing cramps in his calves the last few times he went jogging, and wanted to talk to me about it.

"I don't understand why my legs are cramping," he said. "I've been drinking lots of water."

Considering that it was the middle of an unusually hot summer, and Fred usually jogged in the afternoon, I suspected he might have a potassium deficiency from all the sweating caused by the physical activity in the hot sun.

As a therapeutic experiment, I handed Fred a glass of water and three potassium tablets.

"Try these," I said.

"Sure, what are they?" Fred asked.

"Potassium," I replied. "I think you may be a little low because of this intense heat we are having."

After Fred took the tablets and drank the water, we sat down to talk.

About five minutes later, Fred said, "My cramps are gone! It usually takes hours for them to go away."

Our experiment had worked.

I told Fred to increase his intake of bananas and orange juice to prevent further cramping. I also recommended that he drink half a bottle of a sports drink (rich in potassium and other electrolytes) a half hour before jogging, and the other half immediately after. His cramps did not return for the rest of the summer.

## A VITAL SUBSTANCE

Potassium is critical to life as it is required for the proper functioning of cells, including heart muscle cells. It interacts with sodium and other charged particles (magnesium, calcium, and others) known as electrolytes. Sodium and potassium are both positively charged, and compete with each other to get inside cells, which are negatively charged. This "ionic dance" creates the electricity that sustains life. So, think of potassium as an important part of your "cell's battery."

Adequate levels of potassium are required to prevent high blood pressure, muscle cramps, and for normal heart function. Potassium is also required for muscle contraction; nerve conduction; glucose, protein, and carbohydrate metabolism; kidney and adrenal function; and water balance.

A high amount of potassium can be lost through excessive sweating, frequent urination (caused by diuretic medications), and vomiting or diarrhea. Diseases such as untreated diabetes can also lead to excessive potassium loss.

Magnesium deficiency also contributes to potassium loss. To get the best use out of potassium, you need to make sure you get adequate amounts of magnesium from whole grains and green leafy vegetables.

A deficiency of potassium can lead to muscle cramps and weakness, irregular heartbeat, fatigue, mental confusion, irritability, and impaired growth.

## BALANCING OUR DIETS

The Recommended Daily Allowance (RDA) for anyone over 10 years old is 2,000 milligrams daily. Potassium is found in many different foods, but particularly in fruits and vegetables. Good sources include carrots, avocados, tomatoes, apples, bananas, and oranges.

Dulse, a type of seaweed, is particularly high in potassium. Meat, fish, and milk are also good sources of potassium.

It is not only the total amount of potassium that is important, but also the balance with sodium. Many people are aware of the importance of reducing sodium (table salt) intake, but it is equally as important to increase potassium intake. Fruits and vegetables provide a high ratio of potassium to sodium.

According to nutritional researchers, most North Americans have a potassium-to-sodium ratio of less than 1:2. Experts recommend a potassium-to-sodium ratio of 5:1. Many fruits and vegetables have a potassium-to-sodium ratio of at least 50:1 and many times as high as 100:1. For example, bananas have a potassium to sodium ratio of 440:1, while oranges have a ratio of 260:1.

## DOSAGE

It is best to increase potassium intake through foods, thus consuming other helpful vitamins and minerals as well. Another common way to increase potassium and reduce sodium is to use salt substitutes (such as Nu-Salt®, No Salt®, or Morton® Salt Substitute), which are mainly composed of potassium chloride.

Most multivitamins contain potassium and help increase the daily intake. Potassium is also available as a supplement. Supplements are not allowed to contain more than 99 milligrams per dose. A dose of 500 to 3,000 milligrams is used by doctors for the therapeutic treatment of hypertension.

Remember, a diet rich in potassium and low in sodium will require a much lower dosage of potassium supplements. Consult a nutrition-oriented doctor to find the dosage of potassium that is correct for you.

## WHAT ARE THE SIDE EFFECTS?

Some people should never take potassium unless they are advised to do so by their doctor. If you have kidney disease, you should not take potassium supplements without specific instructions from your doctor. Also, potassium supplements should not be used without a doctor's recommendation by people who are taking digoxin, ibuprofen, or naproxin, or potassium-depleting diuretics (such as lasix and thiazide diuretics), and cisplatin (chemotherapy drug).

Too high a dosage of potassium supplements can cause nausea, vomiting, diarrhea, and ulcers.

## POTASSIUM
### RECOMMENDATIONS FROM THE NATURAL PHYSICIAN FOR . . .

### ❧ High Blood Pressure

Potassium is one of the most important minerals needed to prevent and treat high blood pressure. Studies have shown that taking potassium supplements significantly reduces systolic and diastolic blood pressure. Be aware that it is important to reduce sodium in the diet while increasing potassium. This is done by avoiding foods high in sodium, such as processed and packaged foods, canned foods, crackers, cheeses, and luncheon meats.

A number of people with high blood pressure have salt sensitivity. This means that even a small amount of sodium will drive up their blood pressure. (Other important vitamins and minerals to include for hypertension are calcium, magnesium, CoQ10, and vitamin C.)

### ❧ Muscle Cramps

As was shown earlier, muscle cramps and spasms, especially when caused by dehydration, are relieved by taking potassium. I recommend potassium if a patient has repeated muscle cramps that are not helped by increasing water intake, and taking calcium and magnesium.

### ❧ Stroke Prevention

Potassium helps to lower blood pressure, which is one of the leading risk factors for stroke. An 8-year study of 43,738 men, ages 40 to 75, found that those who consumed the highest amount of potassium (as well as calcium and cereal fiber) had a reduced risk of stroke.

# Prayer

Shawn Mitchell, head pastor of New Venture Christian Fellowship in Oceanside, California, as well as chaplain for the San Diego Chargers, experienced the tragedy of his younger brother Andre succumbing to an aggressive form of kidney cancer in 1998.

Pastor Mitchell realized that he, too, should be tested to make sure he did not have cancer. At the time of his brother's death, the pastor realized that he had been experiencing fatigue for some time—and he wanted to make sure everything was okay. In 1999 Pastor Mitchell went through a battery of tests and scans.

Pastor Mitchell learned that the scans had detected a growth—what appeared to be a tumor—on one of his kidneys. His doctor recommended exploratory surgery to ascertain the extent of the growth and to remove it as soon as possible.

The news was stunning. Married, and the father of a young boy, Pastor Mitchell was gripped with the realization that he had the potential diagnosis of cancer.

Later, Pastor Mitchell would recall the moment when he broke down in tears, only moments before he was supposed to give a sermon. Even so, he found he was able to mount the pulpit, and once in front of the congregation, he began to preach his prepared sermon.

To his amazement, someone in the congregation requested to pray for his healing. One long-time member stood up and said he had heard that the pastor might have a serious cancer, and requested the opportunity for the congregation to pray for his healing. The service came to a halt as the congregation invited the preacher to come down from his pulpit and join them. Pastor Mitchell was surprised by the suggestion, but appreciative of the congregation's care. As he walked into the middle of the congregation, many of the parishioners laid hands on him while praying for his recovery.

Pastor Mitchell had been scheduled for exploratory surgery within days—and the doctor did a follow-up scan to pinpoint the location of the tumor. Two days later, a call came from the doctor, reporting on the new scan. Since the Pastor was not at home, his wife took the call. Her dread and fear quickly changed to relief when she heard the doctor's first words.

"Something has happened—your husband has a textbook-perfect kidney. We can't explain it, but the repeat scan shows that the growth is not there now."

The doctor admitted that neither he nor any of the other doctors at the hospital could explain the results of the scan. But the evidence was there for all to see—where once there had been a tumor, it was gone. The tumor that was previously so apparent had completely disappeared.

Tests and scans were repeated. A number of other doctors joined the team that examined the results with intense thoroughness. All agreed: There were no signs of cancer in Pastor Mitchell's body. Pastor Mitchell was shown the first scans, where the growth on the kidney was large and obvious—then, the subsequent scans, which were normal. Since no medical treatment had been attempted between the two scans, none of the doctors could conjure any explanation for the "miraculous cure."

On his final visit to the doctor, Pastor Mitchell stated, "I know how this happened. The Lord answered our prayers."

## WHAT'S GOING ON?

As I write, Pastor Mitchell has been tested at regular intervals. There are no signs that the kidney growth has returned.

Not so very long ago, a story like this would have been greeted by most rational, scientific medical doctors with incredulity or, at the very least, cynical disbelief. Now, even the most research-oriented doctor is much more likely to admit that there's good research and some very compelling arguments for the power of prayer. Many conventional and complementary practitioners have also accepted that prayer is a powerful weapon in the battle against disease and a tool that can be utilized more effectively than "great bedside manner" for the optimization of health.

There is no doubt in my own mind that prayer is good medicine. In fact, I recommend that patients pray, and I pray for them. Like other doctors and practitioners, I've discovered that I do indeed get a higher rate of response to treatment and healing if I make a conscious decision to pray for all my patients.

## PRAYER WHEN YOU NEED IT

Perhaps the best thing about prayer is that you never need to wait for an appointment. Long before there were doctors—as we use that term today—people have used prayer for healing. Even today, whenever I see a new poll about religion in America, the results show that most Americans do use prayer in their daily lives.

Sometimes, we pray for others; often, it's for ourselves. Dr. Larry Dossey, author of *Healing Words: The Power of Prayer and the Practice of Medicine,* refers to these two types of prayers as petitionary and intercessory. Depending on the studies—and Dr. Dossey cites many of them—both types of prayer are effective.

But studying and measuring the health benefits of prayer is a challenging enterprise, as you can well imagine. How can you control the amount of belief that someone feels? Surely, if someone gives up control to a "higher being," that could be a great stress reliever, and we know that stress is an important factor in health.

What we do know, however, is that people need more than just physical healing. According to Dr. Dossey, who reviews the studies on prayer, "The evidence is simply overwhelming that prayer functions at a distance to change physical processes in a variety of organisms, from bacteria to humans. These data . . . are so impressive that I have come to regard them as among the best-kept secrets in medical science."

My recommendation is simple—a daily routine of prayer, offered in faith, to enhance health and wellness. Prayer can be used to prevent illness, maintain good health, and heal the most serious of diseases.

# Progesterone

"Please tell me you have something else other than horse urine to help my hot flashes!" said Leanne, a 49-year-old artist.

"Oh, you know all about Premarin®," I replied.

Leanne nodded. Her gynecologist had told her all about the synthetic forms of progesterone—with the trade names Premarin® and Provera®—and after asking a few questions, Leanne realized that Premarin® is made from substances taken from horse urine. She was also alarmed by some reports that synthetic hormones could raise the risk of breast cancer.

"I asked my doctor if she thought I looked like a horse," said Leanne. "Plus, breast cancer is the last thing I want."

"I have never prescribed Premarin® or Provera® and likely never will. Tell me more about what you have been experiencing."

"It really isn't all that bad. I have three to four hot flashes during the day and then sometimes at night. Other than that, I can't complain."

"Have you had a bone density test lately?" I asked.

"Yes, and the doctor said it looked good," replied Leanne.

I also asked Leanne about her family history to determine whether there was any record of breast, uterine, or other types of cancer in the family. She told me that both her grandmother and aunt had died of breast cancer.

"Any problems with depression, anxiety, low libido, insomnia, vaginal dryness?" I asked.

"Not really," replied Leanne.

"Have you tried herbal or other natural supplements for your menopausal symptoms?"

"I saw a herbalist who recommended a few different herbal menopausal formulas, but they didn't seem to stop the hot flashes," Leanne said.

By the end of the examination, I had concluded that natural progesterone would be good for Leanne to try. I explained to her that the term "natural" was the best possible description of what it actually was. "This is exactly the same progesterone that your body produces."

Leanne had heard of it. She said that some of her friends had used it with positive results. She was ready to give it a try.

Two weeks after Leanne started using a natural progesterone cream, she reported a decrease in the number of hot flashes. Before long, they were only occurring at rare intervals.

## HORMONAL WORKINGS

Progesterone is one of two main female hormones, the other being estrogen. (Actually, men have progesterone, too.) A cascade of biochemical events causes the production of progesterone by the corpus luteum in the ovary, by the placenta when a woman is pregnant, and by the adrenal glands during menopause. (In men, the production task goes to the adrenal glands and testes.) In the conversion process, cholesterol is turned into the hormone pregnenelone, which is then converted into progesterone.

The progesterone secreted by the adrenal glands also acts as a precursor for the formation of estrogen, testosterone, and corticosteroids.

Progesterone is secreted by the ovaries just prior to ovulation. It helps maintain normal function in the endometrium of the uterus. It also works to maintain a balance with estrogen to regulate the menstrual cycle and prevent side effects related to "estrogen dominance," a condition caused when estrogen levels are too high relative to the progesterone levels. Progesterone is an important precursor hormone for the synthesis of other hormones.

Progesterone has many important functions, including the following:

- It protects against fibrocystic breasts.
- It's a natural diuretic—that is, it helps the body rid itself of excess water.
- It helps turn fat (lipids) into energy.
- It acts as a natural antidepressant.
- It helps thyroid hormone action.
- It normalizes blood clotting.
- It can help restore the sex drive.

- It helps normalize blood-sugar levels.
- It normalizes zinc and copper levels.
- It restores proper cell oxygen levels.
- It has a thermogenic (temperature-raising) effect.

In addition, it has a number of protective effects, helping to guard against endometrial cancer and breast cancer. It may slow the advance of osteoporosis, and it also has antiinflammatory effects.

## THE QUEEN BEE OF HORMONES

All things considered, progesterone is an extremely important hormone, and not the least of its functions is its role in balancing estrogen. Imagine a scale, with estrogen on one side and progesterone on the other. The body produces these two hormones to maintain balance and for proper biochemical and hormonal activities.

Many women in our society have a progesterone deficiency, which tilts the balance with their estrogen levels. One reason that researchers have discovered is that many women have a problem with xenoestrogens. These are estrogenlike compounds found in such things as pesticides, herbicides, fungicides, cosmetics, and many materials derived from petroleum products such as plastics. Once in the body, xenoestrogens attach to estrogen receptors and mimic the action of estrogen.

Another reason for relatively low levels of progesterone in women is that many women do not ovulate regularly. Since most progesterone is released when ovulation occurs, there's a shortage of this hormone when ovulation is infrequent. This is a major problem related to conditions such as polycystic ovary syndrome (PCOS) and irregular menstrual cycles.

For women reaching the age of menopause, an imbalance of progesterone and estrogen levels is predictable. Progesterone levels drop more dramatically than estrogen levels during menopause.

## NATURAL VERSUS SYNTHETIC

More doctors are beginning to realize that there is a difference between synthetic and natural progesterone. Simply put, the term natural progesterone refers to progesterone that is identical to what you find in the human body (termed as bioidentical). Synthetic progesterone, which has been labeled progestin, refers to progesterone that is synthetically created and is not identical to the progesterone in the human body.

Progestins are the synthetic hormones found in most pharmaceutical products for menopause and for PMS. They're also in birth-control pills. They are known to cause many different side effects.

Most holistic doctors prefer to use natural progesterone as it appears to be much safer than the synthetic version. Potential side effects of Provera®, for instance, include water retention, weight gain, and irritability. Some women also experience spotting or breakthrough bleeding between menstrual cycles. Others have breast tenderness, blood clots, headaches, nausea, and high blood pressure.

## DOSAGE

Natural progesterone is available commercially as a transdermal cream that is applied to the skin in areas with high capillary density for absorption. The areas of the skin where it's best applied include the forearms (palm side), breasts, cheeks, and bottom of feet (as long as there are no calluses). It is a good idea to rotate sites with each application.

The advantage of this is that this direct absorption bypasses the liver. Conventional progesterone pills require more metabolism by the liver, which increases the risk of liver toxicity and degrades the progesterone into metabolites so the concentration is not so high. The disadvantage is that the absorption and utilization varies depending on the woman and it is not known whether it prevents the buildup of the endometrium in women taking estrogen therapy.

Through trial and error, and with the help of a doctor knowledgeable in natural hormone replacement, you can find the dose right for you and your condition. Saliva hormone testing is recommended to evaluate and monitor your hormone levels.

In considering natural progesterone products, you may become aware of the "wild yam cream" sold by a number of companies and promoted as having natural progesterone in them. In fact, however, many of these wild yam creams contain no progesterone at all. Your body cannot convert the diosgenin in wild yam cream into progesterone; it needs to be done in a lab. Thus, the term "wild yam scam" has been used to describe these types of products.

The dosage and scheduling of natural progesterone varies depending on what condition is being treated. When you buy natural progesterone cream commercially, make sure to purchase a product that contains actual progesterone. Look for natural progesterone creams that contain 960 milligrams per two ounces. Thus, one-quarter teaspoon of natural progesterone cream is equivalent to 20 milligrams of progesterone.

This typically works out to one-quarter teaspoon applied to the skin twice daily, or one-half teaspoon applied daily. See the recommendations for specific dosing schedules.

Another source of natural progesterone is oral microionized progesterone (OMP), which comes in capsule form. It has been shown to prevent endometrial hyperplasia when taken in conjunction with estrogen. OMP is available only with a doctor's prescription. The dosage varies depending on what condition is being treated, and needs to be adjusted depending on the woman.

There are other delivery mechanisms for progesterone as well. For example, sublingual progesterone comes in tablet and drop form, taken orally. You hold the tablet under your tongue until it dissolves.

Find a physician experienced in natural hormone replacement if you want to use natural progesterone. Every woman is different and requires a different dosage; there is no "typical dosage."

## WHAT ARE THE SIDE EFFECTS?

Even though natural progesterone is "natural," it is still a hormone and must be used correctly to avoid side effects. Herbal, nutritional, and homeopathic therapies should be used as a first line of treatment for hormone balance as they are inherently safer. However, natural progesterone is needed in certain cases.

Overall, natural progesterone appears to be very safe when used properly. However, I have seen women experience symptoms such as increased breast tenderness and irritability when the dosage is too high.

Women who use natural progesterone to relieve menopausal symptoms can experience a period of spotting over the course of one to three months; this usually stops when the body adjusts to the progesterone. If the bleeding does not stop after three months, consult your doctor.

I recommend that women who are taking hormones (natural or synthetic) should also take supplemental phytonutrients such as calcium-d-glucarate and indole 3 carbinol to help the liver break down the metabolites of these hormones effectively.

# PROGESTERONE
## Recommendations from the Natural Physician for . . .

### Autoimmune Conditions

A number of my female patients with autoimmune conditions, such as rheumatoid arthritis and lupus, showed improvement after being on a hormone-balancing program.

I have found natural progesterone quite effective for women who want to continue using Premarin®. It has a balancing effect, reduces inflammation, and improves circulation for these women. Research has shown that synthetic estrogen replacement can worsen lupus.

### Endometriosis

Natural progesterone has helped quite a few women manage this sometimes difficult-to-treat condition by acting as an estrogen balancer. (Estrogen stimulates endometrial tissue growth.) Apply one-quarter teaspoon of the cream twice daily for three weeks and then discontinue during menses (one week). Some women require a different medication schedule prescribed by a knowledgeable doctor. It can take up to six months of use to notice improvements.

### Fibrocystic breasts

Natural progesterone helps most women with this condition. The dosage is one-quarter teaspoon to one-half teaspoon applied twice daily from ovulation to the day before menses. It should be applied to the breast for direct benefits.

It works even better if you take a daily dosage of 800 IU of natural vitamin E and essential fatty acids such as flaxseed or fish oil and evening primrose oil.

### Menopause

Many doctors tell their female patients who are going through perimenopause and menopause that their hot flashes and other symptoms are caused by a decrease in estrogen. Although estrogen does decline, progesterone drops much more dramatically (to almost zero), and is more likely responsible for a lot of the symptoms. Many women find that natural progesterone works extremely well to manage their perimenopausal and menopausal symptoms. It helps with hot flashes, mood swings, and low libido to name a few.

Menopausal women should apply one-quarter teaspoon of natural progesterone twice daily for two to three weeks a month. Perimenopausal women who are still having a menses should discontinue using it during the five to seven days when they're having their period.

Postmenopausal women should apply one-quarter teaspoon one to two times daily for three weeks a month.

Women who are taking a hormone replacement (e.g., Premarin®) and wish to use natural progesterone can do so by applying one-quarter teaspoon twice daily on the days they take Premarin®. The dosage of Premarin® often needs to be reduced by half or more when it is used with natural progesterone. Consult with your doctor about dosage issues.

### Migraine Headaches

I have had women use natural progesterone to prevent migraine headaches that are tied to their menstrual cycles. I have them apply a quarter teaspoon twice daily three to four days before their menses, or three to four days before the time they usually get the migraine headaches.

### Osteoporosis

Natural progesterone may be helpful in the prevention and treatment of osteoporosis. One

*(continued)*

researcher has found that natural progesterone increases bone density in women.

The dosage for postmenopausal women is one-quarter teaspoon of natural progesterone cream applied twice daily for three weeks of the month. For those women who are peri-menopausal, the dosage is the same except that it is taken for two weeks before the menses (days 15 to 26).

### ❧ Ovarian Cysts

Natural progesterone can be effective for shrinking ovarian cysts. Have a knowledgeable doctor prescribe the correct dose specifically for you.

### ❧ Pregnancy Complications

Natural progesterone vaginal suppositories are often used by obstetricians and fertility specialists for pregnant women who have a history of miscarriage. It is used during the first trimester.

### ❧ Premenstrual Syndrome (PMS)

For women who do not respond to nutritional, herbal, and homeopathic treatments for PMS, I recommend applying one-quarter teaspoon of natural progesterone twice daily beginning in the middle of the cycle (day 15). I usually advise continuing the applications twice daily until one day before the start of their period, then stop.

However, if the PMS symptoms begin near ovulation (near day 14), apply one-quarter teaspoon daily from days 8 to 14 and then a quarter teaspoon twice daily until one day before the menses starts. Stop using it when your period begins.

It can also be helpful for acne associated with menses.

### ❧ Uterine Fibroids

More than 50 percent of all women have uterine fibroids. The goal of natural treatment of uterine fibroids is to slow down, halt, or shrink their growth until menopause (when estrogen levels decrease). Natural progesterone can be quite helpful in managing this condition. Apply one-quarter teaspoon to one-half teaspoon twice daily for three weeks of the month. Discontinue during menses.

### ❧ Vaginitis

Women who are prone to vaginal yeast infections may have an estrogen/progesterone imbalance. Some cases respond well to natural progesterone. Apply one-quarter to one-half teaspoon of progesterone cream twice daily for one week before your period begins.

# Propolis

Another miracle of nature, propolis is a very popular health product in Europe and is becoming better known in North America. Bees gather propolis from the buds and barks of certain trees and carry it to the hive, where they are met by other worker bees that help them unload this precious material. The worker bees add salivary secretions and wax flakes, then spread the finished product on the beehive walls, from the entrance all the way to the individual chambers. Hence, propolis is also referred to as "bee glue."

The propolis within the beehive actually does more than glue the walls together. Researchers have found that propolis actually prevents disease in the colony by inhibiting the growth of microbes such as bacteria, viruses, and fungi. As bees enter and exit the hive, they brush against the propolis, which acts like an instant decontaminant. Everything inside and outside the hive, including the interior cells where the queen lays her eggs, is covered with a thin coating of propolis.

Propolis is also used as an embalming agent for bugs or insects that have invaded the hive. The Greek translation of propolis is fitting as it means "for or in defense of the city."

Propolis is one of the most powerful topical antimicrobial agents humans can use.

## THE PROPERTIES OF PROPOLIS

Although I was aware of propolis, I never understood all of its medicinal effects until I heard them described by Jan Slama, a Canadian herbal scientist and researcher. Citing all the European research that had been done with this product, he spoke passionately and enthusiastically about the almost-miraculous antiseptic properties of this bee-manufactured substance.

Knowing that Jan Slama is a reliable source, I immediately decided that it was time to start paying more attention to propolis and its potential benefits for my patients. I reviewed the medical literature to confirm Jan's findings and quickly discovered that hundreds of investigations had been conducted to probe the medicinal properties of propolis.

Hippocrates, the Greek widely regarded as the first "modern" physician, was one of the first to recommend propolis. He said it would heal ulcers of the skin and digestive tract. In *The History of Plants,* written by John Gerard in 1597, propolis was praised for its ability to provide quick and effective healing for several of the conditions mentioned by Hippocrates, as well as other conditions. Ancient Egyptians also used propolis for a variety of different ailments. Propolis has a history of use for cancer in Japan.

Until recently, most clinical information on propolis has come from Europe, though a few studies are now being conducted in the United States, sparked by rising interest in this natural product. Most of the research has focused on immune-stimulating and topical, antimicrobial qualities. However, researchers are also exploring the antioxidant properties of bee propolis, as well as considering its possible uses as a cancer treatment, antiinflammatory, and dental product. It may also prove useful for surgical recovery and—in a throwback to Hippocrates's original recommendations—as a palliative for ulcers of the skin and digestive tract.

## ACTIVE INGREDIENTS

There are over 150 active components in propolis. Researchers now think that the substances called flavonoids—responsible for its bright yellow color—are responsible for most of its therapeutic activity. These are the same healing flavonoids that are found in such plants as ginkgo, grapes, as well as many other herbs and foods that have human health benefits.

But scientists have been interested to note that the flavonoids found in propolis are totally unlike those found in plants. Their unique biochemical make-up might account for the powerful therapeutic activity of propolis.

In addition, bee propolis contains a class of chemicals known as phenols that seem to be responsible for many of its antimicrobial effects. The bee product also has B vitamins and amino acids, more essential components of human health. Finally, it contains an essential oil that likely contributes to its medicinal effects.

## DOSAGE

Propolis is available commercially in the following forms.

### ∾ *Capsules*

I recommend capsules to enhance immunity. The typical adult dosage is 500 to 1,000 milligrams daily.

### ∾ *Tincture*

This form can be taken internally to enhance immunity, especially if you have a sore throat or upper respiratory tract infection. The dose is 1 to 3 milliliters taken three times daily. It can also be diluted in water—10 parts water to 1 part propolis—and applied topically.

### ✍ *Throat Spray*

A few companies offer propolis in a spray form. This is ideal for throat and mouth infections.

### ✍ *Cream*

This form is ideal for preventing skin infections if you have a cut, scrape, or other type of small wound.

## WHAT ARE THE SIDE EFFECTS?

Propolis is not known to have any toxicity to humans, but some people may have an allergic reaction. The most frequent reaction is dermatitis when propolis is applied topically. If you notice skin inflammation, sometimes accompanied by bumps and itchiness, it might be caused by the propolis. (Paradoxically, bee propolis is also used in Europe for the treatment of contact dermatitis.)

If you take an oral dose, you need to be cautious about the possibility of a severe allergic reaction, although only a few cases have been reported. To see if you are sensitive, apply a small amount on your skin or tongue. If no sensitivity or allergy is observed in 4 hours, you can take a regular dose.

It is recommended that individuals sensitive to balsam of Peru or poplar bud exudates (major source of propolis for bees in Europe) avoid the use of bee propolis.

---

## PROPOLIS
### RECOMMENDATIONS FROM THE NATURAL PHYSICIAN FOR . . .

#### ✍ *Dental Conditions*
Propolis has demonstrated benefit for common dental conditions such as gingivitis, mouth ulcers, and periodontal disease. This has led to its inclusion in a number of European dental-care products such as toothpastes and mouthwashes. Russian and Bulgarian researchers have found that the alcohol extract (tincture) of propolis has weak local anesthetic activity, so it helps to numb the gums for pain relief.

#### ✍ *Digestive Conditions*
Propolis is commonly used in Europe for the treatment of peptic ulcers and ulcerative colitis. Because the flavonoids have antiinflammatory properties, they are thought to have a healing effect on internal digestive organs, including the stomach and intestines.

*(continued)*

### ❧ Herpes

Genital herpes is a prevalent, sexually-transmitted disease that is carried by over 45 million Americans. Antiviral drugs such as acyclovir are prescribed by conventional doctors to suppress the outbreak of herpes lesions.

I find natural therapies to be very effective for this condition, and they have the advantage of carrying few or no side effects. In one study involving 90 men and women, investigators compared an ointment made of Canadian propolis to the pharmaceutical acyclovir. (Both were compared with a group that got no treatment at all.) The participants were examined on the third, seventh, and tenth days of treatment by doctors at seven different medical centers.

When doctors accumulated their results, they found that improvement in the propolis group far outpaced the acyclovir group. (Those who got no treatment at all lagged even farther behind.) The authors concluded that propolis ointment appeared to be more effective than both acyclovir and placebo ointments in healing genital herpetic lesions, and in reducing local symptoms.

This study is important because it provides scientific proof of propolis in the treatment of genital herpes. People with this condition can dramatically benefit from propolis if they suffer an outbreak. It would be interesting to have a similar study where people with genital herpes not only used propolis to heal acute outbreaks, but also took propolis internally for long-term immune system support to prevent outbreaks.

### ❧ Infections

One of the unique characteristics of propolis is its broad-spectrum antimicrobial effects. By this I mean the ways it can defend the body against bacteria, viruses, parasites, and fungus.

Propolis has been called "Russian penicillin," giving a nod of credit to research Russian scientists have done on this substance. Though many of the antibacterial properties have only been demonstrated in test-tube studies, it's interesting that propolis has been shown to improve the effects of certain antibiotics. In some cases, antibiotics were 10 to 100 times more effective in destroying bacteria when propolis was added to the mix. Also, test-tube studies have shown that antibiotics such as erythromycin and tetracycline became more effective against disease-resistant bacteria if their power was enhanced with propolis. In fact, these antibiotics were unable to fight the disease-resistant bacteria strains until the medicines were combined with propolis. It's now been shown that propolis helps prevent bacteria cells from dividing and forming more of those disease-causing cells.

A similar effect has also been demonstrated with propolis and antifungal medications. The propolis actually boosts the power of the medications. Propolis has also been shown in animal studies to activate antibody formation and increase the activity of macrophages, immune cells that help protect our bodies by gobbling up invading microbes.

### ❧ Wound Healing

Propolis has incredible healing effects when it's applied to topical wounds. Russian and European doctors use it routinely for the healing of surgical wounds. Compared with conventional therapies, topical use of propolis provides up to an 80 percent faster healing rate for burns, ulcers, and surgical wounds.

The bee product actually has two distinct properties important to wound healing. First, propolis accelerates tissue healing. Second, it prevents wound infection. In a remarkably revealing study of 42 hospitalized people who were suffering from burns, doctors found that topical application of napkins saturated with propolis were enormously helpful to the patients. In fact, the average length of hospital treatment was 11 days less among those who got the propolis applications, as compared with those who didn't.

# Pulsatilla

Hundreds of my patients and family members have benefited from this remedy.

Pulsatilla is the homeopathic preparation from the pulsatilla plant, also known as the windflower. The leaves on pulsatilla are very soft, almost velvety. According to homeopathic physicians, that's a good description of the personality types who can benefit from this healing remedy—that is, people who have very gentle spirits and personalities, who are very sensitive to the feelings of others, and go the extra mile to avoid hurting anyone else's feelings. Their own feelings are hurt easily.

Being well-liked is extremely important to a pulsatilla type. Like the windflower, they can be easily swayed by more domineering types. Depending on what an influential person around them thinks or what the majority of a group feels, their decisions and opinions can be easily altered. This is analogous to the lightweighted flowers of pulsatilla that move in different directions depending on which way the wind is blowing.

Jolene is a good example of the constitutional type requiring pulsatilla. During our visit, she broke down in tears several times because her relationship with her boyfriend was not going smoothly. He would get mad at her when she wanted to go out with her friends and so she would cancel plans with her friends who she missed being with. At the same time, her friends would get upset with her for never going out with them and would criticize her boyfriend for being so controlling. Jolene felt like she was in a no-win situation. In conventional medicine, of course, the influence of personality and relationships are rarely taken into account when making a diagnosis. But as Jolene talked about her feelings, she also mentioned that her PMS was becoming increasingly worse over the past year. She would get very weepy and moody, she craved chocolate, and she suffered from intense menstrual cramps.

## BALANCING ACT

Pulsatilla is one of the top hormone-balancing remedies, and given Jolene's personality, I decided that the remedy would probably be right for her. Over the next two months, Jolene took the pulsatilla as I recommended. She found that her PMS symptoms dramatically improved. Even after her menstrual cycle was over, she felt that her general mood had stabilized. (Interestingly enough, she also started to become more assertive with her boyfriend and months later I found out that she had broken off their relationship and was feeling in much more control of her life.)

Pulsatilla is also one of the important grief remedies. Death of a loved one, broken relationships, and other traumatic events that lead to grief are inevitable in life. Pulsatilla helps those who have longstanding issues with grief move in the direction of emotional healing.

Pulsatilla is one of those homeopathic remedies that parents or caretakers of children should have in their "home remedy kit." It's easy to spot the children who can be helped with this remedy. Loving and cuddly, they always want to be held. Often, they are shy around strangers and take a lot of time to adapt to new kids or situations. In a group of children, the "pulsatilla type" tends to be timid—they're followers rather than leaders.

Even body temperature is distinctive among the adults and children who fit the pulsatilla picture. A pulsatilla type tends to be on the warm side. If you find that you get warm easily—compared to other people—and you feel uncomfortable in a warm room, you may be a pulsatilla type. Also, you probably prefer to have a window open and feel better when you can breathe in fresh air. (Another sign: You throw off the covers at night, or like to sleep with your feet exposed to the night air.)

Pulsatilla is also one of the most important acute remedies. It can be very effective in cases of respiratory ailments such as asthma, ear infections, bronchitis, sinus infections, and conjunctivitis.

## DOSAGE

For acute treatment I recommend the 30C potency two to four times a day or as needed for relief of symptoms. For chronic use, take a 6C or 30C potency one to two times daily for a couple of weeks. If you see improvement, then just use the remedy whenever needed.

## WHAT ARE THE SIDE EFFECTS?

Side effects are rare, though I have seen cases where the symptoms get worse when a patient takes the remedy too frequently. If that happens, just take the remedy less often until symptoms start to improve again.

# PULSATILLA
## RECOMMENDATIONS FROM THE NATURAL PHYSICIAN FOR . . .

### ❧ Anxiety

I find many women who have problems with anxiety benefit from this remedy. I believe there are two reasons why this is so. First, the constitutional types that resonate with this remedy are usually very concerned about other people's feelings toward them, and much of their anxiety is actually fear of the unknown. Do others *really* like and accept them?

Second, I have found that hormone imbalance, specifically estrogen and progesterone balance, can lead to increased feelings of anxiety. So pulsatilla simultaneously helps the anxiety that's associated with imbalances in hormone levels.

### ❧ Arthritis

Pulsatilla is a more common remedy for women than for men, and it seems to be especially effective with women who have arthritis. One of the reasons that pulsatilla helps certain cases of arthritis is that it is a hormone balancer. Recent research has shown that hormone imbalance and the use of synthetic hormones is associated with various types of arthritis in women.

I would prescribe pulsatilla if a woman has arthritic pains that move around to different parts of the body—what doctors call "wandering" or "migratory pains." Also, I prescribe it if the patient tells me her arthritis feels better with warm applications such as a hot shower, heating pad, or a hot tub.

### ❧ Asthma

Asthma can be associated with a great many factors—stress, pollution, and nutritional deficiencies, to name a few. I have helped many patients cut down or get off their asthma inhalers or reduce the use of steroid medications by prescribing the homeopathic remedy pulsatilla. It is especially rewarding when this remedy helps young children who have asthma, because it gives them a chance to lead a more normal lifestyle.

Before you give pulsatilla to a child who has asthma, however, I recommend discussing the symptoms with a homeopathic doctor. No asthma medications should be stopped without the guidance of the doctor who prescribed them.

### ❧ Bladder Infection

I have found pulsatilla to be effective in curing chronic cases of bladder infections in women. It has a tonic effect on the urinary tract. Also, hormone imbalance can make a woman susceptible to bladder infections, and pulsatilla can correct this problem.

### ❧ Bronchitis

You may have experienced a case of bronchitis where you felt feverish, coughing up yellow or green mucus, and had trouble falling asleep due to the cough. Pulsatilla helps to eradicate the infection and ease the cough.

*(continued)*

When parents call in the evening and tell me their child has a bad cough that is preventing the child from sleeping, I always consider pulsatilla the remedy of first choice if a child fits the pulsatilla type. After a dose or two, the child goes to sleep and wakes up with a less severe cough.

### Conjunctivitis

Many years back my sister called me when her family was on holidays. One of my nephews woke up with one eye "stuck closed" from a yellowish discharge. My sister wanted to know which remedy I'd recommend for his eye infection.

Pulsatilla did the job, clearing up the infection within 24 hours.

Nor was this an isolated incident. Recently, my wife, son, and I were taking a vacation together. The evening before our return, my son's eye was infected with yellow-green mucus that caused his eyelashes to stick closed. We knew we would be traveling for at least eight hours the next day, and it would be a miserable trip if my son was dealing with the discomfort of an eye infection the whole way. So I gave him a dose of pulsatilla before he went to bed that night. He awoke the next morning with a 90 percent improvement. After another dose that morning, the infection was completely cleared.

### Depression

I have had seen many cases where pulsatilla helped both men and women recover from longstanding cases of depression. The "pulsatilla type" is someone who gets some relief of depression when comforted. The person tends to consume sweets, especially chocolate, during periods of emotional despair. Pulsatilla helps to correct the underlying biochemical causes of depression.

### Endometriosis

Since it is such a great hormone balancer, pulsatilla is one of the major remedies to consider for women who have endometriosis. The remedy can work at a deep level and in some cases totally alleviate this serious condition.

### Headache

Cynthia, a quiet and shy 35 year old, came to me for natural treatment of chronic migraine headaches. After taking her history, it became obvious to me that her headaches were hormone related. The migraine headaches occurred during the first three days of her menstrual period.

Cynthia's doctor had recommended that she take birth-control pills to prevent or cure the migraines—but before she went that route, Cynthia came to me for a holistic approach. Her symptom picture, and her personality, suggested that pulsatilla would be effective.

He headaches were less intense after the first month of treatment with pulsatilla. She was free of the headaches by her second menstrual period. A few more months on the remedy, and her chronic headaches were history.

### Menopause

Along with the remedies lachesis and sepia, pulsatilla is one of the three most prescribed reme-

(continued)

dies for menopause. Characteristic symptoms include hot flashes, general increase in body temperature (even the women who generally "felt chilly" before menopause may stick out their feet or throw off the covers at night). When the pulsatilla type is in menopause, she may also have a strong craving for sweets and chocolate, and probably feels an increase in mood swings, particularly feelings of weepiness and sadness.

### ✣ Menstrual Cramps

Pulsatilla is a top homeopathic remedy to cure the excruciating menstrual cramps from which so many women suffer. Also known as dysmenorrhea, menstrual cramps occur in about 25 percent of the patients I see. But treatment is highly effective with many of these patients.

It all goes back to hormone imbalance. If the hormones are balanced, the cramps won't occur in the first place. Pulsatilla helps to alleviate acute menstrual cramps and cures the chronic susceptibility as well.

### ✣ Orchitis

Orchitis refers to inflammation of the testicles. This condition is typically a complication that occurs among young men after they've had the mumps, because the virus gets carried to the testicles. Pulsatilla is one of the most important remedies for clearing up this condition.

### ✣ Psoriasis

In cases where someone is a pulsatilla type, the remedy can greatly improve this aggravating skin disease. I have had a number of cases respond to pulsatilla.

### ✣ Sinusitis

You can take pulsatilla if you have a case of sinus infection or inflammation where yellow-green mucus forms.

### ✣ Varicose Veins

Pulsatilla can help your circulation and also help improve varicose veins. The remedy is particularly recommended if you have varicose veins that have a deep blue color or the kind that form during pregnancy.

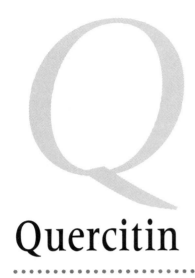

# Quercitin

"My asthma is acting up again, I think it's this darn pollen."

As soon as Holly told me that, I asked what she had been taking. She named a number of pharmaceutical items as well as supplements. But quercitin was not among them.

I urged her to pick up some quercitin from her local health food store. I knew that the quercitin would act as a natural antihistamine to alleviate the allergies, which were causing her asthma to flare up.

Two days later, I had another call from Holly.

"I'm taking the quercitin, but it doesn't seem to make a difference," she said.

"Let's double the dose to 3,000 milligrams a day," I said.

Sure enough, a day later, she called and reported that her symptoms started to subside. She now finds that 1,500 milligrams daily keeps her asthma symptoms at bay.

## QUERCITIN QUESTIONS

Quercitin is one of the many types of flavonoids. Flavonoids are plant pigments that give fruits and flowers much of their color. They also have potent medicinal effects on the body. There are thousands of different flavonoids, each having a slightly different molecular makeup. (Many people are familiar with the citrus bioflavonoids, often found in vitamin C supplements.) Quercitin is found in many different plants and is the most common of all the flavonoids. Studies also show it to be the most active of all the flavonoids.

Common food items that contain quercitin include apples, onions, tea, berries, and brassica vegetables (such as kale, turnips, Chinese cabbage), as well as many seeds and nuts. It is also found in herbs such as ginkgo biloba and St. John's Wort.

Quercitin is the major flavonoid in the human diet. The estimated average daily dietary intake of quercitin by an individual in the United States is 25 milligrams.

Quercitin has several different functions in the body. It acts as an antioxidant. This prevents oxidative damage of LDL cholesterol (a process that initiates atherosclerosis), skin, and nerve tissue. It acts as an antiinflammatory. It has an inhibiting effect on enzymes related to inflammation (e.g., lipoxygenase and cyclooxygenase) and other inflammatory chemicals such as prostaglandins. It also prevents the release of histamine, thus having an antiinflammatory and antiallergy effect. Quercitin also enhances the action of vitamin C.

Quercitin is also proving to be valuable for cardiovascular protection, cancer prevention, ulcers, allergies, cataracts, and antiviral activity.

## DOSAGE

For acute inflammation I generally recommend a dosage of 500 to 1,000 milligrams taken three times daily. There is some information showing that quercitin is not well absorbed, so it is important to use this dosage to achieve therapeutic results. For general prevention one can take 500 milligrams daily.

## WHAT ARE THE SIDE EFFECTS?

Quercitin is very safe. The only reactions I have seen are in people who are sensitive to citrus, and use quercitin in a formula containing vitamin C or citrus bioflavonoids. Some have reported mouth sores, headaches, and digestive upset.

## QUERCITIN
### RECOMMENDATIONS FROM THE NATURAL PHYSICIAN FOR . . .

 **Allergies**

Quercitin is often recommended in high dosages for the relief of environmental allergies, particularly allergies to pollen. By inhibiting the

release of the inflammatory chemical histamine, quercitin acts like a pharmaceutical antihistamine to prevent allergic symptoms. Some prac-

*(continued)*

titioners recommend it for people with food sensitivities as well.

Quercitin is helpful for conditions such as sinusitis, arthritis, and inflammatory bowel disease.

### ∿ Cancer Prevention and Treatment

Quercitin has been shown to have anticancer effects in test-tube and animal studies. Human studies are underway with quercitin to see how effective it is for human cancers. Most of the studies used very high dosages, and often given intravenously. Quercitin has been shown to increase the effectiveness of the chemotherapy drug cisplatin, as well as protect the kidney cells from the toxicity of this drug.

### ∿ Cardiovascular Protection

Quercitin is one of the many valuable antioxidants that helps to protect the heart and cardiovascular system.

It protects LDL cholesterol from being oxidized. This is important to prevent free-radical damage to the blood vessel walls and protect against plaque buildup. It also protects vitamin E that is incorporated into LDL to act as an antioxidant.

Quercitin prevents the aggregation of platelets so that circulation is improved and reduces the chances of blood-clot formation.

One study looked at the relationship of dietary flavonoid intake and risk of coronary heart disease in men between the ages of 65 and 85. Researchers found that the risk of heart disease mortality decreased significantly as flavonoid intake increased. It should be noted that the flavonoid-containing foods most commonly eaten in this study contained a high amount of quercetin—tea, onions, and apples.

### ∿ Diabetes

Aldose reductase is an enzyme that plays a part in the formation of diabetic cataracts, neuropathy, and retinopathy. This enzyme converts glucose to sorbitol, which in the case of a diabetic cataract builds up in the lens of the eye. Quercetin has been shown to be a strong inhibitor of human lens aldose reductase.

### ∿ Digestive Disorders

Since quercitin has antiinflammatory effects, it is often incorporated into the treatment protocol of patients with inflammatory bowel disease such as Crohn's disease and ulcerative colitis. It is also thought to be helpful in repairing leaky gut syndrome, a situation where malabsorption takes place in the small intestine.

Quercitin is also used in the treatment of ulcers. It has been shown to inhibit the growth of *Heliobacter pylori*, a bacterium implicated in many cases of ulcers.

# R

# Rhus Toxicodendron

· · · · · · · · · · · · · · · · · · · · · · · · · · · · · · · · · · · · · · · · · · · · · · · · · · · · · · · · · · · · ·

Todd, a 60-year-old retired farmer, came to see me for his arthritis. He was very much into natural therapies. He pulled out a bag of supplements that he had tried for his osteoarthritis. They included glucosamine sulfate and about 12 other supplements as well.

"I hope you have something else that can help me," he said. "I'm taking all these supplements and even so, it's getting hard to walk."

He also complained of the expense of the supplements, which were costing him about $150 every month.

After asking Todd about all the symptoms he experienced, I recommended rhus toxicodendron (commonly called rhus tox).

He asked me two questions: "Is this going to work?" and, "How much is the medicine going to cost me?"

"It should help reduce the joint pain and stiffness," I replied, "even in the first couple of weeks. As far as cost goes, you can buy a month's supply at the health food store for about seven dollars."

"Seven dollars, that's all it costs?" he questioned.

"That's it," I replied.

I suggested that Todd stop taking all the other supplements, as he had not noticed any improvement in his condition. I advised him to take only the rhus tox.

When he came to my office for a follow-up visit six weeks later, Todd reported a 70 percent improvement in his arthritic symptoms.

## PALLIATIVE FROM A POISON

Rhus tox is the homeopathic dilution of poison oak. We know this as a plant that causes a nasty, blistering rash. However, this homeopathic is one of the best skin remedies for relieving symptoms in people who have touched poison ivy. It is also effective in treating eczema, where the skin is very itchy and feels better after the application of very hot water.

I have also used this for people with shingles. The itching, burning pain of the shingles blisters can be relieved in a few days with rhus tox.

## DOSAGE

The typical dosage for rhus tox is 30C potency taken two to three times daily for a day or two for conditions such as stiffness from overexertion. For long-term use for eczema or arthritis, I generally start with a lower dose such as 6C taken two to three times daily.

## WHAT ARE THE SIDE EFFECTS?

While rhus tox has few side effects, some people may experience skin irritation. People with chronic eczema or arthritis may experience a flare-up of their condition at the beginning of treatment. This is usually a sign that the remedy is working (known as a healing aggravation).

If you do have a flare-up and you begin taking the rhus tox less frequently, you'll probably notice that the flare-up subsides. Soon after, you'll probably notice an improvement in your condition.

If you are not sure whether you should use rhus tox, consult a homeopathic practitioner.

# RHUS TOXICODENDRON
## RECOMMENDATIONS FROM THE NATURAL PHYSICIAN FOR . . .

### ❧ Arthritis

Rhus tox is commonly used for osteoarthritis and rheumatoid arthritis. This is probably the right remedy for you if you notice certain characteristics about your symptoms: they are worse in the morning, improve with motion and activity during the day, and then get worse again at night while in bed.

Rhus tox is also a good remedy if these arthritic symptoms flare up before a storm or in damp weather. It's probably the right remedy for you if hot baths and showers also provide joint pain relief.

### ❧ Flu

Rhus tox is a good remedy for the type of flu that makes your joints and muscles stiff.

### ❧ Herpes

Cold sores on the mouth or face, or genital herpes outbreaks can be helped greatly with rhus tox.

### ❧ Shingles

This dormant chicken-pox virus erupts when the immune system is weakened. Many elderly people suffer from excruciating pain that is often not relieved with conventional medicines. Rhus tox has worked wonders in several cases I have treated.

### ❧ Strains

Rhus tox should be used when ligaments and tendons are strained. It helps speed up the recovery process. Athletes should have a supply of rhus tox available at all times.

### ❧ Urticaria

Urticaria is a fancy way of saying hives. For hive breakouts that do not require emergency treatment (such as when the throat closes), rhus tox helps to relieve the itching and works to heal the lesions more quickly. It is also effective for relieving itching caused by mosquito bites.

# SAMe

It was Sandy's first visit. A 40-year-old legal assistant, she had been suffering from on-and-off depression for more than ten years.

"I've tried everything," she told me. Her list included St. John's wort, B vitamins, hypnosis, homeopathy, acupuncture, counseling. She refused to try antidepressant drugs—otherwise, those would have been on her list as well.

"What about SAMe?" I asked, pronouncing it "Sammy."

"What is it?"

"It's the abbreviation for S-adenosylmethionine, which is a substance naturally found in the cells of your body. There's some impressive research showing it helps depression and osteoarthritis. It is what we call a methyl donor."

The term methyl donor was obviously unfamiliar to her, so I went on to explain that SAMe could activate chemical reactions in the body. Among other things, it contributed to the way the brain used neurotransmitters to influence mood.

Sandy called me five days after starting SAMe and told me that she was doing better. I encouraged her to keep taking it, knowing that a positive response after five days of supplementation could well be a placebo effect, especially in someone who had a 10-year-old depression problem.

One month later, though, when Sandy returned to my clinic, she declared she had a new friend. "His name is Sammy."

She was thrilled to be feeling so much better. A year later, when she saw me again, Sandy continued to do very well on SAMe as her sole treatment for her depression.

## FOR LOOSER LIMBS

I also recommend SAMe when patients have osteoarthritis, a common condition that affects almost everyone over the age of 50.

Troy, a 55-year-old carpenter, was a good example of what SAMe can do for this condition. When he came in the first time, the severe osteoarthritis in his knees and hips forced him to walk stiffly. He commented on how his joints "creaked" like an old wooden floorboard. Troy said his knees were always quite swollen and painful when he woke up in the morning.

Troy's chiropractor had him on some good supplements including glucosamine sulfate, vitamin C and other antioxidants, and MSM. For exercise, he swam five times a week. But after a year of taking these supplements and pursuing this regular exercise regimen, he still didn't feel much improvement.

Troy wondered whether it was just a matter of giving the supplements more time to work. But I told him that he should have noticed significant benefits within a few months. To speed up the process, I recommended that, for one thing, we work on his diet, since he might have digestive problems that were getting in the way of his improvement. I also had him stop taking his current supplements and start with SAMe.

The next time I saw Troy, three months later, he said that his joint pain had improved and the swelling had gone down. From observing his mobility, I judged that there had been a 70 percent improvement, at least.

## WHAT MAKES SAMe RUN?

Needless to say, when something works, I stay with it—and I'm now a pretty strong advocate of SAMe for both depression and osteoarthritis. But how can one supplement address such different conditions?

Our bodies manufacture SAMe by combining the amino acid methionine with ATP (adenosine triphosphate, also known as the "energy molecule"). When this reaction occurs, the resulting compound becomes a "methyl donor," meaning that it can transfer a group of one carbon and three hydrogen atoms ($CH_3$).

Numerous biochemical reactions require this "methylation" reaction—which helps to explain why it can be used for such different conditions. By taking SAMe as a supplement, you're essentially making sure that the "raw materials" are available for crucial chemical reactions to take place.

Some researchers have speculated that our bodies lose their ability to manufacture or utilize SAMe as we get older. Also, it appears that some people may have a genetic defect that prevents their bodies from utilizing the chemical very efficiently. (This could help explain why depression, in some cases, seems to be passed along genetically in families.) Vitamin $B_{12}$ and folic acid deficiency can also interfere with the body's production of SAMe.

After SAMe donates its methyl group, it is converted to another substance called SAH (S-adenosyl-homocysteine). SAH then donates its sulfur group to other molecules, which is very important for a number of body processes, especially detoxification and cartilage formation.

## THE LURE OF THE NEW

The popularity of SAMe has increased most sharply during the past decade or so, although it's been available commercially, at least in Europe, since 1975.

Before commercial introduction, SAMe was tested in 1973 as a treatment for people with schizophrenia. It didn't have a significant impact on the symptoms of schizophrenia, but during the treatments, doctors observed that schizophrenia patients became less depressed when given SAMe.

Thousands of studies have now been done with SAMe, mainly related to its use for osteoarthritis and depression. There is also research showing that it is effective for fibromyalgia and cirrhosis of the liver. It is an approved prescription drug in Italy, Spain, Russia, and Germany.

Interestingly, SAMe outsells Prozac in Italy, even though insurance companies only pay for Prozac. While its popularity may not be quite that high in the United States, SAMe can now be found in virtually every health food store and pharmacy in North America. In all likelihood, SAMe's popularity will increase even more as its price steadily decreases.

## DOSAGE

Most people will notice benefits when taking between 400 to 1,200 milligrams of SAMe on a daily basis. Many of my patients find that between 400 to 800 milligrams works well as a long-term dosage. The key is to find the dosage that works best for you.

SAMe is generally available in 200-milligram tablets. Make sure it is enteric-coated, which is critical for maintaining stability. It is generally available in 200 milligram tablets. It should be taken a half hour before meals. I usually recommend that people take 800 micrograms of folic acid and 1,000 micrograms of $B_{12}$ every day to help their bodies with the metabolism of SAMe—and some SAMe formulas already contain these two additional nutrients. If not, take a high potency 100-milligram B-complex vitamin.

(The B-complex has other benefits as well. The $B_{12}$, folic acid, and $B_6$ included in a B-complex vitamin also help prevent depression and osteoporosis, so it's a perfect complement to SAMe.)

## WHAT ARE THE SIDE EFFECTS?

SAMe is very safe. When extremely high dosages were given to animals, there were few signs of toxicity—and lower doses used in human studies have not shown any adverse reactions. As a matter of fact, in comparison tests, the people taking a placebo had more side effects than the people who were taking SAMe. (As in all scientific studies of this kind, neither group knew whether it was taking a real supplement or an inactive placebo.)

High dosages have sometimes been given intravenously without any harm. Oral dosages of 3,600 milligrams per day also produced no side effects in humans.

Rarely, some people find that taking SAMe on an empty stomach causes heartburn. If this happens, take it with meals or just try taking a different brand. If you get diarrhea or stomach upset at higher-than-recommended dosages, you can simply reduce the dosages; the symptoms will go away.

It is recommended that people with bipolar depression do not use SAMe or only do so under the guidance of a medical professional.

Pregnant or breast-feeding women should only use SAMe under a doctor's supervision. To date, there aren't any studies to indicate that SAMe can cause pregnancy problems or harm the unborn baby, but it is not known whether SAMe can be guaranteed safe for long-term use. My feeling is that it would be safer for the baby than pharmaceutical antidepressants, as SAMe is a normal constituent in the body.

SAMe has been used by psychiatrists in conjunction with pharmaceutical antidepressants. This approach helps the patient to feel better more quickly. Many antidepressant drugs take a full month to have an effect while SAMe can help in days. Also, people who continue on the pharmaceutical medication can usually reduce their dosage. European physicians commonly recommend a combination.

However, if you are on pharmaceutical medications, be sure to consult with your physician before starting SAMe. Your doctor will want to be able to monitor your progress and, of course, will need to decide whether your drug therapy may need to be reduced. It's also important to never stop taking a pharmaceutical antidepressant "cold turkey" when starting SAMe, as this could lead to worsening of symptoms.

Some researchers urge caution if you're taking MAO (monoamine oxidase) inhibitor antidepressants, as they suspect there may be some problem combining the MAO's with SAMe. This combination has not been well researched.

Some researchers feel that SAMe supplementation can lead to the buildup of homocysteine in the body, which is a substance associated with the risk of heart attack. Actually, the opposite may be true. SAMe increases the activity of an enzyme (cystathione-beta-synthetase) that converts homocysteine into the beneficial antioxidant glutathione. In any event, taking B vitamins as I recommended prevents the build up of homocysteine.

# SAMe
## RECOMMENDATIONS FROM THE NATURAL PHYSICIAN FOR . . .

### ∾ Depression

I recommend starting at 400 milligrams daily for two weeks. Stay at this dosage if you notice improvement. If there is little to no improvement, then increase the SAMe dosage to 800 milligrams daily for another two to four weeks. Some people may need to use up to 1,200 milligrams to notice an effect. This is fine as toxicity is not a concern.

There are different theories as to how SAMe works to alleviate depression. One is that it increases the cellular levels of phosphatidylserine, which is a substance found in very high concentration in brain cells. It improves cell-to-cell communication, allows the efficient passage of nutrients into cells, and helps remove waste products. Phosphatidylserine has been shown to help relieve depression.

The other thing SAMe accomplishes is the increase of concentration of the neurotransmitters responsible for controlling mood such as norepinephrine, dopamine, and serotonin. Researchers believe that, at the same time, SAMe improves the way your brain cells receive these important neurotransmitters. While the exact mechanism is unknown, the benefits are certainly related to the methyl-donor effect, which allows for biochemical reactions to occur more normally in the brain.

Several studies have shown that people with severe depression have markedly low levels of SAMe. When the published clinical studies on SAMe between the years of 1973 and 1992 were analyzed, researchers found a total of 38 studies that showed the effectiveness of the supplement. When SAMe was compared with a placebo and with pharmaceutical antidepressants, it was found to be more effective than the placebo and just as effective as the class of drugs known as tricyclic antidepressants.

A 1994 study at the University of California Irvine Medical Center compared the effectiveness of SAMe with the pharmaceutical antidepressant desipiramine. This double-blind study found that 62 percent of the people taking SAMe and 52 percent of those taking desipiramine improved significantly.

Given all the potential side effects of traditional antidepressants, it makes sense that natural compounds such as SAMe and St. John's wort be used as a first line of treatment. If you are currently taking pharmaceutical antidepressants, I recom-

*(continued)*

mend working with a doctor to add SAMe to your protocol. Medications always have side effects, and if you can reduce the dosage, you're likely to reduce or eliminate at least some of the effects.

SAMe works at a much deeper level than drug therapy. With the methyl-donor mechanism, it opens the door to more biochemical reactions. Drug antidepressants, by contrast, force a chemical change to take place.

### ❧ Fibromyalgia

SAMe does seem to have some benefit for fibromyalgia, though the results aren't likely to be so dramatic as they are for the treatment of depression and osteoarthritis. In one double-blind fibromyalgia study, 44 patients received either 800 milligrams of SAMe or a placebo. The SAMe group showed significant improvement, with less pain, relief from fatigue, less morning stiffness, and improved mood. However, there was no difference between the groups in respect to tender points and muscle strength.

Another double-blind study found that SAMe improved trigger-point pain and depression. It appears that SAMe has some effect on fibromyalgia symptoms and significantly relieves depression associated with fibromyalgia.

I recommend 800 milligrams daily as the average dosage for this condition. Some people may need to use higher amounts and some may only need 400 milligrams.

### ❧ Liver Problems

The highest concentration of SAMe is found in the liver. It is involved in various detoxification pathways, including the proper metabolism of estrogen. It also is involved in the production of bile salts that help to digest fats.

When people get cirrhosis of the liver (most commonly from alcoholism), they have depleted levels of SAMe, which is necessary for bile production and detoxification. With more SAMe,

there's an increased level of glutathione—a beneficial substance that becomes depleted when liver function is impaired. (Glutathione is one of the most important antioxidants for detoxification.)

Since SAMe can be helpful in preventing liver degeneration, it's also a treatment for hepatitis.

For conditions like cirrhosis and hepatitis, it's important to consult an experienced doctor or practitioner before taking SAMe at any dosage. If you don't have these conditions, you can take SAMe as a general aid in detoxification, since it helps your liver remove impurities.

For cirrhosis, I recommend 800 to 1,200 milligrams daily. This can be taken indefinitely, with the consent of your doctor. For general liver and detoxification support, the dosage is 200 to 400 milligrams daily.

### ❧ Osteoarthritis

Osteoarthritis is the most common type of arthritis, where symptoms include stiffness, pain, and swelling of the joints. SAMe is known as a "chondroprotective agent," meaning that it prevents damage and degeneration of cartilage. Specifically, SAMe prevents the breakdown of substances called proteoglycans.

Proteoglycans hold water in the cartilage, which helps keep it flexible. These substances also help to keep the joints lubricated, thus preventing friction, and reducing wear and tear. Similar to glucosamine sulfate, SAMe has been shown in animal and human studies to increase cartilage production, which is critical in counteracting the effects of osteoarthritis.

In the largest study on SAMe and osteoarthritis, researchers followed the progress of 20,641 people who took SAMe for eight weeks. Patients took 400 milligrams three times daily for the first week, 400 milligrams twice daily for the second week, and 200 milligrams twice daily during the third to eighth weeks. Seventy-one percent of SAMe users

*(continued)*

reported "good" or "very good" benefits, while only 9 percent reported poor outcomes.

Several studies have compared SAMe with popular NSAID (nonsteroidal antiinflammatory medications such as Advil® or ibuprofen). In general, SAMe was as effective in relieving pain, stiffness, and other symptoms common to osteoarthritis. One of the major advantages of SAMe as compared with standard drug treatment is that it does not carry the risk of side effects. With NSAIDs you can get internal bleeding, liver damage, and kidney problems—but SAMe produces none of these side effects.

There's another benefit to taking SAMe. If you have conventional treatment with an NSAID, aspirin, or steroids, there's a good chance you actually speed up the destruction of cartilage even though you may be relieving some of the pain. All the conventional drugs have that effect—but SAMe does the opposite, actually helping to build healthier, more flexible cartilage. Along with a good diet and exercise, therefore, SAMe is a primary treatment for reducing osteoarthritis symptoms and regenerating cartilage.

Start at 800 milligrams daily for the first month and then cut back to 400 milligrams as a maintenance dose. Since SAMe is one of the more expensive supplements, many patients start at 400 milligrams. If you can get a good response at that level, there's no reason to go higher.

# Saw Palmetto

The old adage is "a dog is a man's best friend." If you were to talk to men over age 50, that saying may be changed to "saw palmetto is a man's best friend."

Saw palmetto *(Serenoa repens)* is an incredible herb for treatment of prostate enlargement, also known as benign prostatic hypertrophy (BPH). This common condition affects 50 percent of men over the age of 50—and close to 90 percent of men in their 80's have a problem with BPH. Youth is no guarantee of immunity, however. Nearly one out of every ten men between the ages of 25 and 30 have BPH. Common symptoms of prostate enlargement include:

- Need to urinate more frequently, especially at night
- Delay in urination
- Slow stream of urine flow
- Incomplete emptying of the bladder
- Increased incidence of prostatitis (prostate infection)
- Increased incidence of bladder infections

The prostate is a walnut-shaped gland located beneath the bladder. It surrounds the neck of the bladder and encircles the urethra (the passageway from the bladder through the penis). If the prostate gland starts to enlarge, it puts pressure on the bladder wall, urethra, and the sphincter muscles that control the flow of urine out of the bladder—hence, the increased difficulty with urination. Since urine flow is impeded, there's a greater likelihood of infections.

# A FLUID ROLE

The function of the prostate is to secrete prostatic fluid that creates a favorable environment for sperm to live. As a man ages and his hormones fluctuate, testosterone levels decline while other hormones such as estrogen increase. Specialists surmise that the prostate enlarges because, as men get older, a lot of testosterone is converted to a substance known as dihydrotestosterone (DHT). The enzyme responsible for this conversion of testosterone to DHT is 5-alpha reductase. It is believed the activity of this enzyme increases as men age, so that DHT levels increase. DHT is implicated in the stimulation of the growth of prostate cells.

Recently, researchers have also given attention to the role of estrogen and its role in prostate enlargement. Some researchers feel that prostate cell growth is largely a result of the balance among estrogen, testosterone, and DHT.

It is interesting to note that the enzyme aromatase converts testosterone to a potent form of estrogen known as estradiol, which causes cells to grow and multiply. It is believed that this enzyme activity increases as men get older. As estrogen levels increase, hormones such as progesterone and prolactin may play roles as well.

One study showed that the combination of saw palmetto and the herb nettles helps shrink enlarged prostate tissue. While no definitive explanation has been agreed upon, hormone balance seems to play a role.

My patient Michael, a 54-year-old real estate entrepreneur, would agree that saw palmetto can work wonders for a man's prostate. Though he originally came to see me for a problem with insomnia, I quickly determined that he wasn't sleeping well because he had to get up three or four times every night to urinate. Once awake, he then had trouble getting back to sleep. On further questioning, I found out that he also had dribbling after urination—another symptom of BPH. In other words, Michael's waking up at night was actually a symptom of prostate enlargement.

Blood work and a prostate exam helped to confirm the diagnosis of BPH. Within four weeks of taking saw palmetto extract, Michael was just getting up twice a night, as opposed to the three or four wakenings he'd had previously. Three months later, after continued use of saw palmetto, he was getting up no more than once a night.

## A BERRY TONIC

The credit for medicinal use of saw palmetto goes to Native Americans who (as far as we know) were the first to make a tonic for the prostate and urinary system out of saw palmetto berries. American settlers adopted saw palmetto for their own uses, and before long it was also being used in Europe, where it is still a very popular treatment for prostate enlargement and urinary tract infections. (Some European doctors also recommend it as an aphrodisiac.) Saw palmetto is native to Florida, Georgia, Louisiana, and South Carolina.

Saw palmetto berry contains about 1.5 percent oil that is high in fat-soluble fatty acids and sterols. It also contains flavonoids, carotene, essential oil, enzymes, and phytosterols. Saw palmetto berry extracts with a standardized fatty-acid content are approved by both the German and French governments for the treatment of BPH.

Research has shown that saw palmetto helps the prostate in a number of ways. Among its many activities in the body, saw palmetto:

- Inhibits the activity of the enzyme 5-alpha reductase, thus reducing the conversion of testosterone to DHT
- Blocks DHT from binding to prostate cells
- Reduces the effects of estrogen and progesterone on the prostate cells
- Causes smooth muscle relaxation (theoretically allowing the urethra to open more effectively and prevent the backup of urine)
- Reduces inflammation and edema by inhibiting the effects of inflammatory-producing chemicals called prostaglandins
- Alters cholesterol metabolism in the prostate
- Modifies the levels of sex hormone binding globulin (SHBG)

Although saw palmetto is mainly used to benefit the prostate, it is also used by herbalists for:

- Acne, which is highly influenced by hormones
- Prevention of bladder infections related to BPH
- Premature balding, which is related to the conversion of testosterone to DHT

- Polycystic ovary syndrome, which typically is characterized by DHEA and testosterone excess
- Prostatitis-inflammation and infection of the prostate
- Prostate cancer, which is influenced by hormonal factors

## DOSAGE

The saw palmetto extracts that I recommend contain 85 to 95 percent fatty acids and sterols. The total dosage should be 320 milligrams daily.

I tell my patients to give saw palmetto extract a "trial run" of at least 4 weeks, but that's a minimum. In some men it can take up to two months before improvements begin.

## WHAT ARE THE SIDE EFFECTS?

The only reported side effect is stomach upset in a small percentage of users. If you have that problem, try taking the herb with meals.

## SAW PALMETTO
### RECOMMENDATIONS FROM THE NATURAL PHYSICIAN FOR . . .

#### ∾ *Acne*

While I don't know of any studies on saw palmetto as a treatment for acne, some herbalists have seen positive results. I include saw palmetto in acne formulas that contain other herbs such as vitex, burdock root, and milk thistle. The combination has helped some teenagers who have serious cases of acne. In theory, saw palmetto reduces hormonal stimulation of the sebum glands, so fewer pustules form.

#### ∾ *Baldness*

Recently, some advertisers have been touting products that help balding men regrow their hair, and the ads mention a "special herb" that prevents high levels of DHT from building up in the scalp. That herb could only be saw palmetto. I haven't seen reports of studies on saw palmetto and baldness, and I would not expect dramatic effects—but on the other hand, I have not seen any evidence to refute the claims.

#### ∾ *Benign Prostatic Hypertrophy (BPH)*

I find that saw palmetto helps over 80 percent of men with BPH who take the full dosage for 4 to 6 weeks. Saw palmetto also combines well with the herb *Pygeum africanum* for an effective treatment. To be even more aggressive with treatment, I ask

*(continued)*

men to take some extra zinc (50 to 100 milligrams with a few milligrams of copper), and the supplement(s) calcium d-glucarate plus indole 3 carbinol (for their hormone-metabolism properties). In addition, essential fatty acid sources such as flaxseed/flaxseed oil, and pumpkinseed/pumpkinseed oil are effective for BPH.

Alternatively, you may be able to find a ready-made formulation that includes saw palmetto blended with herbs such as *Pygeum africanum* and nettle root. Another helpful supplement included in some formulations is cernilton, a rye pollen extract, which has also been shown in studies to be effective for BPH as well as prostatitis.

In one study involving 1,098 men over the age of 50, researchers compared the results of taking saw palmetto extract (320 milligrams) with a prescription dosage of the drug Proscar (5 milligrams daily). After a 6-month trial, researchers were able to report that the treatments were equally effective in reducing the symptoms of BPH. However, the men taking the prescription pharmaceutical Proscar had far more problems with sexual dysfunction, complaining of lowered libido, impotence, and ejaculatory disorders.

Based on studies like this, saw palmetto clearly shows the same benefits without the drawback of negative side effects.

The prestigious *Journal of the American Medical Association (JAMA)*—the bible of conventional medicine—summed up the findings in a number of reports on the healing effects and the safety of saw palmetto extract in men with prostate enlargement. When the authors reviewed 18 scientifically controlled trials involving 2,939 men with BPH, they concluded that, indeed, saw palmetto was just as effective as Proscar, and the side effects were fewer.

### ❧ Bladder Infections

Bladder infections and urinary tract infections are much more likely to occur in men who have BPH. As urine flow is impeded and slowed down, bacteria are more likely to thrive and cause infection in the bladder and urinary tract. By reducing the prostate congestion and improving urination, saw palmetto treats the underlying condition that often leads to bacterial infection.

### ❧ Polycystic Ovarian Syndrome

This condition involves hormone imbalance. Women who have this syndrome may begin to grow facial hair, gain weight, experience menstrual irregularities, and have ovulation problems. Higher-than-normal levels of the hormones DHEA and testosterone are found in some women with this condition. Herbalists theorize that saw palmetto may be helpful because it blocks the effects of these hormones. I doubt it would be effective by itself, but it's worth trying in herbal hormone-balancing formulas.

### ❧ Prostate Cancer

There are no studies looking at saw palmetto's effect on prostate cancer. My view is that it would not hurt and may have some benefit as part of a comprehensive approach. After all, saw palmetto may prevent excess hormone stimulation of the prostate cells, so perhaps it reduces the stimulus for cell growth. Fortunately, saw palmetto does not appear to affect the PSA marker (test marker for prostate cancer), so there is no conflict in using it.

### ❧ Prostatitis

Congestion and inflammation of the prostate leads to a condition known as prostatitis. This can cause serious pain in the prostate gland—pain that can be felt in other areas of the body such as the low back, abdomen, and testis. (Doctors call this "referred pain," since it affects body areas that are separate from the actual pain site.) Saw palmetto helps to reduce the congestion and alleviate prostatitis when used on a long-term basis. (The rye pollen extract cernilton has been shown in studies to treat prostatitis even more effectively than saw palmetto.)

# Schussler Cell Salts

"Dr. Mark, I picked up the kali phos 6x that you recommended for my nerves. On the bottle it said 'Schussler Cell Salt.' What does that mean?" asked Florence, a patient of mine.

"Schussler cell salts refer to a group of homeopathic remedies that was developed by Dr. Schussler of Germany in the late 1800s. His research led him to believe that twelve inorganic minerals were the key constituents of cells. He referred to these twelve minerals as tissue builders and said that healthy cells contain normal amounts of these minerals. He theorized that disease occurs when there is a deficiency or imbalance of these cell salts. By taking the indicated cell salt or combination of salts, the proper structure and function of the cells could be restored. Healthy cells make for a healthy person. In your case, you are stimulating your cells to use potassium more effectively, which benefits your nervous system."

## SIMPLE, BUT EFFECTIVE

There are more than a thousand homeopathic remedies. Each one has its own set of symptoms on which it is used. The Schussler cell salts are a simplified system that complements the other homeopathic remedies. As you will see, they are easy for the public and homeopaths to use. What is more important, they work!

Have you ever taken a mineral like magnesium to help reduce or prevent muscle cramps, and find that it does not help?

You may not be getting the benefit from the magnesium at the cellular level, no matter how much you are taking. In a case like this, I find that taking the cell salt, or the homeopathic form of the deficient mineral, works quickly to alleviate the condition. The cell salt stimulates a biochemical change at the cellular level, which then gives the desired result.

## DOSAGE

Cell salts are used like other homeopathic remedies—and as with other homeopathics, they come in pellet, tablet, or liquid form. The most common potency available commercially is 6x.

Cell salts are best taken 10 to 20 minutes before or after you have any drink or meal. For an infant, you can crush a cell salt tablet and place it on the child's tongue. Or you can mix the tablet with an ounce of purified water and place a few drops in the child's mouth using a dropper or teaspoon. Children like the sweet taste of the pellets and tablets.

When you do take cell salts, however, you'll probably want to avoid strong odors, such as the fragrance of eucalyptus or essential oils.

For acute conditions, cell salts should be taken every 15 minutes or 2 hours, depending on the severity of the condition. For chronic conditions, cell salts are usually taken one to three times daily. Since they are of a low potency, they can be used on a long-term basis.

As described below, one type of cell salts—or a combination of them—can be taken to treat a particular symptom or condition. For example, mag phos helps to relieve muscle spasms. If a person is also experiencing nerve pain, then kali phos could be used as well. These different types of cell salts can either be taken at the same time or in alternating doses throughout the day.

There are also some formulas that combine all the cell salts together in one formula. These are commonly known as bioplasma. They may be used preventatively or to recover from various chronic illnesses.

## WHAT ARE THE SIDE EFFECTS?

Side effects are not an issue with cell salts. They either help or do nothing at all.

## SELECTING THE APPROPRIATE CELL SALT

A list of various cell salts follows, with the conditions for which each is used.

### ✍ *Calcarea Fluorica (Calc Fluor)*

This cell salt is involved in the formation of connective tissue, making it important for the skin, ligaments, and tendons. It is also found in bones. I recommend it for the following conditions:

Abnormal spine curvature

Brittle teeth and sore gums

Hard nodules of the breast or other tissues

Hemorrhoids

Spine that "goes out" easily (including during pregnancy)

Sprains and strains

Varicose veins, weak ligaments, tendons, and joints

## ❧ Calcarea Phosphorica (Calc Phos)

This is the main cell salt for bone health. Interestingly, calcium phosphate is an important enzyme required for bone formation. Calc phos helps in bone formation. I recommend it for the following conditions:

Arthritis

Fractures

Growing pains

Osteoporosis

Teething

## ❧ Calcarea Sulphurica (Calc Sulph)

This cell salt is a wound- and skin-healer. (It is especially recommended when there is a yellow discharge from the skin.) I recommend it for the following conditions:

Abscess

Acne

Boils

Bronchitis

Post-masal drip

## ❧ Ferrum Phosphoricum (Ferrum Phos)

This cell salt is homeopathic iron bound to phosphate. It is required for red blood cell formation and function. I recommend it for the following conditions:

Anemia treatment and prevention (iron deficiency)

Bleeding (acute and chronic)

**409**

Fever and infection

Heavy menstruation

## ❧ *Kali Muriaticum (Kali Mur)*

This cell salt helps to dissolve mucus. I recommend it for the following conditions:

Fluid in the ears

Sore throat (with white mucus being produced)

## ❧ *Kali Phosphoricum (Kali Phos)*

This is the primary cell salt for nervous tissue, including the brain. I recommend it for:

Anxiety and nervousness

Depression

Fatigue

Nerve injury

Poor memory and lack of concentration

## ❧ *Kali Sulphuricum (Kali Sulph)*

This is another remedy for skin and mucous membrane discharges (especially where there is a yellow discharge). I recommend it for:

Bronchitis

Eczema

Psoriasis

## ❧ *Magnesia Phosphorica (Mag Phos)*

This is the primary cell salt for the muscles—both internal and external. It also has a tonic effect on the nervous system as well. It can help with:

Anxiety and nervousness

Hyperactivity

Menstrual cramps

Muscle spasms and cramps

Seizures

Stomach cramps

Toothache

### ∾ *Natrum Muriaticum (Nat Mur)*

This cell salt regulates water balance within the cells and tissues. I recommend it for the following conditions:

Cold sores

Depression

Dry skin

Edema

Grief

Hayfever

Skin rash from sun exposure

### ∾ *Natrum Phosphoricum (Nat Phos)*

This is the cell salt that is an acid-base balancer of the cells. I recommend it for the following conditions:

Bladder infections

Heartburn

Muscle soreness

Vaginitis

### ∾ *Natrum Sulphuricum (Nat Sulph)*

This remedy has a balancing effect on the fluids of the body. In addition, it tonifies the liver and digestive tract. I recommend it for:

Asthma

Head injury

Hepatitis

**411**

Newborn jaundice

Swelling

### ❧ Silica

This cell salt is found in the connective tissue, skin, glands, and bones. It acts as a tissue cleanser. I recommend it for the following conditions:

Acne

Asthma

Boils

Brittle hair and nails

Sinusitis

# Selenium

· · · · · · · · · · · · · · · · · · · · · · · · · · · · · · · · · · · · · · · · · · · · · · · · · · ·

Humans require very small amounts of the trace mineral selenium, yet it is involved in some very important functions in the body. Specifically, selenium is necessary for the production of antioxidant enzymes that remove toxic waste products formed from oxidative reactions.

Selenium works synergistically with vitamin E to prevent oxidative damage of cell membranes. Vitamin E works more effectively in the presence of selenium.

Selenium is also important for preventing heart disease, cancer, inflammatory conditions such as rheumatoid arthritis, and cataracts. It plays a role in the production of thyroid hormone, and it's needed during pregnancy for the growing baby.

Selenium binds to heavy metals such as mercury and may reduce their toxicity.

The Recommended Daily Allowance (RDA) for men and women is 55 micrograms. Foods containing selenium include wheat germ, Brazil nuts, oats, liver, whole wheat bread, broccoli, red grapes, onions, and egg yolks.

Unfortunately, though these foods contain the nutrient, the actual concentrations are unpredictable. That's because the level of selenium in food depends on levels of selenium in the soil where the food was grown. Since soil's selenium levels vary from region to region, the broccoli raised in California is very likely to have a different concentration from the broccoli raised in New Jersey.

But there are also selenium supplements, and they are generally well absorbed. Selenomethionine and selenium-enriched yeast are good forms.

The greatest risks for those with selenium deficiency appear to be heart disease, cancer, and lowered immune function. Possibly the best evidence of this comes from a study of the residents of Nianning County, China. There, the soil is deficient in selenium, and most of the food that's consumed in that area comes from the same region. Children and women of childbearing age who lived in this area had an abnormally high rate of a rare form of heart disease called Keshan disease. It was later discovered that the selenium deficiency made the children and women susceptible to a viral infection that caused the heart disease. Selenium supplementation significantly reduced the prevalence of this disease in these people.

## DOSAGE

I recommend a dosage of 200 micrograms as an adult supplement. For those with viral infections, I recommend a dosage of 400 to 600 micrograms daily.

## WHAT ARE THE SIDE EFFECTS?

Toxicity can occur with dosages above 900 micrograms. A toxic dosage may interfere with sulfur metabolism, preventing you from absorbing sulfur in ways that are necessary for your health. Side effects of toxicity can include depression, nausea, vomiting, and nervousness. If you notice a garlic odor on your breath (even though you haven't been eating garlic) or if you perspire excessively, these symptoms might be a sign of toxicity. Also, you should be aware of any signs of hair loss or changes in the appearance of your fingernails.

Children and infants should not take separate selenium supplements unless instructed to do so by a physician. Some selenium may be included in multivitamin supplements for children, but this is acceptable since the controlled doses are very small.

# SELENIUM
## RECOMMENDATIONS FROM THE NATURAL PHYSICIAN FOR . . .

### AIDS

People with AIDS tend to have low levels of selenium. That shortage puts a stress on the immune system, because selenium is needed to avoid oxidative stress. Selenium should be taken with other major antioxidants to optimize immune function.

### Cancer

Several studies have shown that low levels of selenium are associated with an increased risk of cancer. This is especially true for stomach, esophageal, colon, rectal, and prostate cancers. Interestingly, garlic, onions, broccoli, and whole grains are recommended to prevent cancer, and all of them are good sources of selenium. As I've mentioned, selenium concentrations vary in these foods, but of course they also have other nutrients and phytochemicals that seem to help prevent cancer.

Smokers may benefit from increased selenium intake.

### Cataracts

Cataracts are the result of free-radical damage to the lens of the eye. Studies have shown that people with cataracts generally have low levels of selenium, so I recommend supplementation—both for prevention and treatment—to help provide antioxidant support.

### Heart Disease

In his book *The Antioxidant Miracle,* Lester Packer states that research by Dr. Raymond Shamberger of the Cleveland Clinic has shown "that people who live in states with the lowest selenium content were three times more likely to die of heart disease than those who lived in states that were more selenium rich." The states that were found to have selenium-deficient soil include Connecticut, Illinois, Ohio, Oregon, Massachusetts, Rhode Island, New York, Pennsylvania, Indiana, Delaware, and District of Columbia. For people living in those areas, I would recommend 200 micrograms of supplementation.

### Hepatitis C

I recommend selenium supplementation for those with hepatitis C to help keep this viral infection of the liver under control.

### Immunity

Selenium is important for the immune system, particularly the function of lymphocytes and macrophages. One study found that 200 micrograms of selenium given to people with normal blood selenium levels resulted in a significant increase in immunity. It increases the ability of immune cells to kill cancer cells and various pathogens.

### Prenatal Infant Growth

Selenium appears to be important for proper fetal growth and is included in prenatal multivitamins.

### Rheumatoid Arthritis

Selenium helps to reduce the production of inflammatory chemicals and supports the function of vitamin E in preventing joint inflammation and destruction.

### Skin

Selenium helps to prevent oxidative damage to the skin. It appears to help prevent skin cancer, but does not help once the cancer has already developed.

### Sudden Infant Death Syndrome (SIDS)

Selenium deficiency may be a factor in sudden infant death syndrome. Breast-feeding mothers can provide adequate selenium for their infants by taking a multivitamin that contains this nutrient.

# Sepia

Tiffany, a 25-year-old housewife and mother of three, came to my office with a problem that seemed to be turning her life into an unrelenting torment: severe premenstrual syndrome. In fact, she was so upset by what was happening that she began crying as we talked.

She explained that she had always suffered from PMS, but the symptoms had become much more extreme since the birth of her last child. Her husband concurred. From his perspective, her PMS seemed to last the entire month.

Through her tears, she went on to confess that she had been struggling with depression and constantly felt tense and irritable, especially during the week before her menstrual cycle. What bothered her most was how short-tempered she had become with her kids, snapping at them for "normal" childhood mischief. She could not understand why she was acting this way, and her feelings of guilt were now beginning to overwhelm her.

Physically, Tiffany felt burned out. Her energy was at an all-time low. She experienced some improvement emotionally and physically after exercise, but the relief was temporary. She was constantly chilly, and some recent blood tests revealed that her thyroid function was close to being underactive. She also experienced extreme bloating just before the start of her menstrual flow.

All of this turmoil was putting a strain on her relationship with her husband. Not only was the communication between them breaking down, but Tiffany's libido had dwindled to almost nothing. She confessed that she actually felt repulsed by the thought of having sexual relations.

## THE CRITICAL BALANCING ACT

As extreme and general as her condition sounded, however, when Tiffany mentioned one particular symptom—a craving for pickles—I realized immediately that her solution would be simple and specific: a homeopathic remedy, made from the ink of the cuttlefish, called sepia.

Very early in my clinical practice, I learned how valuable sepia can be for women. In fact, it has turned out to be one of the most effective natural therapies I've

## Do You Need Sepia?

In homeopathy, the following signs often indicate that a person can be helped by taking sepia. If you have a few or more of these signs, it may be helpful.

*Mental*
- irritability
- sarcastic demeanor
- feeling better when alone, worse with company
- episodes of crying without knowing why they occur
- poor memory and concentration
- low libido

*Head*
- left-sided headaches
- cracking of lips

*Digestive*
- constipation
- hemorrhoids
- gas and bloating
- empty sensation in stomach not relieved by eating
- craving for sour foods (pickles, vinegar)

*Urinary*
- urine leak while laughing, sneezing, or exercising

*Genital*
- chronic vaginitis
- uterine prolapse
- genital warts
- scanty or irregular menses

*Chest*
- Loss of fullness and flatness in breasts

*Skin*
- dryness
- psoriasis

*General*
- chills
- symptoms grow worse between 2 P.M. and 5 P.M.
- problems ever since using the birth-control pill, pregnancy, miscarriage

ever come across for treating hormone-related conditions. PMS, menopause, irregular menstrual cycles, ovarian cysts, fibrocystic breast syndrome, hormonal headaches, and many other conditions related to hormonal imbalance all respond wonderfully to sepia.

I explained to Tiffany that the underlying cause of her problem was most likely a hormonal imbalance. It's common for a woman's hormones to "get out of whack" after a pregnancy, and hormones are such powerful chemicals that when they fall out of balance, they can negatively affect the neurotransmitters of the brain, causing mental and emotional difficulties. Many women also find that the thyroid becomes sluggish after pregnancy, which can also cause problems with thinking, weight gain, chilliness, and constipation.

## RELIEF AT LAST

The terrible feelings of guilt that had plagued Tiffany disappeared like vapor when she learned that she wasn't to blame for the way she had been feeling and behaving. Her problems clearly had a physical basis. We started her on sepia, and week-by-week she saw improvement. First, her energy began to increase. After three weeks, her husband noticed that she was growing calmer. Her body temperature also slowly increased over time, indicating that her thyroid function was improving.

Last of all, her libido began to reassert itself. The last time I met with her, she had resumed sexual relations with her husband. She had not yet returned completely to normal in this part of her life, but she was headed in the right direction, and she described her marital relationship as "much better."

What pleased and relieved Tiffany most, however, was that she felt so much more patient with her children.

## DOSAGE

I recommend starting with a lower potency of sepia, usually 6C taken two times daily, but many health food stores and pharmacies carry the 30C potency—which is generally safe—that can be used as well. Try the remedy for one week. If you notice improvements in your mood, energy, or physical symptoms, continue daily use for another two weeks. Then use it only as needed.

## WHAT ARE THE SIDE EFFECTS?

Occasionally, I see women who experience an initial aggravation of symptoms with this remedy if they take too high of a dosage or take it too frequently. If this happens, simply cut back to one dose every two or three days, or switch to a lower potency.

---

# SEPIA
## RECOMMENDATIONS FROM THE NATURAL PHYSICIAN FOR . . .

### ❧ Birth-Control Pill Side Effects

Sepia is an excellent medicine to use when a woman has stopped taking birth-control pills and begins to experience hormonal imbalances such as an irregular menstrual cycle, water retention, tender breasts, headaches, and irritability.

### ❧ Bladder Infections

Sepia is one of the better remedies to use for women who are susceptible to chronic bladder infections. Hormonal changes, such as seen in menopause, lead to changes to the tissues of the bladder wall that can make a woman more susceptible to a bladder infection.

### ❧ Depression

Hormonal imbalance can lead to depression. Sepia can help improve depression that often accompanies irritability.

### ❧ Fertility

Hormone imbalance is one of the major causes of infertility, and sepia can be of benefit to

*(continued)*

women who have this problem. A history of miscarriages is an indication for using sepia.

### Fibrocystic Breast Syndrome

Breast cysts that enlarge or become more tender on a cyclical basis can be helped by using sepia. I have seen this remedy clear up many cases within three to five months.

### Genital Warts and Herpes

Sepia is one of the more common remedies for the natural treatment of genital warts and genital herpes.

### Hypothyroid

I have found sepia to help a number of women with low thyroid function. Imbalances with estrogen and progesterone can suppress normal thyroid function. Sepia appears to balance estrogen and progesterone and thus free up thyroid activity.

### Irregular Menstrual Cycles

Along with pulsatilla, sepia is one of the most common remedies for women who experience irregular menstrual cycles. It is also one of the most effective remedies for amenorrhea (no menstrual cycle).

### Libido

One of the classic symptoms that can be helped by sepia is an unexplained dwindling of libido. Women requiring this remedy state they have developed a sexual aversion to their husband or partner but are not sure why. Taking the remedy does not increase libido immediately but usually helps after a few months of treatment.

### Menopause

Sepia is very effective in helping to reduce the symptoms of menopause, including hot flashes, irritability, depression, vaginal dryness, and low libido.

### Migraine Headaches

Headaches that occur at about the same time each month, especially in relationship to the menstrual cycle, can show great improvement, or disappear altogether, after balancing the hormones by using sepia.

### Nausea During Pregnancy

Sepia is an excellent remedy for ailments that occur during pregnancy, including nausea, which usually worsen during the time from 3 P.M. to 5 P.M. Craving for pickles or vinegar are indications for sepia, too.

### Ovarian Cysts

Many women needlessly suffer from ovarian cysts, which really is a condition of hormonal imbalance. Sepia is one of the main remedies for this condition (along with pulsatilla, lachesis, lycopodium, and folliculinum).

### PMS

Symptoms of extreme irritability, increased craving for chocolate or sweets, breast tenderness, and water retention can all be helped by sepia.

### Prostate Enlargement

This is one of the few male conditions that sepia can relieve. Symptoms include dribbling after urination and the sensation that "a ball is in the rectum."

### Psoriasis

Sepia is one of the more common remedies to use for psoriasis. It has greatly helped several of my female patients.

### Raynaud's Syndrome

Hormones also influence blood circulation. Sepia is a good remedy for this condition (hands and feet that turn pale white or blue after brief exposure to cold), especially when other signs of hormonal

*(continued)*

imbalance are present. Raynaud's syndrome some- ally as a result of hormonal changes that occur
times starts after taking birth-control pills or hor- after pregnancy or during menopause. Sepia can
mone replacement therapy (HRT). help prevent this problem.

### ∾ Sinusitis

### ∾ Vaginitis

Chronic sinusitis is another condition that sepia
can alleviate.

Vaginitis, characterized by a white, offensively
odorous discharge, can be helped by sepia,
especially when the condition is chronic. Vaginal
dryness during or after menopause is another
indication for sepia.

### ∾ Urinary Incontinence

Women requiring sepia can sometimes leak urine
while laughing, sneezing, or exercising. I have found
this remedy works especially well for women who
develop incontinence during menopause.

### ∾ Varicose Veins

I have seen sepia help cases of varicose veins
that became a problem during menopause.

### ∾ Uterine Prolapse

Sagging of the uterus occurs when the ligaments that hold it in place become too lax, usu-

# Sitz Bath

"I'll get started on the diet and medicines you prescribed right away. Is there anything else I should do?" asked Bill, a 54-year-old high school teacher, who came to
see me for his hemorrhoids.

"Yes, there is," I said, "and it will help give you some immediate relief. I want
you to take a sitz bath."

"A sitz bath? I haven't heard that term since I was a teenager," replied Bill.

"Some of these old therapies are the most effective," I responded. "Plus, it
doesn't cost you anything."

"I like that part. How do I do this sitz bath?" asked Bill.

"It's pretty simple."

I explained that I was actually recommending a hot sitz bath alternated with
a cold one—so he would need two plastic or metal tubs, both large enough to sit
in comfortably.

"Fill one tub with hot water—between 100 and 106 degrees Fahrenheit—but make sure it's not too hot—just tolerable. Fill the second tub with cold water—as cold as you can stand."

I recommended that he sit in the hot tub for three to five minutes, then sit in the cold bath for about thirty seconds. "Do this three or four times. Make sure the last tub you are in is the cold one. Then get out and dry off."

I had an additional recommendation as well. "Add an ounce of witch hazel to the water in each tub."

"I'm not looking forward to that cold tub," said Bill.

"I hear you; but it's the cold that really helps improve the circulation to the hemorrhoids and relieves a lot of the congestion and pain. So it is the more important part of the treatment."

"How many times should I do this?" asked Bill.

"Take the sitz bath every day for the next week, and then you should take two to three a week for a month after that."

Bill called, three days later, to tell me that the burning pain from his hemorrhoids had improved. He also mentioned that the bleeding had stopped after the second treatment.

## SOOTHING WATER

The alternating sitz bath is a form of hydrotherapy. Using water as a medium to carry heat or cold, one can manipulate circulation to the pelvis and organs of the lower abdomen. With increased blood flow to this area, you're also bringing in the immune cells and nutrients that are carried in the blood—all of which helps to promote healing. Pain and inflammation are reduced as circulation improves.

Of course, you can try a single-temperature sitz bath, using either hot or cold water. But in most cases I recommend the alternating sitz bath because it does a better job of improving circulation.

## DOSAGE

For acute conditions, take a sitz bath one to two times daily. For chronic conditions, sitz baths can be taken two to seven times a week. I recommend resting after the sitz bath. You'll probably want to avoid physical activity for an hour or two afterward, until blood flow returns to normal.

# WHAT ARE THE SIDE EFFECTS?

Sitz baths are as safe as regular baths. Of course, you need to be careful getting in and out of the tubs—and anyone who needs assistance should have a partner or helper nearby.

Don't take a sitz bath if you have any kind of bleeding condition, including heavy menstrual flow. Also, I don't advise a sitz bath if you have acute urinary tract infections, because the infections can get worse with prolonged soaking in hot or cold water.

---

## SITZ BATH
### RECOMMENDATIONS FROM THE NATURAL PHYSICIAN FOR . . .

### ❧ Chronic Urinary Tract Infections

The alternating sitz bath can help relieve chronic urinary tract infections. It improves the flow of immune cells that prevent microbes from overgrowing.

One reminder, however: Sitz baths should not be used for *acute* urinary infections. If you have one kind of infection but aren't sure which it is, be sure to check with your doctor before you start treating yourself with alternating sitz bath.

### ❧ Constipation

The alternating sitz bath stimulates circulation and the nerve impulses to the colon and rectum. Thus, it tonifies the muscles and nerves that initiate bowel movements.

### ❧ Hemorrhoids and Fissures

If you use the procedure I've described here, an alternating sitz bath can be extremely effective for the relief and treatment of these conditions.

### ❧ Pelvic Congestion and Inflammation

By improving circulation to the lower abdomen and pelvis, many different conditions can be relieved. Of course, it is important to see your doctor to find out what is causing the discomfort.

### ❧ Prostatitis

Inflammation or infection of the prostate gland is common among men with benign prostate enlargement. The alternating sitz bath can provide relief from pain, and it may help combat infection in the prostate area.

### ❧ Vaginal Infections

An alternating sitz bath can help provide relief from a vaginal infection while you are being treated by your doctor.

# Soy

· · · · · · · · · · · · · · · · · · · · · · · · · · · · · · · · · · · · · · · · · · · · · · · · · · · · · · · · · · · · · ·

Soy *(Glycine max)* is a prime example of good eating that's good medicine. It's a staple of many diets throughout Southeast Asia, and as its many health properties are being uncovered and cooks are using it in more recipes, I find more soy sneaking into supermarkets as well as health food stores. It comes in many forms—from the newly popular soy burgers in many varieties and flavors to the traditional soybean product, tofu, which has been part of Asian diets for thousands of years.

I recommend soy to my patients to prevent heart disease, because there's no question that it lowers LDLs, the "bad" kind of cholesterol. But I also recommend it because soy can help prevent some kinds of cancer and can help prevent the onset of osteoporosis or delay its progress. Soy also reduces menopausal hot flashes and relieves PMS. It can help increase levels of the good bacteria *bifidobacteria,* too.

## PEAS IN A POD

A member of the pea family—and, therefore, a legume—the soybean is native to Southeastern Asia. More than 2,500 different varieties are cultivated.

Soybeans are rich in calcium, iron, zinc, B vitamins, and fiber. They are a great source of protein. Commercial soy foods such as tofu, as well as most of the soy-based products sold in supermarkets, are highly digestible.

Soy is a staple of the Chinese diet and has been used in that culture as a food and medicine for thousands of years. The Chinese discovered how to ferment soy to make it digestible, and it became a staple throughout Korea, Japan, and Southeast Asia.

Soy arrived in Europe in the 1700s; it was in the United States by the 1800s, brought by Chinese immigrants. It was also popular among Seventh-Day Adventists, who were largely vegetarian. Dr. Harvey Kellogg (founder of Kellogg's® cereals) became an advocate of soy foods and recommended that people eat soy in place of meat products.

## FRESH FROM THE FERMENT

Soy foods come in many different forms. Among the traditional, fermented soy foods are tempeh and miso, as well as the now-common tofu. These represent the forms of soy that are used in population studies where researchers try to pinpoint the dietary benefits of soybeans.

Another popular food product—though not in the "fermented" category—is soy milk. If you have a problem with the lactose in cow's milk, you can safely drink soy milk without any side effects, so it's particularly appealing to people who are lactose intolerant. With calcium-enriched soy milk available, soy milk has nearly all the benefits with none of the lactose-problems that come with "regular" milk.

Soy protein powders (isolates) are used by people looking for nonanimal protein sources. Soy protein powder is also a popular supplement for athletes and for anyone who's active. It helps aid muscle recovery and acts as an energy source.

Roasted soy nuts and toasted soy flour are also popular.

## ALL ABOUT ISOFLAVONES

Soy isoflavones are unique components that have caught the attention of researchers and the media. Chemically, isoflavones resemble the hormone estrogen. Thus, they are referred to as phytoestrogens (plant estrogens). But even though they resemble powerful hormones, the plant forms are much weaker, carrying about one-thousandth the potency of estrogen.

This is thought to be a good thing. Soy isoflavones may block strong or toxic estrogens from binding to receptor sites on hormone-dependent tissues such as the breast, uterus, and prostate. By occupying these sites and effectively taking the place of the more powerful forms, the phytoestrogens help prevent cancer growth.

Isoflavones, which are available in supplement form as well as in foods, are key compounds in decreasing cholesterol levels.

## DOSAGE

Fermented soy foods should be eaten liberally for their health-protective qualities. Next best? Take fermented soy protein powders that have standardized isoflavone content and drink plenty of soy milk.

You also have a third option, which is getting isoflavone capsule supplements. Though the supplements aren't so good a source as food, this may be the most practical way to increase intake of soy isoflavones (although the least-studied). Supplements are available in 50-milligram capsules, and the usual dosage is 50 to 150 milligrams daily.

Look for foods and supplements that are nongmo (meaning they are not genetically engineered). Also, look for soy products that list the isoflavone content.

Not all of them do. (For example, some soy protein isolates have had the isoflavones removed by alcohol extraction.) There are other healthful components in soy, but we know that isoflavones are important active substances, so you want to make sure they're included in whatever soy product you're buying.

## WHAT ARE THE SIDE EFFECTS?

Some people have a sensitivity reaction to soy, which can cause digestive upset. For some people, the side effect is preventable, as long as they take digestive enzymes before eating a meal that has soy in it—or even during the meal.

I have found that some children's eczema and reoccurring ear infections are brought on or worsened by soy products.

Raw soy beans (soy flour, or protein powders made from raw or unfermented or unroasted soybeans) should not be consumed on a regular basis, as they may be harmful to the pancreas and thyroid.

There is speculation that the isoflavones in soy formula for infants and children may be a problem, but the American Academy of Pediatrics still endorses use of the formula. More research will be needed to determine what problems, if any, the formula may cause. Moderate intake appears to be fine.

---

## SOY
### RECOMMENDATIONS FROM THE NATURAL PHYSICIAN FOR . . .

### ༖ Cancer

Many researchers feel that soy as a food works wonders to prevent many different forms of cancer. The death rate among women in China who have breast cancer is one-fifth what it is in the United States. The mortality from cancer in Japan is one-fourth of the United States', and it's just one-tenth in Korea.

People in these countries eat many other plant foods that also account for the decreased susceptibility. But when researchers have focused on soy, they've found that it seems to

be a key ingredient in preventing death from breast cancer in those countries.

People in Japan often consume an average of 200 milligrams of isoflavones daily as compared with the 1 to 3 milligrams Americans consume. Interestingly, in the populations of people who have moved from Japan to the U.S., rates of cancer and prostate cancer have soared toward the same levels as Americans who have been raised on the classic Western diet comprised of many high-fat foods and fewer plant foods. Clearly, there is a strong dietary connection.

*(continued)*

---

424

Many epidemiological studies suggest that soy as a food has a cancer-prevention effect. Soy consumption is associated with a decreased risk of breast, colon, rectum, lung, prostate, and stomach cancers.

Isoflavones seem to be the important cancer-preventing compounds. They have been shown to possess potent antioxidant activity and hormone-balancing qualities, both of which are believed to be important in preventing cancer.

Soybeans also contain protease inhibitors, and although most are lost through cooking, the small amount left appears to protect cell DNA from damage.

In addition, soy contains other potential anticancer compounds such as phytosterols, saponins, and phenolic acids.

While the significance of diet is clearly evident, however, we don't know much about the effectiveness of soy isoflavone supplements. I haven't seen any conclusive information about whether soy isoflavone supplements will prevent cancer, and we still haven't determined whether they're helpful in treating the disease.

### ∾ Cholesterol and Heart Disease

Soy has been shown to lower total cholesterol and LDL cholesterol, whether eaten as a food or taken in the form of isolated isoflavone supplements. As a matter of fact, the FDA approved the claim by manufacturers that a food containing 6.25 grams of soy protein had cardiovascular benefits. It was found that 25 to 50 grams of soy protein consumed on a daily basis can reduce cholesterol levels.

An analysis of 29 studies found that just 31 to 47 grams of isolated soy protein or texturized soy protein decreased total cholesterol by 9 percent and LDL cholesterol by 13 percent.

### ∾ Menopause

Soy is helpful for some women in reducing hot flashes and vaginal dryness. In one study, women were given 160 milligrams of isoflavones daily for three months. They experienced a significant reduction in their menopausal hot flashes and other menopausal symptoms.

### ∾ Osteoporosis

One study of postmenopausal women found that soy protein with high isoflavone content improved bone mineral density in the lumbar spine. Also, soy is a protein source that does not lead to urinary calcium excretion, as does protein from animal foods.

# Spirulina

The longer I practice natural medicine, the more I am impressed with the visible benefits of some specific nutritional supplements. From my experience with patients, and based on nutritional studies, there is no doubt that most people benefit from taking vitamins and minerals. Not only can a vitamin or mineral supplement help prevent deficiencies, it can also help to therapeutically treat existing conditions.

However, we still have a lot to learn about the bioavailability and absorption of the active components in these supplements. How much of the active or beneficial components are actually taken into the body? How quickly can we experience the benefits? We don't have much information about nutrient interactions. That is, we still have to determine what are the positive and negative interactions when certain vitamins and minerals are combined together.

But we do have some limited knowledge. For example, we know that vitamin C enhances iron absorption. We also know that iron hinders calcium absorption. So if you're taking a supplement that's high in iron, it makes sense that you'd also try to get more vitamin C to make sure you absorb as much iron as possible.

But while we're continuing to learn more about the vitamins and minerals we need—and how best to get them—we also know that many of the processes of absorption are almost infinitely complex. Rather than trying to "create" the perfect supplement, or the exact mix of vitamins, minerals, enzymes, and phytonutrients, we also need to consider whole foods for their healing powers.

One potent whole food actually comes in supplement form—and it's called spirulina. This is called a whole food supplement because the actual plant itself, rather than its chemical or nutrient components, are contained in the supplement pill, capsule, powder, or other form. In the case of spirulina, nature seems to have provided a particular combination of nutrients and disease-fighting substances that is greater than the sum of its parts. That is, we don't know the most active or effective ingredients in this whole-food supplement, but we do know that it carries health benefits that are definitely worth enjoying.

## SINK AND SWIM

Spirulina (rhymes with "ballerina"), is a blue-green algae that grows wild in warm-water alkaline volcanic lakes. It has long been a staple food for Mexicans going back to Aztec civilization. The two most common species used for human consumption include *Spirulina maxima* and *Spirulina platensis*.

Spirulina is also an important food for people in Eastern and Central Africa. For example, the people in the nation of Chad in Africa consume 9 to 13 grams of spirulina in each meal.

Today, commercial algae farms cultivate spirulina that is exported to millions of people in over 70 countries. The United States is the world's largest producer of spirulina followed by Thailand, India, and China.

Spirulina has great nutritional value. Between 62 and 71 percent of the plant is comprised of amino acids, and all are the essential amino acids. It is also a remarkable source of protein, and the protein is highly bioavailable, meaning it can be readily absorbed in the body with no harmful effects.

Spirulina contains beta carotene and a blend of the other carotenoids, as well as chlorophyll and the essential fatty acid GLA. It's also said to be the world's richest source of vitamin $B_{12}$.

## MOODY BLUE

One important component is phycocyanin, a phytonutrient that gives spirulina its dark blue-green color. Phycocyanin has been shown in animal studies to stimulate the production of red blood cells.

The probable reason why the bioabsorption is so great is that spirulina contains a soft cell wall composed of proteins and complex sugars that can be easily digested.

More than 100 published scientific references help support the case for the health benefits of spirulina. Some studies demonstrate that spirulina seems to possess anticancer effects and antiviral properties. Also, animal studies show that it is a powerful tonic for the immune system.

Spirulina activates many of the different immune cells, including macrophages, T-cells, B-cells, and natural killer cells. It also activates the organs involved with immune function such as the spleen, liver, bone marrow, lymph nodes, tonsils, and thymus gland. Naturopathic physicians often recommend it to treat high cholesterol, hypertension, and diabetes. It's also a popular product for detoxification.

Like other blue-green algae, spirulina is thought to help bind heavy metals, which is necessary before they can be excreted out of the body. In addition, it has been shown to increase the presence of beneficial bacteria such as *Lactobacillus* and *Bifidus* by acting as a "food" for these friendly flora.

Spirulina is also an important food supplement for children. It is used to prevent blindness in malnourished children. A recognized treatment for radiation sickness, it was given to children in the area of Chernobyl after the nuclear reactor.

## DOSAGE

Spirulina comes in many different forms: capsules, tablets, flakes, and powders. The average intake for adults is 2,000 to 3,000 milligrams per day. The typical children's dosage is 500 to 1,500 milligrams daily. I often recommend spirulina in a formula with other "super green foods" such as wheatgrass and chlorella.

## WHAT ARE THE SIDE EFFECTS?

The safety of spirulina has been well researched. There have been extensive safety studies with animals and humans since the 1970s. It was found to have no toxic side effects.

Spirulina is well tolerated with only occasional reports of allergies or sensitivity reactions. Reputable companies make sure the spirulina has not been taken from water where they might have absorbed heavy metals such as lead, mercury, aluminum, and arsenic. Good quality products are also tested to make sure the spirulina has not been contaminated by algal toxins from other blue-green algae.

Since raw material suppliers cultivate their own spirulina, they can control and test for heavy metals and algal toxins.

Spirulina does not increase the flare-ups of gout in people who are susceptible. That's surprising, because spirulina is high in nucleic acids and protein—which, theoretically, increase the flow of uric acid, one of the contributing factors in gout attacks. But even when spirulina is consumed in high dosages (such as 50 grams a day), it doesn't cause problems for people who have gout.

## SPIRULINA
### RECOMMENDATIONS FROM THE NATURAL PHYSICIAN FOR . . .

### ⌘ Anemia

Anemia is the deficiency of red blood cells. It can have various causes such as blood loss; insufficient bone-marrow production; or deficiencies of $B_{12}$, folic acid, or iron. Phycocyanin, a phytonutrient found in spirulina, has been shown in animal studies to stimulate production of stem cells by the bone marrow. Stem cells are immature cells, which later mature into red and white blood cells.

Spirulina also contains $B_{12}$. If absorption is sufficient, supplementing with spirulina may help prevent B12-deficiency anemia, which is a concern for strict vegetarians.

### ⌘ Cancer

Spirulina and its extracts have shown to have anticancer activity in animal studies. Spirulina stimulates natural killer cells and similar anti-immune components of the immune system that can help fight cancer cells. Laboratory studies also show that spirulina polysaccharides can work to repair genetic material that has been damaged from toxins or from radiation.

It may also help people who have mouth cancer. In one study, tobacco chewers who had a type of mouth disease called oral leukoplakia were given 1 gram a day of spirulina for one year. Nearly half of those who took the supplement showed marked improvement, while only 3 out of 43 in the non-supplement group had any reversal of symptoms.

### Cholesterol

Animal and human studies have shown spirulina to reduce high cholesterol. A study looked at the effect of spirulina supplementation on 30 healthy men with high levels of cholesterol, triglyceride, and LDL. One group of men consumed 4.2 grams daily for 8 weeks and researchers found a 4.5 percent decrease in cholesterol levels. For such a short period of time, that is considered to be a significant decrease in cholesterol.

### Detoxification

I have found spirulina to be a great supplement for helping patients with detoxification. The protein content also helps to stabilize blood sugar.

### Immunity

As mentioned, spirulina stimulates many components of the immune system. Special extracts of spirulina have also shown potent antiviral activity. One type of spirulina known as *Spirulina platensis* was shown to inhibit the HIV virus (HIV-1) in a test-tube study. Another study found a spirulina extract known as Calcium Spirulan inhibited the replication of several viruses. Among the viruses that it helped control were herpes simplex type 1, cytomegalovirus, measles, mumps, influenza A, and HIV-1.

### Malnourishment and Vitamin A Deficiency

Many authorities have recommended that spirulina be used on a large scale to combat world hunger because of its good nutritional value and cost effectiveness. Spirulina supplementation with children has been studied since the early 1970s with impressive results.

In a 1-year program, 5,000 preschool children who lived in a rural area near Madras, India were fed spirulina regularly. At the start of the program, all the children had the symptom of advanced vitamin A deficiency known as Bitot's spots. (This is a superficial foamy patch on the eye conjunctiva that mainly occurs in advanced vitamin A deficiency). During the program, the children consumed 1 gram of spirulina daily for at least 150 days. In many of the children, the Bitot's spots went away, indicating the vitamin A deficiency had been corrected. Whereas 80 percent of the children had the spots at the beginning of the program, only 10 percent showed any sign of Bitot's spots by the time the program was ended.

This is an important finding, as vitamin A deficiency is the leading cause of blindness, and among children who have severe vitamin A deficiency, the death rate can be as high as 50 percent.

In another study of 400 school children, researchers found that spirulina increased their vitamin A status to the same level as those who were administered pure vitamin A. Beta carotene (and perhaps some of the other carotenoids) from spirulina have a high bioavailability and are converted to vitamin A very effectively. Because spirulina contains essential amino acids—which few plant foods do—you get the vitamin A as well as the amino acids, all in one.

### Radiation Poisoning

As I've mentioned, spirulina was used to treat the children of Chernobyl who were suffering from radiation sickness as the result of eating food grown on radioactive soil. Since radiation sickness can produce bone-marrow damage, children with the sickness cannot produce enough red blood cells. They have a deficient immune system because the white blood cells are depleted, but along with that, they also become anemic because of the underproduction of red blood cells. This causes a susceptibility to allergies, infections, and cancer.

Remarkably, spirulina stimulates the production of both red and white blood cells. Children fed 5 grams of spirulina tablets daily have been shown to make dramatic recoveries, a striking contrast to the children who did not have access to spirulina.

# St. John's Wort

. . . . . . . . . . . . . . . . . . . . . . . . . . . . . . . . . . . . . . . . . . . . . . . . . . .

"I've been on Prozac for over a year now. I seem to be doing fine. I have my moments where I feel depressed, but don't we all?" said Tony, a 49-year-old money manager.

"Yes, that's part of life," I replied.

"My wife and I are concerned about side effects from Prozac. She feels it's the reason why my libido is so low. I'm worried about that as well as what I have read in the papers. I've heard it can sometimes cause suicidal depression!"

"Do you feel suicidal at times?" I asked.

"No, that was never a problem," replied Tony.

Then I asked, "Have you talked to your other doctor about getting off the Prozac?"

"Sort of. I brought it up and he kind of brushed me off, saying if I'm feeling good why go off it."

"Interesting. So you want to get off the Prozac?" I asked.

"Yes, I feel like this is a good time. Have you gotten other patients off Prozac?" asked Tony.

"I sure have." I went on to tell him how some patients were able to "wean themselves" off Prozac by using St. John's wort *(Hypericum perforatum).*

"I was going to ask you about that," said Tony. "My friend Tim says that St. John's wort works better than drugs to prevent depression."

"For some people it does. The other bonus is that it doesn't have the side effects like reduced libido," I replied.

"My wife will be happy when she hears that," said Tony with a smile.

I then explained that it is very important that he be monitored closely while switching over from the Prozac. Stopping the Prozac too rapidly could cause a rebound effect, sending him into very severe depression as his brain is deprived of the accustomed medication.

Tony was weaned off the Prozac over the next two months. It turned out to be a smooth transition for him. To prevent a reoccurrence of his depression, I also recommended he see a counselor to address underlying emotional problems. I felt these were at the root of his history of depression.

## AN ANCIENT HERBAL HEALER

North Americans have been using St. John's wort for the treatment of mild to moderate depression for the past 15 years. This trend began when clinical research from Germany was publicized. Supplement companies helped to broadcast the information, which was readily picked up in the media. Today, St. John's wort is one of the top ten best-selling herbs in the United States. In Germany, St. John's wort outsells pharmaceutical antidepressants.

More than 30 clinical studies have been done on St. John's wort, and several more are still underway, including some under the auspices of the National Institutes of Health.

St. John's wort is grown in many different areas, including North Africa, Europe, western Asia, Canada, Australia, China, and the United States (especially northern California and southern Oregon). The characteristic bright yellow flowers contain a red pigment, known as hypericin, which is one of the active constituents. When you get a "standardized" preparation of St. John's wort, it is standardized to hypericin. (That is, the preparation contains the percentage of hypericin that's stated on the label.)

The Latin translation of hypericum means "over an apparition." This refers to the belief that the scent of the herb would drive away evil spirits. Ancient Europeans believed that St. John's wort protected one against evil and disease.

Physicians in ancient times, such as Hippocrates and Dioscorides, used St. John's wort for depression as well as for burns, wounds, sciatica, ulcers, and poisonous reptile bites.

## BACK TO THE ORIGINS

The name "St. John's wort" is believed to come from Christian tradition. There are different theories as to how the name came about. One is that the plant blooms around St. John's Day, which is June 24. Another is that red spots appeared on the leaves during the anniversary of St. John's beheading. These were thought to symbolize his blood. Yet another is that if you put the herb under your pillow, St. John would appear in a dream and bless you, and prevent a loved one from dying the following year.

As with many herbs, St. John's wort appears to have many different active constituents. Early research focused on the standardization of products to hypericin. In recent years there has been a movement toward the standardization to another active substance, hyperforin.

It is also believed that flavonoids play an important role in the antidepressant action of this herb. Other important constituents include essential oils and pseudohypericin.

At least one study has shown that a combination of constituents is responsible for the potent antidepressive effect. It is interesting to note that isolated extracts of hypericin and hyperforin are not effective antidepressants by themselves. Both need to be present, as they are in St. John's wort.

St. John's wort appears to act like SSRI (selective serotonin reuptake inhibitors) antidepressants such as Prozac and Zoloft, as well as tricyclic antidepressants, such as amitryptiline and imipramine. It causes an increase in the neurotransmitter serotonin, a powerful chemical that is responsible for good moods. It has also been shown that St. John's wort increases the neurotransmitters dopamine and norepinephrine, which are also responsible for moods.

There are studies that have suggested that St. John's wort affects GABA receptor sites (a neurotransmitter known for its calming effect) and lowers the stress hormone cortisol.

## DOSAGE

For the treatment of depression, I recommend 300 milligrams of an extract to be taken three times daily. I recommend a product containing 3% to 5% hyperforin and 0.3% hypericin. People usually notice improvement within two to six weeks.

The tincture can also be used. I recommend taking 30 drops (approximately 0.5 milliliters) three times daily.

The oil is used topically for skin conditions.

## WHAT ARE THE SIDE EFFECTS?

St. John's wort has a good safety rating. However, one study reported that some people experienced digestive upset, fatigue, restlessness, and allergic reactions using St. John's wort extract.

A number of researchers have reported that St. John's wort may cause the skin to be sensitive to light. There have been a few reports of people's skin burning more easily, or of their eyes becoming more sensitive to light. I don't think it is a side effect to be overly worried about. If you have light skin, be more cautious in the sun; cover up with light clothing, and wear a hat as well as sunglasses.

I do not recommend St. John's wort for children unless it is used with the guidance of a doctor. There have been no studies done on children. However, if a child does need additional therapy beyond counseling, then St. John's wort seems like a better choice to me than a pharmaceutical antidepressant.

It is best to avoid this herb during pregnancy and while breast-feeding.

Do not combine St. John's wort with your pharmaceutical antidepressant as it could potentially lead to serious side effects. You need to be gradually weaned off your medication under a doctor's care.

Also, this herb should not be used if you are using the following medications: digoxin, cyclosporine, theophylline, warfarin, or the AIDS drug Indinavir.

# ST. JOHN'S WORT
## RECOMMENDATIONS FROM THE NATURAL PHYSICIAN FOR . . .

### ∾ Anxiety

St. John's wort has been found to be as effective as pharmaceuticals in treating anxiety.

### ∾ Bruises, Burns, and Wounds

St. John's wort has a long history of use for the treatment of bruises, burns, and wounds. The oil is applied topically and provides soothing relief as well as prevents secondary bacterial infections. It also helps to relieve nerve injuries and nerve pain. European herbalists also use the oil for the treatment of eczema.

### ∾ Depression

St. John's wort has been the subject of some of the best and most intensive clinical and scientific research among all the herbs in the world. I find that it is helpful in about 70 percent of people who take it for depression. This is quite a high response rate, whether a pharmaceutical or

natural therapy is used. In a review of 23 European clinical studies involving 1,700 patients, researchers found that St. John's wort was significantly more effective than placebo and equally as effective as standard drug therapy for mild to moderate depression.

Several studies have shown comparable effects when St. John's wort has gone head-to-head with pharmaceutical antidepressants. This includes two studies with the antidepressant imipramine. In the first study people took either 900 milligrams of St. John's wort or 75 milligrams of imipramine per day for 6 weeks. The St. John's wort users had a slightly better improvement and experienced fewer and milder side effects as compared with the imipramine group.

A similar study compared the two therapies but used double the amount of dosages. This study also looked at people with moderate to severe depression. People took either 1,800 mil-

*(continued)*

ligrams of St. John's wort or 150 milligrams of imipramine for 6 weeks. Improvements in depression were about equal. Again, side effects were more common in those taking imipramine. This study was important because it examined people with moderate to severe depression. Most studies have been done on people with mild to moderate depression. Further studies will clarify the value of St. John's wort for severe depression.

Overall, I would recommend that doctors start antidepressant therapy with St. John's wort instead of with pharmaceutical antidepressants. My reasoning for this is that St. John's wort has proven to have less risk of side effects. For people who do not respond to adequate trials and dosages of St. John's wort, pharmaceutical treatment can be considered.

Like pharmaceutical medications, St. John's wort works most effectively when combined with counseling, hormone balancing, nutritional therapy, exercise, and other holistic therapies that treat the underlying cause of the depression.

Some people have been diagnosed with "genetic depression" and told they must take pharmaceutical antidepressants, that natural therapies would not be strong enough. I have found that St. John's wort and other natural therapies are strong enough for "genetic depression."

### ❧ Seasonal Affective Disorder (SAD)

This is a condition where people experience depression and mood changes as the result of reduced light exposure during the winter. One small study showed that people who took St. John's wort in combination with either bright light or dim light therapy experienced significant improvement in SAD.

### ❧ Viral Infections

The constituents hypericin and pseudohypericin have shown in test-tube studies to have strong antiviral activity against herpes simplex virus—both Type 1 (mouth) and Type 2 (genital)—as well as influenza virus A and B, and Epstein–Barr virus.

# Sulphur

· · · · · · · · · · · · · · · · · · · · · · · · · · · · · · · · · · · · · · · · · · · · · · · · · · · ·

"I've had this rash all over my back and arms. One doctor calls it eczema and the next one calls it dermatitis."

There was confusion in Jeff's voice—but also a fair degree of outrage. A 40-year-old construction worker who had been trying to beat this problem for five years, he was obviously in search of some reliable answers.

"I've used creams and lotions," he recalled. "They usually help for a week or so, but after that, the rash comes back. It itches like mad. Sometimes I think it'll drive me crazy. I have problems getting to sleep as it is—and the itching always gets worse at night."

After we had discussed his dilemma for a few minutes, I inquired whether he was the type of person who often felt too warm.

"Oh yeah, it can be freezing outside and I won't need a coat. I sweat like a pig when it's warm out."

"Well, I'm going to prescribe homeopathic sulphur for you. It should help to clear up that rash for good."

"I'm ready to try anything," said Jeff.

When I saw Jeff six weeks later, his rash was completely gone. We were both impressed. He was sleeping better, too.

"It's hard to believe those little white pellets could make such a difference," Jeff commented.

"Welcome to the world of homeopathy!" I replied.

## MINERAL MAGIC

Sulphur is a mineral that's present in the foods we eat and the water we drink. It appears to be important for detoxification and for joint health. Historically, sulphur baths have been used as a means of detoxification and for healing. Homeopathic sulphur, a highly diluted preparation of this mineral, is one of the most important medicines used by homeopaths today.

Homeopathic sulphur affects many of the organs of the body. Specifically, it improves liver function and detoxification. It also has a profound effect on the entire digestive tract, stimulating healing. More important, sulphur works at the cellular level to stimulate cellular detoxification.

Homeopathic sulphur is used most commonly for skin ailments. This includes rashes, eczema, psoriasis, boils, cradle cap, and many other dermatological conditions. It is also an excellent remedy for digestive conditions such as ulcers, diarrhea, flatulence, and inflammatory bowel disorders. Sulphur is also a common homeopathic remedy for insomnia and headaches.

## WHAT CHARACTER

Each homeopathic remedy has its own set of characteristics, and seems to work best with people who fit a particular description. The sulphur "constitutional" picture is unique. There are generally two types of people requiring this remedy. First is the philosophical type. Described as a deep thinker who likes to let people know how smart he or she is, this philosophical type tends to be unkempt—since outward appearance is not important to him or her—and a loner.

The other sulphur "type" is more outgoing and social. This person loves to be around other people and is extroverted. Women who fit the constitutional type tend to be quick witted, leaders in their field, and, quite often, the leaders of their group or business. Children requiring sulphur are usually outgoing and are very curious, wanting to know how everything works and always asking "why?"

People requiring sulphur are almost always on the warm side. They sweat easily, prefer cool rooms, and often sleep with no blankets on (especially children).

They also tend to be thirsty, especially for ice-cold drinks.

There's also a profile for appetite. The sulphur type will have food cravings for sweets, spicy foods, fats, and alcohol, especially beer. I often see the strong craving for spicy foods with people who fit the sulphur constitutional type.

People requiring this remedy often are night people. They like to stay up late at night and prefer to sleep in when the morning comes.

## DOSAGE

If you need to clear up a rash that you've had only recently, I recommend taking two pellets of 30C potency twice daily for two to three days.

When taking sulphur as a constitutional remedy to strengthen the body as a whole, you can take two pellets of a 6C or 12C potency twice daily for two weeks and then stop. If you notice improvement, take the remedy as needed in the future for a few days as a "tune up."

## WHAT ARE THE SIDE EFFECTS?

Homeopathic sulphur is extremely safe. Side effects are uncommon. Some people with longstanding rashes or skin eruptions who take the remedy too frequently or in too high a potency may see their skin problems worsen. This occurs because the body is detoxifying too quickly. When they stop taking the sulphur, this reaction will stop. They may not even need to take it anymore as the detoxification process will have been initiated. From then on, they can take the sulphur less frequently (e.g., once every two days instead of daily) or use a lower potency (e.g., 6C instead of 30C).

# SULPHUR
## Recommendations from the Natural Physician for ...

### ❧ Attention Deficit Disorder

One 12-year-old boy I treated for this condition was completely cured by this remedy without other types of therapies.

I sometimes recommend sulphur for the related condition, Attention Deficit Hyperactivity Disorder.

### ❧ Digestive Ailments

Sulphur is indicated for many digestive disorders. Homeopathic doctors have found that it's especially likely to be effective if a person is prone to flatulence that has an odor like "rotten eggs."

Sulphur is commonly used for acute or chronic bouts of diarrhea, especially where there is burning. The diarrhea often occurs first thing in the morning. It is a common homeopathic for colitis, ulcers, and Crohn's disease.

### ❧ Fatigue

Sulphur can be an excellent remedy to bring the energy levels back up if the person fits the "constitutional type." It improves energy production through improved cellular detoxification.

### ❧ Headache

Sulphur is effective for headaches that occur only on the weekend and feel better after cold applications.

### ❧ Insomnia

Sulphur can be helpful for those who fall asleep for a few hours, then wake up and cannot fall asleep again. Peculiarly, those who are helped by sulphur prefer to sleep on their left side.

### ❧ Low Back Pain

Sulphur may help relieve a weak low back that is going out all the time, and also reduce the frequency of episodes.

### ❧ Menopause

Sulphur helps to cool down a person. It will bring relief from hot flashes associated with menopause.

### ❧ Skin Eruptions

The most common use of sulphur is for the various types of skin eruptions that people experience. These can range from a simple rash to a severe case of eczema, acne, or boils.

You'll know that there's a good chance of being helped with sulphur if the skin eruption is very red, inflamed, and extremely itchy. In fact, the itch can be so bad that you want to scratch it until it bleeds. The skin condition is worse from heat, bathing, touching wool, and at nighttime.

For nearly anyone with these conditions, sulphur soothes the skin and relieves the itching and sensitivity.

### ❧ Sore Throat

Sulphur can relieve a burning sore throat or chest infection. It's most likely to be helpful if you have the kind of burning sore throat or chest infection that feels better when you have ice-cold drinks, especially if you're very feverish.

# Symphytum

Symphytum is the homeopathic preparation of the herb comfrey, which has the interesting common name "bone-knit." That's precisely what the remedy and the herb can do—help heal broken bones.

Of course, if you've broken a bone, the first thing you do is go directly to the emergency room for evaluation and treatment. (On the way to the emergency room, however, I'd advise taking some arnica to help with the pain.) Once there, the bone will be set and put into a cast—and you might have surgery, if that's necessary. Homeopathic care comes later.

I encourage patients to come and see me after a fracture has been evaluated and set in a cast—but not before. Homeopaths in the past have reported that symphytum heals the bone so quickly that it should not be given until the fracture is set. (If the bone heals in the wrong position, then it would need to be rebroken and reset again!)

While helping to stimulate healing of the fracture, symphytum also reduces the pain. Other painkillers might still be needed, but at least the homeopathic remedy helps to take the edge off the pain. (At the same time, I often recommend other complementary treatments for fractures, including acupuncture and magnet therapy.)

Many people who take symphytum are surprised at how quickly their fractures begin healing—and so are their doctors. Some doctors have observed that fractures heal 50 percent faster among people who take symphytum during the healing process.

## DOSAGE

The typical dosage is a 30C potency taken twice daily for one week. Practitioners of homeopathy may give a single dose of a high potency such as 200C, 1M, or higher.

# WHAT ARE THE SIDE EFFECTS?

I have not read about or seen any side effects with symphytum.

## SYMPHYTUM
### RECOMMENDATIONS FROM THE NATURAL PHYSICIAN FOR . . .

#### ᗡ᠍ *Eye Injury*

Symphytum is a remedy to consider when there is blunt trauma to the eye or to the orbit (the bone that surrounds the eye). Typically, I'll try arnica first; if that doesn't give relief, I recommend symphytum instead.

#### ᗡ᠍ *Fracture*

While symphytum is the most common homeopathic remedy for healing fractures, homeopathic calc phos should be considered in the small percentages of cases where the bones do not unite together even after using symphytum. Not only does symphytum speed bone healing, it also helps to heal the soft tissue that covers the bone (the periosteum). It also helps treat pain, whether or not a fracture has occurred, such as when a soccer player has been kicked in the front of the lower leg.

In the case of fractures, however, it's important to note that symphytum should be accompanied by other natural remedies that encourage bone healing. I encourage patients to make sure they are on a proper diet and getting the nutrients that are required for bone healing, with special emphasis on calcium-rich foods such as broccoli, orange juice, and almonds. At the same time, it's important to avoid food products that cause the loss of calcium and other bone minerals. These culprits include caffeinated beverages such as soda and coffee.

I encourage people to avoid eating large amounts of red meat and to stop smoking. (For quicker bone healing, some of the most beneficial vitamins and minerals include calcium, magnesium, vitamin C, vitamin K, B vitamins, silica, and boron. I usually recommend a comprehensive bone formula or a high-potency multivitamin and a separate calcium/magnesium supplement, supplying at least 1,000 milligrams of calcium and at least 500 milligrams of magnesium.)

# Tea Tree Oil

"This toe fungus just won't go away," said Marlene, a 33-year-old patient of mine. "I tried a couple of antifungal creams for it and there was no improvement. One doctor recommended a prescription for an antifungal medication that you take internally, but after reading that it could damage my liver, I said forget it."

"Let me take a look." It didn't take long to ascertain that she had a very mild case. "Tea tree oil should clear that up," I suggested.

"Is that something I need a prescription to get?"

"Oh no, you can get it at any health food store as well as many pharmacies."

We discussed some of its properties, and then I described how to use it.

"First you need to cut your nails really short so that the tea tree oil can come in contact with the fungus. Then each morning and evening wash your feet with tea tree soap. Dry your feet, and then apply a few drops of tea tree oil to those three toes that have the fungus. You can use a cotton swab to apply it. Over the next four weeks the fungus should be killed by this treatment. The area of skin where you apply it will become dry and slough off."

"That's all I have to do?" asked Marlene.

"Pretty much. But I also want you to stay away from sugar products."

"So you think that will clear this up?"

"It should."

Another possibility was to use a bleach solution, but I would reserve that for a more serious case of the fungus. I suspected it wouldn't be necessary as long as she followed my initial recommendations.

Two months later Marlene was back for a return visit.

"Take a look," she said as she showed me her feet. "The tea tree oil really did work. I've been recommending it to my friends who have the same problem."

## A TREASURE FROM DOWN UNDER

Tea tree oil *(Melaleuca alternifolia)*, also referred to as ti tree oil, or cajeput oil, has become very popular for its antiseptic and healing properties to the skin. This oil comes from the leaves of the Australian *Melaleuca alternifolia* tree, and early settlers in Australia made tea from these leaves—which explains the origin of its most common name. But even before the arrival of Europeans, Aborigines of the area were well aware of the medicinal benefits of the oils from this tree.

Most of the research on the medicinal effects of tea tree oil has focused on *Melaleuca alternifolia* in the New South Wales area of Australia.

The first scientific investigations of tea tree oil began in Sydney in 1922 when a government chemist noticed the antiseptic effects of tea tree oil. Though the oils were potent, he observed, they were nontoxic and nonirritating. His initial investigations were followed up by numerous studies, especially in the years between 1922 and 1930. The benefits of this oil became so well established that it was included as standard medical issue in the Australian Army during World War II.

## ALL STEAMED UP

*Melaleuca alternifolia* oil is extracted from the leaves using a steam-distillation process that extracts only the essential oils. There are approximately 100 chemicals in tea tree oil. Two of the key active constituents are terpinen-4-ol and cineole.

A standard for tea tree oil was established in 1985. It requires a minimum content of 30% terpinen-4-ol and less than 15% cineole. Higher quality oils contain 40% to 47% terpinen-4-ol and 2.5% cineole. The balance between these two constituents is important, with a high-quality product having oils high in terpinen-4-ol and low in cineole. The oil has natural antiinflammatory, analgesic, antiseptic, and healing properties. It destroys bacteria, fungus, and viruses.

Tea tree oil can be used topically for almost any skin condition. Examples include acne, athlete's foot and fungal infections of the skin, boils, bruises, burns, cold sores, cuts, dandruff, insect bites, rashes, lice, and warts.

It can also be used for gingivitis and vaginitis.

# DOSAGE

Make sure to get a product that is 100 percent *Melaleuca alternifolia* oil. An organic product is best. Tea tree oil is generally used in one of three ways: topically, oral rinse, or inhaled.

### ∾ *Topically*

When used topically, the oil is placed on the skin. The oil itself can be used, or you can use a cream or gel formula. It can also be used in baths.

Do not apply tea tree oil on infants' skin. Do not use tea tree oil near the eyes.

### ∾ *Oral Rinse*

When using it as an oral rinse, dilute a few drops in water, gargle, and spit out. It can be used for conditions like gingivitis, toothaches or tooth infections, and sore throat.

### ∾ *Inhaler*

To inhale it, add a few drops of tea tree oil to a mister or steamer. You can also put a few drops on a tissue and smell it.

**Note:** Tea tree oil also makes a good disinfectant for washing clothes. Look for laundry detergents made with tea tree oil or add 5 to 10 drops in your washing machine with each load of laundry.

# WHAT ARE THE SIDE EFFECTS?

Tea tree oil is very safe for topical use. It is generally nonirritating and nontoxic. It has a pH balance that is almost neutral, so it is not caustic. As with any substance, however, some people could be sensitive to tea tree oil; it is not common but it has been reported in the literature. You can test your sensitivity by putting a couple of drops on your skin before going to bed and seeing if an irritation occurs by morning.

Pure undiluted tea tree oil should not be applied to the skin of children or pregnant or lactating women. These people should use a commercial cream or gel.

# TEA TREE OIL

## Recommendations from the Natural Physician for . . .

### ❧ Acne

Tea tree oil has become popular as a treatment for acne. It is applied most commonly as a gel or cream. One study showed that a 5 percent tea tree oil gel extract was comparable to benzoyl peroxide in the treatment of mild to moderate acne. Tea tree oil users experienced fewer side effects (dryness, burning, redness, and itching). Another technique is to dab the oil on the pimples with a cotton swab before bedtime.

### ❧ Athlete's Foot and Toe Fungus

Fungal infections of the feet (athlete's foot), toes, and toenails (onychomycosis) are very common and can be stubborn to treat. Tea tree oil has become a popular treatment for this problem.

One study compared 100 percent tea tree oil to the antifungal topical drug clotrimazole for the treatment of toenail fungus for a period of 6 months. Results indicated very similar results with the two treatments.

I usually have patients trim their toenails, wash feet with soap or tea tree soap, and then apply tea tree oil to the infected area. This needs to be repeated on a daily basis for weeks and sometimes months to eradicate the infection. Another technique is to add 10 drops of tea tree oil to 1 quart of warm water. Soak the feet for 10 minutes and then dry the feet thoroughly with a towel and hair dryer. Continue the treatment for at least six weeks.

Tea tree oil can also be used to combat foot odor (bromhidrosis).

### ❧ Cold Sores

Tea tree oil can be dabbed onto the sores at the first signs of an outbreak. This will keep the lesions under control and prevent the infection from spreading.

### ❧ Lice

Approximately 12 million cases of head lice infestation are discovered each year, mostly in preschool- and elementary school-aged children. Lice are extremely small parasites that live and feed on skin. For those seeking a natural, nontoxic approach to this irritating condition, try the following:

Mix 1 1/2 teaspoons of tea tree oil and 1 1/2 teaspoons of lavender oil into 4 ounces of olive oil or 4 ounces of your child's shampoo. Massage this mixture into the hair and scalp. Do not rinse. Cover the head with a shower cap until morning and then comb the hair with a fine-tooth comb. Add 5 drops of tea tree oil to the comb before using it to get out the eggs. Rinse hair and then blow dry for 5 to 10 minutes. (This helps to destroy the eggs.) Repeat this procedure for 7 days.

Tea tree oil can also be used in a shampoo to help treat dandruff.

### ❧ Mouth and Gum Infections

Tea tree oil is used for mouth and gum infections, including gingivitis and tooth abscess. Use it as a gargle by adding 3 drops of tea tree oil to 1 ounce of warm water. It can also be purchased commercially as a mouthwash. This treatment can also be used daily for bad breath.

### ❧ Skin Infections and Eruptions

Tea tree oil is excellent for the topical treatment of skin infections. It has been shown to be effective against many different types of bacteria and fungus, including *Staphylococcus aureus*, *Candida albicans*, and many others. It can be used in cream or gel form to treat skin infections such as acne, impetigo, and boils. It also helps to alleviate the infection and

*(continued)*

443

inflammation caused by insect bites. Its soothing and antiinflammatory properties make it helpful for burns and rashes such as eczema.

### ✎ Vaginitis

Tea tree oil solutions have been shown to be effective for vaginitis caused by *Candida albi-*

cans and trichomonas. This treatment should be done only under a doctor's care.

### ✎ Warts

Tea tree oil can be applied topically to warts as it has antiviral properties. It is especially useful for plantar warts.

# Turmeric

Nutritional science is very focused on the medicinal effects of common herbs and spices. Incredibly, many of these "food items" have powerful medicinal effects. Turmeric *(Curcuma longa)* has created a lot of excitement in the natural medicine world. It exhibits excellent antiinflammatory and antioxidant effects. It also appears to have cancer-protective effects, promotes digestion, and protects the liver and cardiovascular system.

Turmeric is a member of the ginger family. The rhizome is the part that is used and is cured (boiled, cleaned, sun-dried, and polished). It has long been cultivated in India, China, and other tropical countries. India is the major producer of turmeric, responsible for 94 percent of the world's production.

Turmeric has been used in Asian culture throughout the ages for many different purposes including as a spice, dye, food preservative, and medicine. Many of the medicinal uses have come out of Ayurvedic and Chinese medicines—treating liver disease, digestive problems, painful menstruation, and as a poultice for sprains and arthritis. In the West, it has become a major ingredient in curry powder, and it's also a coloring agent for prepared yellow mustard.

## MELLOW YELLOW

Turmeric has many different active constituents. One group of these constituents that is thought to be important for its antioxidant and antiinflammatory properties is curcuminoids. Curcuminoids give turmeric its bright yellow-orange color (which makes for a good dye).

Curcumin is one of the curcuminoids that has been the focus of a lot of research. Its antioxidant activity is comparable to that of vitamins C and E. Similar to capsaicin in cayenne, curcumin depletes substance P so that pain messages are not sent through the nerves.

Turmeric also contains volatile oils, which contribute to its medicinal effects.

## NATURAL BENEFITS

It is not fully understood how turmeric reduces inflammation in the body. Researchers feel that curcumin and the volatile oils play a major role in this. Studies confirm that these turmeric extracts have potent antiinflammatory effects.

For example, one study examined 40 men with swelling and tenderness of the spermatic cord following surgery for a hernia or hydrocele. At the end of the 6-day study, it was found that curcumin was nearly identical to the antiinflammatory medication phenylbutazone in reducing inflammation.

Turmeric and its constituent curcumin also reduce cholesterol levels and increase the good HDL cholesterol. It reduces the levels of lipid peroxides (oxidants that can initiate atherosclerosis). The turmeric inhibits platelet aggregation, which is thought to prevent the risk of stroke.

## DOSAGE

Turmeric is excellent to use in the diet. As a supplement, the typical adult dosage is 450 to 600 milligrams of curcumin, but you can take up to two grams a day. Use it liberally as a spice in food.

## WHAT ARE THE SIDE EFFECTS?

Turmeric is quite safe as a spice and supplement. However, pregnant women should not use it in supplement form. Also, people with gallstones should check with their doctors before using it, as it stimulates bile production. People taking blood-thinning medications should check with their doctors before using turmeric as a supplement.

# TURMERIC
## RECOMMENDATIONS FROM THE NATURAL PHYSICIAN FOR . . .

### ∾ *Arthritis*

Turmeric extract is commonly found in arthritis supplements to reduce pain and inflammation. A study of people with rheumatoid arthritis found that taking 1,200 milligrams of curcumin per day for two weeks significantly improved morning stiffness, joint swelling, and walking ability.

This is important because natural antiinflammatories like curcumin do not have the toxicity that standard conventional antiinflammatory drugs have. I like to use nutritional formulas containing curcumin to reduce pain and inflammation while treating the underlying cause of the disease—such as poor digestion, nutritional deficiencies, diet, hormone imbalance, stress, and lack of exercise.

### ∾ *Cancer*

Turmeric and curcumin suppress the cancer-causing effects of mutagens and carcinogens such as tobacco smoke and other chemicals. A study of smokers who took a supplement of 1.5 grams of turmeric a day had reduced urinary excretion of mutagens (substances that cause damage to cell DNA which can lead to cancer formation).

### ∾ *Digestive and Liver Problems*

Turmeric has a long history of use for digestive problems. It stimulates bile production and reduces intestinal gas. Also, curcumin protects the liver cells from toxins as a result of its antioxidant properties. It is also used to lower elevated liver enzymes. For these reasons, it is often included in digestive formulas that target the liver and gallbladder.

### ∾ *Infection*

Studies have shown that turmeric inhibits the growth of several bacteria as well as fungi. I especially recommend it for respiratory tract infections and for hepatitis.

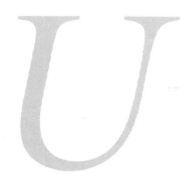

# Uva Ursi

· · · · · · · · · · · · · · · · · · · · · · · · · · · · · · · · · · · · · · · · · · · · · · · · · · · · ·

"I think I have a urinary tract infection. I feel burning when I go to the bathroom and feel feverish today."

Karen, my 25-year-old patient, also looked feverish—and a quick check with the thermometer confirmed that she had a low-grade fever. My suspicions were confirmed when the nurse came by a few minutes later with the results of the urinalysis. The report indicated that there were bacteria in her urine—a moderate amount, but still, they were there.

I let Karen know that I'd send out for a culture just in case she needed antibiotics. "But I really want to avoid antibiotics if possible," I went on.

Karen agreed with me. She'd had yeast infections in the past, and if she took antibiotics there was a good chance the drug would lead to a new flare-up. (Antibiotics knock out the "good" bacteria that help control yeast as well as the "bad" bacteria that cause infection—and yeast can begin to thrive if they aren't naturally controlled by your body's healthy supply of bacteria.)

"I know antibiotics could bring back that yeast problem," Karen acknowledged. Clearly, neither of us thought antibiotics were a good idea.

"The trick is to get the infection under control in the first forty eight hours," I told her. "We especially want to make sure this infection doesn't spread to the kidneys."

"Should I drink cranberry juice?" asked Karen.

"Unsweetened cranberry juice would be fine to take, but I find it works better for the prevention of urinary tract infections rather than actually treating them."

I had other recommendations. "I want you to drink lots of water, at least eight tall glasses a day. And I don't want you eating any sugar products while we're treating you for this. Sugar can suppress the immune system. Also, I want you to take some herbs that help to eradicate the infection."

At that point, I told her about uva ursi. I also told her my experience with it—that I had seen evidence that it could help eradicate bacteria in the urinary tract very quickly.

During the next two days, Karen reported that the burning she experienced during urination was dramatically reduced. A week later, she had a repeat urinalysis, and the test didn't turn up any signs of infection.

I kept Karen on uva ursi—as well as a number of other bacteria-fighting herbs—for another week. I just wanted to make sure the infection was completely gone. Only when the urinalysis continued to be negative did we decide to stop the treatment.

## BERRY USEFUL

Uva ursi *(Arctostaphylos uva ursi)*, also known as bearberry, is one of the best herbs for treatment of urinary tract infections. The leaves, long used by practitioners of herbal medicine, have antiseptic effects. The leaf extract is also a diuretic, helping to remove excess liquids from the body. As a popular home remedy, uva ursi was traditionally used for treatment of bladder and kidney infections, and kidney stones. It was also recommended for treatment of bronchitis.

In my own practice, I most often recommend it for treatment of urinary tract infections, bladder infections, and even kidney infections. Uva ursi is considered to be an astringent. It is slightly sweet tasting and has cooling and drying properties.

Uva ursi leaves contain a substance known as arbutin, which is converted to hydroquinone. This acts as an effective antimicrobial agent.

Uva ursi also works to make the urine more alkaline, which improves the effectiveness of hydroquinone. But there are many other active substances as well—including flavonoids, tannins, phenolics acids, volatile oil, resin, and gallic and egallic acid.

## DOSAGE

For acute urinary tract infections, the dosage is 500 milligrams of the capsule (10% to 20% arbutin) or 60 drops (1 milliliter) of the tincture taken four times daily. It should not be taken with anything that will acidify the urine.

## WHAT ARE THE SIDE EFFECTS?

Because the effects of uva ursi have not been thoroughly researched as yet, I do not recommend that pregnant or breast-feeding women take it without the advice of a doctor. It should also not to be given to children under age 12.

Digestive upset, such as nausea and vomiting, can occur in some people. Those with kidney disorders should not use it. Very high dosages may cause tinnitus (ringing in the ears), vomiting, delirium, difficulty breathing, convulsions, and loss of consciousness. Do not take more than the recommended dosage as given in this section unless you are seeing a practitioner who is familiar with the herb.

---

## UVA URSI
### RECOMMENDATIONS FROM THE NATURAL PHYSICIAN FOR . . .

**∾ Kidney Stones**

A number of physicians and researchers have reported that uva ursi can be helpful for the prevention of kidney stones.

**∾ Urinary Tract Infections**

I recommend uva ursi for any infection of the urinary tract. I usually combine it in formulas with herbs such as echinacea, goldenseal, buchu, marshmallow, and usnea. A number of companies produce variations on this formula for people who have urinary tract infections.

# V

# Valerian

· · · · · · · · · · · · · · · · · · · · · · · · · · · · · · · · · · · · · · · · · · · · · · · · · · · · · · · · · · · · · · · · · · · ·

There were lots of reasons why Steve couldn't sleep. A 40-year-old lawyer who worked long, grueling hours under intense pressure, he'd always had trouble winding down after work. He'd also recently been through a divorce. This was a man with a lot on his mind—and it all conspired to throw a monkey wrench into his sleep patterns.

Wisely enough, he had talked to a doctor. But he was reluctant to accept the doctor's advice.

"My sister said Valium could be dangerous," he admitted.

I was not at all surprised to hear him mention one of the most often-prescribed drugs for anxiety. But I was quick to reassure him that there were many other options.

"There are a lot of natural approaches we could use to help with the anxiety and insomnia. Are you seeing a counselor?" I asked.

"Yes, just started last week," replied Steve.

"Good, that will be very helpful. While you are working on the emotional issues, I'd like to recommend a natural medicine to help you cope better. My first choice is the herb valerian for a situation like yours. It does not have significant side effects."

I also observed that it wasn't "dangerous" in the way that Valium could be. No one, in my experience, had ever become addicted to valerian—while new cases of Valium-addiction were cropping up every day.

Several days after he left the clinic, Steve reported that the valerian was working for him. He was taking it nightly to help him sleep, and he'd found that it also helped to reduce anxiety during the day.

## FROM SEIZURES TO SHELL SHOCK

Valerian *(Valeriana officinalis)* was used by the ancient Greeks and Romans to treat menstrual cramps, seizures, digestive problems, and other common health conditions. Europeans used it during the sixteenth century for anxiety and insomnia, and it was also prescribed to ease digestion.

After World War I, physicians favored it for treatment of shell shock. Then during World War II, when England endured the bombings, Londoners would take valerian to help them sleep.

Valerian is used in Ayurvedic medicine for the treatment of hysteria, neurosis, and epilepsy. It's considered a "warming herb" in Chinese and Ayurvedic medicines. Early American physicians, known as the Eclectics, learned of the use of valerian from English colonists. Today, valerian is approved for over-the-counter distribution in pharmacies throughout Germany, France, Belgium, Italy, and Switzerland—countries where doctors regularly prescribe the herbal remedy.

## TRAVELS WITH VALERIAN

Though it was first found in northern Asia and Europe, today *Valeriana officinalis* is cultivated in many parts of the world, including North America. The roots and rhizomes are collected for medicinal use.

Over 200 species of valerian are used to treat a very wide range of ailments that include not only insomnia, anxiety, and stress, but also pain, hypertension, menstrual cramps, muscle spasms, and stress-related digestive disorders.

It is not clear how valerian works to promote relaxation. According to one theory, valerian has an effect that's similar to Valium's, but without the side effects of Valium such as impaired mental function. Another theory holds that valerian contains the neurotransmitter GABA, which has a calming effect on the brain, or that it somehow influences GABA concentrations in the brain.

Also, some researchers believe that valerian has an effect on serotonin levels similar to antidepressant drugs such as Prozac. Volatile oils, valepotriates, valeric acid, and velerenic acid are all constituents of valerian that may contribute to its sedative effects. In the most recent experiments, however, scientists have focused on the effects of valeric acid.

## DOSAGE

If you're using valerian to treat insomnia, take the herb 30 to 60 minutes before you go to bed. You can take it two to four times throughout the day for treatment of stress and anxiety.

The recommended dose of tincture is 30 to 60 drops (0.5 to 1.0 milliliter). If you prefer the capsule or tablet, I recommend between 300 and 500 milligrams. Valerian also makes a tea, though some people strenuously object to its flavor.

Valerian combines well with the herbs scutellaria, kava, lemon balm, and passionflower for relaxation.

## WHAT ARE THE SIDE EFFECTS?

While valerian does not, generally, produce the "hangover effect" that people usually get from Valium, some people seem to be very sensitive to it and may feel very groggy after taking valerian. I've also noticed that a small percentage of people find it stimulating.

These reactions would be considered completely understandable in traditional Chinese medicine. Valerian is a warming herb, so if you take it by itself, the herb may cause too much "heat." This would explain why it overstimulates those who already—again, in Chinese medicine terms—are constitutionally warm.

A small number of people may experience stomach upset. If you take a dose that's too high, you may have symptoms that include blurred vision, change in heartbeat, headache, nausea, and uneasiness. Lowering the dose will probably alleviate these side effects, but by all means, avoid taking high doses if you intend to drive or operate machinery.

Valerian should never be combined with tranquilizers or antidepressant medications—and you should never discontinue these prescription medications without consulting your doctor. If you're taking medications, be sure to talk to your doctor before you take any dose of valerian.

## VALERIAN
### Recommendations from the Natural Physician for . . .

**∾ Anxiety and Depression**

One study found the combination of valerian and St. John's wort to be equivalent to the antidepressant drug amitryptiline, but without the side effects such as dry mouth and lethargy.

**∾ Digestive Problems**

Valerian can be helpful for digestive conditions associated with stress, such as irritable bowel syndrome (IBS).

**∾ Hypertension**

I like to add valerian to herbal hypertension formulas to help relax the nervous system. Stress and anxiety can play major roles in high blood pressure for some people.

**∾ Insomnia**

I find that valerian works well for many people to help alleviate insomnia. Those who have sleep disturbance due to anxiety and stress seem to be particularly well served by this herb, and several clinical studies confirm that valerian is effective for insomnia.

In a scientifically controlled study that involved 121 people who had insomnia, researchers studied the effects of 600 milligrams of valerian that was administered in tablet form. Not knowing whether they were getting the herbal treatment or an inactive placebo, all participants took tablets one hour before bedtime for 28 days. When the results were analyzed, researchers saw that people who took valerian reported significant improvement in their feelings of being rested after sleep. They also reported better sleep quality than those taking the placebos, with better dream recall and less daytime fatigue.

Reported side effects in the study were rare.

**∾ Menstrual Cramps**

Valerian has been historically used to help relieve the pain of menstrual cramps. It is commonly included in menstrual cramp formulas.

**∾ Muscle Spasms**

I readily recommend valerian for relief from muscle spasms in combination formulas.

**∾ Stress**

While valerian does not treat the cause of someone's stress, it can be used to help calm the nervous system so that one can cope more effectively and deal with the underlying cause.

# Vanadium

Paul, a new patient of mine, had just been diagnosed with Type 2 diabetes.

"What's the deal with vanadium?" he asked me bluntly.

I wasn't surprised. It had been in the news. One of Paul's relatives had mentioned it to him—but he wasn't about to try it without doing his homework first. So he had come to me.

Quickly, I gave him a rundown of this trace mineral and what it was said to do. "Trace mineral simply means that you require it in very tiny amounts," I explained. "There have been a few studies in recent years showing that it helps to lower elevated blood-sugar and cholesterol levels."

"Should I use it instead of chromium?" asked Paul.

"I wouldn't advise it. But if someone has diabetes, it makes sense to take chromium *along with* vanadium. Both help to normalize blood-sugar levels. In fact," I added, "many blood-sugar–related nutritional formulas already contain vanadium."

Understandably enough, vanadium started to gain attention as the evidence mounted that this substance could help with blood sugar and cholesterol metabolism. Animal studies show that high dosages improve the mineralization of bones and teeth, adding calcium and other minerals that improve bone density.

There is still a lot more to learn about the role of vanadium in the human body. For instance, though we know it helps lower blood-sugar levels, the mechanism that makes that happen is still under investigation.

There's some speculation, about vanadium, too. One theory holds that vanadium helps insulin transport glucose more effectively in the cells.

But whatever the exact role of vanadium, researchers feel that this trace mineral is probably an essential nutrient for humans.

Food sources of vanadium include shellfish, mushrooms, dill, black pepper, soy, corn, and cereals.

# DOSAGE

Studies have used a form of vanadium that's combined with another substance to create vanadyl sulfate, which is an excellent form for absorption. The usual dose used in studies is 300 milligrams per day of vanadyl sulfate. With regard to elemental vanadium, up to 100 micrograms daily is thought to be safe.

# WHAT ARE THE SIDE EFFECTS?

There is not a lot known about the side effects of vanadium and there have not been any long-term human studies to investigate adverse effects. Digestive upset was the main side effect in one human study where vanadyl sulfate was used. If you're taking a diabetes medication, it's essential to consult with your doctor before you start taking vanadium.

## VANADIUM
### RECOMMENDATIONS FROM THE NATURAL PHYSICIAN FOR . . .

**∾ Type 2 Diabetes**

This is the only condition for which vanadium seems to be a particularly effective treatment. Small human studies involving vanadium have all been done with people who have noninsulin-dependent diabetes (Type 2). The most recent study involved 16 people with Type 2 diabetes, who were studied before and after they had been treated for 6 weeks with vanadyl sulfate at three different dosages (75, 150, and 300 milligrams). The signs of blood-sugar problems decreased significantly in those taking 150 and 300 milligrams of vanadyl sulfate.

# Vitamin A

"Is there anything else I can take for this bronchitis? The herbs I've been using just don't seem to be working," said Simon, a 29-year-old patient of mine.

"Yes, let's get you on some vitamin A. Take 50,000 IU for the next two days and let's see how you do."

A few days later, Simon called to report that he was doing much better. "The vitamin A seems to be working."

I have so often seen marked improvement using vitamin A—particularly for respiratory tract infection—that I agree that this deserves the name of "antiinfective vitamin."

Vitamin A, which is also called retinol, is important for normal growth and development. It can improve vision, and it also provides benefits for the immune system. I've recommended this vitamin to improve health of epithelial tissue, which includes mucus membranes, lining of the digestive system, lungs, urinary tract, vagina, and skin. In addition, it has antioxidant activity.

Vitamin A also benefits the brain and nervous system. Researchers have also discovered that children need vitamin A in order to learn properly. That's an important fact, with global implications, since an estimated 190 million children worldwide have a vitamin A deficiency.

## GETTING ALL A'S

Food sources of vitamin A include beef liver, chili peppers, carrots, sweet potatoes, parsley, kale, spinach, mangoes, broccoli, and squash. Milk and butter are commonly fortified with vitamin A, as well.

Carotenoids, such as beta carotene, found in foods or taken as a supplement, are converted into vitamin A—so any orange or yellow-colored fruit or vegetable, or any dark-green type of lettuce—is potentially a good source of vitamin A because it's a source of carotenoids.

The Recommended Daily Allowance (RDA) of vitamin A is as follows:

Under 1 year: 1,875 IU (375 RE)

1–3 years: 2,000 IU (400 RE)

4–6 years: 2,500 IU (500 RE)

7–10 years: 3,500 IU (700 RE)

Males 11 years to adult: 5,000 IU (1,000 RE)

Females 11 years to adult: 4,000 IU (800 RE)

**Note:** RE stands for retinol equivalent, which is just one kind of common, comparative measurement of this particular nutrient.

Severe vitamin A deficiency can cause a wide range of health problems, from eye inflammation and blindness to impaired growth, weight loss, improper tooth and bone formation, and reduced resistance to infection. While most people in the United States have access to plenty of foods that can provide vitamin A, some people do suffer from deficiencies because their bodies don't absorb the nutrient properly or because they're on very low-fat diets.

Vitamin A is especially important for growth and development and proper immune function in children. Vitamin A supplements are associated with a significant reduction in mortality. When given to impoverished children who had been deprived of the nutrient, vitamin A literally saves lives.

## DOSAGE

Multivitamin supplements often contain vitamin A or beta carotene in the amount of 1,500 to 5,000 IU. (If it's in the form of beta carotene, it's converted into vitamin A once you take the supplement.) This is adequate to take as a preventative dosage.

Higher amounts may be needed for therapeutic levels to treat specific diseases. For example, 50,000 IU is usually recommended for the short-term treatment of a respiratory tract infection.

I wouldn't advise any higher dosages unless you're under the guidance of a nutrition-oriented doctor. It's especially important to not take high dosages for long periods of time.

Vitamin A is best taken with meals for better absorption.

## WHAT ARE THE SIDE EFFECTS?

Vitamin A is a fat-soluble vitamin and gets stored in the tissues. High amounts taken over prolonged periods of time can result in toxicity.

An overdose of vitamin A can produce symptoms of vomiting; joint pain; abdominal pain; bone abnormalities; dry, cracking skin; headache; gingivitis; irritability; and fatigue. Symptoms disappear after you stop taking the supplement.

Tolerance to high vitamin A dosages varies. For example, 50,000 IU taken by an adult for several months or years may result in toxicity. If you're taking any amount higher than the RDA, I recommend consulting with a doctor.

Pregnant women should be extremely cautious. Vitamin A can cause birth defects if you take a very high dose. It is advised that pregnant women take vitamin A supplements below a dosage of 5,000 IU.

People with liver diseases such as cirrhosis or hepatitis should use vitamin A with caution as it can build up to toxic levels more easily.

Children can safely handle the amounts found in a children's multivitamin. They should not use vitamin A supplements on a long-term basis, however, unless under the supervision of a doctor.

## VITAMIN A
### RECOMMENDATIONS FROM THE NATURAL PHYSICIAN FOR . . .

### ❧ Acne

High dosages of vitamin A can be helpful for acne but should be used only under the direction of a nutrition-oriented doctor, as side effects can become a problem. When other supplements—such as vitamin E, zinc, and selenium—are used, a much lower dosage of vitamin A can be taken so that side effects are not an issue.

The common acne drug Accutane is actually a synthetic version of vitamin A.

### ❧ AIDS

Anyone with AIDS may benefit from vitamin A supplementation. One study found that vitamin A deficiency is associated with many people who are HIV positive. Researchers have found that vitamin A can improve the immune function—in particular, raising the concentration of CD4 T-cells.

### ❧ Dry Eyes

Practitioners of natural medicine find that vitamin A eyedrops can help alleviate dry eyes. Check with your local pharmacist for the special eyedrops known as Aquasol A.

### ❧ Night Blindness

If you have trouble with night blindness, the condition could be related to a vitamin A deficiency. For people who are having this problem, I usually recommend zinc in combination with vitamin A. An ideal combination is 5,000 to 10,000 IU daily of vitamin A along with 50 milligrams of zinc.

### ❧ Respiratory Tract Infections

I have found that vitamin A works well for respiratory tract infections such as bronchitis and pneumonia. It is particularly good to help improve immune function against viral infections.

# Vitamin C

"It's winter time again. I wonder how many colds and infections Jeremy and Tim will get?" pondered Samantha, the mother of two boys in grade school.

"Do they get sick a lot in the winter?" I asked.

"Yes, it seems like they come down with something every other week," replied Samantha.

"Why don't you give them each some extra vitamin C? I know they already take a children's multivitamin, but I have found that a little extra vitamin C—100 to 200 milligrams—can make a big difference in reducing the amount of colds and infections for kids in the winter. They'll love the chewable vitamin C. Just make sure they rinse their mouths with water afterwards because the acidity can be hard on their gums and tooth enamel."

I went on to recommend vitamin C for Samantha and her husband as well. "You two can take an extra 500 milligrams each day," I noted. "It won't hurt and it will probably be helpful."

Five months later, Samantha reported that her boys had considerably fewer colds and sick days as compared with other winters. She also noted that she had fewer episodes of sinusitis since taking the vitamin C.

## C CHANGE

Vitamin C (ascorbic acid) is one of the most widely used supplements in the world. Interestingly, while most animals can manufacture their own vitamin C, humans need to get it from their diet or as a supplement.

Many animals have an enzyme that converts glucose to vitamin C. Goats, for example, can produce up to 13,000 milligrams of vitamin C a day. Unfortunately, a number of animals lack this ability, including humans, guinea pigs, a type of fruit-eating bat from India, and a songbird called the red vented bulbul.

Historically, humans experienced great suffering before learning about vitamin C. Severe vitamin C deficiency caused scurvy, a condition that devastated people who didn't have access to fresh fruits or vegetables (the best natural sources of vitamin C). Sailors on long voyages, who went months without eating fresh food, often had all the symptoms—bleeding gums, skin hemorrhage and easy bruising, weakened bones, poor wound healing, susceptibility to infection, and depression. Numerous shipboard deaths were attributed to scurvy, even before the cause was known.

As far back as 1227, an explorer by the name of Gilbertus de Aguilla began advising sailors to carry fruits and vegetables on trips to avoid scurvy. But this was considered off-the-cuff advice until, in the mid 1700s, a British physician by the name of James Lind conducted an experiment and found that sailors who ate lemons and oranges were able to reduce the effects of scurvy.

Vitamin C was first isolated from the red pepper in 1928 by Albert Szent-Gyorgi. For this he was awarded the 1937 Nobel Prize for Medicine.

Today, new attributes of vitamin C are still being discovered.

## Getting Your Vitamin C

Vitamin C is found mainly in plant foods, particularly in fruits and vegetables. Citrus fruits, tomatoes, peppers, dark green leafy vegetables, broccoli, kale, strawberries, and potatoes are all rich in vitamin C. The Recommended Dietary Intake (RDI) for vitamin C are as follows:

| | |
|---|---|
| Infants: | 6 months and younger—40 milligrams |
| | 7–12 months—50 milligrams |
| Children: | 1–3 years—15 milligrams |
| | 4–8 years—25 milligrams |
| Males: | 9–13 years—45 milligrams |
| | 14–18 years—75 milligrams |
| | 19 and older—90 milligrams |
| Females: | 9–13 years—45 milligrams |
| | 14–18 years—65 milligrams |
| | 19 and older—75 milligrams |
| Pregnant women: | 18 years and younger—80 milligrams |
| | 19 years and older—85 milligrams |
| Lactating mothers: | 18 years and younger—115 milligrams |
| | 19 years and older—120 milligrams |

**Note:** Smokers should add an additional 35 milligrams to their RDI.

While you'll never be deficient in vitamin C if you meet these minimum levels, your needs for optimum health may actually be higher. For example, if you're exposed to environmental pollutants or already have a disease that requires extra vitamin C—such as heart disease, arthritis, cataracts, or cancer—you should take more. Vitamin C is nontoxic and very safe for people who can benefit greatly from higher dosages.

# HOW IT WORKS

Vitamin C is an important antioxidant. A water-soluble antioxidant, it protects cells and cholesterol from oxidative damage. It helps to regenerate vitamin E in the body and is one of the few supplements that can elevate red blood cell levels of glutathione, another one of the body's potent antioxidants. It also prevents premature aging of the skin, cataract formation, and many other conditions related to free-radical damage.

It is also critical for the liver's ability to detoxify substances that get into the body. It does this by acting as an antioxidant and increasing the levels of glutathione.

As is true of many antioxidants, vitamin C is important for reducing the risk of heart disease. Vitamin C prevents oxidation of cholesterol, which is a major factor in the formation of atherosclerosis.

Vitamin C is required for the production of collagen. This is a type of protein that forms the connective tissue that holds our skin together. Collagen is also an important component of cartilage, tendons, ligaments, bone, and blood vessels.

Also, vitamin C strengthens the capillaries and may be helpful for those who bruise easily. It generally helps people to recover from bruises more quickly.

The immune system requires vitamin C to work properly. The late Dr. Linus Pauling touted vitamin C as a cure for the common cold, and a number of studies have since shown that it does help prevent and reduce the severity and length of the common cold.

Vitamin C is very concentrated in white blood cells, the most critical components of the immune system. This vitamin increases the activity of those cells and improves antibody response—that is, the way those cells fight against invading microbes. Vitamin C also increases interferon—an antiviral chemical produced by the body that is required to manufacture protective hormones and also needed to help fight cancer.

## DOSAGE

The dosage for vitamin C depends on the individual. People who regularly consume fruits and vegetables generally do not require vitamin C supplements. A general recommendation for adults requiring supplements is 500 milligrams daily.

For those with conditions such as cancer, weakened immunity, diabetes, and cataracts, a much higher dosage is recommended. For acute infections such as the common cold, you can take 500 to 1,000 milligrams every two to three hours. Most people can take 2,000 milligrams daily without side effects. Doctors can use intravenous vitamin C for the treatment of serious conditions such as cancer or hepatitis.

It is best to take vitamin C in divided doses during the day.

Vitamin C works synergistically with other antioxidants such as vitamin E. Therefore, it makes sense to take it as part of antioxidant or multivitamin formulas.

Vitamin C is available in capsule, crystal, powder, and tablet forms. Most people do fine with regular ascorbic acid. However, the combination of vitamin C with bioflavonoid mixtures is more effective, providing that there is an adequate amount of bioflavonoids. For example, 250 to 500 milligrams of bioflavonoid milligrams complex per 500 milligrams of vitamin C will improve the effects of vitamin C.

Some people are sensitive to regular vitamin C. The acidity upsets their stomach or causes heartburn. This is a problem for people who have general citrus fruit sensitivity. If you have this problem, I recommend taking buffered vitamin C, where the acidity is reduced by combining calcium, potassium, sodium, or magnesium with ascorbate. The calcium ascorbate form is probably the best. (Another option that works well is to use Ester-C®, although this is more expensive.)

Skin creams and topical liquid serums that contain vitamin C are now available. These products fight wrinkling of the skin. Look for a product that contains 10 percent vitamin C stated on the label.

## WHAT ARE THE SIDE EFFECTS?

Vitamin C is nontoxic. However, if people ingest too much, they suffer diarrhea and digestive upset. This is reversible when the dosage is reduced.

If you need to take high dosages of vitamin C, you can try increasingly larger doses every day. You'll know you've reached the maximum level of toleration if you start to have diarrhea. If that occurs, just cut back the dose to a more comfortable level. The diarrhea stops immediately. This is known as "bowel tolerance."

There has been concern about high dosages of vitamin C causing kidney stones. This appears to be unwarranted. In fact, one study showed that men who consumed 1,500 milligrams daily were less likely to get kidney stones than those who consumed less than 250 milligrams. Urinary oxalate—the mineral that goes into the make-up of kidney stones—doesn't increase unless you're taking more than 4,000 milligrams daily, which would be a very high dose.

---

# VITAMIN C
## RECOMMENDATIONS FROM THE NATURAL PHYSICIAN FOR . . .

### ❧ Allergies and Asthma

If you're allergic to environmental pollutants, you may also be more prone to getting asthma. Vitamin C works to reduce the allergenic response, though I usually find it works best in combination with other antioxidants. Anyone with asthma is more susceptible to respiratory tract infections, but you can reduce the risk by supporting the immune system with vitamin C. Anyone with asthma, including children, should take vitamin C and antioxidant supplements.

In one study, people with asthma received 1,000 milligrams of vitamin C for 14 weeks, and their health was compared with others with asthma who were taking a placebo. Those receiving vitamin C had 73 percent fewer asthma attacks than those receiving placebo. Also, the asthma attacks the vitamin C users had were less severe than the ones experienced by people taking the placebo.

Another study, done in Italy, analyzed the diets and respiratory health of 19,000 children ages 6 to 7. Children who consumed the most vitamin C-rich fruit were 36 percent less likely to experience wheezing.

### ❧ Arthritis

Vitamin C has natural antiinflammatory properties that make it effective for all different types of arthritis. It is required for the production of cartilage and prevents joint destruction due to its antioxidant properties. I find it most helpful when used as part of an antioxidant formula or nutritional arthritis formula.

### ❧ Cancer

Many studies show that a diet rich in vitamin C is protective against many different types of cancer. Vitamin C protects the genetic material in cells—

*(continued)*

their DNA—from damage. This is significant because researchers think DNA damage is one of the leading reasons why people have cancer.

Vitamin C also supports proper functioning of the white blood cells and immune cells, which help keep cancer cells in check. In addition, it is an important component of general detoxification. To the extent that you can detoxify your liver and other body organs, you help to metabolize or "burn up" some of the cancer-causing chemicals and excrete them from your body.

Many nutrition-oriented doctors recommend vitamin C-rich foods, supplementation, and even intravenous treatments.

### ∾ Cataracts

Vitamin C is important in preventing cataract formation. It prevents oxidation in the lens of the eye, and the oxidation process is what contributes to formation of cataracts.

### ∾ Common Cold

Many studies have confirmed that vitamin C reduces the length and severity of the common cold. I find it works best when people load up on it at the first signs of symptoms and take it consistently for the next 48 hours.

### ∾ Diabetes

Vitamin C and glucose compete to get into the cells, and glucose usually wins. Thus, people with diabetes who are prone to diabetes often have a vitamin C deficiency. If you have diabetes, you need to eat foods that are rich in vitamin C, and you may need to take supplements as well to help prevent such complications as poor wound healing, bruising, and high cholesterol. For anyone with diabetes, I'd recommend a minimum dose of 500 milligrams of vitamin C, taken twice daily.

### ∾ Gallstones

An increasing amount of research is showing that vitamin C reduces the risk of developing gallstones. It activates an enzyme that breaks down cholesterol into bile acids—which is significant because gallstones occur when your blood is too highly saturated with cholesterol. In one study that included more than 13,000 women, researchers found that those who consumed the greatest amount of vitamin C had a 39 percent lower risk of developing gallstones.

### ∾ Gingivitis

If you have gum inflammation and your gums seem to bleed easily, it's an indication that you might be suffering marginal vitamin C deficiency. Extra supplements can help improve this condition.

### ∾ Glaucoma

This disease is characterized by increased pressure within the eyeball. Vitamin C is one of the supplements that has been shown to help decrease the pressure.

### ∾ Heart Disease

Numerous studies have demonstrated that vitamin C reduces the risk of cardiovascular disease. It prevents the oxidation of LDL cholesterol and lipoproteins, which are often the precursors of atherosclerosis or "hardening of the arteries." Vitamin C also raises the good HDL cholesterol.

A higher level of vitamin C is also associated with lower blood pressure. Since elevated blood pressure is one of the greatest risk factors for heart disease, the more you can bring it down, the better.

Third, vitamin C strengthens the collagen in the artery walls, which means that the walls become sturdier and less susceptible to scarring. (Cholesterol buildup seems to be worst—and

*(continued)*

the danger of blockage the greatest—in areas where the artery walls have been scarred.)

In a UCLA study, researchers discovered that men who took 300 milligrams of vitamin C each day had a 45 percent lower risk of heart disease than men who took less than 49 milligrams daily. This well-publicized study, published in *The Journal of the American Medical Association* in 1997, first looked at the short-term effect of a high-fat meal on the arteries. Researchers found that healthy people who were given a high-fat meal and supplementation of 1,000 milligrams of vitamin C and 800 IU of vitamin E had no negative effects in blood flow through the arteries. By comparison, those who ate a high-fat meal *without* taking these two supplements had blood flow that was negatively affected for up to four hours after eating the fatty meal.

### ∾ Hepatitis

Vitamin C is commonly recommended by nutrition-oriented doctors for people with hepatitis, especially the B and C types. It activates the immune system's white blood cells, which helps keep the hepatitis virus under control.

### ∾ Infections

Vitamin C can be used as an adjunctive therapy for pretty much any type of infection as it supports normal functioning of the white blood cells.

### ∾ Macular Degeneration

The antioxidant properties of vitamin C make it important for the prevention of this eye disease.

### ∾ Male Infertility

Vitamin C protects against DNA sperm damage and prevents sperm cells from clumping together. One study examined a group of men with infertility due to sperm agglutination (clumping). Some were given 500 milligrams of vitamin C twice daily. Within three weeks, researchers found that the sperm clumping was reduced, and thus the number of normal cells increased.

There was another interesting result. Pregnancy occurred in the wives of all the men who took the vitamin C for two months. No pregnancies occurred in the wives of the men who were not given vitamin C.

### ∾ Osteoporosis

Vitamin C is necessary for proper bone health. It is one of the many vitamins required to prevent and treat osteoporosis, as well as to heal fractures.

### ∾ Pregnancy Complications

Vitamin C appears to be one of the important nutrients for preventing preeclampsia, a condition that can be potentially fatal to the mother and infant.

### ∾ Stress

Vitamin C is one of the more important nutrients to help your body cope with stress. It not only acts as an antioxidant and improves immune status, it is also involved in the production of stress hormones by your adrenal (stress) glands.

### ∾ Sunburn

As an antioxidant, vitamin C helps to retard some of the harmful effects of the sun's ultraviolet rays. This makes it useful when taken internally and used topically.

### ∾ Wounds

I find that skin wounds such as cuts, burns, and even bedsores heal more quickly if you take extra vitamin C supplements.

### ∾ Wrinkles

New research is showing that vitamin C creams may be helpful in reducing wrinkles.

# Vitamin D

• • • • • • • • • • • • • • • • • • • • • • • • • • • • • • • • • • • • • • • • • • • • • •

"Here's what I'm taking for my bones. What do you think?"

Marla had placed a number of supplements on my desk, including calcium, magnesium, ipriflavone, and boron. All of these were appropriate, but I had one more to recommend—vitamin D.

There were two reasons for my recommendation. Marla already had mild osteoporosis and she lived in northern Canada. When people live that far north, they usually need supplementation for reasons I was about to explain to her.

"Right now you are getting only 200 IU a day. You need closer to 800 IU. Remember, you're spending a lot of time indoors during the winter and when that happens, you just don't get enough sunlight. Sunlight is converted in your skin to vitamin D. So keep doing what you are doing with your diet, exercise, and supplements, and boost your vitamin D."

There are two main forms of vitamin D—vitamin $D_2$ (ergocalciferol), and vitamin $D_3$ (cholecalciferol). vitamin $D_2$ is the type added to milk and other foods. The type that's most commonly used in nutritional supplements, it is derived from plant foods.

Vitamin $D_3$ is found in animal foods such as fish, oils, and eggs. This is also the kind that's produced by human skin when your skin is exposed to sunlight.

## Getting Your D's

People can become deficient in vitamin D from poor dietary intake. Strict vegetarians may be more prone to such deficiency.

A number of different kinds of fish are particularly good food sources of vitamin D, including salmon, herring, mackerel, and sardines. Other sources are butter, egg yolks, and vitamin D-fortified milk. Most plant sources are low in vitamin D, but you can glean some from mushrooms and dark green leafy vegetables.

Fifteen minutes of direct sunlight daily is recommended. Be aware that sunscreen blocks the UV rays from activating vitamin D synthesis.

The Recommended Daily Allowance for vitamin D is as follows:

Infants under one year of age: 300 IU

Children ages 1–10: 400 IU

Males 11–24 years: 400 IU

Males 25 and older: 200 IU

Females 11–24 years: 400 IU

Females 25 and older: 200 IU

Pregnant women: 400 IU

## IN HIGH DEMAND

Vitamin D has several functions. Most important, it promotes calcium absorption and enhances bone mineralization. But it also performs a kind of "blood rescue" function. If blood levels of calcium are too low, a form of vitamin D, synthesized in the kidneys, helps draw some calcium and phosphorous from the bones and deliver these crucial minerals to the blood, bringing blood-calcium levels up to snuff.

Since the liver and kidneys are involved in the activation of vitamin D, diseases of these organs can cause vitamin D deficiency-related diseases.

The symptoms of severe vitamin D deficiency are quite extreme. Children can get a condition called rickets, evidenced by bowed legs, knock-knees, softening of the skull bones, spinal curvature, and increased joint size. In adults, a deficiency can result in osteomalacia, which means softening of the bone. This is more common in people who are not exposed to sunlight or women who have had a number of closely spaced pregnancies—which can deplete a mother's reserves of vitamin D.

It also appears that people lose some of their ability to produce vitamin D from sunlight as they get older. Studies show that people over the age of 61 produce only one-fourth the amount of vitamin D from ultraviolet rays as do people who are under 31 years of age.

Children, especially, need to get enough vitamin D, as good bone density in childhood is associated with a reduced likelihood of developing osteoporosis when they grow into adulthood.

It has also been shown that breast-fed infants who received vitamin D supplements during the first year of life had increased bone density in later childhood.

## DOSAGE

With osteoporosis so prevalent in our society, it is important to get adequate amounts of this bone-enhancing vitamin. The typical recommendation has been a dosage of 400 IU of vitamin D. It is now being recommended that adults with signs of osteoporosis take 800 IU daily. This is especially important for the elderly, for those who are beginning to show signs of osteoporosis (a bone density test will tell the story), or if members of your family have had osteoporosis.

People in nursing homes and people who are hospitalized are particularly susceptible to a deficiency and must take vitamin D supplements.

Certain drugs are known to cause vitamin D deficiency, including anticonvulsants, cimetidine (Tagamet®), corticosteroids, heparin, and diuretics.

A multivitamin containing vitamin D is recommended for children. It should contain 200 to 400 IU of vitamin D.

## WHAT ARE THE SIDE EFFECTS?

Prolonged supplementation of vitamin D above dosages of 1,200 IU may result in side effects such as calcification of internal organs, soft tissue damage, kidney damage, kidney stones, digestive upset, and headaches.

If you have hyperparathyroidism or sarcoidosis, you should not take vitamin D supplements unless your doctor instructs you to do so.

Certain cautions should be observed if you are taking certain drugs. If you're taking cholesterol-lowering drugs—such as cholestyramine and colestipol—that prevent bile acid reabsorption then you shouldn't take vitamin D within an hour *before* you take the medications, nor within 6 hours *after* taking the medication. Also, don't take mineral oil within two hours of taking vitamin D—*either* before or after. You should also not take any vitamin D supplements at any time if you're taking the drug verapramil.

---

# VITAMIN D
## RECOMMENDATIONS FROM THE NATURAL PHYSICIAN FOR . . .

### ᴓ *Osteoporosis*

Though vitamin D is always necessary for good health, it's particularly critical for prevention and treatment of osteoporosis.

Several studies have shown that the combination of calcium and vitamin D is more effective in slowing bone loss or increasing bone density than calcium alone. One study examined 249 healthy postmenopausal women with an average age of 61. All the women received a calcium supplement, bringing their total combined dietary intake to 800 milligrams a day. Half the women received 400 IU of vitamin D and the other half a placebo. Bone density was measured three times over the course of one year. The group receiving the calcium only (calcium citrate malate) had no bone loss over the course of the year. The women who received additional vitamin D supplementation along with the calcium had a significant gain in bone density of the spine.

Lactating mothers should take 400 IU of vitamin D.

# Vitamin E

"My doctor said I could take vitamin E if I wanted to. He said there would be no harm in doing so but that it would likely not be of much benefit either," said Joe, a 45-year-old teacher who was concerned about preventing heart disease. He had an important reason for being concerned about this particular health problem. His father had died of a heart attack at the age of 53.

"I would say those cautions are a little outdated," I observed. "Vitamin E is not a magic bullet, but it is one of the best—if not *the* best—vitamins to take to help prevent heart disease."

"How much should I take?"

I noted that the multivitamin he was already taking contained 200 IU of vitamin E. My recommendation was an additional, separate supplement containing 400 IU of natural vitamin E, bringing the total to 600 IU daily. (Vitamin E is measured in International Units, typically expressed as "IU.")

"Why 600 IUs? Isn't that too high?"

"There's no danger taking 600 IUs," I replied. "I find that somewhere between 400 and 800 IU is a good dosage for someone with a high susceptibility to heart disease."

There was no way I could guarantee that Joe would outlive his father. But given the strong evidence that vitamin E can be helpful as a preventative for heart disease, Joe was reassured to be taking a supplement that was rarely prescribed in his father's day.

## THE E IN GREENS

Vitamin E was first discovered in 1922 when researchers found that an unknown substance in green lettuce prevented rats from miscarrying. It was later isolated in wheat germ oil in 1936. Vitamin E is often referred to as alpha-tocopherol, which is the most biologically active form of the tocopherols.

The term tocopherol translated from Greek means "to bear children." Therefore, vitamin E has been referred to as the "fertility" or "antisterility" vitamin.

Vitamin E is very important as the body's most important fat-soluble antioxidant. It prevents cell membranes and cholesterol from becoming damaged by the process of oxidation, which is similar to the chemical process that leads to rusting in metal and rotting in fruit and vegetables. Vitamin E is important for a healthy immune system, cardiovascular disease protection, and cancer prevention.

People with certain diseases, such as diabetes and Parkinson's disease, should always have extra vitamin E supplementation—and there's ample research to support this view. But there are, in addition, many other conditions for which vitamin E can be helpful, ranging from arthritis to skin wounds.

Athletes require additional antioxidant support from the free radicals generated by exercise. Vitamin E is important for reducing muscle inflammation and soreness from strenuous exercise.

A severe vitamin E deficiency is rare in North America, except in infants who are born prematurely and in adults who require kidney dialysis. But people who have cystic fibrosis may lack vitamin E because they can't absorb it properly, and vitamin E deficiencies have also shown up in some people who have genetic disorders such as sickle cell disease.

Symptoms of a vitamin E deficiency can include nerve problems, muscle weakness, anemia, and poor coordination. More commonly, people in our society experience less overt symptoms of vitamin E deficiency—the kinds of slow-developing problems that tend to lead to health problems over prolonged periods of time. These include heart disease, skin problems, and a weakened immune system.

## GETTING YOUR VITAMIN E

Vitamin E is found in the fats of vegetables. Polyunsaturated vegetable oils such as wheat germ oil contain high amounts of the tocopherols. Interestingly, vitamin E is found in nature in foods that contain high amounts of polyunsaturated fatty acids (such as safflower oil, corn oil, and soybean oil), which help protect the foods against rapid oxidation. Theoretically, then, we would get vitamin E from commercial vegetable oils—but unfortunately they're so altered in processing that they have little vitamin E left by the time they reach the shelves of the store. The same holds true for most grains, which start out with vitamin E, but are depleted as they're processed into the flours that are used in most breads and other baked goods.

Vitamin E is also found in nuts, seeds, whole grains, legumes, and dark green leafy vegetables. Animal products, however, are poor sources of vitamin E.

Tocotrienols are also a part of the vitamin E family and are found in foods such as cereal bran, rice bran, wheat bran, and oat bran.

## DOSAGE

I recommend that adults get an average of 400 IU natural vitamin E daily. Some people (those with a history of heart disease or cancer) may require a higher dosage such as 800 IU daily.

Vitamin E works better in the presence of vitamin C, lipoic acid, and coenzyme Q10.

More research is being done on "mixed vitamin E." Different types of tocopherols found in mixed vitamin E include alpha, beta, gamma, and delta.

The dosage for tocotrienols for a healthy person ranges from 20 to 80 milligrams daily. Those with high cholesterol may need dosages as high as 400 milligrams. (Tocotrienols can be purchased as a separate supplement for people needing very high dosages.)

Always choose the natural form, which is d-alpha tocopherol, as opposed to the synthetic version, which is d'l-alpha tocopherol. So, if it has an "l" in it, then "leave" it alone. Although it costs more, the natural form is more available to your body tissues.

Vitamin E is available in what is called the dry form—an oil-free powder that is water-soluble. According to the Shute Institute, a leading center for vitamin E research, the dry form is particularly well absorbed.

## WHAT ARE THE SIDE EFFECTS?

Vitamin E is quite safe when used at a dosage of 1,200 IU and lower, although studies have shown it to be safe even at 2,000 IU. The major caution for vitamin E is for those taking blood-thinning medications. If you're taking coumadin as a blood thinner, or if you regularly take aspirin for any reason, consult with your doctor first before taking a vitamin E supplement.

I find that my patients who take these medications can safely take vitamin E in lower dosages such as 200 to 400 IU, as long as they are monitored with blood-clotting tests.

# VITAMIN E

## RECOMMENDATIONS FROM THE NATURAL PHYSICIAN FOR . . .

### ✍ Acne

I have found that vitamin E helps teenagers and adults with mild to moderate acne.

### ✍ AIDS

Vitamin E is an extremely important antioxidant for people with AIDS. Studies have shown that those with this disease are often deficient in vitamin E and that taking vitamin E helps to slow down the progression of the disease.

### ✍ Alzheimer's Disease

Although the cause of Alzheimer's disease is unknown, research is showing that free-radical damage in brain cells accelerates progression of this disease. Vitamin E protects against cell oxidation.

In a study done in the late 1990s, researchers found that vitamin E supplementation reduced the risk of reaching the most severe stages of Alzheimer's disease as compared with those taking standard drug therapy or placebo. I recommend vitamin E and the other major antioxidants for those who have or are suspected of having this disease.

### ✍ Angina

Vitamin E is recommended by nutrition-oriented doctors to help prevent and treat angina. I always combine it with other heart-healthy nutrients such as CoQ10, magnesium, and herbs such as hawthorn, ginkgo, and cactus.

### ✍ Arthritis

Vitamin E appears to have a natural antiinflammatory effect and can be helpful for persons suffering from different types of arthritis, particularly rheumatoid arthritis.

### ✍ Burns, Wounds, and Scars

Vitamin E promotes the healing of burns and wounds to the skin. It is excellent to take internally and to apply externally to prevent scarring or reduce newly formed scars. You can open up a capsule of the mixed form of vitamin E gel capsules to apply to scars or purchase creams that are rich in vitamin E.

### ✍ Cancer

Studies have shown that people with low vitamin E levels are more susceptible to different types of cancers. Vitamin E appears to be especially important for the prevention of prostate and lung cancer.

Tocotrienols have been shown to be important for the prevention and treatment of cancer, especially breast cancer. Gamma tocopherol has been shown to be important for the prevention of lung cancer for those who smoke.

### ✍ Carotid Stenosis

Tocotrienols appear to be one of the few effective options to surgery for carotid stenosis, the buildup of plaque that narrows the carotid artery blood flow to the brain. The surgery for carotid stenosis (carotid endarterectomy) is quite dangerous, with a 1 in 10 risk of stroke and death. So it's much preferable to try to avoid the necessity of such surgery by taking tocotrienols.

In one 4-year study, people with severe carotid stenosis were given either tocotrienols or a placebo. Analysis with ultrasound showed that 94 percent of those taking tocotrienols improved or stabilized. None of those given placebo improved, and half got worse. This

*(continued)*

**471**

study offers some hope for a nonsurgical treatment for this serious condition.

### ᔆ Cataracts

Cataracts occur as the result of oxidation of the lens in the eye. Vitamin E is one of the important antioxidants that can help to prevent this condition.

### ᔆ Diabetes

Vitamin E has been shown to improve glucose tolerance in people who have diabetes. In addition, it helps to protect against nerve damage associated with free radical damage caused by the disease.

### ᔆ Eczema

Vitamin E taken both internally and applied externally can be helpful to reduce eczema.

### ᔆ Fibrocystic Breast Syndrome

I have found that women with this condition respond very well to a dosage of 800 IU of vitamin E.

### ᔆ Heart Disease

The most popular use of supplemental vitamin E is for the prevention of heart disease. Vitamin E prevents the oxidation of cholesterol, which is a leading culprit in the buildup of atherosclerotic plaque in the arteries.

Polls of cardiologists have shown that nearly 50 percent take vitamin E themselves. The Cambridge Heart study of 2,000 patients with heart disease found that those who took between 400 to 800 IU of vitamin E had a 77 percent decrease in cardiovascular disease over a year's time. In a Nurses Health study involving 87,000 women, doctors learned that women who took vitamin E for two years or more had a 41 percent reduction in the risk of heart disease.

Women taking 200 IU had more protection than those taking 100 IU.

A further study was conducted with 11,000 seniors, ages 67 to 105, over a 9-year period. Doctors found that those who took a vitamin E supplement of 400 IU daily had a 41 reduction in heart disease. Results were even better when people took vitamin C in addition to vitamin E.

Vitamin E also helps to reduce another important marker of cardiovascular disease. C-reactive protein is an inflammatory marker—and inflammation of the blood vessels sets the stage for artery disease. Elevated C-reactive protein levels are associated with a 4.5 times increased risk of having a heart attack. Vitamin E also reduced another marker of inflammation known as interleukin-6 by 50 percent.

Vitamin E has natural blood-thinning properties; this is thought to be why it helps to improve circulation as well as prevent strokes. In one study, where people took 600 IU of vitamin E daily for two weeks, researchers found immediate evidence that the vitamin delayed blood clotting—a good indication that it was acting as a blood thinner.

### ᔆ High Cholesterol

Vitamin E prevents the oxidation of cholesterol, particularly the "bad" LDL cholesterol. It also increases the "good" HDL cholesterol in young adults who have abnormally low HDL levels.

Rice bran tocotrienols are proving to be powerful in their ability to lower cholesterol (especially LDL) and increase the protective HDL cholesterol.

Many researchers feel that tocotrienols are a much better choice than cholesterol-lowering drugs, which can be toxic to the liver and cause other side effects. A dosage of 400 milligrams of tocotrienols is recommended for those with abnormal cholesterol levels. *(continued)*

### ∾ Infections

Vitamin E is one of the many nutrients required for a healthy immune system. People with chronic infections such as hepatits or those with susceptible immune systems may benefit from taking vitamin E supplements.

### ∾ Macular Degeneration

Studies have shown that vitamin E can help prevent and improve this eye disease, which is a leading cause of blindness.

### ∾ Menopause

Vitamin E helps to reduce hot flashes as well as vaginal dryness in menopausal women. Studies have shown that vitamin E in dosages of 400 to 800 IU reduces the frequency of hot flashes.

Also, taking a vitamin E supplement during this transitional time is important as the risk of heart disease increases greatly with the hormonal changes.

### ∾ Multiple Sclerosis

I recommend that people suffering from this autoimmune disease take a vitamin E supplement to help prevent relapses.

### ∾ Parkinson's Disease

Researchers speculate that free radicals—the electrically charged molecules that speed up oxidation—play an important role in Parkinson's disease. Since vitamin E is one of the antioxidants that helps control free-radical activity, it should be included in a comprehensive treatment program.

### ∾ Peripheral Vascular Disease

As a natural blood thinner, vitamin E helps to improve blood flow to the hands and feet.

# Vitex

"My menstrual cycle is out of control! It's been irregular for the last five years."

When I asked Sherry, a 24-year-old nurse, to explain what she meant, she described a menstrual cycle that did, indeed, seem out of control. One month her menstrual flow might last twenty days; the next month, only seven.

"Sometimes I go a month or two without a period," she continued. "It's so frustrating! My gynecologist wants to put me on the birth-control pill and that's the last thing I want to take. I want to get pregnant in the near future. Anyway, a friend of mine told me that you helped her out with a similar problem. She said that you could balance hormones naturally."

"Yes, usually. Are there any other hormone-related symptoms or conditions you have?" I suspected that she might also have PMS, ovarian cysts, or other problems.

"I have mood changes and breast tenderness for three or four days each month. My husband calls me the PMS monster during this time. I have had cysts show up on my pelvic ultrasounds in the past. Do you have different treatments for all these things?" Sherry asked.

"It's all pretty much the same treatment," I said. "Once we balance your hormones, most of these problems should clear up."

I wanted Sherry to appreciate that hormones are very powerful chemicals. If they were out of balance, some major problems could occur, exactly like the ones she was having.

"Based on what you've told me about your menstrual pattern, it appears that you are not ovulating regularly," I observed.

"That's what my gynecologist said, too," replied Sherry.

I explained that while the birth-control pill often helps to regulate the menstrual cycle—because of the estrogen and progesterone it contains—it does not help ovaries to ovulate. In fact, it actually prevents ovulation.

"So we need to regulate your cycle and make sure you're ovulating regularly," I concluded. "I have had good results in cases like this with the herbal extract vitex, commonly called chasteberry. It helps to increase the pituitary gland's release of luteinizing hormone, which then stimulates the ovaries to ovulate. You get a release of progesterone once this happens, so that ultimately you have a balance between estrogen and progesterone, and the menstrual cycle balances out."

"And it will also help my fertility because I will be ovulating," Sherry added.

"Yes. In fact, I have found it helps some cases of infertility related to anovulation (no ovulation)."

Sherry began taking vitex extract every day.

By the second month, her period was lighter than usual and she was less irritable than she had been during previous cycles. After five months of continuous use, Sherry began having regular menstrual cycles. Each period occurred once a month and lasted about 5 days. Also, she no longer had a problem with breast tenderness.

I asked Sherry to continue taking vitex for another five months.

Soon after, she reported that she was pregnant. I cannot say she became pregnant because of vitex—as there is no way to prove that—but I do know that vitex has definitely helped other women who wanted to become pregnant.

# A HISTORY OF HELPING

*Vitex agnus-castus,* also known as chasteberry or chaste tree, is the most important herb for women in western and European herbal therapy. If I were limited to one herb for women's health, vitex would be the one I would pick, as it is so versatile. It can help acne, fibrocystic breast syndrome, infertility, lactation, menopausal hot flashes, menstrual disorders, ovarian cysts, and premenstrual syndrome. In other words, it is a woman's best herbal friend.

The long history of medicinal use dates back to the fourth century B.C., when Hippocrates wrote about the capabilities of this remarkable herb. In fact, the terms "chasteberry or chaste tree" were originally applied to this plant because people believed that it somehow made chastity easier. To Ancient Greeks, vitex was an appropriate symbol of chastity to display during festivals that honored the goddess Demeter.

Later, the Christian Church adopted a similar type of symbolism. Vitex was the plant of choice for the pathway to the monastery that monks would follow during their initiation. The herb was thought to restrain the libido of monks who might go astray. (Whatever its effect on men, however, vitex has no reported dampening effect on *women*'s libido.) The practice of planting vitex along the monastery pathways continues to this day in Italy.

Another common name for vitex is "monk's pepper." The vitex fruit smells like pepper and was used as a spice on monastery meals.

Vitex does not contain hormones. Rather, it acts on a part of the brain known as the hypothalamus and the pituitary gland (located in the brain) to increase the production of luteinizing hormone (LH). LH is responsible for stimulating the ovaries to ovulate.

When ovulation occurs, there is a release of progesterone during the second half of the cycle. This is important to maintain a balance with estrogen. Many women do not ovulate on a regular basis, and therefore have a relative higher elevation of estrogen to progesterone, referred to as "estrogen dominance." By helping to normalize progesterone levels, vitex promotes hormone balance. This is why it is effective for so many female conditions, which are in large part caused by an estrogen–progesterone imbalance.

Also, vitex has been shown to lower levels of prolactin. This hormone, which is also secreted by the pituitary gland, is associated with PMS, irregular menstrual cycles, and infertility.

# DOSAGE

I most often use the capsule form of vitex. I have had good results with a dosage of 80 to 240 milligrams (usually one to three capsules) of a 0.6% aucubin extract. Products containing 0.5% agnuside are also frequently used. There is no agreed-upon standardization for vitex. It is generally recommended that the product contain 30 to 40 milligrams of the dried fruit, and that it be taken daily.

Clinical studies have used 40 drops of a standardized tincture extract taken once a day in the morning, so that's probably the minimum dose for effectiveness. However, I sometimes recommend 40 drops of the tincture form to be taken three times daily.

Vitex is best used on a long-term basis. Women may notice improvements within two menstrual cycles; however, it often needs to be taken for a minimum of four to six months. Long-standing conditions such as infertility, amenorrhea, irregular menstrual cycles, or endometriosis may require vitex supplementation for a year or longer.

# WHAT ARE THE SIDE EFFECTS?

Vitex is quite safe. In rare cases, there may be mild digestive upset, nausea, headaches, and skin rash. Vitex should not be taken by women who are also taking birth-control pills. Also, you should not take vitex if you're also taking drugs that block dopamine receptors, such as haloperidol.

So far, we don't know whether vitex interferes with hormone replacement that is given for menopause, so caution should be used. I have, at times, had women use vitex who were on hormone replacement, and none of them reported problems.

As with most herbs, it is best avoided during pregnancy, although some herbal practitioners recommend it for the first trimester for women who have a history of miscarriage due to progesterone deficiency.

Some women experience an "adjustment phase" with vitex during the first few months of use. During this phase, the cycle shortens or lengthens. Menstrual flow can become lighter or heavier than what it was previously. This "adjustment phase" almost always normalizes after three to four months of use.

# VITEX

## Recommendations from the Natural Physician for . . .

### ॐ Acne

Acne is a hormone-dependent condition. As a hormone balancer, vitex is especially effective in reducing menstruation-related acne.

I have also found it to work well for teenage acne, for both boys and girls. They can usually see improvement in a few months.

### ॐ Amenorrhea

Vitex is one of the most specific herbs to use for amenorrhea. It has been used mainly in cases of secondary amenorrhea (where there has been menstrual flow in the past but it has stopped).

There can be different causes of amenorrhea—lack of ovulation being one of them. This is the type that vitex is indicated for, since vitex increases the production of LH by the pituitary gland to stimulate ovulation and progesterone production.

Vitex also reduces elevated levels of the hormone prolactin by binding to dopamine receptors of the pituitary gland, where prolactin is secreted. A study of 52 women who did not ovulate due to high prolactin levels found that vitex extract taken for three months reduced prolactin levels. As a result, the progesterone levels were normalized as well as the cycle itself.

### ॐ Fibrocystic Breasts and Breast Pain

Benign breast cysts are very common, and women frequently turn to their gynecologists when they have cysts. Often, the first sign is an increase in sensitivity or pain right before menstruation. This is thought to be a result of estrogen dominance.

I have found vitex to eliminate or improve benign breast cysts and cyclical breast pain. Again, this usually takes up to three months to be effective and up to six months for some women.

A study of 104 women who suffered from premenstrual breast pain found that vitex extract significantly reduced breast pain. Improvements were noticed within two cycles. (Vitamin E and essential fatty acid, such as evening primrose oil, are very helpful as well.)

### ॐ Infertility

Vitex is indicated for cases of infertility resulting from insufficient progesterone production (which means there's no ovulation) and due to high prolactin levels. I have seen it help women begin to ovulate when they were previously unable to do so. Work with your doctor to incorporate vitex into a treatment protocol for infertility.

### ॐ Menstrual Disorders

The hormone-balancing effects of vitex make it a superior herb for a wide variety of menstrual disorders. This includes painful periods, medically known as dysmenorrhea. It does not work well for the acute relief of dysmenorrhea, but is excellent for long-term treatment to correct the hormone imbalance that is causing the problem.

Also, it helps with irregular menstrual cycles that are too long or too short. I particularly like vitex for young teenage girls who suffer from abnormal menstrual cycles or dysmenorrhea. It seems like a much better option than the birth-control pill.

Speaking of the birth-control pill, vitex is commonly used by herbalists to normalize the menstrual cycle after a woman has discontinued using the pill and then suffers from menstrual irregularity.

*(continued)*

One study of women with menstrual disorders found that vitex improved cases of polymenorrhea (too frequent) as well as cases of women with menorrhagia (excessive bleeding).

## Lactation

Vitex has long been used to increase milk supply during lactation. Recently, I had a female patient who stopped breast-feeding a few days after the birth of her child because she was put on medication. A week later, she had problems resuming breast-feeding because her milk production had greatly diminished. I recommended vitex. Over the next ten days, it helped to reestablish her milk flow.

A study of 353 breast-feeding mothers with poor milk production found that vitex supplementation for seven days resulted in significant improvement.

## Menopausal Hot Flashes

Vitex has been used by European doctors to help relieve hot flashes for women going through the transition of menopause. I normally prescribe it in a menopausal formula that contains herbs such as black cohosh.

## Ovarian Cysts

Ovarian cysts, another condition related to hormone imbalance, can often be eliminated with vitex. A separate condition known as polycystic ovary syndrome can also be helped with regular vitex supplementation.

## PMS

Balancing hormones is the key to treating the underlying cause of PMS. Most of the research on vitex has been done with regard to premenstrual syndrome. Again, it helps to reduce high levels of prolactin and to lower the levels of progesterone—both of which are associated with PMS.

One survey involved over 1,500 women with premenstrual syndrome who supplemented with vitex extract. The women took 40 drops of vitex for an average of 166 days. Fifty-seven percent of the patients reported improvement, and another 33 percent reported complete relief of symptoms. The physicians reported positive results in 92 percent of the cases.

In another study, 127 women were given 200 milligrams of vitamin $B_6$ or vitex extract for three menstrual cycles. While both groups had good responses, the women using vitex had a greater overall decrease of symptoms, especially breast tenderness, bloating, and depression. Overall, 77 percent of the vitex group had improvement compared with improvement of these symptoms in 61 percent of those taking vitamin $B_6$.

As you can see from these studies, natural and nontoxic therapies such as vitex and vitamin B are quite effective. I consider them nature's "PMS busters." I certainly favor their use over conventional therapies for PMS, which include the birth-control pill, diuretics, antidepressants such as Prozac, and tranquilizers such as Xanax.

Vitex works well for PMS if you take the herb by itself, and I consider it essential in any PMS formula. As a matter of fact, if a PMS formula does not contain vitex, then I would advise you don't bother purchasing it.

## Uterine Fibroids

Vitex is one of the better herbs to use for uterine fibroids. It helps to keep the fibroids from enlarging in mild to moderate cases. If a woman can keep the symptoms at bay until she is past menopause, the fibroids will shrink on their own, due to the decrease of estrogen. While I don't recommend vitex as a general preventative, I will recommend it in some cases.

Fortunately, most fibroids do not cause symptoms. For severe cases, we recommend natural progesterone. In a small number of cases, surgery is required.

# W

# Water

I remember a span of about three weeks during medical school when I experienced dull headaches, dizziness, and lethargy. It seemed like my thinking was cloudy. While I couldn't explain all these symptoms, I assumed that mounting stress of my classes, plus all the hours I'd been working in the clinic, were beginning to take their toll.

Then, one day, when I decided I was tired of feeling this way, I sat down and analyzed everything I had been doing. I was eating pretty well and exercising a reasonable amount. It seemed very unlikely that I was suffering any kind of nutritional deficiency.

But even while I contemplated possible explanations, I happened to notice someone getting a glass of water at a nearby watercooler. Then it occurred to me. Many of my symptoms suggested dehydration. It was just possible that I was experiencing these symptoms because I wasn't consuming enough water.

As I reviewed my actions of the last few days, I realized I'd really had very little water—possibly two tall glasses a day, total. That wasn't nearly enough, considering that I was exercising regularly, under stress, and mentally active. I decided that was a good time to start doing exactly what I was recommending to many patients—drinking more water.

With the phrase "physician heal thyself" dancing in my head, I immediately resolved to triple the amount of water I was consuming. After that small revelation, I started drinking approximately six 8-ounce glasses a day.

My symptoms disappeared over the next three days. It was a long, round-about route, but I'd been forced to the simple rediscovery that water is one of the fundamental necessities of good health. Few of us are regularly in danger of dying of thirst—but I suspect that many of us are seriously slowed down by unrecognized thirstiness.

## WAITER, MORE WATER!

As we all probably learned in school, water is composed of two hydrogen molecules and one oxygen molecule. More than half of our total body weight is water, and a newborn is about three-quarters fluids and one-quarter solid, living human matter.

The brain, surprisingly, is the most concentrated reservoir. There, the concentration of water is almost 85 percent.

About two-thirds of the water in our systems comes from those glasses of fluids that we drink. The rest comes from food and from the leftover "disposables" of cellular metabolism.

Our bodies are really the middle of a streambed. While the water is coming in through various pathways, it's exiting in the urine (60%), evaporating from skin (20%), hissing out through the respiratory tract (15%), and departing in stool (5%).

Water is involved in every single biochemical activity in the body and is required as a solvent for many processes. It is an important component of blood (plasma) and fluids inside and outside the cells. All the tissues of the body—including cartilage and skin—are unquenchable water drinkers. The medium of water is a traveling roadshow, where electrolytes move around, enabling the cells to perform their duty as they generate electrical activity. You need water for detoxification, because waste products course their way out of the body through the multitude of aqueducts—veins, arteries, glands, and organs—that pump, feed, and carry fluids from place to place. Throwing in some thermostatic responsibilities, water also provides a means for temperature regulation.

## BODY LUBE

Humans have a thirst mechanism that is activated when our body is becoming low in reserves of water. Researchers have noted that there is often a long delay between the time when your body actually becomes dehydrated and the moment when you experience the sensation of thirst. In other words, by the time you feel thirsty, you're *already* somewhat dehydrated.

I've already mentioned the symptoms of dehydration that I experienced myself, but there are others. Thirst, naturally, is one—and any time your mouth feels dry or "sticky," you probably need fluids. Dark urine is another sign.

Many people are in a constant, low-grade state of dehydration. They won't faint, nor do they need to be hospitalized. But that low-grade dehydration can sap vitality and contribute to many of the symptoms I've noted.

Of course, there are situations that lead, almost automatically, to dehydration. If you're in a hot climate, exercising heavily, and not drinking very much, your water reserves drop fast. But excessive sodium intake—eating a lot of salty foods, including heavily processed food products—will draw water out of the tissues. (I am always reminded of the effects of sodium a couple hours after eating sushi with soy sauce, or foods containing lots of sodium.)

## THE DEHYDRATORS

If you drink a lot of beverages containing caffeine—coffee and soda, for instance—you're sure to have some dehydration unless you also drink lots of water. Alcoholic beverages also have a dehydrating effect.

Any medication that's described as a diuretic, or drugs that have diuretic side effects, will require you to compensate for water loss by getting more fluids every day.

Conditions I see that are related to insufficient water intake include headaches, dizziness, heart palpitations, high blood pressure, irritability, cloudy thinking, skin rashes, kidney pain, and fatigue. Other physicians have noted even more conditions associated with dehydration, ranging from colitis and rheumatoid arthritis to obesity, asthma, and allergies.

Of course, while I'm recommending that people drink sufficient water, I'm acutely aware that many are concerned with the quality of their drinking water. Thousands of people suffer from parasites and other infections related to contaminated water each year. Industrial pollutants and chemicals are traceable in many sources of drinking water. Even the chemicals used to purify water—such as chlorine—have in some cases been linked to cancers such as bladder cancer and, possibly, aggravating asthma. Heavy metal contamination such as lead, mercury, and aluminum are problems as well.

I advise people to invest in a high-quality filtration system or drink tested bottled water. I also recommend having your local water tested.

## DOSAGE

Drink at least six to eight 8-ounce glasses of water daily. If you drink coffee, consume one 8-ounce glass of water for every cup of coffee you drink.

If the weather is hot, drink a glass or two before exercising, and have more than eight glasses during the day.

People on detoxification programs often need to increase their water intake to help flush toxins out of the body.

## WHAT ARE THE SIDE EFFECTS?

In rare cases, too much water consumption may place stress on your heart or kidneys. If you have kidney or heart disease, consult with your doctor before drinking larger-than-normal amounts of water.

You may feel bloated if you haven't been drinking very much water and then abruptly increase your water intake. The bloating comes from swallowing extra air—but it won't take long for your body to adjust to increased water intake.

## WATER
### RECOMMENDATIONS FROM THE NATURAL PHYSICIAN FOR . . .

### ✋ *Cloudy Thinking*

I call this symptom "brain fog," and most people know instantly what I mean. The mind is not clear, and you find it hard to concentrate. I have seen these symptoms improved with increased water consumption.

### ✋ *Dizziness*

Unexplained dizziness may be related to dehydration. Water is required for normal blood pressure. When you're dehydrated, your circulation may be poor, which deprives cells of needed nutrients. Dizziness is one outcome.

*(continued)*

### ❧ Fatigue

Unexplained fatigue can be a result of dehydration. Many people notice increased energy when they drink more water.

### ❧ Headaches

Patients with chronic, low-grade headaches are often dehydrated. It is often described as a fuzzy sensation in the head.

### ❧ Heart Palpitations

Occasionally a patient reports a history of heart palpitations. These episodes may improve or cease completely when water intake increases.

### ❧ High Blood Pressure

You'd think that anyone consuming lots of water would be raising their own blood pressure, but the opposite is true. When you're dehydrated, your body tries to compensate by increasing blood pressure. So for anyone with high blood pressure (hypertension), it's important to increase water intake.

### ❧ Irritability

There are many reasons for irritability, of course, but if you think dehydration might be one possible cause, there's a quick way to find out—just start drinking a lot more water, and see if your mood improves.

### ❧ Kidney Pain

A number of patients experience kidney pain when they are not drinking enough water. Any kind of kidney pain should be taken seriously. But while you should see the doctor and explain your symptoms, it's also advisable to increase your intake of water. It can't do any harm—and that just might turn out to be the explanation of the problem.

### ❧ Skin Rashes

The skin is a major organ of detoxification. If you're not getting enough water in your system to aid detoxification, you can begin to develop skin rashes of many sorts. Increase water consumption, and you'll help expel some of the accumulated toxins in the body. This is the quickest "first aid" I can think of for treatment of skin rashes.

### ❧ Weight Gain and Edema

Your body will retain water if you are chronically dehydrated. This condition, called edema, contributes to weight gain as well. Thus, increased water consumption is an important therapy for helping these conditions.

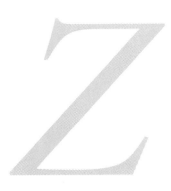

# Zinc

Jim was concerned about his son's acne.

"Is there anything you can give him?" Jim asked me. "Randy is seventeen years old now, and we actually thought his acne would start to get better. But it's not."

"There are lots of good natural treatments," I answered. "But I'd start by giving him zinc."

I explained that I'd seen zinc help in many cases of teenage and adult acne, and I recommended that Randy start at a high dosage.

"Have him take 30 milligrams three times daily, with meals, for a month. Then cut back to 50 milligrams a day as a maintenance dosage. You should also make sure he gets a few milligrams of copper to maintain a balance with zinc."

"That high dosage won't harm him in any way, will it?" asked Jim.

"No. We prescribe dosages like that all the time. The studies show that long-term usage of dosages of 150 to 200 milligrams daily can cause toxicity problems, and I'm not recommending a dosage near that high," I replied.

After taking the zinc supplement for two months, Randy noticed a marked improvement in his skin. Although his acne still broke out at times, it was much less noticeable and the daily blemishes were greatly improved.

# THE QUALITIES OF ZINC

Zinc is a mineral with many important functions. Found in all the cells of the body, it's known as a cofactor—that is, a substance required for numerous enzymatic reactions, including detoxification.

It is important for the synthesis and activity of many hormones such as thymic hormone, growth hormone, and insulin, as well as testosterone and other sex hormones. It is necessary for proper immune function and wound healing. It is also needed for protein and DNA synthesis.

Zinc is needed for proper vitamin A metabolism. It is involved in bone formation and in taste.

There are several reasons why people may develop zinc deficiencies. Poor dietary intake is one reason. For example, vegetarians may be more prone to zinc deficiency, as zinc in plant foods is not so bioavailable as in animal products.

Other factors come into play such as genetic susceptibility and some problems with absorption. We also know that certain medications, such as ACE inhibitors like captopril, enalapril, and lisinopril that are commonly used to lower blood pressure, can cause zinc deficiency. Other problematic drugs are aspirin and the birth-control pill.

The elderly are more prone to a deficiency because digestive powers decrease as we age, and our bodies don't absorb zinc so well. Alcoholics are at risk for zinc

## When Zinc Is Missing

Severe nutritional deficiencies are not that common—but I often see people who have marginal or subclinical deficiencies. Symptoms and conditions associated with zinc deficiency include the following:

- Poor wound healing
- Lowered immunity; susceptibility to infections
- Poor skin and nail health (nails may have white spots)
- Fatigue
- Loss of taste and smell
- Poor growth and development
- Blood sugar imbalance
- Anorexia; reduced appetite
- Delayed sexual development and maturation
- Night blindness (due to involvement with vitamin A metabolism)
- Infertility
- Skin abnormalities
- Dandruff
- Impaired nerve conduction
- Hair loss
- Prostate enlargement
- Birth malformations
- Psychiatric illness

deficiency, and so is anyone with a metabolic disease such as diabetes. When people have diseases of the digestive tract such as Crohn's disease or Celiac disease, and just have general malabsorption—caused by leaky gut syndrome, for instance—they may have impaired mineral absorption.

## GETTING YOUR ZINC

The recommended daily allowance is 15 milligrams per day for adult males and 12 milligrams for adult females. Good food sources include fish and seafood such as oysters and other shellfish. Red meat is also high in zinc.

Eggs and milk also contain ample amounts of zinc. Plant foods such as whole grains and cereals, legumes, nuts, and seeds (particularly pumpkin seeds) contain good amounts of zinc, but the mineral isn't so bioavailable as the zinc that comes from animal products.

Breast milk contains a good supply of zinc, so infants are well protected.

## DOSAGE

Adults can benefit from supplementing with an extra 15 to 30 milligrams daily of zinc. Most high-potency multivitamins contain this amount.

Children under one year of age can use a pediatric multivitamin that contains up to 5 milligrams. Children over the age of one can take a children's multivitamin that contains 5 to 15 milligrams in each daily dose.

For specific conditions, such as wound healing or acne, higher dosages of up to 100 milligrams daily may be required for a limited amount of time.

Avoid the use of zinc sulfate, which is not readily absorbed. I recommend other formulas such as zinc picolinate, zinc monomethionine, zinc citrate, and zinc chelate.

**Note:** If you are taking a calcium supplement, take it at a different time from when you take your zinc supplement. The calcium may hinder zinc absorption.

## WHAT ARE THE SIDE EFFECTS?

Zinc is actually quite a safe supplement, though some people may experience digestive upset if they take zinc on an empty stomach.

High dosages of 150 to 200 milligrams or more, taken over a long period of time, might cause depressed immunity. But I don't recommend taking such high doses anyway, even if you're treating a condition such as severe acne.

One concern is the possibility of developing copper anemia if you are taking high dosages of zinc without taking copper. In the absence of copper, red blood cells change shape; when that happens, they don't carry oxygen so efficiently.

# ZINC
## RECOMMENDATIONS FROM THE NATURAL PHYSICIAN FOR ...

### ❧ Acne

Zinc is involved in the metabolism of testosterone. As that "male hormone" is metabolized, it is converted to a metabolite hormone known as DHT (dihydrotestosterone). High levels of DHT are associated with the development of acne, because it increases sebum production. Zinc works to reduce the conversion and also promotes skin healing. Many studies have shown that zinc is beneficial for acne treatment, and at least one indicated that zinc is as effective as tetracycline.

### ❧ AIDS

People with AIDS are prone to several nutritional deficiencies. Zinc is one of the critical minerals for the immune system, therefore an essential supplement if you have AIDS.

### ❧ Alzheimer's Disease

Zinc may be helpful in slowing the progression of Alzheimer's disease. In a study that included ten people who had Alzheimer's, researchers found that supplementation with zinc helped eight of the people improve memory and communication.

### ❧ Atheroslcerosis

Zinc appears to be one of the many nutrients that helps to prevent atherosclerosis.

### ❧ Birth Complications

Zinc is important during pregnancy because it is required for cell division. A deficiency of zinc is linked to conditions such as premature birth, low birth weight, growth retardation, and preeclampsia. A good prenatal multivitamin should help prevent a zinc deficiency when used in combination with a balanced diet.

### ❧ Burns, Cuts, and Wounds

Zinc is needed for cell division and protein synthesis, both of which are required for skin and wound healing. Burns, cuts, and other skin traumas can be relieved with zinc supplements. By taking supplements, you can also speed healing.

### ❧ Common Cold

Several studies have shown that zinc lozenges reduce the severity and duration of the common cold, and also help to relieve sore throats that accompany a cold. It is helpful to take zinc lozenges containing 15 to 25 milligrams of elemental zinc at the first signs of a cold. I find they are particularly good for healing a sore throat.

### ❧ Eating Disorders

Zinc is involved in producing stomach acid as well as stimulating a normal appetite. Studies

*(continued)*

**487**

have shown that people with anorexia and bulimia have deficient zinc levels and may benefit from zinc supplements. Holistic practitioners recommend zinc as part of a comprehensive protocol for people with these eating disorders.

### ❧ Macular Degeneration

Zinc is important in maintaining normal vision. One study of 155 people with macular degeneration found that 45 milligrams of zinc per day significantly slowed the rate of visual loss.

The macula is the portion of the eye that is responsible for fine vision, and when there's degeneration in that area, the sight begins to go. In fact, macular degeneration is the leading cause of blindness in the aged. There are two main types—"dry" and "wet." Nutritional therapy is mainly used for the dry type.

I usually recommend combining zinc supplementation with other important supplements including vitamin C, selenium, carotenoids, taurine, lutein, and the herbs ginkgo and bilberry.

### ❧ Male Infertility

Men who are deficient in zinc may have decreased testosterone and sperm production. Studies have shown that zinc supplements increase sperm counts and testosterone in men who previously had deficiencies that prevented conception.

In one study, 11 men who were infertile were treated with 55 milligrams of zinc daily for 6 to 12 months. They showed an increase in sperm count and motility—and three of the men's wives became pregnant during the study.

### ❧ Prostate Enlargement

Zinc is an effective treatment for prostate enlargement. The mineral inhibits the enzyme 5-alpha reductase, which converts testosterone to dihydrotestosterone (DHT). Since high levels of DHT are believed to promote prostate enlargement, I generally prescribe 90 to 100 milligrams daily for men with this condition. After two months, I recommend reducing the zinc dosage to a maintenance level of 50 milligrams.

### ❧ Wilson's Disease

Zinc is one of the primary treatments for this genetic disease in which copper accumulates in the liver and body, causing brain damage. High doses of zinc help to hinder copper absorption.

# References by Section

## ACIDOPHILUS

- "... It is amazing to realize that *acidophilus* and the other friendly flora are part of the one hundred trillion bacteria that live together in the human digestive system." Mitsuuoka T., Intestinal flora & aging. *Nutrition Reviews* Dec 1992; 50:438–446.

- "... Fructooligosaccharide ... inhibits parasites and toxic bacteria from attaching to the digestive tract." Tomomatsu H., Health effects of oligosaccharides. *Food Tech* October 1994:61–65.

- "... Sources of this unique good bacteria promoter include bananas, barley, garlic, honey, chicory, fruit, wheat, onions, soybeans, and tomatoes." Williams Ch et al., Influence of dietary neosugar on selected bacterial groups of the human faecal microbiota. *Microb Ecol Health Dis* 1994; 7:91–97.

- "... Acidophilus produces an acidic environment, which inhibits the reproduction of many harmful bacteria. In addition they produce substances called bacteriocins, which act as natural antibiotics to destroy harmful microorganisms." Barefoot SF, Klaenhemmer TR, Detection and activity of lactacin B, a bacteriocins produced by lactobacillus acidophilus. *Appl Environ Microbiol* 1983; 45:1808–1815.

- "... Acidophilus and other members of the friendly flora activate the immune system by increasing antibody response in the mucosal tissues." Perdigon G, Vintini E, Alvarez S, Medina M, Medici., Study of the possible mechanisms involved in the mucosal immune system activation by lactic acid bacteria. *J Dairy Sci* 1999 Jun; 82(6):1108–1114.

- "... This is of particular importance for colon and breast cancer prevention." Shahaniand, Anticarcinogenic and immunological properties of dietary lactobacilli. *Journal of Food Protection* 1990; 53:740–710.

- "... One study showed it beneficial for those with constipation who had colitis, irritable bowel syndrome, and other various disorders." Rettger LF et al., *Lactobacillus Acidophilus. Its Therapeutic Application.* New Haven, CT: Yale U. Press, 1935.

- "... Numerous studies have shown that acidophilus and other good bacteria are helpful to prevent and treat cases of infectious diarrhea." Fernandes CF et al., Control of diarrhea by Lactobacilli. *J Appl Nutr* 1988; 40(1):32–41.

- "... A study looking at a group of children suffering from food allergies showed evidence of Lactobacillus and Bifidobacteria deficiency." Kuvaeva I et al., The microecology of the gastrointestinal tract and the immunological status under food allergy. *Nahrung* 1984; 28(6–7):689–693.

- "... It is well known that 75 percent of adults (except those of northwest European descent) have a deficiency of this enzyme and thus cannot break down milk sugar products effectively." *The Merck Manual,* Seventeenth Edition. Merck Laboratories, 1999, p. 298.

# ALOE

- " . . . The combination may allow a person with AIDS to use lower dosages of AZT, which would reduce the risk of toxicity and side effects." Murray, M, *The Healing Power of Herbs.* Rocklin, CA: Prima Publishing, 1995, p. 34.

- ". . . The injection of acemannan was shown in one study to be very effective as an injection against feline leukemia virus." Murray, M, *The Healing Power of Herbs.* Rocklin, CA: Prima Publishing, 1995, pp. 33–34.

- ". . . The oral ingestion of aloe vera extract for 6 months was found to be effective in the treatment of asthma." Shida T et al., Effect of aloe extract on peripheral phagocytosis in adult bronchial asthma. *Planta Medica* 1985; 51:273–275.

- ". . . One study found a special form of acemannan gel to be more effective than a conventional medication (Orabase) in speeding the healing of canker sores." Plemons JM, Rees TD, Binnie WH, et al., Evaluation of acemannan in the treatment of recurrent apthous stomatitis. *Wounds* 1994; 6(2):40–45.

- ". . . A study on 31 children with canker sores found it to be effective for 80 percent of the children." Andriani E, Bugli T, Aalders M, Castelli S, De Luigi G, Lazzari N, Rolli GP, The effectiveness and acceptance of a medical device for the treatment of aphthous stomatitis. Clinical observation in pediatric age. *Minerva Pediatr* 2000 Jan–Feb; 52(1-2):15–20.

- ". . . A single-blind, placebo-controlled clinical trial in Thailand involved 77 people who had just been diagnosed with diabetes mellitus (Type 2)." Yongchaiyudha S et al., Antidiabetic activity of Aloe vera L. juice. I. Clinical trial in new cases of diabetes mellitus. *Phytomedicine* 1996; 3(3):241–243.

- ". . . One double-blind study, placebo-controlled study found that a 0.5% aloe vera cream used for 4 weeks was significantly more effective than placebo in relieving psoriasis lesions." Syed TA, Ahmad SA, Holt AH, et al., Management of psoriasis with Aloe vera extract in a hydrophilic cream: A placebo-controlled, double blind study. *Tropical Medicine and International Health* 1996; 1(4):505–509.

- ". . . One of aloe's constituents known as emodin may destroy the bacteria *H. Pylori,* which is implicated in causing stomach ulcers." Wang HH, Chung JG, Ho CC, Aloe-emodin effects on arylamine n-acetyltransferase activity in the bacterium Heliobacter pylori. *Planta Medica* 1998; 64:176–178.

# AMINO ACIDS

- ". . .Specific amino acids act as precursors of neurotransmitters . . . Other amino acids act directly as neurotransmitters." Braverman E., *The Healing Nutrients Within.* New Canaan, CT: Keats Publishing, 1997, p. 9.

# ARSENICUM

- ". . . According to Dana Ullman, coauthor of *Everybody's Guide to Homeopathic Medicines,* over 70,000 registered homeopaths practice in India. Britain is home of the Royal London Homeopathic Hospital, and the Royal Family has been under homeopathic care since 1930.

In France, more than 6,000 physicians practice homeopathy and over 18,000 pharmacies sell homeopathic remedies." Cummings S, Ullman D, *Everybody's Guide to Homeopathic Medicines*. Los Angeles: Jeremy P. Tarcher, Inc, 1984.

- ". . . One of the few studies on arsenicum album was done on rats that were given arsenic." Cazin JC, Cazin M, Gaborit JL, Chaoui A, Boiron J, Belon P, Cherruault Y, Papapanayotou C, A study of the effect of decimal and centesimal dilutions of arsenic on the retention and mobilization of arsenic in the rat. *Hum Toxicol* 1987 Jul; 6(4):315–320.

- ". . . A randomized double-blind clinical trial comparing homeopathic medicine with placebo in the treatment of acute childhood diarrhea was conducted in Leon, Nicaragua, in July 1991." Jacobs J, Jimenez LM, Gloyd SS, Gale JL, Crothers, D Treatment of acute childhood diarrhea with homeopathic medicine: A randomized clinical trial in Nicaragua. *Pediatrics* 1994 May; 93(5):719–725.

## ASHWAGANDHA

- ". . ." 3000 milligrams of purified ashwagandah powder or placebo was given to 101 normal healthy male volunteers, ages 50–59 for one year." Kuppurajan K, et al. *J Res Ayu Sid* 1, 247, 1980. As cited in Bone K and Mills S, *Principles and Practice of Phytotherapy*. London: Church Livingstone, 2000, p. 600.

- ". . . A double-blind trial for 60 days involved 58 healthy children ages 8–12 years." Venkataraghavan S, Seshadri C, Sundaresan TP, et al., The comparative effect of milk fortified with ashwagandah, ashwagandah and punarnava in children: A double-blind study. *J Res Ayur Sid* 1980; 1:370–385.

- ". . . A double-blind, placebo-controlled cross-over study of 42 people with osteoarthritis were randomized to receive a formula containing ashwagandah (also boswellia, turmeric, and zinc) or placebo for three months." Kulkarni RR, Patki PS, Jog VP, et al., Treatment of osteoarthritis with a herbomineral formulation: A double-blind, placebo-controlled, cross-over study. *J Ethnopharmacol* 1991; 33:91–95.

## ASTRAGALUS

- ". . . . the interferon levels remained elevated for two months after astragalus supplementation ended." Yunde H, Guoliang M, Shuhua W, et al., Effects of radix astragali seu hedysari on the interferon system. *Chinese Medical Journal* 1981; 94(1):35–40.

- ". . . astragalus improved the activity of damaged cells to a higher activity than normal cells that were taken from people who had no cancer." Mavlit G, Ishii Y, Patt Y, et al., Local xenogenic graft-vs-host reaction: A practical assessment of T-cell function among cancer patients. *Journal of Immunology* 1979; 123(5):2185–2188.

- ". . . a toxic chemical often used to study the protective effects of the liver." Zhang ZL, Wen QZ, Liu CX, Hepatoprotective effects of astragalus root. *Journal of Ethnopharmacology* 1990; 30:145–149.

- ". . . experienced fewer and less severe colds after taking astragalus as a nasal spray or as a tablet." Chang HM, But PPH, *Pharmacology and Applications of Chinese Materia Medica*, Vol. 2. Hong Kong: World Scientific, 1987.

- ". . . effective in the treatment of chronic bronchitis." Yunde H, Guoliang M, Shuhua W, et al., Effects of radix astragali seu hedysari on the interferon system. *Chinese Medical Journal* 1981; 94(1):35–40.

## B-COMPLEX

- ". . . In a 1998 study, researchers compared riboflavin (400 mg) and placebo in 55 patients with migraine in a randomized trial of 3 months' duration." Schoenen J, Jacquy J, Lenaerts M, Effectiveness of high-dose riboflavin in migraine prophylaxis. A randomized controlled trial. *Neurology* 1998 Feb; 50(2):466–470.

- ". . . avoid the use of time-released niacin, which can be toxic to the liver." McKenney JM et al., A comparison of the efficacy and toxic effects of sustained vs immediate release niacin in hypercholesterolemic patients. *JAMA* 1994; 271:672–677.

- ". . . In one double-blind study, 84 percent of the women undergoing $B_6$ treatment experienced reduction of PMS symptoms including headaches, swelling, bloating, depression, and irritability." Barr W, Pyridoxine supplements in the premenstrual syndrome. *The Practitioner* 1984; 228:425–427.

- ". . . Studies have shown it to be helpful in strengthening the nails. In one study of people with brittle nails, biotin supplementation at 2,500 micrograms daily resulted in improvement in two-thirds of the users." Hochman LG, Scher Rk, Meyerson MS, Brittle nails: Responses to daily biotin supplementation. *Cutis* 1993; 51(4):303–305.

## BILBERRY

- ". . . if you are on blood-thinning medication let your doctor know that you are taking bilberry and that it has a blood-thinning effect comparable to the drug dipyridamole." Morazzoni P, Magistretti MJ, Activity of Myrtocyan, an anthocyanosides complex from Vaccinium myrtillus(VMA), on platelet aggregation and adhesiveness. *Fitoterapia* 1990; 61(13):13–21.

- ". . . the combination of bilberry (360 milligrams) and vitamin E (100 milligrams) daily for four months prevented the progression of cataracts in 97 percent of 50 people with mild senile cataracts." Bravetti GO, Fraboni E, Maccolini E, Preventive medical treatment of senile cataract with vitamin E and Vaccinium myrtillus anthocyanosides: Clinical evaluation. *Annali di Ottalmologia e Clinica Oculista* 1989; 115:109–116.

- ". . . study that looked at 51 pregnant women who took bilberry extract. Bilberry significantly improved the pain, burning, and itching associated with their hemorrhoids." Teglio L, Mazzanti C, Tronconi R et al., Vaccinium myrtillus anthocyanosides (Tegens) in the treatment of venous insufficiency of lower limbs and acute piles in pregnancy. *Quadeni di Clinica Osterica e Ginecologica* 1987; 42(3):221–231.

- ". . . Bilberry extract demonstrated significant improvements in their speed of adaptation speed ability to light changes." Paronzini S, Indemini P, Modifications of the macular recovery tests in normal subjects after administration of anthocyanosides. *Bolletino de Pculistica* 1988; 67(4):185–188.

- ". . . more recent study found no improvement in night visual acuity with the supplementation of bilberry." Muth E, Laurent OD, Jasper P, *Altern Med Rev* 2000; 5(2):164–173.

- ". . . In the same study looking at bilberry supplementation and its benefit in reducing hemorrhoid symptoms with pregnant women, it was also shown to improve varicose veins as well." Teglio L, Mazzanti C, Tronconi R et al., Vaccinium myrtillus anthocyanosides (Tegens) in the treatment of venous insufficiency of lower limbs and acute piles in pregnancy. Quadeni di Clinica Osterica e Ginecologica 1987; 42(3):221–231.

## BLACK COHOSH

- ". . . hormone LH (lutenizing hormone) is lowered with black cohosh supplementation." Duker EM et al., Effects of extracts from Cimicifuga racemosa on gonadotropin release in menopausal women and ovariectomized rats. *Planta Medica* 1991; 57:420–424.

- ". . . dosages than I recommend may result in headaches and dizziness." Harnischfeger G, Stolze H, Black cohosh. *Notabene Medici* 1980; 10:446–450.

- ". . . inhibited the cancer cells from proliferating." Nesselhut T et al., Examination of the proliferative potential of phytopharmaceuticals with estrogen-mimicking acting in breast carcinoma. *Arch Gynecol Obstet* 1993; 254:817–818.

- ". . . the breast cancer cells whose growth is dependent on estrogen were *not* stimulated by black cohosh. Zava D, Dollbaum C, Blen M, Estrogen and progestin bioactivity of foods, herbs, spices. *Proc Soc Experi Biol Med* 1998; 217:369–378.

- ". . . 83 percent had improvement in their depression with 46 percent no longer having any symptoms of depression left." Stolze H, An alternative to treat menopausal symptoms. *Gyne* 1982; (3)1:14–16.

- ". . . that black cohosh relieved anxiety and depression more effectively in menopausal women than the anti-anxiety drug diazepam." Warnecke G, Influencing menopausal symptoms with a phytotherapeutic agent. *Die Medizinische Welt* 1985; 36:871–874.

- ". . . heart palpitations, ringing in the ears, and insomnia." Stolze H. An alternative to treat menopausal symptoms. *Gyne* 1982; (3)1:14–16.

- ". . . proves the effectiveness of black cohosh over estrogen replacement." Stoll W, Phytopharmacon influences atrophic vaginal epithelium: Double-blind study—Cimicifuga vs. estrogenic substances. *Therapeutikon* 1987; 1:23–30.

- ". . . twenty-eight were able to make the switch to black cohosh without being given additional hormones." Petho A, Menopausal complaints: Changeover of a hormone treatment to a herbal gynecological remedy practicable? *Arzliche Praxis* 1987; 38(47):1551–1553.

## BOSWELLIA

- ". . . One review of 11 German clinical studies looked at 260 people who did not respond well to conventional treatments." Etzel R, Special extract of Boswellia serrata (H15) in the treatment of rheumatoid arthritis. *Phytomedicine* 1996; 3(1):91–94.

- ". . . Boswellia does not cause this cartilage degradation but actually reduces the breakdown of cartilage building blocks known as glycosaminoglycans." Reddy GK, Chandraksan G, Dhar SC, Studies on the metabolism of glycosaminoglycans under the influence of new herbal antiinflammatory agents. *Biochem Pharm* 1989; 38:3527–3534.

- ". . . A six week study found boswellia extract to be as effective as the drug sulfasalazine in causing remission of ulcerative colitis symptoms in a study involving 42 people." Gupta I, Parihar A, Malhotra P et al., Effects of Boswellia serrata gum resin in patients with ulcerative colitis. *Eur J Med Res* 1997; 2:37–43.

## BROMELAIN

- ". . . The combination of bromelain and antibiotics was given to 53 hospitalized patients with the following conditions: pneumonia, bronchitis, skin staphylococcus infection, thrombophlebitis, cellulitis, pyelonephritis (kidney infection), and abscesses of the rectum." Neubauer RA, A plant protease for potentiation of and possible replacement of antibiotics. *Exp Med Surg* 1961; 19:143–160.

- ". . . In addition to this study, another group of 106 cases was treated with bromelain alone, with results comparable to those obtained with antibiotic treatment." Neubauer RA, A plant protease for potentiation of and possible replacement of antibiotics. *Exp Med Surg* 1961; 19:143–160.

- ". . . A specially prepared bromelain cream has been shown to eliminate burn debris and speed up the healing of burned skin." Houck JC, Chang CM, Klein G, Isolation of an effective debriding agent from the stems of pineapple plants. *Int J Tissue React* 1983; 5:125–134.

- ". . . Resolution of cancerous masses and a decrease in metastasis was reported." Gerard G, Anti-cancer therapy with bromelain. *Agress* 1972; 3:261–274.

- ". . . Bromelain in doses of over 1000 mg daily has been combined with chemotherapy drugs such as 5-FU and vincristine, and has been reported to result in tumor regression." Nieper HA, A program for the treatment of cancer. *Krebs* 1974; 6:124–127.

- ". . . In one study, bromelain administered at a dosage of 400 to 1,000 milligrams per day to 14 patients with angina resulted in the disappearance of symptoms in all patients within 4 to 90 days." Nieper HA, Effect of bromelain on coronary heart disease and angina pectoris. *Acta Med Empirica* 1978; 5:274–278.

- ". . . since it has been shown to dissolve arteriosclerotic plaque in rabbit heart arteries." Taussig SJ, Nieper HA, Bromelain: Its use in prevention and treatment of cardiovascular disease, present status. *J IAPM* 1979; 6:139–151.

- " . . . An early clinical trial on bromelain was conducted on 74 boxers with bruises on the face, lips, ears, chest, and arms." Blonstein JL, Control of swelling in boxing injuries. *Practitioner* 1960; 185:78.

- ". . . The bromelain-takers took an average of 1.5 days to be pain free, compared with an average of 3.5 days for those who went without it." Tassman GC, Zafran JN, Zayon GM, Evaluation of a plant proteolytic enzyme for the control of inflammation and pain. *J Dent Med* 1964; 19:73–77.

# BUTCHER'S BROOM

- ". . . A study was done with 40 people with chronic venous insufficiency." Rudofsky G, Improving venous tone and capillary sealing. Effect of a combination of Ruscus extract and hesperidine methyl chalcone in healthy probands in heat stress. *Forschr Med* 1989; 107(19):52–55.

# CALCIUM

- ". . . According to the Merck Manual, 75 percent of adults have some degree of lactase deficiency." *The Merck Manual*, Seventeenth Edition, 1999, p. 298.

- ". . . Greater than 24 ounces of whole cow's milk daily after the first year of life is a risk factor for iron deficiency because this milk has little iron, may replace foods with higher iron content, and may cause occult (hidden) gastrointestinal bleeding." O Pizarro F, Yip R, Dallman PR, Olivares M, Hertrampf E, Walter T, Iron status with different infant feeding regimens: Relevance to screening and prevention of iron deficiency. *J Pediatr* 1991; 118:687–692.

- ". . . It has been proven that caffeine (coffee and soda), alcohol, and sugar all promote the urinary excretion of calcium." Stengler Angela, Stengler Mark, *Build Strong Bones*. Green Bay, WI: Impakt Communications, 1998, pp. 11–12.

- ". . . *The New England Journal of Medicine* reported that postmenopausal women who added 1,000 milligrams of calcium to their normal daily diets experienced a 43 percent reduction in bone loss when compared with [controls]." Reid IR et al., Effects of calcium supplementation on bone loss in postmenopausal women. *New Engl J Med* 1993; 12:S11–S16.

- ". . . Along with magnesium and vitamin $B_6$, calcium supplementation has been shown to help alleviate premenstrual syndrome." Bernstein D et al., Calcium carbonate and the premenstrual syndrome: Effects of premenstrual and menstrual symptoms. Premenstrual Syndrome Study Group. *Amer J Obstet Gynecol* August 1998; 179(2):444–452.

# CAROTENOIDS

- ". . . A six-year Harvard study of 48,000 male physicians found that men who consumed tomato-rich foods (tomatoes, tomato sauce, and pizza) at least ten times a week had a 35 percent decreased risk of prostate cancer as compared with those men who ate less than 1.5 weekly servings." Giovannucci E et al., Intake of carotenoids and retinol in relation to risk of prostate cancer. *J Natl Cancer Inst* 1995; 87:1767–1776.

- ". . . One research review looked at the intake of tomatoes and tomato-based products and blood lycopene levels in relation to the risk of various cancers." Giovannucci E, Tomatoes, tomato-based products, lycopene, and cancer: Review of the epidemiologic literature. *J Natl Cancer Inst* 1999 Feb 17; 91(4):317–331.

- ". . . This study looked at 30 men with localized prostate cancer who were scheduled to undergo surgical removal of the prostate." Kucuk O et al., Lycopene supplementation in men with prostate cancer reduces grade and volume of preneoplasia and tumor, decrease serum PSA and modulates biomarkers of growth and differentiation.

- "... A recent study showed that high lutein diets were associated with a 17 percent decrease in colon cancer risk, and young people with a diet high in lutein had a 34 percent lower risk of colon cancer." Slattery ML et al., *American Journal of Clinical Nutrition* 2000; 71:575–582.

- "... One study showed that eating a diet rich in carotenoids may reduce the risk of angina." Ford ED, Giles WH, Serum vitamins, carotenoids, and angina pectoris: Findings from the National Health and Nutrition Examination Survey III. *Annals of Epidemiology* 2000; 10:106–116.

- "... A survey of 876 elderly individuals showed that those whose intake of these two carotenoids was high were 56 percent less likely to develop age-related macular degeneration." Seddon JM et al., Dietary carotenoids, vitamin A, C, and E, and advanced age-related macular degeneration. *JAMA* 1994; 272:1413–1420.

- "... A study of 528 people ages 65 to 85 years old found that persons with high blood levels of beta carotene, lycopene, and alpha carotene had significantly better lung function than those with low levels of these nutrients." Grievink L et al., Serum carotenoids, a-tocopherol, and lung function among Dutch elderly. *American Journal of Respiratory and Critical Care Medicine,* 2000; 161:790–795.

- "... A recent study showed that 25 milligrams of a natural carotenoid complex protected against sunburn after eight weeks of supplementation." Stahl W et al., Carotenoids and carotenoids plus vitamin E protect against ultraviolet light induced erythema in humans. *American Journal of Clin Nutrition,* 2000; 71:795–798.

## CAYENNE

- "... [One] study has shown that capsaicin actually inhibits the growth of the bacteria *H. Pylori,* which is implicated in many cases of stomach ulcers." Jones NL, Shabib S, Sherman PM, Capsaicin as an inhibitor of the growth of the gastric pathogen Heliobacter pylori. *FEMS Microbiology Letters* 1997; 146:223–227.

- "... When researchers tried the cream with 49 patients who had moderate to severe diabetic neuropathy, it was found that 90 percent of the people who took capsaicin had pain reduction by the eighth week of use." Scheffler NM, Sheitel PL, Lipton MN, Treatment of painful diabetic neuropathy with capsaicin 0.075 percent. *Journal of the American Podiatric Medical Association* 1991; 81(6):288–293.

- "... In a study of 23 patients who had mastectomies for breast cancer, researchers found that a cream with 0.075% capsaicin significantly reduced pain levels." Watson CP, Evans RJ. The postmastectomy pain syndrome and topical capsaicin: A randomized trial. *Pain* 1992; 51:275–279.

## CHAMOMILE

- "... In all, colic disappeared in 57 percent of the babies who were given the formula." Weizman Z, Alkinrawi S, Goldfarb D et al., Efficacy of herbal tea preparation in infantile colic. *Journal of Pediatrics* 1993; 122:650–652.

- "... One study found chamomile to be effective in speeding the healing of skin abrasions after tattoos were surgically removed with abrasive materials." Glowania HJ, Raulin C,

Swoboda M, The effect of chamomile in healing wounds: A clinical, double-blind study. *Zeit fur Hautrankheiten* 1987; 17(62):1262–1271.

- "... Animal studies have demonstrated the anti-ulcer effects of chamomile." Szelenyi I, Isaac O, Thiemer K, Pharmacological experiments with compounds of chamomile/III. Experimental studies of the ulcer-protective effect of chamomile. *Planta Medica* 1979; 35:218–227.

# CHROMIUM

- "... Chromium has been shown to lower total cholesterol and triglycerides by about 10 percent in people with Type 2 diabetes and also those who do not have diabetes. It also increases the good cholesterol HDL." Lee NA, Reasner CA, Beneficial effect of chromium supplementation on serum triglyceride levels in NIDDM. *Diabetes Care* 1994; 17:1449–1452. 1994. Also, Press RI, Geller J, and Evans GW. The effect of chromium picolinate on serum cholesterol and apolipoprotein fractions in human subjects. *Western J Med* 1993; 152, 41–45.

- "... Researchers examined 29 overweight individuals who also had a family history of diabetes." William Cefalu, M.D, director of the Diabetes Comprehensive Care and Research Program at the Bowman Gray School of Medicine, Wake Forest University. Fifty-seventh Annual Scientific Session of the American Diabetes Association Meeting in Boston, June 23, 1997.

# COENZYME Q10

- "... The body manufactures CoQ10 from the amino acid tyrosine. This synthesis requires the action of vitamins C, $B_2$, $B_6$, $B_{12}$, folic acid, niacin, and pantothenic acid." Folkers K, Relevance of the biosynthesis of coenzyme Q10 and of the four bases of DNA as a rationale for the molecular causes of cancer and a therapy. *Biochem Biophys Res Commun* 1996 Jul 16; 224.

- "... Five cases of metastatic breast cancer have been documented in which there was complete reversal of metastasis with high doses of CoQ10 (390 milligrams). Lockwood K, Moesgaard S, Yamamoto T, Folkers K, *Biochem Biophys Res Commun* 1995 Jul 6; 212.

- "... Coenzyme Q10 has a stabilizing effect on the electrical conductivity of the heart, so it helps prevent arrhythmia." Ohinishi S et al. The effect of Coenzyme Q10 on premature ventricular contraction. In *Biomedical and Clinical Aspects of Coenzyme Q10,* vol 5, Folkers K, Yamamura Y. Amsterdam: Elsevier Science Publishing, 1986, pp. 257–266.

- "... Their two year survival rate was 62 percent compared with a second group of people who only had conventional therapy." Judy WV et al. Myocardial effects of Co-enzyme Q10 in primary heart failure. In *Biomedical and Clinical Aspects of Coenzyme Q,* vol.4. Folkers K and Yamamura Y. Elsevier science Publ, Amsterdam, 1984, pp. 353–367.

- "... Beta blockers are a class of drugs that deplete CoQ10 as well." Kishi T, Kishi H, Folkers K, Inhibition of cardiac CoQ10 enzymes by clinically used drugs and possible prevention. In *Biomedical and Clinical Aspects of Coenzyme Q,* Vol. I. Folkers K and Yamamura Y (eds). Amsterdam: Elsevier/North Holland Biomedical Press, 1977, pp. 47–62.

- "... Coenzyme Q10 works as an antioxidant to protect the heart from the damaging effects of this chemotherapy agent." Kishi T, Makino K, Okamato T, et al., Inhibition of myocardial respiration by psychotherapeutic drugs and prevention by Coenzyme Q. In *Biomedical and Clinical Aspects of Coenzyme Q*, Vol. 2. Yamamura Y, Folkers K, and Ito Y. (eds). Amsterdam, Elsevier/North-Holland Biomedical Press, 1980, pp. 139–145.

- "... Dr. Folkers has shown in two small studies that CoQ10 improved physical performance...." Folkers K, Simonsen R, Two successful double-blind trials with Coenzyme Q10 (vitamin Q10) and muscular dystrophies and neurogenic atrophies. *Biochem Biophys Ata*, 1995; 1271(1):281–286.

- "... Coenzyme Q10 has been shown to improve the fertility potential of sperm." Lewin A et al., The effect of coenzyme Q10 on sperm motility and function. *Mole Apects Med* 1997; 18(suppl):213–219. Also, Angelitti A.G.. Colacicco L, Calla C, et al., Coenzyme Q: Potentially useful index of bioenergetic and oxidative status of spermatozoa. *Clin Chem*, 1995; 41:217–219.

## CRANBERRY

- "... [A] 1998 study in *The New England Journal of Medicine* demonstrated that cranberry prevents the fimbriae (analogous to arms and hands of bacteria) from attaching to the urinary tract walls." Howell AB, Vorsa N, Marderosian AD, et al., Inhibition of the adherence of P-fimbriated Escerichia coli to uroepithelial-cell surfaces by proanthocyanadin extracts from cranberries. *New England Journal of Medicine* 1998; 339(15):1085–1086.

- "... A 1994 study in *The Journal of the American Medical Association* found that regular consumption of cranberry juice significantly reduced the frequency of bacteria and pus in the urine of elderly women." Avorn J, Monane M, Gurwitz JH, et al., Reduction of bacteriuruia and pyuria after ingestion of cranberry juice. *JAMA* 1994; 271(10):751–754.

## DANDELION

- "... According to Dr. Bernard Jensen, author of *Foods That Heal*, 'dandelion greens have more vitamin A than almost any other vegetable.' Jensen B, *Foods That Heal*. Garden City Park, NY: Avery Publishing, 1998, p. 140.

- "... The German Commission E states that dandelion is a safe herb for women to use during pregnancy or while breast-feeding." Blumenthal M et al., *The Complete German Commission E Monographs*. Austin, TX: American Botanical Council, 1998, p. 118.

- "... One of the benefits of dandelion leaf as a diuretic is that it does not cause the loss of potassium." Racz-Kotilla E, Racz G, Solomon A, The action of Taraxacum officinale extracts on the body weight and diuresis of laboratory animals. *Planta Medica* 1974; 26:212–217.

## D-GLUCARATE

- "... In one study, supplementing 2 percent of the animals' diet with d-glucarate produced dramatic results...." Walaszek Z et al., Potential use of D-Glucaric acid derivative in cancer prevention. *Cancer Letters* 1990; 54:1–8.

- "... seemed to prevent certain types of cancers in animals." Walaszek Z. Chemopreventive properties of D-glucaric acid derivatives. *Cancer Bulletin* 1993; 45:453–457.

# DHEA

- "... The study included men between the ages of 40 and 70. There was an inverse relationship found between the levels of DHEA and heart disease." Feldman HA, Johannes CB, McKinlay JB, Longcope C, Low dehydroepiandrosterone sulfate and heart disease in middle-aged men: Cross-sectional results from the Massachusetts Male Aging Study. *Ann Epidemiol* 1998 May; 8(4):217–228.

- "... There was an inverse relationship found between the levels of DHEA and heart disease." Moriyama Y, Yasue H, Yoshimura M, Mizuno Y, Nishiyama K, Tsunoda R, Kawano H, Kugiyama K, Ogawa H, Saito Y, Nakao K, The plasma levels of dehydroepiandrosterone sulfate are decreased in patients with chronic heart failure in proportion to the severity. *J Clin Endocrinol Metab* 2000 May; 85(5):1834–1840.

- "... A longitudinal study showed a relationship between low serum DHEA levels in HIV-infected men and a more rapid progression to AIDS." Mulder JW et al., Dehydroepiandrosterone as predictor for progression to AIDS in asymptomatic human immunodeficiency virus type infected men. *Journal of Infectious Diseases* 1992; 165:413–418.

- "... Researchers from the University of Vienna who tracked the results of DHEA replacement therapy in a group of 40 men found that the hormone was helpful for impotence (erexctile dysfunction)." Reiter WJ, Pycha A, Schatzl G, Pokorny A, Gruber D, Huber JC, Marberger M, Dehydroepiandrosterone in the treatment of erectile dysfunction: A prospective, double-blind, randomized, placebo-controlled study. *Urology* 1999; 53(3):590–595.

- "... Researchers evaluated DHEA and cortisol levels in patients with ulcerative colitis and Crohn's disease." Straub RH, Vogt D, Gross V, Lang B, Schölmerich J, Andus T, Association of humoral markers of inflammation and dehydroepiandrosterone sulfate or cortisol serum levels in patients with chronic inflammatory bowel disease. *Am J Gastroenterol* 1998; 93(11):2197–2202.

- "... In one study, some women with systemic lupus erythematosus were given 200 milligrams of DHEA daily, and others were given a placebo." van Vollenhoven RF, Engleman EG, McGuire JL, Dehydroepiandrosterone in systemic lupus erythematosus. Results of a double-blind, placebo-controlled, randomized clinical trial. *Arthritis Rheum* 1995 Dec; 38(12):1826–1831.

# ECHINACEA

- "... With the courage of his convictions upon him, ..." Elingwood F, *American Materia Medica, Therapeutics,and Pharmacognosy.* Chicago, Illinois, 1919. Reprinted by Eclectic Medical Publications, Portland, OR, in 1983.

- "... Researchers in a German study, found clear evidence that echinacea helps to promote good immune cells ..." Jurcic K et al., Two test subject studies for the stimulation of granulocytes phagocytosis by echinacea-containing preparations. *Zeit Phytother* 1989; 10(2):66–70.

- "... An antibacterial formula containing echinacea (along with two other herbs—thuja and baptisia)." Stolze H and Forth H. A Treatment with Antibiotics can be optimized by Additional Immunostimulation. *Der Kassenarzt* 1983;(23)50:43–48.

- "... One clinical study looked at the effectiveness of *Echinacea purpurea* for 120 patients ..." Heisel O et al., Echiniguard treatment shortens the course of the common cold: A double-blind, placebo-controlled clinical trial. *Eur J Clin Res* 1997; 9:261-268.

- "... In a study of 180 men and women between the ages of 18 and 60, researchers compared three different groups." Braunig B et al., Echinacea purpurea radix. For Strengthening the Immune Response in Flu Like Infections. *Zeit Phytotherapie* 1992; 13:7–13.

- "... Sports medicine specialists studied the effect of echinacea on men who participated in triathlons ..." Berg, A et al., Influence of Echinacin (EC31) treatment on the exercise-induced immune response in athletes. *J Clin Res* 1998; 1:367–380.

- "... A review of 4,958 clinical cases focused on the effectiveness of echinacea ointment." Bergner P, *The Healing Power of Echinacea and Goldenseal*. Rocklin, CA: Prima Publishing, 1997, pp. 97–98.

- "... Reoccurring vaginal yeast infections can be quite troublesome for women." Coeugniet E, Kuhnast R, Recurrent candidiasis: Adjuvant immunotherapy with different formulations of echinacin. *Therapiewoche* 1986; 36:3352.

- "... One clinical study looked at the effectiveness of *echinacea purpurea* for 120 patients who had the initial symptoms of the common cold." Schoenberger D. The influence of immune stimulating effects of a pressed juice from echinacea pupurea on the course and severity of colds, results of a double blind study. *Forum immunolgie* 1992; 8:2–12.

- "... A group of 206 women who used echinacea during pregnancy. ..." Gallo M et al., Pregnancy outcomes following gestational exposure to echinacea, a prospective controlled study. The Motherisk Program, Division of Clinical Pharmacology, Hospital for Sick Children and the University of Toronto, and the Canadian College of Naturopathic Medicine, 1999.

- "... An animal study that appeared in 1999 suggested that echinacea might adversely affect fertility. ..." Ondrizek RR et al., Inhibition of human sperm motility by specific herbs used in alternative medicine. *J Assist Reprod Genet* Feb 1999; 16:87–91.

# ENZYMES

- "... The results of his clinical trial showed that a treatment protocol consisting of diet, nutritional supplements (which included mega doses of animal-derived pancreatic enzymes), and detoxification was significantly more successful than conventional therapy (chemotherapy) for inoperable pancreatic cancer." Gonzalez NJ, Isaacs LL, Evaluation of pancreatic proteolytic enzyme treatment of adenocarcinoma of the pancreas, with nutrition and detoxification support. *Nutr Cancer* 1999; 33(2):117–124.

# EVENING PRIMROSE OIL

- "... Researchers in one study looked at the effects of GLA on 84 people who had Type 2 (adult-onset) diabetes." Keen H, Payan J, Allawi J, et al., Treatment of diabetic neuropathy with gamma-linolenic acid. *Diabetes Care* 1993; 16(1):8–15.

- "... Studies have shown that their mothers also have a history of eczema. .." Buscino L, Ioppi M, et al., Breast milk from mothers of children with newly developed eczema has low levels of long chain polyunsaturated fatty acids. *J Allergy Clin Immunol* 1993; 91:1134–1139.

- "...A study of 52 adults with eczema found that evening primrose oil was very effective in reducing skin redness and damage." Humphreys F, Symons JA, Brown HK, et al., The effect of gamolenic acidon adult atopic eczema and premenstrual exacerbation of eczema. *European Journal of Dermatology* 1994; 4:598–603.

- "...It helps reduce symptoms of irritability and depression ..." Horrobin DF, The role of essential fatty acids and prostaglandins in the premenstrual syndrome. *J Reprod Med* 1993; 28:465–468.

# EXERCISE

- "...A study of over 72,000 female nurses found that women who walk briskly five or more hours a week cut their risk of heart attack by 50 percent." Manson JE, Hu FB, Rich-Edwards JW et al., A prospective study of walking as compared with vigorous exercise in the prevention of coronary artery disease in women. *N Engl J Med* 1999; 341(9):650–658.

- "...A study reported in the *Journal of Epidemiology* showed that those who participated in exercise, sports, and physical activity experienced a decrease in depression, anxiety, and malaise." Farmer ME et al., Physical activity and depressive symptomatalogy: The NHANES 1 epidemiologic follow-up study. *Am J Epidemiol* 1988; 1328:1340–1351.

# FAT REDUCTION

- "...The average American consumes 125 pounds of sugar a year." Sanchex A et al., Role of sugars in human neutrophilic phagocytosis. *American Journal of Clinical Nutrition* 1973; 26:1180–1184.

# FEVERFEW

- "Otherwise, as one study has shown, the migraines may recur as soon as the herbal treatments are discontinued." Johnson ES, Kadam NP, Hylands DM, et al., Efficacy of feverfew as a prophylactic treatment of migraine. *British Medical Journal* 1985; 291:569–573.

- "...A 1998 study looked at 59 people who suffered migraine headaches." Murphy JJ, Heptinstall S, Mitchell JRA, Randomized double-blind placebo controlled trial of feverfew in migraine prevention. *The Lancet* July 23, 1988; 189–192.

# FIBER

- "...Table 4 ..." Marlett J, Cheung T. Database and quick methods of assessing typical dietary fiber intakes using data for 228 commonly consumed foods. *J Am Diet Assoc* 1997; 97:1139–1147.

- "...Women on vegetarian diets have been shown to have up to 50 percent lower levels of free estrogen in their blood than women who eat meat ..." Goldin B.R. et al., Estrogen patterns and plasma levels in vegetarian and omnivorous women. *New Engl J Med* 1982; 307:1542–1547.

- "... Some oat bran studies have been shown to produce very little improvement in cholesterol levels, while others show up to a 21 percent reduction in serum cholesterol." Lovegrove JA, Clohessy A, Milon H, Williams CM, Modest doses of beta-glucan do not reduce concentrations of potentially atherogenic lipoproteins. *Am J Clin Nutr* 2000 Jul; 72(1):49–55.

- "... Whyte J, McArthur R, Toppping D, et al., Oat bran lowers plasma cholesterol levels in mildly hypercholesterolemic men. *Am J Clin N* 1983; 37:699.

- "... For example, cultures that consume a high-fiber diet (100 to 170 grams per day) have a transit time of 30 hours. In comparison, the low-fiber American diet (10 to 20 grams per day) have a transit time that exceeds 48 hours." Pizorno J, *Total Wellness*. Rocklin, CA: Prima Publishing, 1998, pp. 120–121.

# FISH OIL

- "... A 4-year study of the Mediterranean diet found that people could reduce their risk of heart attack by as much as 70 percent." de Longeril M et al., *Circulation: Journal of the American Heart Association* 1999; 99:733–785.

- "... [You] can take a garlic supplement to help neutralize this potential effect of the fish oil." Morcos NC, Modulation of lipid profile by fish oil and garlic combination. *J Natl Med Assoc* 1997 Oct; 89(10):673–678.

- "... DHA supplementation has been shown to decrease aggression while a child is under stress." Hamazaki T et al., The effect of docosahexanoic acid on aggression in young adults: A placebo-controlled, double-blind study. *Jnl Clic Invest* 1996; 97:1129–1133.

- "... One study found that many patients were able to go off their antiinflammatory drugs while supplementing fish oil and experienced no relapse in their rheumatoid arthritis." Kremer JM, Lawrence DA, Petrillo GF, Litts LL, Mullaly PM, Rynes RI, Stocker RP, Parhami N, Greenstein NS, Fuchs BR, et al., Effects of high-dose fish oil on rheumatoid arthritis after stopping nonsteroidal antiinflammatory drugs. *Arthritis Rheum* 1995 Aug; 38(8):1107–1114.

- "... [You] can expect to stay on it for at least 12 weeks before it begins to yield benefits." Kremer JM, N-3 fatty acid supplements in rheumatoid arthritis. *Am Jnl Clin Nutr* 2000 Jan; 71(1 Suppl):349S–351S.

- "... Studies show that children who eat oily fish more than once a week have one-third the risk of getting asthma as children who do not eat fish or eat lean fish on a regular basis." Hodge L et al., Consumption of oily fish and childhood asthma risk. *MJA* 1996; (164):137–140.

- "... In one study of ulcerative colitis, people who took fish-oil supplements (high in omega-3's) were able to cut their steroid medications in half." Stenson WF, et al., Dietary supplementation with fish oils in ulcerative colitis. *Ann Int Med* 1992; 116:609–614.

- "... [It's] been shown that they resume normal kidney function more quickly when omega-3–rich fish oil is supplemented." DeCaterina R et al., N-3 fatty acid and renal disease. *Am Jnl of Kidney Diseases* 1994; 24(3):397–415.

# FLAXSEED

- ". . . Flaxseed has approximately 48 to 64 percent omega-3's, 16 to 34 percent omega-6's, and 18 to 22 percent omega-9 fatty acids." Gursche, S, *Fantastic Flax.* Burnaby, British Columbia: Alive Books, 1999.

- ". . . [Researchers} compared the health of women who had diets that included flaxseed and, in some cases, wheat bran as well." Haggans CJ, Travelli EJ, Thomas W, Martini MC, Slavin JL, The effect of flaxseed and wheat bran consumption on urinary estrogen metabolites in premenopausal women. *Cancer Epidemiol Biomarkers Prev* 2000 Jul; 9(7):719–725.

- ". . . With its excellent fiber and lignan content, flaxseed has been shown to protect against colon cancer as well." Sung MK, Lautens M, Thompson LU, Mammalian lignans inhibit the growth of estrogen-independent human colon tumor cells. *Anticancer Res* 1998 May–Jun; 18(3A):1405–1408.

# FOOD SENSITIVITY

- ". . . In this study, the test proved accurate and reproducible when compared against conventional tests." Tseui J et al., A food allergy study utilizing the EAV acupuncture technique. *Am J Acupuncture* 1984; 12(2):105.

# GARLIC

- ". . . Long-term use of garlic helps to protect the elasticity of the aorta." Breithaupt-Grogler K, Ling M, Boudoulas H, Belz GG, Protective effect of chronic garlic intake on elastic properties of aorta in the elderly. *Circulation* 1997 Oct 21; 96(8):2649–2655.

- ". . . Population studies have shown that garlic reduces the risk of cancer of the colon, esophagus, and stomach." Steinmetz KA, Kushi LH, et al., Vegetables, fruit, and colon cancer in the Iowa women's health study. *Am J Epidiol* 1994; (139):1–5. Also, Dorant E, Vander Brandt PA, et al., Garlic and its significance for the prevention of cancer in humans: A critical review. *Br J Cancer* 1993; 67:424–429.

- ". . . In an overview of 16 prominent garlic studies, including a total of 952 people, researchers concluded that garlic lowered total cholesterol levels by 12 percent after 1 to 3 months of treatment." Silagy C, Neil A, Garlic as a lipid-lowering agent–A meta-analysis. *Journal of Royal College of Physicians* 1994; 28(1):39–45.

- ". . . Garlic has also been shown in studies to reduce the oxidation of cholesterol. . . ." Steiner M, Lins RS, Changes in platelet function and susceptibility of lipoproteins to oxidation associated with administration of aged garlic extract. *Journal of Cardiovascular Pharmacology* 1998; 31(6):904-908. Also, Phelps S, Harris WS., Garlic supplementation and lipoprotein oxidation susceptibility. *Lipids* 1993; 28(5):475–477.

- ". . . [Garlic] has been shown to have mild blood-pressure–lowering effects." Silagy C, Neil A., A meta-analysis of the effect of garlic on blood pressure. *J Hypertens* 1994; (12):463–468.

- ". . . Garlic has a direct effect on the blood's clotting activities." Josling P, Walpera A, Grunwald J (eds.), The action of garlic in the pathogenesis of atherosclerosis: Selected abstracts from the 4th and International Congress on Phytotherapy. *Eur J Clin Res* 1992; 3A:1–12.

- ". . . Garlic also lowers fibrinogen. . . ." Josling P. Walpera A, Grunwald J (eds.), The action of garlic in the pathogenesis of atherosclerosis: Selected abstracts from the fourth and International Congress on Phytotherapy. *Eur J Clin Res* 1992; 3A:1–12.

## GENTIAN ROOT

- ". . . According to Dr. Rudolf Weiss, 'The bitter taste (of gentian) persists even in a dilution of 1:20,000. It is the most important of all European bitters . . .'" Weiss R, *Herbal Medicine.* Beaconsfield, England: Beaconsfield Arcanum, 1988, p. 40.

- ". . . One study involving 205 people found that gentian root capsules gave quick and dramatic relief of constipation, flatulence, appetite loss, vomiting, heartburn, abdominal pain, and nausea." Mills S, Bone K, *Principles and Practice of Phytotherapy.* London: Churchill Livingstone, 2000, p. 40.

## GINGER ROOT

- ". . . Fresh ginger has a warming effect on the exterior of the body, while the dried ginger is apt to be recommended for warming the middle of the body." Bensky D, Gamble A, *Chinese Herbal Medicine. Materia Medica,* revised ed. Seattle, WA: Eastland Press, 1993, pp. 300–301.

- ". . . In 19 of the 27 women who took ginger for nausea and vomiting, both symptoms became less frequent within four days of treatment." Fischer-Rasmussen W, Kjaer SK, Dahl C, et al., Ginger treatment of hyperemesis gravidarum. *European Journal of Obstetrics and Gynecology*, and Reproductive Biology 1990; 38:19–24.

- ". . . A study in 1982 revealed that ginger was superior to the drug Dramamine® for reducing motion sickness." Mowrey DB, Clayson DE, Motion sickness, ginger, and psychophysics. *Lancet* 1982; I:655–657.

- ". . . .[Some] excellent research done in 1994—involving 1,741 people-confirmed that ginger was indeed very effective in treating motion sickness." Grontved A, Brask T, et al., Ginger root against seasickness. *Acta Oto-Laryngol* 1988, 105:45–49.

## GINKGO BILOBA

- ". . . [Ginkgo] exerts antioxidant activity in the brain, eyes, and cardiovascular system." Ferrandini C, Droy-Lefaix MT, Christen Y, *Ginkgo Biloba Extract (Egb 761) as a free radical scavenger.* Paris: Elsevier, 1993.

- ". . . [They found] a 57 percent increase in blood flow among those who were regularly taking ginkgo." Jung F, Mrowietz C, et al., Effect of ginkgo biloba on fluidity of blood and peripheral microcirculation in volunteers. *Arzneim-Forsch Drug Res* 1990; 40:589–593.

- ". . . [Less] than one percent of those who take it—have reported mild digestive upset." DeFeudis FV, *Ginkgo biloba extract (Egb 761): Pharmacological activities and clinical applications.* Paris: Elsevier, 1991, pp. 143–146.

- ". . . [M]easurable improvements in memory, attention, and mood." Hofferberth B, The efficacy of Egb 761 in patients with senile dementia of the Alzheimer's type: A double blind, placebo controlled study on different levels of investigation. *Hum Psychopharmacol* 1994; 9:215–222.

- "... [Gingko] can help alleviate [intermittent claudication within] 3 to 6 months if you take daily dosages of 120 to 160 milligrams." Schneider B, Ginkgo biloba extract in peripheral arterial disease. Meta-analysis of controlled clinical trials. *Arzneim-Forsch Drug Res* 1992; 42:428–436.

- "... The improvements were even more dramatic." Schubert H, Halama P, Depressive episode primarily unresponsive to therapy in elderly patients. Efficacy of Ginkgo biloba extract (Egb 761) in combination with antidepressants. *Geriatr Forsch* 1993; 3:45–53.

- "... [T]aking this herb might produce some positive effects." Bascher V, Steinert W, Differential diagnosis of sudden deafness and therapy with high dose infusions of ginkgo biloba extract. *Vertigo, Nausea, Tinnitus, and Hypoacusia in Metabolic Disorders.* Amsterdam: Elsevier Science Publishing, 1988, pp. 575–582.

- "... [U]sing 60 milligrams of ginkgo per day regained potency." Sikora R et al., Ginkgo biloba extract in the therapy of erectile dysfunction. *J Urol* 1989; 141:188A.

- "... [S]ignificant change can occur as rapidly as 8 to 12 weeks." Voberg G, Ginkgo biloba extract(GBE): A long term study of chronic cerebral insufficiency in geriatric patients. *Clin Trials J* 1985; 22:149–157. Also, Rai GS, Shovlin C, and Wesnes K: A double blind, placebo-controlled study of Ginkgo biloba extract (Tankan) in elderly outpatients with mild to moderate memory impairment. Curr Med Res Opin 12:350–355, 1991. Also Mancini M, Agozzino B, and Bompani R. Clinical and therapeutic effects of Ginkgo biloba extract(GBE) versus placebo in the treatment of psychoorganic senile dementia of arteriosclerotic origin. *Gaz Med Ital* 1993; 152:69–80.

- "... [Gingko] can be helpful in alleviating breast tenderness and fluid retention." Tamborini A, Taurelle R, Value of standardized Ginkgo biloba extract (Egb 761) in the management of congestive symptoms of premenstrual syndrome. *Rev Fr Gynecol Obstet* 1993; 88:447–457.

- "... [Providing] the same antioxidant benefits that help protect normal body cells from the effects of rapid aging." Halpern G, *Ginkgo: A Practical Guide.* Garden City Park, NY: Avery Publishing, 1998, pp. 143–144.

# GINSENG

- "... Animal and human studies have shown that it supports and strengthens the function of the adrenal glands." Shibata S, Tanaka O, Shoji J, et al., Chemistry and pharmacology of Panax. In: Wagner H, Hikino H, Farnsworth NR (eds.), *Economic and Medicinal Plant Research. Vol. 1* London: Academic Press, 1985.

- "... *Panax* ginseng has a balancing effect on the stress hormones...." Tokorozawa, Saitama, Japan. Department of Obstetrics and Gynecology, National Defense Medical College. Effect of Korean red ginseng on psychological functions in patients with severe climacteric syndromes. *Int J Gynaecol Obstet* Dec. 1999; 169–74.

- "... Rg1 has been shown to stimulate brain and central nervous system activity, allowing increased energy and improved intellectual performance." Shibata S, Tanaka O, Shoji J, et al., Chemistry and pharmacology of Panax. In: Wagner H, Hikino H, Farnsworth NR (eds.), *Economic and Medicinal Plant Research. Vol. 1.* London: Academic Press, 1985.

- "... In one trial with 49 elderly people, the results demonstrated that 1,500 milligrams of *Panax* (red) ginseng improved coordination and reaction time. ..." Fulder S, Kataria M, Gethyn-Smith B, A double-blind clinical trial of Panax ginseng in aged subjects. Presented at the Fourth International Ginseng Symposium, Daejon, Korea, September 18–20, 1984.

- "... In addition, all three types of ginseng have been shown to have good antioxidant activity, which is also thought to slow the aging of cells." Kitts DD, Wijewickreme AN, Hu, C, Antioxidant properties of a North American ginseng extract. *Mol Cell Biochem* 2000, Jan; 203(1–2):1–10.

- "... A placebo-controlled, double-blind 20-week trial with male athletes supplementing 200 milligrams of a standardized Chinese ginseng extract found that it increased performance significantly." Forgo I, Schimert G, The duration of effect of the standardized ginseng extract G115 in healthy competitive athletes (in German). *Notobene Medici* 1985; 15(0):636–640.

- "... In a study of Siberian ginseng, 12 male athletes were given either the herb or a placebo." Asano K, Takahashi T, et al., Effect of Eleutherococcus senticosus extract on human working capacity. *Planta Med* 1986; 37:175–177.

- "... Athletes who take Siberian ginseng generally notice improved performance and quicker recovery from workouts and competition." McNaughton L, A comparison of Chinese and Russian ginseng as ergogenic acids to improve various facets of physical fitness. *Int Clin Nutr Rev* 1989; 9:32–35.

- "[Researchers] showed that this component of ginseng had a suppressive effect on the growth of prostate cancer cells." Liu WK, Xu SX, Che CT, Anti-proliferative effect of ginseng saponins on human prostate cancer cell line. *Life Sci* 2000 Aug; 67(11):1297–1306.

- "... Another study compared the effects of American ginseng and estrogen on breast cancer cells." Duda RB, Zhong Y, Navas V, Li MZ, Toy BR, Alavarez JG, American ginseng and breast cancer therapeutic agents synergistically inhibit MCF-7 breast cancer cell growth. *J Surg Oncol* 1999 Dec; 72(4):230–239.

- "... One Russian clinic studied the effects of Siberian ginseng on 80 women undergoing chemotherapy and radiation treatment for breast cancer." Brown D, *Herbal Prescriptions for Better Health*. Rocklin, CA: Prima Publishing, 1996, p. 75.

- "... A [2000] study done by the University of Toronto found that American ginseng reduced blood-sugar levels in people with Type 2 diabetes." Vuksan V et al., American ginseng (Panax quinquefolius L) reduces postprandial glycemia in nondiabetic subjects and subjects with type 2 diabetes mellitus.

- "... [One] Chinese study looked at the effects of Chinese ginseng on heart function." Chung Kuo Chung Hsi I Chieh Ho Tsa Chih, Effects of red ginseng on the congestive heart failure and its mechanism. *Research Section for Cardiovascular Diseases,* Yanbian Medical College, 1995 Jun; 15(6):325–327.

# GLANDULARS

- ". . . . According to naturopathic physician Michael Murray, the spleen produces two immune-enhancing compounds known as tuftsin and splenopentin." Murray MT, *Encyclopedia of Nutritional Supplements*. Rocklin, CA: Prima Publishing, 1996, p. 402.

## GLUCOSAMINE SULFATE

- ". . . In a study that involved 252 doctors and 1,506 patients, each patient was given 1,500 milligrams of glucosamine sulfate every day for about 7 weeks." Tapadinhas MJ et al., Oral Glucosamine sulfate in the management of arthrosis: Report on a multi-centre open investigation in Portugal. *Pharmatherapeutica* 1982; 3:157–168.

- ". . . In fact, there's evidence that NSAIDs and aspirin actually destroy cartilage by suppressing the cells and enzymes that should help to build it!" Shield MJ, Antiinflammatory drugs and their effects on cartilage synthesis and renal function. *European Journal of Rheumatology and Inflammation* 193:13(1):7–16. Also, Brandt K. Effects of Nonsteroidal antiinflammatory drugs on chondrocyte metabolism in vitro and in vivo. *American Journal of Medicine* November 20 1987; 83(5a):29–35. Also, Rainsford KD, Mechanisms of NSAIDs on joint destruction in osteoarthritis. *Agents and actions—supplements.* 1993; 44:39–43. Also, Dingle JT, Cartilage maintenance in osteoarthritis: Interaction of cytokines, NSAID and prostaglandins in articular cartilage damage and repair. *Journal of Rheumatology-Supplement* March 1991; 28:30–37.

## GREEN TEA

- ". . . Researchers have found that if you want the most protective effect of this kind, you should drink green tea before any meal that might contain nitrites and nitrates." Wang H, Wu Y, Inhibitory effect of Chinese tea on N-nitrosation in vitro and in vivo. *IARC Scientific Publications* 1991; 105:546–549.

- ". . . Lastly, green tea polyphenols prevent certain enzymes (specifically, cytochrome P450) in the liver from activating carcinogens during the detoxification process." Bu-Abbas A, Clifford MN, Walker R et al., Selective induction of rat hepatic CYP1 and CYP4 proteins and of peroxisomal proliferation by green tea. *Carcinogenesis* 1994; 15(11):2575–2579.

- ". . . One study looked at 472 women in various stages of breast cancer (labeled I, II, or III. . . ." Nakachi K, Suemasu K, Suga K et al., Influence of drinking green tea on breast cancer malignancy among Japanese patients. *Japanese Journal of Cancer Research* 1998; 89:254–261.

- ". . . [A] group of Japanese researchers concluded that green tea is potentially beneficial to anyone who takes it to help prevent cancer." Fujiki H, Yoshizawa S, Horiuchi T et al., Anticarcinogenic effects of (-)epigallocatechin gallate. *Preventive Medicine* 1992; 21:503–509.

- ". . . Animal studies have shown that green tea polyphenols, especially EECG, prevents cholesterol from being absorbed from food into the body." Ikeda I, Imsato Y, Sasaki E et al., Tea catechins decrease micellar solubility and intestinal absorption of cholesterol in rats. *Biochimia et Biophysica Acta* 1992; 1127:141–146.

- ". . . A study of 1,371 Japanese men showed that a high consumption of green tea (more than 10 cups daily) was associated with lower total cholesterol levels." Imai K, Nakachi K, Cross sectional study of effects of drinking green tea on cardiovascular and liver diseases. *British Medical Journal* 1995; 310:693–696.

- ". . . Green tea was also shown to reduce the oxidation of LDL cholesterol, which is implicated in the initial development of atherosclerosis." Miura S, Watanabe J, Tomita T et al., The inhibitory effects of tea polyphenols (flavan-3-ol derivatives) on Cu2+ mediated oxidative modification of low density lipoprotein. *Biological & Pharmaceutical Bulletin* 1994; 17(12):1567–1572.

- ". . . According to *The Green Tea Book,* "Green tea promotes a healthy digestive tract by altering the intestinal environment to make it favorable to the growth of the friendly bacteria and less favorable to the growth of undesirable bacteria." Mitscher L, *The Green Tea Book.* Garden City Park, NY: Avery Publishing, 1998, p. 119.

- ". . . One Japanese study demonstrated that a special green-tea extract improved the levels of the good bacteria *Lactobacilli* and *Bifidobacteria* in nursing home patients." Goto K, Kanaya S, Nishikawa T et al., Green tea catechins improve gut flora. *Ann Long-Term Care* 1998; 6:1–7.

- ". . . In one study with human subjects, researchers found that green tea polyphenols decreased plaque deposits even when the volunteers just took the green tea, without bothering to brush or floss their teeth." Ooshima T, Minami T, Aono W et al., Reduction of dental plaque deposition in humans by oolong tea extract. *Caries Research* 1994; 28:146–149.

## GUGGUL

- ". . . One 12-week study demonstrated that 1,500 milligrams of guggulipid had average reductions in serum cholesterol of nearly 22 percent, while triglycerides were reduced about 25 percent in people who took it regularly." Nityanand S, Srivastava JS, Athana OP, Clinical trials with guggulipid: A new hypolipidemic agent. *Journal of Association of Physicians of India* 1989; 37(5):323–328.

- ". . . One study showed that guggulipid works best for people who have high-cholesterol readings of the type IIb (increased LDL, VLDL, and triglycerides) and type IV (increased VLDL and triglycerides)." Agarwal RC, Singh SP, Saran RK et al., Clinical trial of guggulipid—A new hypolipidemic agent of plant origin in primary hyperlipidemia. *Indian Journal of Medical Research* 1986; 84:626–634.

## GYMNEMA SYLVESTRE

- ". . . [This herb] contains resins, saponins, stigmasterol, quercitol, and the amino-acid derivatives betaine, choline, and trimethylamine." Kapoor LD, *Handbook of Ayurvedic Medicinal Plants.* Boca Raton, FL: CRC Press, 1990, pp. 200–201.

- ". . . Two animal studies found gymnema extracts doubled the number of insulin-secreting beta cells in the pancreas and returned blood sugars to almost normal." Prakash AO, Mather S, Mather R, Effect of feeding Gymnema sylvestre leaves on blood glucose in beryllium nitrate treated rats. *J Ethnopharmacol* 1986; 18:143–146. Also, Shanmugasundaram ER, Gopinath KL, Shanmugasundaram KR, Rojendran VM, Possible regeneration of the islets of Langerhans in streptozotocin-diabetic rats given Gymnema sylvestre leaf extracts. *J Ethnopharmacol* 1990; 30:265–279.

- ". . . Gymnema also increases the activity of enzymes responsible for glucose uptake and utilization." Shanmugasundaram KR, Panneerselvam C, Samudram P, Shanmugasundaram ER, Enzyme changes and glucose utilisation in diabetic rabbits: The effect of Gymnema sylvestre, R.Br. *J Ethnopharmacol* 1983; 7:205–234.

- ". . . In a controlled study, a standardized gymnema extract was given to 27 people with Type 1 diabetes, all receiving a dose of 400 milligrams daily for periods ranging from 6 months to 2 1/2 years." Shanmugasundaram ER, Rajeswari G, Baskaran K et al., Use of Gymnema sylvestre leaf in the control of blood glucose in insulin-dependent diabetes mellitus. *J Ethnopharmacol* 1990; 30:281–294.

- ". . . In another study, 22 people with Type 2 diabetes were given 400 milligrams of gymnema extract daily for 18 to 20 months while they also continued to get their usual medication for hypoglycemia." Baskaran K, Ahamath BK, Shanmugasundaram KR, Shanmugasundaram ER, Antidiabetic effect of a leaf extract from Gymnema sylvestre in non-insulin-dependent diabetes mellitus patients. *J Ethnopharmacol* 1990; 30:295–305.

- ". . . Several animal studies have also confirmed the blood-sugar lowering effect of gymnema sylvestre." Srivasta Y, Bhatt HV, Prem AS et al., Hypoglycemic and life-prolonging properties of Gymnema sylvestre leaf extract in diabetic rats. *Isr J Med Sci* 1985; 21:540–542. Also, Okabayashi Y, Tani S, Fujisawa T et al., Effect of Gymnema sylvestre, R.Br. on glucose homeostasis in rats. *Diabetes Res Clin Pract* 1990; 9:143–148. Also, Venkatakrishna-Bhatt H, Srivastava Y, Jhala CI et al., Effect of Gymnema sylvestre, R.Br. leaves on blood sugar and longevity of alloxan diabetic rats. *Indian J Pharmacol* 1981; 13:99.

## HAWTHORN

- ". . . [Researchers] demonstrated that daily doses of 180 milligrams had a significant effect on blood flow to the heart." Hank T, Bruckel MH, Treatment of moderately stable forms of angina pectoris with Crataegutt novo. *Therapiewoche* 1983; 33:4331–4333.

- ". . . One high-quality study, for example, showed that eight weeks of hawthorn extract supplementation improved heart function and symptoms in people who had a moderate degree of congestive heart failure." Weikl A, Assmus KD, Neukum-Schmidt A et al., Crataegus special extract WS 1442. Objective proof of effectiveness for patients with heart failure (NYHA II). *Fortschritte Medizin* 1996; 114(24):291–296.

- ". . . [Researchers] learned that hawthorn extract is just as effective as the drug catopril, a pharmaceutical medication that's custom-designed for people with high blood pressure who are prone to congestive heart failure." Tauchert M, Ploch M, Hubner W-D, Effectiveness of hawthorn extract LI 132 compared with catopril. *Munch Medizinische Wochenschrift* 1994; 136:27–33.

## HORSE CHESTNUT

- ". . . One study of 240 people found that horse chestnut was just as effective as the treatments most often used in conventional medicine . . ." Diehm C, Trampisch HJ, Lange S et al., Comparison of leg compression stocking and oral horse chestnut seed extract therapy in patients with chronic venous insufficiency. *Lancet* 1996; 347:292–294.

# HYDROTHERAPY

- ". . . . [The] judge asked specifically who had helped the patient. The patient replied, "They have all helped me. The doctors, the apothecaries, and Priessnitz. The former helped me to get rid of my money, and Priessnitz, to get rid of my illness." Kirchfeld F, Boyle W, *Nature Doctors*. Portland, OR: Buckeye Naturopathic Press, 1994.

# IPRIFLAVONE

- ". . . A negative study about ipriflavone appeared in the Journal of the American Medical Association (JAMA) . . ." Alexandersen P, Christiansen C, et al., Ipriflavone in the treatment of postmenopausal osteoporosis. *JAMA* 2001; 285:1482–1488.

- ". . . In one study, 15 postmenopausal women were given ipriflavone or a placebo." Melis GB, Paoletti AM, Cagnacci L et al., Lack of any estrogenic effect of ipriflavone in postmenopausal women. *J Endocrin Invest* 1992; 15:755–761.

- ". . . Studies do show that ipriflavone acts synergistically with estrogen to normalize calcitonin secretion." Yamazaki I, Kinoshita M, Calcitonin secreting property of ipriflavone in the presence of estrogen. *Life Sci* 1986; 38:1535–1541.

- ". . . [As of 1997,] long-term safety of ipriflavone for periods ranging from 6 to 96 months . . ." Agnusdei D, Bufalino L, Efficacy of ipriflavone in established osteoporosis and long-term safety. *Calcif Tissue Int* 1997; 61:S23–S27.

- ". . . In one study of 132 women who were taking ipriflavone . . ." Alexandersen P, Toussaint A, Christansen C, et al., Ipriflavone in the treatment of postmenopausal osteoporosis. *JAMA* 2001; 285:1482–1488.

- ". . . In one case, someone who was already taking theophylline had excessive levels of this substance in her blood . . ." Takahashi J, Kawakatsu K, Wakayama T, Sawaoka H, Elevation of serum theophylline levels by ipriflavone in a patient with chronic obstructive pulmonary disease. *Eur J Clin Pharmacol* 1992; 43:207–208.

- ". . . Animal studies have found that ipriflavone may inhibit certain liver enzymes . . ." Monostory K, Vereczkey L, Interaction of theophylline and ipriflavone at the cytochrome p450 level. *Eur J Drug Metab Pharmacokinet* 1995; 20:43–47.

- ". . . One study showed that 1,200 milligrams of ipriflavone daily . . ." Mazzuoli G, Romagnoli E, Carnevale V et al., Effects of ipriflavone on bone remodeling in primary hyperparathyroidism. *Bone Miner* 1992; 19:S27–S33.

- ". . . One study of 23 people on kidney dialysis with decreased bone mineralization . . ." Hyodo T, Ono K, Koumi T et al., A study of the effects of ipriflavone administration in hemodialysis patients with renal osteodystrophy: Preliminary report. *Nephron* 1991; 58:114–115.

- ". . . The most significant study I've run across involved 100 postmenopausal women between the ages of 53 and 65, whom researchers tracked for one year." Moscarin M,

Patacchiola F, Spacca G, Palermo P, Caserta D, Valenti M, New perspectives in the treatment of postmenopausal osteoporosis: Ipriflavone.

- ". . . For example, in one controlled, one-year study, 83 postmenopausal women were divided into three groups." Agnusdei D, Gennari C, Bufalino L, Prevention of early postmenopausal bone loss using low doses of conjugated estrogens and the non-hormonal, bone-active drug ipriflavone. *Osteoporos Int* 1995; 5:462–466.

- ". . . These results have been supported by other human studies as well. Gambacciani M, Ciaponi M, Cappagli B et al., Effects of combined low dose of the isoflavone derivative ipriflavone and estrogen replacement on bone mineral density and metabolism in postmenopausal women. *Maturitas* 1997; 28:75–81. Also, Agnusdei D, Gennari C, Bufalino L, Prevention of early postmenopausal bone loss using low doses of conjugated estrogens and the non-hormonal, bone-active drug ipriflavone. *Osteoporos Int* 1995; 5:462–466.

- ". . . In this study, [32 recently ovariectomized women] received 500 milligrams of calcium and 600 milligrams ipriflavone daily for 12 months." Gambacciani M, Spinetti A, Cappagli B et al., Effects of ipriflavone administration on bone mass and metabolism in ovariectomized women. *J Endocrinol Invest* 1993; 16:333–337.

- ". . . [Researchers] tried a small study of patients who had tinnitus due to otosclerosis." Sziklai I, Komora V, Ribari O, Double-blind study of the effectiveness of a bioflavonoid in the control of tinnitus in otosclerosis. *Acta Chirurgica Hungarica* 1992–93; 33:101–107.

- ". . . When doctors studied 16 patients [with Paget's disease] . . ." Agnusdei D, Camporeale A, Gonnelli S et al., Short-term treatment of Paget's disease of bone with ipriflavone. *Bone Miner* 1992; 19:S35–S42.

## IRON

- ". . . Studies show that approximately 9 percent of all children in the U.S. between the ages of 12 months to 36 months have iron-deficiency anemia." Looker AC, Dallman PR, Carroll MD, Gunter EW, Johnson CL, Prevalence of iron deficiency in the United States. *JAMA* 1997; 277(12):973–976.

- ". . . Iron deficiency may impair the body's ability to manufacture thyroid hormone." Beard JL, Brel MJ, Derr J, Impaired thermoregulation and thyroid function in iron-deficiency anemia. *Am J Clin Nutr* 1990; 52:813–819.

## KAVA

- ". . . One placebo-controlled study looked at 101 people with anxiety who were given an extract of kava three times daily (approximately 70 milligrams of kavalactones per dose)." Volz HP, Kieser M, Kava kava extract WS 1490 versus placebo in anxiety disorders. A randomized placebo-controlled 25-week outpatient trial. *Pharmacopsychiat* 1997; 20:1–5.

- ". . . Researchers found that kava was superior to placebo for short- and long-term effectiveness, and most people improved within two months." Singh NN, Ellis CR, Singh YN et al., A double-blind, placebo-controlled study of the effects of kava (Kavatrol) on daily stress and anxiety in adults. *Alternative Therapies in Health and Medicine* 1998; 4(2):97–98.

- ". . . [It] proved to be just as effective as the anti-anxiety drug oxazepam." Lindenberg VD, Pitule-Schoedel H, DL-Kavain in comparison with oxazepam in anxiety states: Double-blind clinical study. *Frotschritte der Therapie* 1990; 108(2):31–24.

# L-CARNITINE

- ". . . One double-blind, placebo-controlled study of people diagnosed with Alzheimer's disease were given 2,000 milligrams twice daily of ALC or a placebo." Spagnoli A et al., Long-term acetyl-L-carnitine treatment in Alzheimer's disease. *Neurology* 1991; 41:1726–1732.

- ". . . Another double-blind study demonstrated that ALC was effective for the elderly with age-associated memory impairment." Cipolli C, Chiari G, Effects of acetyl-L-carnitine on mental deteoriation in the aged: Initial results. *Clin Ther* 1990; 132:479–510.

- ". . . It has also been shown in studies to be effective for senile depression." Bella R, Biondi R, Raffaele R, Pennisi G, Effects of acetyl-L-carnitine on geriatric patients suffering from dysthymic disorders. *Int J Clin Pharmacol Res* 1990; 10:355–360.

- ". . . [Researchers] found that 22 percent of angina patients given L-carnitine became angina-free during the study." Cherchi A, Lai C, Angelino F et al., Effects of L-carnitine on exercise tolerance in chronic stable angina: A multicenter, double-blind, randomized, placebo-controlled crossover study. *Int J Clin Pharmacol Ther Toxicol* 1985; 23:569–572.

- ". . . Another study looked at what happened when scientists gave L-carnitine supplementation of 2,000 milligrams daily to 100 randomly selected patients with stable angina over a 6-month period." Cacciatore L, Cerio R, Ciarimboli M et al., The therapeutic effect of L-carnitine in patients with exercise-induced stable angina: A controlled study. *Drugs Exp Clin Res* 1991; 17:225–235.

- ". . . In patients with anorexia nervosa, the combination of carnitine and vitamin $B_{12}$ accelerates the gain of body weight and helps normalize gastrointestinal function."

- ". . . The combination of $B_{12}$ with carnitine has been proven helpful for infantile anorexia." Giordano C, Perrotti G, Clinical studies of the effects of treatment with a combination of carnitine and cobamamide in infantile anorexia. *Clin Ter* 1979; 88:51–60.

- ". . . Children with this form of heart disease and who had carnitine deficiency responded favorably to carnitine supplementation." Ino T, Sherwood WG, Benson LN et al., Cardiac manifestations in disorders of fat and carnitine metabolism in infancy. *J Am Coll Cardiol* 1988; 11:1301–1308.

- ". . . [One] study that showed clinical improvement in 12 of 18 people with chronic fatigue syndrome." Plioplys AV, Plioplys S, Amantadine and L-carnitine treatment of chronic fatigue syndrome. *Neuropsychobiology* 1997; 35:16–23.

- ". . . In one study, 21 people with congestive heart failure were given 1,000 milligrams of carnitine twice daily for 45 days along with conventional drugs." Ghidini O, Azzurro M, Vita G, Sartori G, Evaluation of the therapeutic efficacy of L-carnitine in congestive heart failure. *Int J Clin Pharmacol Ther Toxicol* 1988; 26:217–220.

- ". . . Although Down's syndrome is a genetic condition, one 90-day study found that ALC supplementation was beneficial in improving visual memory and attention. . . ." De Falco FA et al., Effect of the chronic treatment with acetyl-L-carnitine in Down's syndrome. *Clin Ther* 1994; 144, 123–127.

- ". . . Anticonvulsant drugs . . . significantly lower carnitine levels." Hug G, McGraw CA, Bates SR, Landrigan EA, Reduction of serum carnitine concentrations during anticonvulsant therapy with phenobarbital, valproic acid, phenytoin, and carbamazepine in children. *J Pediatr* 1991; 119:799–802.

- ". . . So does the drug pivampicillin." Melegh B, Pap M, Molnar D et al., Carnitine administration ameliorates the changes in energy metabolism caused by short-term pivampicillin medication. *Eur J Pediatr* 1997; 156:795–799.

- ". . . L-carnitine may prevent heart complications in people with cancer who receive interleukin-2 immunotherapy and the chemotherapy drug adriamyacin." Lissoni P, Galli MA, Tancini G, Barni S, Prevention by L-carnitine of interleukin-2 related cardiac toxicity during cancer immunotherapy. *Tumori* 1993; 79:202–204.

- ". . . One study of 160 people who recently suffered a heart attack showed significant improvements in blood pressure, heart rate, angina attacks, and other markers of heart function." Davini P et al., Controlled study on L-carnitine therapeutic efficacy in postinfarction. *Drugs Exp Clin Res* 1992; 18:355–365.

- ". . . Studies have also shown that victims of a heart attack are more likely to survive if they take carnitine supplements during the next 24 hours." Singh RB, Niaz MA, Agarwal P et al., A randomised, double-blind, placebo-controlled trial of L-carnitine in suspected acute myocardial infarction. *Postgrad Med J* 1996; 72:45–50. Also, Iliceto S, Scrutinio D, Bruzzi P, et al., Effects of L-carnitine administration on left ventricular remodeling after acute anterior myocardial infarction: The L-Carnitine Ecocardiografia Digitalizzata Infarto Miocardico (CEDIM) Trial. *J Am Coll Cardiol* 1995; 26:380–387.

- ". . . It appears to also have a protective effect on the cell mitochondria for people with HIV using the drug zidovudine (AZT)." Semino-Mora MC, Leon-Monzon ME, Dalakas MC, Effect of L-carnitine on the zidovudine-induced destruction of human myotubes. Part I: L-carnitine prevents the myotoxicity of AZT in vitro. *Lab Invest* 1994; 71:102–112.

- ". . . A few studies have shown that carnitine supplementation can be helpful in improving the immune status (CD4 and CD8 counts) in people with HIV." Moretti S, Alesse E, Di Marzio L et al., Effect of L-carnitine on human immunodeficiency virus-1 infection-associated apoptosis: A pilot study. *Blood* 1998; 91:3817–3824. Also, Cifone M, Alesse E, Di Marzio L et al., Effect of L-carnitine treatment in vivo on apoptosis and ceramide generation in peripheral blood lymphocytes from AIDS patients. *Proc Assoc Am Physicians* 1997; 109:146–153.

- ". . . Carnitine helps fatty acids in the liver." Sachan DS et al., Ameliorating effects of carnitine and its precursors on alcohol induced fatty liver. *Am J Clin Nutr* 1984; 39:738–744. Also, Noto R et al., Free fatty acids and carnitine in patients with liver disease. *Curr Ther Res* 1986; 40:35–39.

- ". . . Supplementation of L-carnitine can improve sperm quality in some patients with idiopathic asthenospermia (defective sperm motility of unknown cause)." Costa M Canale D,

Filicori M et al., L-carnitine in idiopathic asthenozoospermia: A multicenter study. Italian Study Group on Carnitine and Male Infertility. *Andrologia* 1994; 26:155–159.

- ". . . One study showed that women have healthier babies who are less likely to have respiratory distress syndrome if the expectant mothers are given carnitine along with the drug betamethasone during the prenatal period." Kurz C, Arbeiter K, Obermair A et al., L-carnitine–betamethasone combination therapy versus betamethasone therapy alone in prevention of respiratory distress syndrome. *Z Geburtshilfe Perinatol* 1993; 197:215–219.

## LICORICE ROOT

- ". . . [Glycyrrhizin and glycyrrhetinic acid] have been shown in animal studies to increase the body's supply of one of nature's most powerful antiviral agents: interferon." Abe N, Ebina T, Ishida N, Interferon induction by glycyrrhizin and glycyrrhetinic acid in mice. *Microb Immunol* 1982; 26:535–539.

- ". . . One study of 20 people found that a DGL mouthwash improved the symptoms of 15 of the participants by a 50 to 75 percent within 1 day, and complete healing of the sores within 3 days." Das Sk, Gulati AK, Singh VP, Deglycyrrhizinated licorice in apthous ulcers. *J Assoc Physicians India* 1989; 37:647.

- ". . . In a single-blind study of 100 people with peptic ulcers, participants took either DGL . . . or the medication Tagament (cimetidine)." Morgan AG, McAdam WAF, Pacsoo C et al., Comparison between cimetidine and Caved-S in the treatment of gastric ulceration, and subsequent maintenance therapy. *Gut* 1982; 23:545–551.

- ". . . Another study of 874 people also demonstrated that DGL was as effective as antacids and the anti-ulcer drug cimetidine in persons with duodenal ulcers." Kassir ZA, Endoscopic controlled trial of four drug regimens in the treatment of chronic duodenal ulceration. *Irish Medical Journal* 1985; 78(6):153–156.

## LOMATIUM

- ". . . Several earlier in vitro studies have shown lomatium to have direct killing effects on many different types of bacteria and fungus, including *Candia albicans*. It is also believed that phytochemicals found lomatium have the ability to inhibit viruses from replicating." Alstat EK, Lomatium Dissectum—An Herbal Virucide? *Complementary Medicine* 1987; 2(5).

## LYSINE

- ". . . A study was conducted on 45 patients who experienced frequent herpes outbreaks. They received 312 to 500 milligrams of L-lysine for 2 months to 3 years." Griffith RS et al., A multicentered study of Lysine therapy in herpes simplex infection. *Dermatologica* 1978; 156:257–267.

- ". . . Another study found that 1,200 milligrams of L-lysine significantly reduced the recurrence of herpes simplex outbreaks." McCune MA et al., Treatment of recurrent herpes simplex infections with L-Lysine hydrochloride. *Cutis* 1984; 34:366–373.

# MAGNESIUM

- ". . . One study showed that persons with congestive heart failure who had normal levels of magnesium had longer survival rates than those with lower magnesium levels." Gottlieb SS et al., Prognostic importance of serum magnesium concentration in patients with congestive heart failure. *J Am Coll Cardiol* 1990; 16:827–831.

- ". . . It has also been shown that children with insulin-dependent diabetes have lower levels of magnesium than other children." Rohn R, Pleban P, Jenkins L, Magnesium, zinc, and copper in plasma and blood cellular components in children with IDDM. *Clin Chim A* 1993; 215:21–28.

- ". . . One study showed that magnesium a dose of 141.5 milligrams twice daily for one month improved the visual fields of people with glaucoma." Gaspar AZ, Gasser P, Flammer J, The influence of magnesium on visual field and peripheral vasospasm in glaucoma. *Opthalmologica* 1995; 209:11–13.

- ". . . One study examined 55 people with reoccurring kidney stones, who were given 500 milligrams of magnesium daily for up to 4 years." Johansson G et al., Effects of magnesium hydroxide in renal stone disease. *J Am Coll Nutr* 1982; 1:179–185.

- ". . . Studies have shown magnesium to be helpful in preventing preeclampsia. . . ." Husain S, Sibley C, Magnesium and pregnancy. *Min Elect M* 1993; 19:296–307. Also, Rudnicki P, Frolich A, Fishcer-Rasmussen W, Magnesium supplementation in pregnancy induced hypertension and preeclampsia. *Acta Obst Gyn Sc* 1994; 73:526–530.

- ". . . Magnesium levels have been shown to be lower in women with PMS than in those without this condition." Abraham GE, Lubran MM, Serum and red blood cell magnesium levels in patients with premenstrual tension. *Am J Clin Nutr* 1981; 34:2364–2366.

- ". . . One double-blind study found that 200 milligrams per day of magnesium supplementation alleviated PMS symptoms such as breast tenderness, abdominal bloating, weight gain, and swelling of the extremities." Walker AF et al., Magnesium supplementation alleviates premenstrual symptoms of fluid retention. *J Womens Health* 1998; 7:1157–1165.

- ". . . Another study found that magnesium was effective in relieving premenstrual mood changes." Facchinetti F et al., Oral magnesium successfully relieves premenstrual mood changes. *Obstet Gynecol* 1991; 78:177–181.

# MELATONIN

- ". . . More research needs to be done before we can say for sure that melatonin has an 'anti-aging effect,' but it seems to be promising." Maestroni GJ, Conti A, Pierpaoli W, Pineal melatonin, its fundamental immunoregulatory role in aging and cancer. *Annals of the New York Academy of Sciences* 1988; 521:140–48.

- ". . . The antiproliferative effect seems to apply to estrogen-dependent breast cancer and androgen-dependent prostate cancer." Eck-Enriquez K, Kiefer TL, Spriggs LL, Hill SM, Pathways through which a regimen of melatonin and retinoic acid induces apoptosis in MCF-7 human breast cancer cells. *Breast Cancer Res Treat* 2000 Jun; 61(3):229–239. Also, Marelli MM, Limonta P, Maggi R, Motta M, Moretti RM, Growth-inhibitory activity of melatonin on human androgen-independent DU 145 prostate cancer cells. *Prostate* 2000 Nov 1; 45(3):238–244.

- ". . . Also, melatonin has been shown to increase the efficacy of chemotherapy and reduce the toxicity of the treatments." Lissoni P et al., Decreased toxicity and increased efficacy of cancer chemotherapy using the pineal hormone melatonin in metastatic solid tumour patients with poor clinical status. *Eur J Cancer* 1999 Nov; 35(12):1688–1692.

- ". . . It has also been shown to improve the sleep quality of people with chronic schizophrenia." Shamir E, Laudon M, Barak Y, Anis Y, Rotenberg V, Elizur A, Zisapel N, Melatonin improves sleep quality of patients with chronic schizophrenia. *J Clin Psychiatry* 2000 May; 61(5):373–377.

- ". . . I advocate the use of melatonin to help wean people off addictive benzodiazapine drugs that are used for insomnia." Garfinkel D, Zisapel N, Wainstein J, Laudon M, Facilitation of benzodiazepine discontinuation by melatonin: A new clinical approach. *Arch Intern Med* 1999 Nov 8; 159(20):2456–2460.

- ". . . Melatonin has been shown to help normalize the sleeping patterns of blind people." Sack RL, Brandes RW, Kendall AR, Lewy AJ, Entrainment of free-running circadian rhythms by melatonin in blind people. *N Engl J Med* 2000 Oct 12; 343(15):1070–1077.

- ". . . Melatonin may become a common therapy for the prevention and treatment of radiation exposure. One study found that it protected human white blood cells 500 times more effectively than the potent antioxidant DMSO. . . ." Vijayalami BZ, Reiter RJ et al., Melatonin protects human blood lymphocytes from radiation induced chromosome damage. *Mutation Research* 1995; 346(1):23–31.

## MENTAL IMAGERY

". . . [Researchers] explored the effects of visualization, or mental imagery, on immune-system response in people who had depressed white blood cell count." Donaldson VW, A clinical study of visualization on depressed white blood cell count in medical patients. *Appl Psychophysiol Biofeedback* 2000 Jun; 25(2):117–128.

## MILK THISTLE

- ". . . According to the U.S. Environmental Protection Agency, an estimated 2.2 billion pounds of environmental toxins were released into the environment between the years 1987 and 1994. . . ." U.S. Environmental Protection Agency, *1987–1994 Toxic Release Inventory National Report.* Washington, D.C.: Office of Toxic Substances.

- ". . . Treatment with milk thistle is essential for anyone who has been poisoned by eating the deathcap mushroom *(Amanita phalloides)*." Ferenci P, Dragosics B, Dittrich H et al., Randomized controlled trial of silymarin treatment in patients with cirrhosis of the liver. *Journal of Hepatology* 1989; 9:105–113.

- ". . . In a well-controlled study of 105 people with cirrhosis, researchers compared those who took 420 milligrams of silymarin with those who . . . were taking a placebo." Ferenci P, Dragosics B, Dittrich H et al., Randomized controlled trial of silymarin treatment in patients with cirrhosis of the liver. *Journal of Hepatology* 1989; 9:105–113.

- "... In a study of chronic viral hepatitis, silymarin not only lowered elevated liver enzymes, but liver cell damage was also reversed as demonstrated by a liver biopsy." Berenguer J, Carrasco D, Double-blind trial of silymarin versus placebo in the treatment of chronic hepatitis. *Muench Med Wochenschr* 1977; 119:240–260.

- "... A double-blind, placebo-controlled study of 60 people, researchers found that silymarin protected against the long-term use of drugs used for mental illness." Palasciano G, Portincasa P, Palmeri V et al., The effect of silymarin on plasma levels of malon-dialdehyde in patients receiving long-term treatment with psychotropic drugs. *Current Therapeutic Research* 1994; 55(5):537–545.

## MSM

- "... In their book *The Miracle of MSM,* they report that MSM can deliver numerous benefits. . . ." Jacob, S, Lawrence R, Zucker, M, *The Miracle of MSM. The Natural Solution for Pain.* New York: Putnam, 1999, p. 23.

- "... [A study] reported in the *International Journal of Anti-Aging Medicine,* 16 patients ranging in age from 55 to 78 were randomly assigned to two groups." Lawrence RM, Methylsulfonylmethane (MSM): A double-blind study of its use in degenerative arthritis. *International Journal of Anti-Aging Medicine* Summer 1998; 1(1):50.

- "... In one study, 21 patients were assessed by a certified cosmetologist under the direction of a medical doctor. . . ." Lawrence RM, The Effectiveness of the Use of Oral Liginisul MSM (Methylsulfonylmethane) Supplementation on Hair and Nail Health. Preliminary Correspondence, Carol Wood Corporation, 2000.

- "... A similar study, done with Liginisul® MSM, showed similar improvements in nail health." Lawrence RM, The Effectiveness of the Use of Oral Liginisul MSM (Methylsulfonylmethane) Supplementation on Hair and Nail Health. Preliminary Correspondence, CarolWood Corporation, 2000.

- "... All pregnant women should take prenatal vitamins." Preston-Martin S, Pogoda JM, Mueller BA, Lubin F, Holly EA, Filippini G, Cordier S, Peris-Bonet R, Choi W, Little J, Arslan A, Prenatal vitamin supplementation and risk of childhood brain tumors. *Int J Cancer Suppl* 1998; 11:17–22. Also, Botto LD, Multinare J, Erickson JD, Occurrence of congenital heart defects in relation to maternal multivitamin use. *American Journal of Epidemiology* 2000; 151:878–884.

## MULTIVITAMINS

- "... One study examined the effect of a multivitamin on the immune function in the elderly." Chandra RK, Effect of vitamin and trace-element supplementation on immune responses and infection in elderly subjects. *Lancet* 1992; 340:1124–1127.

- "... Another study found that a multivitamin and trace element supplement resulted in stronger immune cell markers, as compared with those who took placebo, whose showed a reduction in immune-cell parameters." Pike J, Chandra RK, Effect of vitamin and trace element supplementation on immune indices in healthy elderly. *Int J Vitam Nutr Res* 1995; 65(2):117–121.

- "... In one study, 60 children ages 12 to 13 were examined for the effect of a multivitamin on intelligence." Benton D, Roberts G, Effect of vitamin and mineral supplementation on intelligence of a sample of schoolchildren. *Lancet* 1988; 1:140–143.

# NETTLE

- "... [Researchers] found that the combination of nettle leaf and a pharmaceutical antiinflammatory (diclofenac) was as effective at relieving the pain of arthritis as a full dose of the drug." Chrubasik S, Enderlein W, Bauer R et al., Evidence for antirheumatic effectiveness of Herba Urtica dioicae in acute arthritis: A pilot study. *Phytomedicine* 1997; 4(2):105–108.

- "... In a randomized, double-blind study, scientists looked into the effects of freeze-dried nettles on people who had hayfever (allergic rhinitis). It was found that after one week of use, 58 percent of the participants were helped by this herbal extract." Mittman P, *Planta Medica* 1990; 56:44–47.

- "... Researchers found that men with BPH could reduce the symptoms of urinary frequency and nighttime urination in the span of ten weeks if they took nettle." Vandierendounck EJ, Burkhardt P, The extract of Radicus Urticae for fibromyadenoma of the prostate with nightly pollakuria. Study for testing the effect of ZY 15095 (Simic®). *Therapiewoche Schweiz* 1986; 10:892–895.

- "... One randomized, double-blind study found the combination of nettle root and saw palmetto worked as effectively as the pharmaceutical drug Finasteride, which is commonly used to reduce the symptoms of BPH." Sokeland J, Albrecht J, A combination of Sabal and Urtica extract vs. Finasteride in BPH. Comparison of therapeutic effectiveness in a 1 year, double-blind study. *Urologe A* 1997; 36(4):327–333.

- "... Another landmark study showed that the combination of saw palmetto and *Pygeum* worked to shrink enlarged prostate tissue." Overmyer M, Saw palmetto shown to shrink prostatic epithelium. *Urology Times* 1999; 27(6):1, 42.

# ONION

- "... Onions have been shown to have strong antioxidant effects." Helen A, Krishnakumar K, Vijayammal PL, Augusti KT, Antioxidant effect of onion oil (Allium cepa. Linn) on the damages induced by nicotine in rats as compared to alpha-tocopherol."

- "... They are a good source of the flavonoid quercitin ..." Hollman PC, Katan MB, Dietary flavonoids: Intake, health effects and bioavailability. *Food Chem Toxicol* 1999 Sep–Oct; 37(9–10):937–942.

- "... Animal studies have shown that phytochemicals within onion such as thiosulfinates and cepaenes inhibit inflammatory compounds associated with inducing asthma." Wagner H, Dorsch W, Bayer T, Breu W, Willer F, Antiasthmatic effects of onions: Inhibition of 5-lipoxygenase and cyclooxygenase in vitro by thiosulfinates and "Cepaenes." *Prostaglandins Leukot Essent Fatty Acids* 1990 Jan; 39(1):59–62.

- "... A French study of 345 women found that risk of breast cancer decreased as consumption of fiber, garlic, and onions increased." Challier B, Perarnau JM, Viel JF, Garlic, onion and cereal fibre as protective factors for breast cancer: A French case-control study. *Eur J Epidemiol* 1998 Dec; 14(8):737–747.

- "The researchers suggested that alluin vegetables, like raw vegetables, may have an important protecting effect not only against stomach cancer, but also against esophogeal cancer." Gao CM, Takezaki T, Ding JH, Li MS, Protective effect of allium vegetables against both esophageal and stomach cancer: A simultaneous case-referent study of a high-epidemic area in Jiangsu Province, China. *J Cancer Res* 1999 Jun; 90(6):614–621K.

- "... Studies have shown that onion reduces elevated blood-sugar levels." Babu Ps, Srinivasan K, Influence of dietary casaicin and onion on the metabolic abnormalities associated with streptozotocin induced diabetes mellitus. *Mol Cell Biochem* 1997 Oct; 175(1-2):49–57.

## PEPPERMINT

- "... Menthol has been shown to be helpful in dissolving gallstones when combined with ursodeoxycholic acid. It's used in a proprietary formulation known as rowachol." Leuschner M, Leuschner U, Lazarovici D, Kurtz W, Hellstern A, Dissolution of gallstones with an ursodeoxycholic acid menthol preparation: A controlled prospective double blind trial. *Gut* 1988 Apr; 29(4):428–432.

- "... One randomized, double-blind, placebo-controlled trial of 110 people with IBS found that peppermint oil improved symptoms of abdominal pain, distention, flatulence, and other symptoms." Liu JH, Chen GH, Yeh HZ, Huang CK, Poon SK, Enteric-coated peppermint-oil capsules in the treatment of irritable bowel syndrome: A prospective, randomized trial. *J Gastroenterol* 1997 Dec; 32(6):765–768.

## PHOSPHATIDYLSERINE

- "... Dr. Paris Kidd ... has reviewed some 3,000 peer-reviewed research papers on PS." Kidd PM, *Phosphatidylserine: The Nutrient Building Block That Accelerates All Brain Functions and Counters Alzheimer's.* New Canaan, CT: Keats Publishing, 1998, p. 8.

- "... In an article in *The Alternative Medicine Review*, ..." Kidd PM, Attention Deficit/Hyperactivity Disorder (ADHD) in Children: Rationale for its integrative management. *Alternative Medicine Review* October 2000; 5:5.

- "... In a 1991 study of phosphatidylserine among people aged 50 to 75, doctors found positive results when they used 100-milligram doses of PS, three times daily." Crook TH et al., Effects of phosphatidylserine in age-associated memory impairment. *Neurology* 1991; 41(5):644–649.

- "... In evaluating this supplement, Dr. Thomas Crook, a leading researcher on the effects of drugs and supplements on memory, concluded... " Crook, TH et al., Effects of phosphatidylserine in Alzheimer's disease. *Psychopharmacology Bulletin* 1992; 28(1):61–66.

- "PS has been shown to improve mood and alleviate depression." Maggioni M et al., Effects of phosphatidylserine therapy in geriatric subjects with depressive disorders. *Acta Psychiatrica Scandinavia* 1990; 81:265–270.

- ". . . PS is also effective in helping athletes adapt to stress caused by exhaustive training." Monteleone P et al., Blunting by chronic phosphatidylserine administration of the stress induced activation of the hypothalamo-pituitary-adrenal axis in healthy men. *European Journal of Clinical Pharmacology* 1992; 41:385–388.

# POTASSIUM

- ". . . Studies have shown that taking potassium supplements significantly reduces systolic and diastolic blood pressure." Cappucio FP et al., Does potassium supplementation lower blood pressure? A meta-analysis of published trials. *J Hypertens* 1991; 9:465–473.

- ". . . An 8-year study of 43,738 men, ages 40 to 75, found that those who consumed the highest amount of potassium . . . had a reduced risk of stroke." Ascherio A et al., Intake of potassium, magnesium, calcium, and fiber and risk of stroke among US men. *Circulation* 1998 Sep 22; 98(12):1198–1204.

# PRAYER

- ". . . According to Dr. Larry Dossey, . . . 'The evidence is simply overwhelming that prayer functions at a distance to change physical processes in a variety of organisms, from bacteria to humans.' " Dossey L, *Healing Words: The Power of Prayer and the Practice of Medicine.* New York: HarperCollins, 1997, p. 3.

# PROGESTERONE

- ". . . Many women find that natural progesterone works extremely well to manage their perimenopausal and menopausal symptoms." Lee J, *What Your Doctor May Not Tell You About Menopause.* New York: Warner Books, 1996, p 72.

# PROPOLIS

- ". . . In one study involving 90 men and women, investigators compared an ointment made of Canadian propolis to the pharmaceutical acyclovir." Vynograd N, Vynograd I, Sosnowski Z, A comparative multi-centre study of the efficacy of propolis, acyclovir and placebo in the treatment of genital herpes. *Phytomedicine* 2000 Mar; 7(1):1–6.

- ". . . In some cases, antibiotics were 10 to 100 times more effective. . . ." Boone, K, Propolis: Nature's agent against infections. *Townsend Letter for Doctors & Patients* 2000, June: 159.

- ". . . In a . . . study of 42 hospitalized people who were suffering from burns, doctors found that topical application of napkins saturated with propolis were enormously helpful to the patients." *Townsend Letter for Doctors & Patients* 2000 June: 162.

# QUERCITIN

- ". . . It has an inhibiting effect on enzymes related to inflammation . . . ." Della Loggia, Ragazzi E, Tubaro A et al., Anti-inflammatory activity of benzopyrones that are inhibitors of cyclo- and lipo-oxygenase. *Pharmacol Res Commun* 1988; 20:S91–S94. Also, Kim HP,

Mani I, Ziboh VA, Effects of naturally-occurring flavonoids and biflavonoids on epidermal cyclooxygenase from guinea pigs. *Prostaglandins Leukot Essent Fatty Acids* 1998; 58:17–24.

- ". . . It also prevents the release of histamine, . . ." Bronner C, Landry Y, Kinetics of the inhibitory effect of flavonoids on histamine secretion from mast cells. *Agents Actions* 1985; 16:147–151.

- ". . . Test tube and animal studies have shown that quercitin is effective against viral infections." Kaul TN, Middleton E Jr, Ogra PL, Antiviral effect of flavonoids on human viruses. *J Med Virol* 1985; 15:71–79.

- ". . . Quercitin has been shown to increase the effectiveness of the chemotherapy drug cisplatin, as well as protect the kidney cells from toxicity of this drug." Hofmann J, Fiebig HH, Winterhalter BR et al., Enhancement of the antiproliferative activity of cisdiamminedichloroplatinum(II) by quercetin. *Int J Cancer* 1990; 45:536–539. Also, Kuhlman MK, Horsch E, Burkhardt G et al., Reduction of cisplatin toxicity in cultured renal tubular cells by the bioflavonoid quercetin. *Arch Toxicol* 1998; 72:536–540.

- ". . . It protects LDL cholesterol from being oxidized." Saija A, Scalese M, Lanza M et al., Flavonoids as antioxidant agents: Importance of their interaction with biomembranes. *Free Radic Biol Med* 1995; 19:481–486. Also, Miller AL, Antioxidant flavonoids: Structure, function and clinical usage. *Alt Med Rev* 1996; 1:103–111.

- Chen YT, Zheng RL, Jia ZJ, Ju Y, Flavonoids as superoxide scavengers and antioxidants. *Free Radic Biol Med* 1990; 9:19–21. Also, DeWhalley CV, Rankin JF, Rankin SM et al., Flavonoids inhibit the oxidative modification of low density lipoproteins. *Biochem Pharmacol* 1990; 39:1743–1749.

- ". . . Quercitin prevents the aggregation of platelets so that circulation is improved and reduces the chances of blood-clot formation." Pace-Asciak CR, Hahn S, Diamandis EP et al., The red wine phenolics trans-resveratrol and quercetin block human platelet aggregation and eicosanoid synthesis: Implications for protection against coronary heart disease. *Clin Chim Acta* 1995; 235:207–219.

- ". . . One study looked at the relationship of dietary flavonoid intake and risk of coronary heart disease in men between the ages of 65 and 85." Hertog MG, Feskens EJ, Hollman PC et al., Dietary antioxidant flavonoids and risk of coronary heart disease: The Zutphen Elderly Study. *Lancet* 1993; 342:1007–1011.

- ". . . Quercetin has been shown to be a strong inhibitor of human lens aldose reductase." Chaudry PS, Cabera J, Juliani HR, Varma SD, Inhibition of human lens aldose reductase by flavonoids, sulindac, and indomethacin. *Biochem Pharmacol* 1983; 32:1995–1998.

- ". . . It has been shown to inhibit the growth of *Heliobacter pylori,* a bacteria implicated in many cases of ulcers." Beil W, Birkholz C, Sewing KF, Effects of flavonoids on parietal cell acid secretion, gastric mucosal prostaglandin production and *Helicobacter pylori* growth. *Arzneimittelforschung* 1995; 45:697–700.

## SAMe

- ". . . To date, there aren't any studies to indicate that SAMe can cause pregnancy problems or harm the unborn baby, but it is not known whether SAMe can be guaranteed for long-term use." Nicastri PL, Diaferi A, Tartagni M, Loizzi P, Fanelli M, A randomized placebo-controlled trial of ursodeoxycholic acid and S'Adenosylmethionine in the treatment of intrahepatic cholestasis of pregnancy. *British Journal of Obstetrics and Gynaecology* 1998:105(11):1205–1207.

- "...When the published clinical studies on SAMe between the years of 1973 and 1992 were analyzed...." Bottigleri T, Hyland K, S-adenosylmethionine levels in psychiatric and neurological disorders: A review. *Acta Scandanavica Neurologica* 1994:89(154):19–26.

- "...When SAMe was compared with a placebo...." Jacobsen S, Danneskiold-Samsoe B, Andersen RB, Oral S-sdenosylmethionine in primary fibromyalgia—Double blind clinical evaluation. *Scandanavian Journal of Rheumatology* 1991:20(4):294–302.

- "...Another double-blind study found that SAMe improved trigger-point pain and depression." Tavoni A, Vitali C, Bonbardieri S, Pasero G, Evaluation of S-adenosylmethionine in primary fibromylagia. A double-blind crossover study. *American Journal of Medicine* November 27, 1987; 83(5a):107–110.

- "...In the largest study on SAMe and osteoarthritis, researchers followed the progress of 20,641 people who took SAMe for eight weeks." Berger R, Nowak H, A new medical approach to the treatment of osteoarthritis. Report of an open phase IV study with ademetionine (gumbaral). *American Journal of Medicine* November 1987; 83(5a):8408.

- "...Several studies have compared SAMe with popular NSAID...." Caruso I, Pietrogrande V, Italian double-blind multicenter study comparing S-adenosylmethionine naproxen, and placebo in the treatment of degenerative joint disease. *American Journal of Medicine* November 20 1987; 83(5a):66–71.

- Muller-Fassbender H, Double-blind clinical trial of S-adenosylmethionine versus ibuprofen in the treatment of osteoarthritis. *American Journal of Medicine* November 20 1987; 83(5a):81–83. Also, Vetter G, Double-blind comparative clinical trial with S-adenosylmethionine and indomethacin in the treatment of osteoarthritis. *American Journal of Medicine* November 20 1987:; 3(5a):78–80. Also, Maccagno A, DiGirogio EE, Caston OL, Sagasta CL, Double-blind controlled clinical trial of oral S-adenosylmethionine versus piroxicam in knee osteoarthritis. *American Journal of Medicine* November 20 1987; 83(5a):72–77.

# SAW PALMETTO

- "...One study showed that the combination of saw palmetto and the herb nettles *(Pygeum)* helps shrink enlarged prostate tissue." Overmyer M, Saw palmetto shown to shrink prostatic epithelium. *Urology Times* 1999; 27(6):1,42.

- "...In one study involving 1,098 men over the age of 50, researchers compared the results of taking saw palmetto extract...." Carraro JC, Raynaud JP, Koch G et al., Comparison of phytotherapy (Permixon) with finasteride in the treatment of benign prostatic hyperplasia: A randomized international study of 1,098 patients. *The Prostate* 1996; 29:231–240.

- "...The prestigious *Journal of the American Medical Association (JAMA)* ...summed up the findings in a number of reports...." Wilt J. et al., Saw palmetto extracts for treatment of benign prostatic hyperplasia: A systematic review. *JAMA* Nov. 11, 1998; 280(18):1604–1609.

- "... One study showed that the combination of saw palmetto and the herb nettles helps shrink enlarged prostate tissue." Overmyer, M, Saw palmetto shown to shrink prostatic epithelium. *Urology Times* 1999; 27(6):1,42.

## SELENIUM

- "... In his book *The Antioxidant Miracle,* Lester Packer states that research by Dr. Raymond Shamberger of the Cleveland Clinic has shown "that people who live in states with the lowest selenium content were three times more likely to die of heart disease than those who lived in states that were more selenium rich." Packer L, Colman C, *The Antioxidant Miracle.* New York: John Wiley and Sons, 1999, p. 143.

- "... One found that 200 micrograms of selenium given to people with normal blood selenium levels resulted in a significant increase in immunity." Kiremidjian-Schumacher L et al., Supplementation with selenium and human immune cell functions. Effect on cytotoxic lymphocytes and natural killer cells. *Biol Trace Elem Res* 1994; 41:115–127.

## SOY

- "... An analysis of 29 studies found that just 31 to 47 grams of isolated soy protein or texturized soy protein decreased total cholesterol by 9 percent and LDL cholesterol by 13 percent." Anderson JW et al., Meta-analysis of the effects of soy protein intake on serum lipids. *New England Journal of Medicine* 1995; 333:276–282.

- "... In one study, women were given 160 milligrams of isoflavones daily for three months." *Journal of Nutrition* 1995; 125(Suppl 3S):567S–909S.

- "... One study of postmenopausal women found that soy protein with high isoflavone content improved bone mineral density in the lumbar spine." Rotter SM et al., Soy protein and isoflavones: Their effects on blood lipids and bone density in postmenopausal women. *American Journal of Clinical Nutrition* 1998; 68:1375S–1379S.

## SPIRULINA

- "... One type of spirulina known as *Spirulina platensis* was shown to inhibit the HIV virus (HIV-1) in a test-tube study." Ayehunie S, Belay A, Hu Y, Baba T, Ruprecht R, Inhibition of HIV-1 replication by an aqueous extract of Spirulina platensis (Arthrospira platensis). Seventh IAAA Conference, Knysna, South Africa, April 17, 1996.

- "... Another study found a spirulina extract known as Calcium Spirulan inhibited the replication of several viruses." Hayashi T, Hayashi K et al., Calcium Spirulan, an inhibitor of enveloped virus replication from a blue-green alga spirulina platensis. American Chemical Society and American Society of Pharmacognosy. *Journal of Natural Products* 1996; 59(1):83–87.

- "... Phycocyanin has been shown in animal studies to stimulate the production of red blood cells." Zhang C et al., The effects of polysaccharide and phycocyanin from spirulina platensis variety on peripheral blood and hematopoietic system of bone marrow in mice. Second Asia Pacific Conference on Alga Biotechnology, April 25–27, 1994, p. 58.

- "... A study looked at the effect of spirulina supplementation on 30 healthy men with high levels of cholesterol, triglyceride, and LDL." Nayaka N et al., *Nutrition Reports International.* Tokai Univ. Pub. 1988; 37(6):1329–1337.

- "... Laboratory studies also show that spirulina polysaccharides can work to repair genetic material that has been damaged by toxins or from radiation." Qishen P et al., Enhancement of endonuclease activity and repair DNA synthesis by polysaccharide of spirulina. *Chinese Genetics Journal* 1988; 15(5):374–381.

- "... In one study, tobacco chewers who had a type of mouth disease called oral leukoplakia were given 1 gram a day of spirulina for one year." Babu M et al., Evaluation of chemoprevention of oral cancer with spirulina. *Nutrition and Cancer* 1995; 24(2):197–202.

- "... In a one-year program, 5,000 preschool children who lived in a rural area near Madras, India were fed spirulina regularly." Seshadri CV, Large scale nutritional supplementation with spirulina alga. All India Coordinated Project on Spirulina. Shri Amm Murugappa Chettiar Research Center, Madras, India, 1993.

- "... Beta carotene (and perhaps some of the other carotenoids) from spirulina have a high bioavailability and are converted to vitamin A very effectively." Annapurna V et al., Bioavailability of spirulina carotenes in preschool children. *Journal of Clinical and Biochemical Nutrition* 1991; 10:145–151.

- "... Children fed 5 grams of spirulina tablets daily have been shown to make dramatic recoveries ...." Evets LB et al., Means to normalize the levels of immunoglobulin E using the food supplement spirulina. Grodenski State Medical University, Russian Federation Committee of Patents and Trade, January 15, 1994.

## ST. JOHN'S WORT

- "... In recent years there has been a movement toward the standardization to another active substance, hyperforin." Laakman G, Schule C, Baghai T et al., St. John's Wort in mild to moderate depression: The relevance of hyperforin for the clinical efficacy. *Pharmacopsychiatry* 1998; 31(suppl):54–59.

- "... [One] study reported that some people experienced digestive upset, fatigue, restlessness, and allergic reactions using St. John's wort extract." Woelk H, Burkard G, Grunwald J, Benefits and risks of the hypericum extract LI 160: Drug monitoring study with 3,250 patients. *Journal of Geriatric Psychiatry and Neurology* 1994; 7(suppl):S34–S38.

- "... The constituents hypericin and pseudohypericin have shown in test-tube studies to have strong antiviral activity against herpes simplex virus—both Type 1 (mouth) and Type 2 (genital)—as well as influenza virus A and B, and Epstein–Barr virus." Brown D, *Herbal Prescriptions for Health & Healing.* Roseville, CA: Prima Publishing, 2000, p. 208.

- "... In a review of 23 European clinical studies involving 1,700 patients, researchers found that St. John's wort was significantly more effective than placebo and equally as effective as standard drug therapy for mild to moderate depression." Linde K, Ramirez G, Mulrow CD et al., St. John's wort for depression—an overview and meta-analysis of randomized clinical trials. *British Medical Journal* 1996; 313:253–258.

- "... People took either 1,800 milligrams of St. John's wort or 150 milligrams of imipramine for 6 weeks." Vorbach EU, Arnoldt KH, Hubner WD, Efficacy and tolerability of St. John's wort extract LI60 versus imipramine in patients with severe depressive episodes according to ICD-10. *Pharmacopsychiatry* 1997; 30(suppl):81–85.

- "... One small study showed that people who took St. John's wort in combination with either bright light or dim light therapy experienced significant improvement in SAD." Martinez B, Kasper S, Ruhrman S et al., Hypericum in the treatment of seasonal affective disorders. *Journal of Geriatrics Psychiatry and Neurology* 1994; (suppl 1):S29–S33.

## TEA TREE OIL

- "... A standard for tea tree oil was established in 1985. It requires a minimum content of 30% terpinen-4-ol and less than 15% cineole." Leung AY, Foster S, *Encyclopedia of Common Natural Ingredients Used in Food, Drugs, and Cosmetics,* Second Edition. New York: John Wiley and Sons, 1995, p. 110.

- "... One study showed that a 5 percent tea tree oil gel extract was comparable to benzoyl peroxide in the treatment of mild to moderate acne." Bassett IB et al., A comparative study of tea tree oil versus benzoyl peroxide in the treatment of acne. *Med J Aust* 1990; 153:455–458.

- "... One study compared 100-percent tea tree oil to the antifungal topical drug clotrimazole for the treatment of toenail fungus for a period of 6 months." Buck DS, Nidorf DM, Addino JG, Comparison of two topical preparations for the treatment of onychomycosis: Melaleuca alternifolia (tea tree) oil and clotrimazole. *J Fam Pract* 38:601.

- An excellent book on tea tree oil is *The Tea Tree Oil Bible: Your Essential Guide* by Dr. Elvis Ali (Ages Publishing).

## TURMERIC

- "... For example, one study examined 40 men with swelling and tenderness of the spermatic cord following surgery for a hernia or hydrocele." Satoskar RR, Shah SJ, Shenoy SG, Evaluation of antiinflammatory property of curcumin in patients with postoperative inflammation. *International Journal of Clinical Pharmacology, Therapy and Toxicology* 1986; 24(12):651–654.

- "... A study of people with rheumatoid arthritis found that taking 1,200 milligrams of curcumin per day for two weeks significantly improved morning stiffness, joint swelling, and walking ability." Deodhar SD, Sethi R, Srimal RC, Preliminary study on antirheumatic activity of curcumin. *Indian Journal of Medical Research* 1980; 71:632–634.

- "... A study of smokers who took a supplement 1.5 grams of turmeric a day had reduced urinary excretion of mutagens (substances that cause damage to cell DNA which can lead to cancer formation)." Polsa K, Raghuram TC, Krishna TP et al., Effect of turmeric on urinary mutagens in smokers. *Mutagenesis* 1992; 2:107–109.

- "... Turmeric and its constituent curcumin also reduce cholesterol levels and increase the good cholesterol. It reduces the levels of lipid peroxides (oxidants that can initiate atherosclerosis)." Soni KB, Kuttan R, Effect of oral curcumin administration on serum peroxides and cholesterol levels in human volunteers. *Indian Journal of Physiology and Pharmacology* 1992; 36(4):273–275.

## VALERIAN

- "... If you take a dose that's too high, you may have symptoms that include blurred vision, change in heartbeat, headache, nausea, and uneasiness." Mills S, Bone K, *Principles and Practice of Phytotherapy.* London: Churchill Livingstone, 2000, pp. 587–588.

- "One study found the combination of valerian and St. John's wort to be equivalent to the antidepressant drug amitryptiline. . . ." Steger W, A randomized, double-blind study to compare the effectiveness of a plant based combination of metabolic substances to a synthetic antidepressant in depressive states. *Zeitschrift Allg Med* 1985; 61:914–918.

- "... and several clinical studies confirm that valerian is effective for insomnia." Donath F, Quispe S, Diefenbach K, Maurer A, Fietze I, Roots I, Critical evaluation of the effect of valerian extract on sleep structure and sleep quality. *Pharmacopsychiatry* 2000 Mar; 33(2):47–53.

- "... In a scientifically controlled study that involved 121 people who had insomnia, researchers studied the effects of 600 milligrams of valerian. . . ." Vorbach EU, Gortelmeyer R, Bruining J, Therapy for insomnia: Efficacy and tolerability of a valerian preparation. *Psychopharmakotherapie* 1996; 3(3):109–115.

## VANADIUM

- "... The most recent study involved 16 people with Type 2 diabetes . . . ." Goldfine AB, Patti ME, Zuberi L, Goldstein BJ, LeBlanc R, Landaker EJ, Jiang ZY, Willsky GR, Kahn CR, Metabolic effects of vanadyl sulfate in humans with noninsulin-dependent diabetes mellitus: In vivo and in vitro studies. *Metabolism* 2000 Mar; 49(3):400–410.

## VITAMIN A

- "... One study found that vitamin A deficiency is associated with many people who are HIV positive." Semba R et al., Increased mortality associated with vitamin A deficiency during Human Immunodeficiency Virus type 1 infection. *Arch Intern Med* 1993; 153:2149–2154.

- "... When given to impoverished children who had been deprived of the nutrient, vitamin A literally saves lives." Fawzi W, Herrera M, Willett W et al., Dietary vitamin A intake and the risk of mortality among children. *Am J Clin N* 1994; 59:401–408.

## VITAMIN C

- "... This appears to be unwarranted. In fact, one study showed that men who consumed 1,500 milligrams daily were less likely to get kidney stones than those who consumed less than 250 milligrams."

- ". . . Urinary oxalate—the mineral that goes into the makeup of kidney stones—doesn't increase unless you're taking 4,000 milligrams daily, which would be a very high dose." Ringsdorf WM, Cheraskin E, Nutritional aspects of urolithiasis. *South Med J* 1981; 74:41–44. Also, Curhan GC et al., A prospective study pf the intake of vitamins C and B6, and the risk of kidney stones in men. *J Urol* 1996; 155:1847–1851.

- ". . . In one study, people with asthma received 1,000 milligrams of vitamin C for 14 weeks . . ." CO et al., High dose ascorbic acid in Nigerian asthmatics. *Trop Geogr Med* 1980; 32:132–137.

- ". . . Another study . . . analyzed the diets and respiratory health of 19,000 children ages 6 to 7." Forastiere F, Pistelli R, Sestini P et al., Consumption of fresh fruit rich in vitamin C and wheezing symptoms in children. *Thorax* 2000; 55:283–288.

- ". . . Vitamin C also supports proper functioning of the white blood cells and immune cells, which help keep cancer cells in check." Loria CM, Klag MJ, Caufield LE et al., Vitamin C status and mortality in U.S. adults. *American Journal of Clinical Nutrition* 2000; 72:139–145.

- ". . . This well-publicized study, published in *The Journal of the American Medical Association* in 1997, first looked at the short-term effect of a high-fat meal on the arteries." Plotnick GD, Corretti MC, Vogel RA, Effect of antioxidant vitamins on the transient impairment of endothelium-dependent brachial artery vasoactivity following a single high-fat meal. *JAMA* 1997 Nov 26; 278(20):1682–1686.

- ". . . In one study that included more than 13,000 women, researchers found that those who consumed the greatest amount of vitamin C had a 39 percent lower risk of developing gallstones." Simon JA, Hudes ES, Serum ascorbic acid and gallbladder disease prevalence among U.S. adults. *Archives of Internal Medicine* 2000; 160:931–936.

- ". . . One study examined a group of men with infertility due to sperm agglutination (clumping). Dawson EB et al., Effect of ascorbic acid on male fertility. *Ann NY Acad Sci* 1987; 498:312–323.

## VITAMIN D

- ". . . It has also been shown that breast-fed infants who received vitamin D supplements during the first year of life had increased bone density in later childhood." Zamora SA, Rizzoli R, Belli DC, Slosman DO, Bonjour JP, Vitamin D supplementation during infancy is associated with higher bone mineral mass in prepubertal girls. *J Clin Endocrinol Metab* 1999 Dec; 84(12):4541–4545.

- ". . . People in nursing homes and people who are hospitalized are particularly susceptible to a deficiency and must take vitamin D supplements." Thomas MK et al., Hypovitaminosis D in medical inpatients. *N Eng J Med* 1998; 338:777–783, Also, Lips P et al., The effect of vitamin D supplementation on vitamin D status and parathyroid function in elderly subjects. *J Clin Endocrinol Metab* 1988; 67:644–650.

- ". . . One study examined 249 healthy postmenopausal women with an average age of 61." Dawson-Hughes B, Dallal GE, Krall EA, Harris S, Sokoll LJ, Falconer G, Effect of vitamin D supplementation on wintertime and overall bone loss in healthy postmenopausal women. *Ann Intern Med* 1991 Oct 1; 115(7):505–512.

# VITAMIN E

- "... The Cambridge Heart Study of 2,000 patients with heart disease found that those who took between 400 to 800 IU of vitamin E had a 77 percent decrease in cardiovascular disease over a year's time." Stephens NG et al., Randomised controlled trial of vitamin E in patients with coronary disease: Cambridge Heart Antioxidant Study (CHAOS). *Lancet* 1996; 347(9004):781–786.

- "... In a Nurses Health Study involving 87,000 women, doctors learned that women who took vitamin E for two years or more had a 41 percent reduction in the risk of heart disease." Stampfer MJ et al., Vitamin E consumption and the risk of coronary artery disease in women. *New Engl J Med* 1993; 328:1444–1448.

- "... A further study was conducted with 11,000 seniors, ages 67 to 105, over a 9-year period." Losonczy KG et al., Vitamin E and vitamin C supplement use and risk of all-cause and coronary heart disease mortality in older persons: The Established Populations for Epidemiologic Studies of the Elderly. *Am J Clin Nutr* 1996 Aug; 64(2):190–196.

- "... Vitamin E has been shown to improve glucose tolerance in people who have diabetes." Devaraj S, Jialal I, Alpha tocopherol supplementation decreases serum C-reactive protein and monocyte interleukin-6 in normal volunteers and type 2 diabetics. *Free Radical Biology and Medicine* 2000; 29:790–792.

- "... [Researchers] found immediate evidence that the vitamin delayed blood clotting." Pignatelli, P et al., *Atherosclerosis, Thrombosis and Vascular Biology* 1999; 2542–2547.

- "... In one 4-year study, people with severe carotid stenosis were given either tocotrienols or a placebo. Analysis with ultrasound showed that 94 percent of those taking tocotrienols improved or stabilized." Bierenbaum ML et al., Antioxidant effects of tocotrienols in patients with hyperlipidemia and carotid stenosis. *Lipids* 1995; 30:1179–80.

# VITEX

- "... [Vitex] increases the production of LH by the pituitary gland to stimulate ovulation and progesterone production." Anmann W, Removing an obstipation using Agnolyt. *Ther Gegenw* 1965; 104:1263–1265.

- "... A study of 52 women who did not ovulate due to high prolactin levels found that vitex extract taken for three months reduced prolactin levels." Milewica A, Gejdel E et al., Vitex agnus castus extract in the treatment of luteal phase defects due to hyperprolactinemia. Results of a randomized placebo-controlled double-blind study. *Arzneim-Forsch Drug Res* 1993; 43:752–756.

- "... A study of 104 women who suffered from premenstrual breast pain found that vitex extract significantly reduced breast pain." Wuttke W et al., Treatment of cyclical mastalgia with a medication containing Agnus castus: Results of a randomized, placebo-controlled, double-blind study. *Geburtshilife und Frauenheilkunde,* 1997; 57:569–574.

- "... One study of women with menstrual disorders found that vitex improved cases of polymenorrhea (too frequent) as well as cases of women with menorrhagia (excessive bleeding)." Bleier W, Phytotherapy in irregular menstrual cycles or bleeding periods and other gynecological disorders of endocrine origin. *Zentrallblatt Gynakol* 1959; 81(18):701–709.

- "...A study of 353 breast-feeding mothers with poor milk production found that vitex supplementation for seven days resulted in significant improvement." Mohr H, Clinical investigations of means to increase lactation. *Deutsche Medizinische Wochenschrift* 1954; 79(41):1513–1516.

- "... One survey involved over 1,500 women with premenstrual syndrome who supplemented with vitex extract." Dittmar FW, Bohnert KJ et al., Premenstrual syndrome: Treatment with a phytopharmaceuticals. *Ther Gynakol* 1992; 5:60–68.

- "... In another study, 127 women were given 200 milligrams of vitamin $B_6$ or vitex extract for three menstrual cycles." Luaritzen CH, Reuter HD et al., Treatment of premenstrual syndrome with vitex agnus castus: Controlled, double-blind study versus pyridoxine. *Phytomedicine* 1997; 4:183–189.

# ZINC

- "... Zinc works to reduce the conversion and also promotes skin healing." Hillstrom L et al., Comparison of oral treatment with zinc sulfate and placebo in acne vulgaris. *Br J Dermatol* 1977; 97:679–684.

- "... [At least one study] indicated zinc is as effective as tetracycline." Michelsson G et al., A double-blind study of the effect of zinc and oxytetracylcine in acne vulgaris. *Br J Dermatol* 1977; 97:561–566.

- "... In a study that included ten people who had Alzheimer's, researchers found that supplementation with zinc helped eight of the people improve memory and communication." Constantinidis J, Treatment of Alzheimer's disease by zinc compounds. *Drug Develop Res* 1992; 27:1–14.

- "... It is helpful to take zinc losenges containing 15 to 25 milligrams of elemental zinc at the first sign of a cold." Mossad SB et al., Zinc gluconate lozenges for treating the common cold: A randomized, double-blind study. *Ann Int Med* 1996; 125:142–144. Also, Halcomb GA, Reduction in the duration of common colds by zinc gluconate lozenges in a double-blind study. *Antimicrob Agents Chmother* 1984; 25:20–24.

- "... In one study, 11 men who were infertile were treated with 55 milligrams of zinc daily for 6 to 12 months." Marmar JL et al., Semen zinc levels in infertile and postvasectomy patients and patients with prostatitis. *Fertil Steril* 1975; 26:1057–1063.

- "... One study of 155 people with macular degeneration found that 45 milligrams of zinc per day significantly slowed the rate of visual loss." Newsome DA et al., Oral zinc in macular degeneration. *Arch Opthalmol* 1988; 106:192–198.

# Quick Cure Finder:
## An A-to-Z Guide to Health Conditions and Therapies

· · · · · · · · · · · · · · · · · · · · · · · · · · · · · · · · · · · · · · · · · · · · · · · · · · · · ·

The following list is a reference guide to help you quickly find solutions to your health problems. Just look up a health condition in the list below, then turn to the specific healing-therapy chapters for complete information about recommendations and dosages.

(Note: This section is solely intended to guide you to healing therapies in the book. For the complete index, please see page 543.)

## A

ABSCESSES: cell salts

ACNE: burdock; cell salts; flaxseed; goldenseal; saw palmetto; tea tree oil; vitamin A; vitamin E; vitex; zinc

AGE-ASSOCIATED MEMORY IMPAIRMENT (AAMI): phosphatidylserine

AGING: ashwagandha; ginseng; melatonin

AIDS: aloe; selenium; vitamin A; vitamin E; zinc

ALCOHOLISM: lachesis; milk thistle; nux vomica; thiamin

ALLERGIES: acupressure; adrenal glandulars; apis; arsenicum album; bee pollen; DHEA; food sensitivity therapy; milk thistle; MSM; nux vomica; quercetin; vitamin C

ALZHEIMER'S DISEASE: gingko biloba; L-carnitine; phosphatidylserine; vitamin E; zinc

AMENORRHEA: vitex

ANEMIA, IRON-DEFICIENCY: ashwagandha; cell salts; ferrum phosphoricum; gentian root; iron; nettle; phytonutrients; spirulina

ANESTHESIA SIDE EFFECTS: ginger root for

ANGINA: amino acids; bromelain; coenzyme Q10; hawthorn; L-carnitine; magnesium; vitamin E

ANOREXIA: L-carnitine

ANTIBIOTIC-ASSOCIATED COLITIS: acidophilus

ANXIETY: aconite; acupressure; amino acids; arsenicum album; Bach Flower Remedies; black cohosh; cell salts; chamomile; exercise; gelsemium; kava; mental imagery; passionflower; phytonutrients; pulsatilla; St. John's Wort; valerian

AORTA ELASTICITY PROBLEMS: garlic

APPETITE, LOSS OF: dandelion for

ARNICA: for head trauma; for sore muscles

ARRHYTHMIAS: coenzyme Q10; hawthorn; L-carnitine; magnesium

ARSENICUM ALBUM: for anxiety

ARTHRITIS: antioxidants; apis; ashwagandha; bee pollen; black cohosh; boswellia; bromelain; cayenne; cell salts; enzymes; evening primrose oil; exercise; feverfew; fish oil; flaxseed; food sensitivity therapy; ginger root; glucosamine sulfate; hydrotherapy; ledum; lycopodium; MSM; nettle; phytonutrients; pulsatilla; rhus toxicodendron; turmeric; vitamin C; vitamin E

ARTHRITIS PAIN: cayenne

ASTHMA: adrenal glandulars; aloe; American ginseng; arsenicum album; cell salts; fish oil; ipecacuanha; lachesis; magnesium; MSM; onions; pulsatilla; quercetin; vitamin C

ATHEROSCLEROSIS: cayenne; coenzyme Q10; guggul; zinc

ATHLETES FOOT: tea tree oil

ATTENTION DEFICIT DISORDER (ADD): evening primrose oil; fish oil; food sensitivity therapy; gingko biloba; sulphur

ATTENTION DEFICIT HYPERACTIVITY DISORDER (ADHD): evening primrose oil; fish oil; food sensitivity therapy; phosphatidylserine; sulphur

AUTISM: food sensitivity therapy

AUTOIMMUNE CONDITIONS: enzymes; food sensitivity therapy; MSM; progesterone

## B

BACK PAIN: horse chestnut; nux vomica

BACTERIAL INFECTIONS: echinacea

BALDNESS: saw palmetto

BEE STINGS: apis

BIRTH-CONTROLL PILL SIDE EFFECTS: sepia

BLADDER INFECTIONS: cell salts; nux vomica; pulsatilla; saw palmetto; sepia

BLEEDING: cell salts; ferrum phosphoricum

BLOATING: food sensitivity therapy; gentian root; ginger root; lycopodium

BLOOD THINNING: green tea

BOILS: cell salts

BONE DENSITY: ipriflavone

BONE PAIN: peppermint

BRAIN INJURY: phosphatidylserine

BREAST CANCER: coenzyme Q10; d-glucarate; green tea

BREAST CANCER PREVENTION: flaxseed; phytonutrients

BREAST PAIN: vitex

BREAST TENDERNESS: evening primrose oil

BREAST-FEEDING: vitex

BREASTS, HARD NODULES OF: cell salts for

BRONCHITIS: astragalus; bromelain; cell salts; food sensitivity therapy; hydrotherapy; ipecacuanha; pulsatilla

BRUISES: bromelain; ledum; St. John's Wort

BURNS: aloe; bromelain; cantharis; phytonutrients; St. John's Wort; vitamin E; zinc

# C

CANCER: arsenicum album; astragalus; bromelain; burdock; coenzyme Q10; enzymes; fiber; fish oil; hydrotherapy; melatonin; mental imagery; phytonutrients; quercitin; spirulina

CANCER PREVENTION: acidophilus; antioxidants; bromelain; carotenoids; d-glucarate; DHEA; flaxseed; garlic; ginseng; green tea; onions; phytonutrients; quercitin; selenium; soy; turmeric; vitamin C; vitamin E

CANDIDA: echinacea; food sensitivity therapy; garlic; gentian root; phytonutrients for

CANKER SORES: aloe

CARDIOMYOPATHY: coenzyme Q10; L-carnitine; magnesium

CARDIOVASCULAR DISEASE: bromelain; hawthorn; phytonutrients

CARDIOVASCULAR DISEASE PREVENTION: antioxidants; bromelain; calcium; carotenoids; cayenne; DHEA; exercise; fish oil; flaxseed; folic acid; garlic; ginger root; green tea; phytonutrients; pyridoxene; quercitin; selenium; soy; vitamin B12; vitamin C; vitamin E

CAROTID STENOSIS: vitamin E

CARPAL TUNNEL SYNDROME: pyridoxene

CARTILAGE DEGENERATION: glucosamine sulfate

CATARACTS: bilberries; gingko biloba; selenium; vitamin C; vitamin E

CHEMOTHERAPY: nux vomica

CHEMOTHERAPY SIDE EFFECTS: ginseng for

CHITOSAN: for weight loss

CHOLESTEROL: amino acids; antioxidants; calcium; cayenne; chromium; fiber; flaxseed; garlic; ginger root; green tea; guggul; niacin; onions; pantothenic acid; phytonutrients; soy; spirulina; vitamin E

CHRONIC FATIGUE SYNDROME: adrenal glandulars; DHEA; gelsemium; L-carnitine

CHRONIC OBSTRUCTIVE PULMONARY DISEASE: fish oil

CIRCULATION: bilberries; cayenne; DHEA; garlic; ginger root; gingko biloba; horse chestnut; lachesis; milk thistle

CIRCULATORY CONDITIONS: calcium; gingko biloba

CIRRHOSIS: liver glandulars; milk thistle; SAMe

CLOUDY THINKING: water

COLD FEET: gingko biloba

COLD SORES: cell salts; lysine; tea tree oil

COLIC: chamomile; enzymes; nux vomica

COLITIS: acidophilus; boswellia; bromelain; fish oil; food sensitivity therapy; lycopodium; nux vomica

COLON CANCER: calcium; lutein

COLON CANCER PREVENTION: onions

COMMON COLD: acupressure; astragalus; echinacea; goldenseal; lomatium; peppermint; vitamin C; zinc

CONCUSSION: arnica

CONGESTIVE HEART FAILURE: amino acids; coenzyme Q10; ginseng; hawthorn; L-carnitine; magnesium

CONJUNCTIVITIS: pulsatilla

CONSTIPATION: acidophilus; acupressure; bitter aloe latex; burdock; dandelion; fiber; flaxseed oil; food sensitivity therapy; gentian root; hydrotherapy; milk thistle; nux vomica; sitz bath

COUGHS: acupressure; licorice root; peppermint

CRADLE CAP: biotin

CROHN'S DISEASE: acidophilus; fish oil; food sensitivity therapy; hydrotherapy; nux, go

CUTS: zinc

CYCLICAL BREAST TENDERNESS: evening primrose oil

## D

DANDRUFF: tea tree oil

DEMENTIA: DHEA; phosphatidylserine

DENTAL CONDITIONS: cell salts for; green tea for; propolis; tea tree oil for

DEPRESSION: amino acids; black cohosh; cell salts; exercise; fish oil; food sensitivity therapy; gingko biloba; ignatia for; kava; milk thistle; phosphatidylserine; phytonutrients; pulsatilla; SAMe; sepia; St. John's Wort; valerian

DETOXIFICATION: antioxidants; burdock; d-glucarate; dandelion; exercise; garlic; green tea; hydrotherapy; licorice root; milk thistle; phytonutrients; spirulina

DIABETES: aloe; antioxidants; biotin; burdock; chromium; coenzyme Q10; dandelion; DHEA; evening primrose oil; exercise; fiber; ginseng; gymnema sylvestre; L-carnitine; magnesium; onions; quercitin; vanadium; vitamin C; vitamin E

DIABETIC NEUROPATHY: cayenne

DIABETIC RETINOPATHY: gingko biloba

DIARRHEA: acidophilus; arsenicum album; bilberries; bilberry; food sensitivity therapy; gelsemium for; ginger root; goldenseal

DIGESTION: astragalus; ginger root; green tea; nux vomica

DIGESTIVE DISORDERS: acidophilus; aloe juice; bromelain; chamomile; enzymes; flaxseed; goldenseal; hydrotherapy; phytonutrients; propolis; quercitin; sulphur; turmeric; valerian

DIZZINESS: water

DOWN'S SYNDROME: L-carnitine

DRUG-ADDICTION RECOVERY: milk thistle

DRY EYES: vitamin A

DRY SKIN: cell salts; flaxseed; flaxseed for; flaxseed oil for

DYSBIOSIS: acidophilus

## E

E COLI: goldenseal

EAR INFECTIONS: aconite; food sensitivity therapy; lachesis

EARACHES: chamomile; ferrum phosphoricum

EARS, FLUID IN: cell salts for

EATING DISORDERS: zinc

ECZEMA: cell salts; evening primrose oil; fish oil; flaxseed; food sensitivity therapy; licorice root; vitamin E

EDEMA: cell salts; dandelion; horse chestnut; nettle; water

EMOTIONAL BLOCKAGES: Bach Flower Remedies; Bach flower remedies; ignatia

ENDOMETRIOSIS: lachesis; progesterone; pulsatilla

ENERGY: bee pollen; DHEA; exercise; ginseng; glandulars; vitamin B12

ENERGY, RECOVERING: flaxseed for

EPSTEIN-BARR SYNDROME: lomatium

ESOPHAGEAL CANCER: beta-carotene

EXHAUSTION: Bach flower remedies

EYE INFECTIONS: goldenseal

EYES, DRY: vitamin A for

EYES, INJURY TO: symphytum for

EYESTRAIN: acupressure; bilberries

# F

FAT MALABSORPTION: phytonutrients

FATIGUE: ashwagandha; cell salts; exercise; food sensitivity therapy; gelsemium; ginseng; iron; licorice root; magnesium; pantothenic acid; phosphatidylserine; sulphur; water

FEARS: Bach flower remedies

FELINE LEUKEMIA VIRUS: aloe

FEMALE INFERTILITY: sepia; vitex

FEVER: aconite; burdock; cell salts; ferrum phosphoricum; hydrotherapy

FIBROCYSTIC BREAST SYNDROME: evening primrose oil; progesterone; sepia; vitamin E; vitex

FIBROMYALGIA: black cohosh; ignatia; magnesium; MSM; SAMe

FISSURES: sitz bath

FLATULENCE: chamomile; dandelion; ginger root; lycopodium

FLU: aconite; acupressure; arsenicum album; echinacea; gelsemium; lomatium; nux vomica; rhus toxicodendron

FOOD ALLERGIES: acidophilus; gentian root; MSM

FOOD POISONING: arsenicum album

FOOD SENSITIVITIES: enzymes; gentian root; reasons

FOOT PAIN: gingko biloba

FRACTURES: cell salts; symphytum

FREE RADICALS: carotenoids

FUNGAL INFECTIONS: echinacea; tea tree oil

# G

GALLBLADDER CONDITIONS: food sensitivity therapy

GALLSTONES: food sensitivity therapy; milk thistle; peppermint; vitamin C

GENITAL WARTS: lomatium; sepia

GINGIVITIS: coenzyme Q10; tea tree oil; vitamin C

GLAUCOMA: bilberries; magnesium; vitamin C

GOUT: dandelion; nettle

GRIEF: Bach flower remedies; cell salts; ignatia; pulsatilla

GROWING PAINS: calcium; cell salts

GUM INFECTIONS: tea tree oil

GUMS, SORE: cell salts for

# H

HAIR HEALTH: MSM

HAIR PROBLEMS: cell salts; nettle; tea tree oil

HANGOVERS: ipecacuanha; nux vomica

HAY FEVER: bee pollen; cell salts; nettle; nux vomica

HEAD INJURY: cell salts

HEADACHES: acupressure; amino acids; food sensitivity therapy; gelsemium; gentian root; hydrotherapy; ipecacuanha; lycopodium; peppermint; pulsatilla; sulphur; water

HEART: coenzyme Q10

HEART ATTACK RECOVERY: hawthorn; L-carnitine

HEART PALPITATIONS: passionflower; water

HEARTBURN: cell salts; food sensitivity therapy

HEMORRHAGE: ipecacuanha; lachesis

HEMORRHOIDS: bilberries; butcher's broom; cell salts; food sensitivity therapy; horse chestnut; sitz bath

HEPATITIS: cell salts; dandelion; liver glandulars; lycopodium; milk thistle; phytonutrients; selenium; vitamin C

HERPES: amino acids; apis; lomatium; lysine; propolis; rhus toxicodendron; sepia

HIV: DHEA; L-carnitine

HIVES: rhus toxicodendron

HORMONE IMBALANCE: d-glucarate; dandelion; licorice root; milk thistle; ovary glandulars; sepia; vitex

HYPERACTIVITY: amino acids; cell salts; fish oil

HYPERPARATHYROIDISM: ipriflavone

HYPERTENSION: amino acids; calcium; dandelion; fish oil; garlic; gingko biloba; hawthorn; lachesis; onions; passionflower; potassium; valerian; water

HYPERTENSION, PREGNANCY INDUCED: calcium for

HYPERTHYROIDISM: lachesis

HYPOGLYCEMIA: chromium; fiber; food sensitivity therapy

HYPOTHYROIDISM: amino acids; iron; pituitary glandulars; sepia; thyroid glandulars

# I

IMMUNE ENHANCEMENT: food sensitivity therapy; phytonutrients

IMMUNE SYSTEM: bee pollen; burdock; echinacea; exercise; lomatium; selenium; spirulina

IMMUNE SYSTEM PROBLEMS: ginseng; spleen glandulars; thymus glandulars

IMPOTENCE: amino acids; DHEA; gingko biloba; lycopodium; testicular glandulars

INCONTINENCE: sepia

INDIGESTION: acupressure; burdock; dandelion; gentian root; milk thistle

INFANTS: soymula and

INFECTION PREVENTION: garlic for; onions for

INFECTIONS: burdock; cell salts; echinacea; hydrotherapy; licorice root; lomatium; phytonutrients; propolis; turmeric; vitamin C; vitamin E

INFECTIONS, SECONDARY: garlic for

INFLAMMATION: boswellia; bromelain; echinacea; ginger root; licorice root; MSM; turmeric

INFLAMMATORY BOWEL DISEASE (IBD): aloe; amino acids; boswellia; DHEA; food sensitivity therapy; licorice root; phytonutrients; quercitin

INJURIES: boswellia; bromelain; enzymes

INSOMNIA: amino acids; chamomile; kava; melatonin; nux vomica; passionflower; sulphur; valerian

INSULIN RESISTANCE: fish oil; gymnema sylvestre

IRRITABILITY: water

IRRITABLE BOWEL SYNDROME (IBS): acidophilus; chamomile; fiber; food sensitivity therapy; gentian root; hydrotherapy; nux vomica; peppermint

## J

JAUNDICE, NEWBORN: cell salts for

JET LAG: melatonin

JOINT PAIN: cayenne

JOINT PROBLEMS: boswellia

JOINTS, WEAK: cell salts for

## K

KIDNEY DISEASE: apis; L-carnitine; phytonutrients

KIDNEY FAILURE: ipriflavone

KIDNEY PAIN: water

KIDNEY STONES: magnesium; pyridoxene; uva ursi

KIDNEY TRANSPLANTS: fish oil

KIDNEYS, DETOXIFYING: burdock for

## L

LACTOSE INTOLERANCE: acidophilus

LEAKY GUT SYNDROME: acidophilus; amino acids

LIBIDO, REDUCED: ginseng; sepia; testicular glandulars

LICE: tea tree oil

LIGAMENTS, WEAK: cell salts for

LIVER DETOXIFICATION: burdock; dandelion; liver glandulars

LIVER DISEASE: L-carnitine; liver glandulars; lycopodium; milk thistle; SAMe; turmeric

LIVER HEALTH: d-glucarate; milk thistle

LIVER PROTECTION: milk thistle

LOW APPETITE: gentian root

LOW BACK PAIN: sulphur

LOW SPERM COUNT: amino acids

LUPUS: DHEA; fish oil

# M

MACULAR DEGENERATION: bilberries; carotenoids protecting against; gingko biloba; vitamin C; vitamin E; zinc

MALE INFERTILITY: coenzyme Q10; L-carnitine; testicular glandulars; vitamin C; zinc

MALNOURISHMENT: spirulina

MANIC-DEPRESSION: lachesis

MEMORY PROBLEMS: ashwagandha; B-complex vitamins; cell salts; flaxseed; gingko biloba; ginseng; L-carnitine; phosphatidylserine; phytonutrients

MENINGITIS: apis

MENOPAUSE: adrenal glandulars; black cohosh; burdock; dandelion; DHEA; exercise; lachesis; passionflower; phytonutrients; progesterone; pulsatilla; sepia; soy; sulphur; vitamin E; vitex

MENSTRUAL CRAMPS: black cohosh; cell salts; chamomile; pulsatilla; valerian

MENSTRUAL DISORDERS: vitex

MENSTRUATION, HEAVY: cell salts for; lachesis for

MENSTRUATION, IRON-DEFICIENCY ANEMIA FROM: ferrum phosphoricum for; iron for

MENSTRUATION, IRREGULAR CYCLES: sepia for

MIGRAINE PREVENTION: magnesium

MIGRAINES: amino acids; feverfew; ipecacuanha; lachesis; progesterone; pulsatilla; riboflavin; sepia

MISCARRIAGE PREVENTION: progesterone; vitex

MITRAL VALVE PROLAPSE: coenzyme Q10; magnesium

MONONUCLEOSIS: gelsemium

MORNING SICKNESS: ginger root; ipecacuanha; sepia

MOSQUITO BITES: ledum

MOTION SICKNESS: ginger root

MOUTH CANCER: beta-carotene; spirulina

MOUTH INFECTIONS: tea tree oil

MOUTH SORES: licorice root

MULTIPLE SCLEROSIS: fish oil; flaxseed; gelsemium; vitamin E

MUSCLE CRAMPS/SPASMS: calcium; cell salts; ignatia; kava; magnesium; potassium; valerian

MUSCLE PAIN: acupressure; arnica; cayenne; cell salts; peppermint

MUSCLE PROBLEMS: boswellia

MUSCLE TENSION: kava

# N

NAIL HEALTH: MSM
NAIL PROBLEMS: cell salts
NASAL CONGESTION: goldenseal
NAUSEA: acupressure; ginger root; ipecacuanha
NECK PAIN: acupressure for
NERVE CELLS, PROTECTING: gingko biloba for
NERVOUSNESS: cell salts
NEURAL TUBE DEFECTS: folic acid
NEUROPATHY: evening primrose oil
NIGHT BLINDNESS: vitamin A; vitamin A for
NIGHT VISION: bilberries; bilberries for

# O

ORCHITIS: pulsatilla
OSTEOARTHRITIS: flaxseed; glucosamine sulfate; MSM; SAMe
OSTEOPOROSIS: amino acids; calcium; cell salts; DHEA; exercise; ipriflavone; lysine; magnesium; progesterone; soy; vitamin C; vitamin D
OSTEOPOROSIS PREVENTION: ipriflavone
OTOSCLEROSIS: ipriflavone
OVARIAN CYSTS: lachesis; progesterone; sepia; vitex
OVARIAN PAIN: apis; lycopodium
OVULATION: vitex

# P

PAGET'S DISEASE: ipriflavone
PAIN: acupressure; aloe; amino acids; arnica; boswellia; feverfew; kava; MSM
PANCREAS: pancreas glandulars
PANIC ATTACKS: kava
PARASITES: goldenseal; MSM
PARKINSON'S DISEASE: vitamin E
PELVIC CONGESTION/INFLAMMATION: sitz bath
PEPTIC ULCERS: licorice root; propolis
PERIODONTAL DISEASE: coenzyme Q10; tea tree oil; vitamin C
PERIPHERAL VASCULAR DISEASE: vitamin E
PHYSICAL TRAUMA: arnica
PNEUMONIA: hydrotherapy
POLYCYSTIC OVARIAN SYNDROME: saw palmetto
POST-SURGICAL PAIN: cayenne
PREDNISONE TAPERING: DHEA
PREECLAMPSIA: calcium; magnesium; vitamin C

PREGNANCY: calcium; iron; nettle; prenatal vitamins

PREGNANCY COMPLICATIONS: vitamin C

PREGNANCY EDEMA: dandelion

PREMATURE EJACULATION: lycopodium

PREMATURE INFANTS: L-carnitine

PREMENSTRUAL SYNDROME (PMS): amino acids; black cohosh; burdock; calcium; dandelion; evening primrose oil; exercise; gingko biloba; ignatia; lachesis; magnesium; passionflower; phytonutrients; progesterone; pulsatilla; sepia; vitex

PRENATAL INFANT GROWTH: selenium

PROSTATE CANCER: d-glucarate; saw palmetto

PROSTATE CANCER PREVENTION: carotenoids; flaxseed; phytonutrients

PROSTATE ENLARGEMENT: nettle; saw palmetto; sepia; zinc

PROSTATE INFECTIONS: cranberries

PROSTATITIS: saw palmetto; sitz bath

PSORIASIS: aloe; cayenne; cell salts; fish oil; food sensitivity therapy; licorice root; pulsatilla; sepia

PUNCTURE WOUNDS: ledum

PYRUVATE: for weight loss

# R

RADIATION EXPOSURE: gingko biloba; ginseng for; melatonin

RADIATION POISONING: spirulina

RASHES: cell salts for; enzymes for; food sensitivity therapy; food sensitivity therapy for; sulphur; water; water for

RESPIRATORY TRACT INFECTIONS: astragalus; bromelain; garlic; goldenseal; hydrotherapy; lomatium; lycopodium; vitamin A

RESTLESS LEG SYNDROME: iron

REYNAUD'S SYNDROME: gingko biloba; sepia

RHEUMATOID ARTHRITIS: apis; cayenne; echinacea; evening primrose oil; fish oil; flaxseed; selenium

# S

SCARS: vitamin E

SCHIZOPHRENIA: fish oil; food sensitivity therapy

SEASONAL AFFECTIVE DISORDER (SAD): St. John's Wort

SEBORRHEIC DERMATITIS: biotin

SEIZURES: cell salts

SHINGLES: apis; cayenne; lachesis; rhus toxicodendron

SINUSITIS: acupressure; bromelain; cell salts; food sensitivity therapy; hydrotherapy; MSM; pulsatilla; sepia

SKIN CANCER PREVENTION: selenium

SKIN CONDITIONS: aloe gel; burdock; cell salts; chamomile; echinacea; hydrotherapy; licorice root; milk thistle; sulphur; tea tree oil

SKIN PROTECTION: carotenoids; coenzyme Q10

SLOW GROWTH: ashwagandha

SMOKING: antioxidants

SORE THROAT: apis; cell salts; ferrum phosphoricum; sulphur

SPINAL PROBLEMS: cell salts

SPRAINS/STRAINS: cell salts; ledum; rhus toxicodendron

STIFF NECK: acupressure

STOMACH CRAMPS: cell salts

STOMACH UPSET: chamomile

STRESS: ashwagandha; chamomile; exercise; ginseng; kava; pantothenic acid; passionflower; phosphatidylserine; valerian; vitamin C

STROKE: gingko biloba

STROKE PREVENTION: potassium

SUDDEN INFANT DEATH SYNDROME (SIDS): selenium

SUNBURN: aloe gel; carotenoids protecting against; vitamin C

SURGERY RECOVERY: bromelain; cayenne

SWELLING: cell salts

SYNDROME X: gymnema sylvestre

SYSTEMIC TOXICITY: garlic

## T

TEETH, BRITTLE: cell salts for

TEETHING: cell salts; chamomile

TENDONS, WEAK: cell salts for

TENSION HEADACHES: acupressure; ignatia; kava; MSM; peppermint

THROMBOPHLEBITIS: bromelain; horse chestnut

THROMBOPHLEBITIS PREVENTION: gingko biloba for

TINNITUS: gingko biloba; gingko biloba for; ipriflavone

TMJ SYNDROME: ignatia

TOE FUNGUS: tea tree oil

TONSILLITIS: ferrum phosphoricum

TOOTH ABSCESS: tea tree oil

TOOTH DECAY PREVENTION: green tea

TOOTHACHE: cell salts

TOXEMIA: apis

TOXICITY, SYSTEMIC: garlic for

TOXINS: ginseng

TRAUMA, EMOTIONAL: Bach Flower Remedies for

TRAVELER'S DIARRHEA: acidophilus

TRIGLYCERIDES: cayenne reducing; chromium; fish oil; garlic; guggul

# U

ULCERATIVE COLITIS: boswellia; fish oil; food sensitivity therapy; hydrotherapy; nux vomica; propolis

ULCERS: acidophilus; aloe; arsenicum album; chamomile; hydrotherapy; licorice root; nux vomica; propolis; quercitin

UPPER RESPIRATORY TRACT INFECTIONS: astragalus

URINARY TRACT INFECTIONS: apis; burdock; cantharis; cranberries; goldenseal; lomatium; saw palmetto; sitz bath; uva ursi; water

URTICARIA: rhus toxicodendron

UTERINE FIBROIDS: progesterone; vitex

UTERINE PROLAPSE: sepia

# V

VAGINAL INFECTIONS: sitz bath

VAGINITIS: acidophilus; cell salts; echinacea; food sensitivity therapy; phytonutrients; progesterone; sepia; tea tree oil

VANADIUM: for diabetes

VARICOSE VEINS: bilberries; bromelain; butcher's broom; cell salts; horse chestnut; lachesis; phytonutrients; pulsatilla; sepia

VEIN CLOTS: bromelain

VERTIGO: gelsemium

VIRAL INFECTIONS: aloe; echinacea; enzymes; phytonutrients; St. John's Wort

VISION: gingko biloba

VITAMIN A DEFICIENCY: spirulina for

VOMITING: arsenicum album; ginger root

# W

WARTS: tea tree oil

WATER RETENTION: dandelion

WEIGHT LOSS: amino acids; chromium; dandelion; green tea; nutritional supplements; water

WILSON'S DISEASE: zinc

WOMEN: sepia

WOUNDS: aloe; amino acids; cell salts; phytonutrients; propolis; St. John's Wort; vitamin C; vitamin E; zinc

WOUNDS, PUNCTURE: ledum for

WRINKLES: vitamin C; vitamin C for

# Index